Gastrointestinal and Hepatobiliary Pathophysiology

Gastrointestinal and Hepatobiliary Pathophysiology

2nd Edition

■ **Suzanne Rose, MD, MSEd** ■

Associate Professor of Medical Education and Medicine,
Division of Gastroenterology
Associate Dean for Undergraduate Medical Education
Mount Sinai School of Medicine
New York, New York

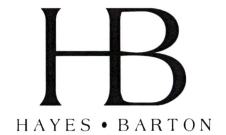

HAYES • BARTON

The authors and publisher have made every effort to ensure that the methods of treatment and drug recommendations are correct at the time of publication. However, new research and new therapies alter approaches constantly and usually there are several methods of diagnosis and treatment available for every condition. We have offered our best approach and advice. Nevertheless, we recommend consulting other sources (textbooks, package inserts, the *Physicians' Desk Reference*, and so on) before deciding on treatment.

Hayes Barton Press, Raleigh, North Carolina 27601-1300
www.hayesbartonpress.com
a division of Vital Source Technologies, Inc.

Second edition, published 2004, and reprint second edition, published 2005, by Hayes Barton Press. First edition published 1998 by Fence Creek Publishing.

ISBN: 1-59377-181-9 (paper)

09 08 07 06 05   3 4 5

Printed in the United States of America

Cover design: Linda de Jesus, Wing and Prayer Design, Springfield, Massachusetts

Cover art: Concepts by Georgia K. Duker, PhD (general organization of GI tract into four layers); and James M. McGill, MD, and Ann Stansfield, PhD (ion transport in biliary epithelial cells); rendered by David Carlson, Visible Productions.

Compositor: Interactive Composition Corporation, Portland, Oregon

Printer: Lightning Source, La Vergne, Tennessee

Distributor: Ingram

Libraries, institution customers, and bookstores my request a pro forma invoice by contacting Hayes Barton Press.
Tel: 919.755.8110
Fax: 919.755.8050
E-mail: nlucas@hayesbartonpress.com

■ DEDICATION ■

To Kenny, my husband, for his love, support, and inspiration.

To Zach and Izzi, our children, for keeping me focused on the priorities in life.

To my Mom, Ryda D. Rose, EdD,
and
my Dad (of blessed memory), Isadore Rose, MD,
for their encouragement and confidence,
and for showing me that education and medicine make a most perfect "marriage."

■ ASSISTANT EDITOR ■

SHARMILA ANANDASABAPATHY, MD, Assistant Professor of Medicine in the Department Medicine, Division of Gastroenterology, at Mount Sinai School of Medicine in New York, contributed by updating and editing the following chapters: Liver Anatomy and Physiology; Liver Metabolism, Physiology of Bile Formation, and Gallstones; Viral Hepatitis; Hereditary Liver Disease; Autoimmune Liver Disease; Pathogenesis and Consequences of Portal Hypertension; Disorders of Cholestasis, Bilirubin Metabolism, and Jaundice; Orthotopic Liver Transplantation; Alcohol and the GI Tract; and Principles of Nutritional Support in the GI Patient.

Contents

Preface

There continues to be an explosion of information in the medical sciences with new and innovative ways to teach and learn medicine. The curriculum revision processes in many medical schools have embraced the integration of information and the incorporation of the skills of knowledge acquisition, information retrieval, and problem solving. Training is much more focused at all levels in medicine in terms of outcomes or competencies.

It has been my good fortune to play a role in curricular change in several medical schools. The first edition of this text was the result of the creation of an integrated Digestion and Nutrition Course at the University of Pittsburgh. I have had the privilege for more than six years to be at the cutting edge of curricular revision at Mount Sinai School of Medicine in my role as Associate Dean for Undergraduate Medical Education. I continue to be amazed at how well students "digest" and synthesize information. The integrative approach to medical education and problem-based learning techniques are giving students skills that will serve them well throughout their professional lives. The purpose of this text is to provide a tool to help students at all stages of their medical career to retrieve information with a similar problem-solving approach.

This text offers state-of-the-art information about the pathophysiologic basis of gastrointestinal and hepatobiliary diseases while encouraging an integrative and problem-solving approach. The reader should be able to absorb information and apply it to solving clinical problems. Although this can provide a superb preclinical text and students will find it useful to review information as they address clinical situations, it will also be useful for house officers, fellows, practitioners of internal medicine and family medicine, as well as for gastroenterologists and hepatologists.

I was amazed by how far knowledge has advanced since the first edition of this book! Although first edition chapters provided the basis for this text, there is updated information in all areas, but especially in inflammatory bowel disease, celiac disease, hepatititis, functional bowel disorders, and pharmacology.

I hope that you find this book valuable in your study of medicine and in your own exploration into the exciting field of gastroenterology and hepatology.

Suzanne Rose
New York, New York
Summer 2004

Acknowledgments

For her expertise, editorial talent, and authorship, I want to thank Sharmila Anandasabapathy, MD, Assistant Professor, Department of Medicine, Division of Gastroenterology, Mount Sinai School of Medicine, who reviewed, edited, and authored updates, for chapters 8, 9, 18, 19, 20, 21, 22, 23, 24, and 29 of the second edition.

I also want to acknowledge the wonderful work of the authors who contributed to the first edition of this text and whose work formed the basis of the second edition: Mark Banchik, chapter 25 (Pathophysiology of Abdominal Pain and Pain Syndromes); John M. Costable, chapter 7 (Management of Water and Electrolytes); Georgia K. Duker, chapter 3 (Anatomy, Histology, and Embryology of the Gastrointestinal Tract); Patricia K. Eagon, chapter 9 (Liver Metabolism, Physiology of Bile Formation, and Gallstones), chapter 22 (Disorders of Cholestasis, Bilirubin Metabolism, and Jaundice), chapter 24 (Alcohol and the GI Tract); Gary W. Falk, chapter 28 (Pharmacology); Sydney D. Finkelstein, chapter 8 (Liver Anatomy and Physiology); David Gabbaizadeh, chapter 13 (Acute and Chronic Pancreatitis); Naresh T. Gunaratnam, chapter 21 (Pathogenesis and Consequences of Portal Hypertension); Lucinda A. Harris, chapter 12 (Small Bowel Disorders); Lillian P. Harvey, chapter 29 (Principles of Nutritional Support in the GI Patient); Matthew Horowitz, chapter 18 (Viral Hepatitis); Richard Kim, chapter 27 (Molecular Biology of GI Malignancies and Overview of Neoplasms of the GI Tract); Jodie Labowitz, chapter 15 (The Mucosal Immune System); Julia M. LaSalle, chapter 6 (Digestion and Absorption); Paul J. Lebovitz, chapter 11 (Peptic Ulcer Disease); James M. McGill, chapter 5 (GI Electrolyte and Fluid Secretion); Javier Minguillán, chapter 19 (Hereditary Liver Disease); Paulo A. Pacheco, chapter 18 (Viral Hepatitis); Patricia L. Raymond, chapter 14 (Functional Bowel Disorders); James C. Reynolds, chapter 2 (Regulation of the Digestive System), chapter 4 (Overview of Gastrointestinal Motility); Robert E. Schoen, chapter 27 (Molecular Biology of GI Malignancies and Overview of Neoplasms of the GI Tract); A. Obaid Shakil, chapter 23 (Orthotopic Liver Transplantation); Charnjit Singh, chapter 17 (Infectious Disorders of the GI Tract); Adam Slivka, chapter 30 (GI Bleeding); Ann Stansfield, chapter 5 (GI Electrolyte and Fluid Secretion); Grace L. Su, chapter 20 (Autoimmune Liver Disease), chapter 21 (Pathogenesis and Consequences of Portal Hypertension); Christina M. Surawicz, chapter 17 (Infectious Disorders of the GI Tract); David C. Whitcomb, chapter 6 (Digestion and Absorption), chapter 13 (Acute and Chronic Pancreatitis); Michele A. Young, chapter 10 (Normal and Disordered Swallowing).

An extra, special word of gratitude to Dr. James C. Reynolds for his confidence in me, his encouragement, and his allowing me my first opportunity to pursue my interests in medical education. I am indebted to many mentors who offered advice, opportunities, and wisdom. My thanks extend to the many incredible students who have touched my life and who continue to inspire me to greater heights of learning and teaching.

I want to thank Nancy Gable Lucas, managing editor at Hayes Barton Press, for her guidance and meticulous work, and Matt Harris, publisher, for his vision and ability to carry out this project.

A very personal appreciation to Rabbi Kenneth A. Stern, my husband, and to Zachary and Isadora, our two children who put up with my various projects: helping me, supporting me, leaving me alone so that I can work, and sharing special moments.

Suzanne Rose
New York, New York
Summer 2004

1

Overview of Gastrointestinal and Hepatobiliary Function

■ LEARNING OBJECTIVES ■

At the completion of this chapter, the reader should be able to:
• Identify epidemiologic factors in the incidence and development of gastrointestinal (GI) and hepatobiliary disorders.
• Assess the importance of the study of disorders of the digestive tract.
• Appreciate the various functions of the organs of the digestive tract.
• Discuss the roles of GI function, including motility, secretion, digestion, and absorption.
• Describe the various functions of the GI tract.

Malnutrition is a leading cause of mortality worldwide and is a problem even in the more affluent Western cultures.

Hepatocellular carcinoma is the leading cause of cancer death worldwide and is related to endemic hepatitis.

CASE STUDY: INTRODUCTION

A 24-year-old woman presented to her family physician with abdominal discomfort relieved with a bowel movement and diarrhea alternating with constipation. She had no significant medical history. The patient denied rectal bleeding, weight loss, or nocturnal symptoms. The physical examination was normal, and limited testing revealed no evidence of thyroid disease or laboratory abnormalities. The patient responded to dietary counseling, reassurance, and increased fiber in her diet.

Introduction

Gastrointestinal (GI) and hepatobiliary disorders account for significant mortality and morbidity in the United States and elsewhere (Table 1-1). Sixty to seventy million people were assessed as affected by digestive diseases in 1985 (according to National Institutes of Health statistics). In that year, 13% of all hospitalizations were for digestive problems. In 1992, $107 billion was spent on digestive diseases, including $87 billion in direct costs and $20 billion in such indirect costs as disability and mortality.

Abdominal pain is the second leading reason for patients to seek a physician. There are many causes of abdominal pain. For instance, peptic ulcer disease affects up to 15% of the population in the United States, and up to 50% suffer from heartburn at least once a month, making anatacids, histamine H_2 blockers, and proton pump inhibitors widely utilized.

In the United States, nearly one-third of all cancers originate in the GI tract. Colon cancer is preventable with screening and health care maintenance, yet it is the second leading cause of cancer mortality.

In the United States, cirrhosis of the liver is the fourth leading cause of death and may result from a variety of causes, including alcohol, infections, autoimmune disorders, and metabolic diseases. Liver transplantation provides treatment for a condition that may otherwise prove fatal.

Gallstones are very common, with a prevalence of 16–22 million people (1976–1987) and accounted for 800,000 hospitalizations in 1987. Newer surgical approaches using laparoscopy has resulted in decreased time in the hospital and shorter recovery times for patients.

Nearly everyone suffers with a GI symptom—whether the symptom is heartburn, abdominal pain, diarrhea, or constipation—at some point in his or her lifetime. It is important to understand the normal physiology to assess the pathophysiologic mechanisms of disease states.

Organs and Their Function

The GI tract begins with the oral cavity and ends with the anus (Fig. 1-1). The role of the GI tract is to accept nutrients, digest and

Table 1-1. Statistics Involving Digestive Disorders

DISEASE	PREVALENCE	HOSPITALIZATIONS
Abdominal wall hernia	4.5 million (1988–90)	640,000 (1980)
Chronic liver disease/cirrhosis	400,000 (1976–80)	300,000 (1987)
Constipation	4.4 million (1983–87)	100,000 (1983–87)
Diverticular disease	2 million (1983–87)	440,000 (1987)
Gallstones	16–22 million (1976–87)	800,000 (1987)
Gastritis/nonulcer dyspepsia	8.5 million (1988)	65,600 (1980s)
Gastroesophageal reflux disease/ esophageal disorders	3%–7% of United States population (1985)	1 million (1985)
Hemorrhoids	10.4 million (1983–87)	316,000 (1983–87)
Inflammatory bowel disease	300,000–500,000 (1987)	100,000 (1987)
Irritable bowel syndrome	5 million (1987)	34,000 (1987)
Peptic ulcer	5 million (1987)	630,000 (1987)
	INCIDENCE	
Viral hepatitis	New cases: Hepatitis A: 32,000 (1992) Hepatitis B: 200,000– 300,000 (1990) Hepatitis C: 150,000 (1991) Hepatitis D: 70,000 (1990)	33,000 (1987)
Infectious diarrhea	99 million new cases (1980)	462,000–728,000 (1987)
Pancreatitis	17 new cases per 100,000 (1976–88)	145,000 (1987)

Source: Information from U.S. Department of Health and Human Services: *Digestive Diseases Statistics*. Washington, DC: National Institutes of Health, 1995, NIH publication no. 95-3873.

absorb them, manage fluid and electrolyte status, and eliminate waste products.

ESOPHAGUS

The esophagus is made up of the upper esophageal sphincter and the body of the esophagus, which is a 20-cm-long empty tube with a transition from predominantly striated (proximally) to predominantly smooth muscle (distally). The role of the esophagus is to serve as a conduit for nutrients from the oral cavity to the stomach so that they may reach the digestive and absorptive regions of the digestive tract. The lower esophageal sphincter separates the esophagus from the stomach. It is tonically contracted at rest to prevent reflux of acid. Inappropriate transient relaxations of this muscle are thought to be the major mechanism for the development of gastroesophageal reflux disease (GERD).

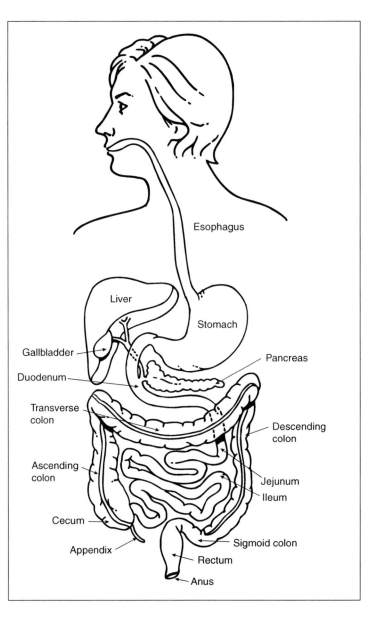

Fig. 1-1. Gastrointestinal Tract

STOMACH

The stomach is divided into four anatomic regions: the cardia, fundus, body, and antrum. The cardia is a relatively short segment of the stomach just below the gastroesophageal junction. The fundus and body serve a reservoir function and regulate the speed of emptying of liquids. The antrum mixes and grinds food and regulates the speed of emptying solids. The pylorus, the muscle separating the stomach from the small intestine, prevents postprandial duodenogastric reflux and helps regulate gastric emptying.

SMALL INTESTINE

The main functions of the small intestine are absorption and secretion. The surface area of the small intestine is 2 million cm^2. The functional unit of the small intestine is the villus. In the human species, the cells lining the villi are renewed every 5–6 days. The villi serve as projections that increase the surface area for absorption in the small intestine. This is analogous to the tiny threaded loops seen on a bath towel that are present to increase the ability to absorb moisture. The additional surface area provided by the villi are important for absorption; when they are not present or the villi are flattened, malabsorption will occur.

There are several portions of the small intestine. Most proximally is the duodenum, followed by the jejunum and then the ileum. Some nutrients and vitamins are absorbed more proximally (e.g., iron, folate), whereas others are absorbed distally (e.g., bile salt, vitamin B_{12}).

Secretion is an important function of the small intestine. Large amounts of fluid and mucus are secreted by the small intestine to facilitate absorption and for protection. Enzyme secretion takes place primarily in the duodenum to facilitate the process of digestion.

LARGE INTESTINE

The large intestine, or colon, serves several functions: maintenance of fluid and electrolyte balance, salvaging the products of intracolonic fermentation, and storage of waste materials until elimination is convenient. Regions of the colon include the cecum, ascending colon, hepatic flexure, transverse colon, splenic flexure, descending colon, sigmoid colon, and rectum. The colon absorbs approximately 1.5 L of fluid a day, mostly in the proximal colon. This results in the daily elimination of 100–200 g of formed stool, usually in one to two bowel movements.

PANCREAS

The pancreas is a complex gland with both exocrine and endocrine functions. The gland consists of acinar, centroacinar, ductal, and islet cells. The exocrine function of the pancreas is to provide enzymes for the digestion of nutrients. The regulation of this process is elaborate, and its disruption can lead to inflammation or destruction of the pancreas. The endocrine pancreas is mostly contained in the islets of Langerhans. Insulin, glucagon, somatostatin, and pancreatic polypeptide are secreted by islet cells.

GALLBLADDER

The gallbladder controls the flow of bile from the liver to the duodenum. Approximately half of the 600–1000 ml bile formed daily enters the gallbladder, where it is concentrated 10-fold. The gallbladder serves many functions, including the acidification, concentration, and storage of bile; release of bile in response to cholecystokinin; regulation of hydrostatic pressure within the biliary tract; and absorption of organic components of bile. Although somewhat controversial, postcholecystectomy patients may experience bile salt diarrhea due to the lack of control of the flow of bile acid. This can be treated with cholestyramine, a bile acid resin.

Two types of electrical activity can be recorded from the smooth muscle of the intestinal tract: slow waves and spike potentials.

Absorption is the process of transferring luminal contents for the purpose of providing energy and building materials for the entire body.

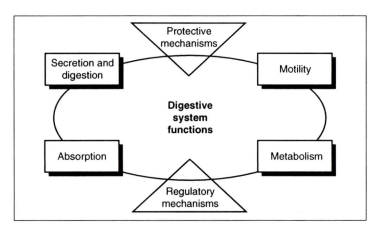

Fig. 1-2. Digestive System Functions

Courtesy of James C. Reynolds, M.D., Drexel University College of Medicine.

LIVER

The liver weighs approximately 1500 g and is divided into four lobes. It is supplied by the right and left hepatic arteries and the portal vein and is drained by the right and left bile ducts. The liver receives 20% of the cardiac output: three-quarters through the portal vein and one-quarter from the hepatic artery. The liver plays a major role in bilirubin metabolism, regulation of hemostasis, protein synthesis and secretion, and drug metabolism.

GI Function

The function of the digestive system is to take food sources from the environment and transport, absorb, and metabolize them, so that they can be used for energy and nutrition (Fig. 1-2).

MOTILITY AND TRANSIT

Transit of material through the digestive tubes results from the interactions of several distinct anatomic and functional units. Slow waves act as the pacing potentials of the gut and control the timing of phasic contractions. Each organ has a characteristic slow-wave frequency.

When depolarization reaches a threshold, spike activity occurs, resulting in influx of calcium (Ca^{2+}) and subsequent muscle contraction. Contractions of the gut have varying influences on transit: Some increase transit, whereas others decrease it. Phasic contractions can be peristaltic (propulsive), antiperistaltic (e.g., vomiting), or segmenting (mixing). Tonic contractions can impede transport (sphincters) or enhance it (gallbladder empties bile).

SECRETION, DIGESTION, AND ABSORPTION

Prior to absorption, ingested nutrients must be broken down into their constituent products through the process of digestion. Digestion is primarily mediated by secretions in the lumen, but it can occur selectively via intracellular mechanisms and via the brush border of small-intestinal epithelial cells.

There are many mechanisms for absorption: passive absorption (down an electrochemical or concentration gradient), solvent drag (neutral cotransport with another ion), cotransport mechanisms (as with glucose or another carrier), and active, receptor-mediated channels (via an active metabolically dependent pump). Absorption can occur anywhere in the small bowel, but certain vitamins and nutrients may be absorbed in specific sites of the small intestine, and therefore certain diseases may result in a selective malabsorption problem. Proximal small bowel disorders, such as celiac disease, may affect absorption of vitamins, iron, and magnesium, whereas disorders of the terminal ileum, such as Crohn's disease, may result in vitamin B_{12} deficiency.

METABOLISM

The GI tract, especially the liver, is the predominant organ system responsible for the metabolic control of nutrients, drug elimination, and synthesis of circulating proteins. Drugs may be broken down by the cytochrome P-450 system in the liver into smaller soluble forms. Detoxification may also take place via glucuronidation.

Mucosal Immunology

The cells lining the luminal intestinal organs are exposed to a hostile environment, including antigens from food and nonfood sources, digestive enzymes, phospholipids, and various solutions at variable pH levels. The epithelium is protected by mucus, and toxic substances are cleared via motility mechanisms and peristalsis.

The mucosal defense system of the GI tract contains a greater mass of reticuloendothelial cells than the spleen. The inflammatory cells of the small intestine constitute a substantial portion of the intestinal wall, approximately 25% by weight of the small intestine. The intestinal immune system consists of various diffuse lymphoid tissues and gut-associated lymphoid tissue (GALT). GALT includes a specialized follicle-associated epithelium known as microfold cells (M cells) in addition to B cells (lymphocytes that may secrete immunoglobulins A, G, or M), plasma cells, and macrophages. The details of the mucosal immune system are reviewed in Chapter 15.

Regulation of the Digestive System

Because of the size of the digestive system (seven organs), the complexity of functions of each organ, and the interaction among different parts of the GI tract, a complex neural and hormonal system is required for the regulation of digestion. The digestive functions are regulated by three different systems: the central nervous system (CNS), the autonomic nervous system, and the enteric nervous system.

The CNS responses may be voluntary, such as in the control of swallowing and the contraction of the external anal sphincter, or involuntary through emotion, stress associations, and conditioned responses. Sensory information may also be interpreted by the CNS. The CNS also modulates function via tonic input from the sympathetic nervous system, which is primarily inhibitory. The parasympathetic fibers serve a primarily stimulatory function via the vagus nerve, particularly in the esophagus and stomach (its role diminishes distally).

The enteric nervous system is an intrinsic, semiautonomous network of nerves that mediate specific events controlled by reflex responses. It is an impressively large system and contains many more neurons than the spinal cord. Cell bodies in the enteric nervous system can reflexively control complex functions in the absence of input from the autonomic or voluntary nervous systems. The myenteric plexus (Auerbach's plexus) and the submucosal plexus (Meissner's plexus) contain the cell bodies of the enteric nervous system.

Enteric hormones regulate the functions of the digestive system. The first such hormone to be discovered, secretin, was identified by Bayless and Starling in 1902. Enteric hormones are released from mucosal endocrine cells, which are derived embryologically from the neural crest. Functions of enteric hormones vary and are often multiple for single hormones. Enteric hormones also influence cell growth.

Neurotransmitters found in the CNS are also located in the enteric nervous system. In addition to classic neurotransmitters like acetylcholine, secretin, and norepinephrine, several recently described transmitters are abundant, including γ-aminobutyric acid and nitric oxide (NO). NO is the leading candidate transmitter for nonadrenergic, noncholinergic inhibition throughout the GI tract. The most abundant class of transmitters in the enteric nervous system and neuroendocrine cells are regulatory peptides. Each peptide may have a variety of functions, depending on the site tested. Regulatory peptides may be released as neurotransmitters, paracrine transmitters, or hormones.

Summary

The GI and hepatobiliary systems perform important functions in the human body. Nutrients must be converted into smaller molecules via the digestive process. These nutrients must be propelled through the digestive system for absorption, and waste must be eliminated. This complex process requires exquisite integrative cooperation and a regulatory and protective mechanism by which to operate. In the ensuing chapters, this book explores the physiologic processes that enable these functions and highlights the complications that occur when the processes malfunction or are disrupted.

CASE STUDY: *RESOLUTION*

The patient presented here was one of the 20% of the entire U.S. population who suffers from irritable bowel syndrome (IBS). Information from the National Digestive Diseases Information

Clearinghouse indicates that, in 1987, IBS affected 5 million people and accounted for 34,000 hospitalizations and 3.5 million physician office visits for complaints consistent with this diagnosis. From 1983 to 1987, approximately 400,000 people were considered disabled because of this diagnosis.

REVIEW QUESTIONS

Directions: For each of the following questions, choose the single best answer.

1 What is the leading cause of cancer death worldwide?

A Lung cancer
B Colon cancer
C Hepatocellular cancer
D Breast cancer

2 In the United States, approximately what percentage of cancers originate in the GI tract?

A 5%
B 10%
C 25%
D 33%

3 The fundus and body of the stomach have which of the following functions?

A They serve a reservoir function and regulate the speed of emptying of liquids.
B They mix and grind food.
C They regulate the speed of emptying of solids.
D They prevent duodenogastric reflux.

4 Which of the following statements concerning the villi is true?

A They are located in the stomach, small intestine, and large intestine.
B They are renewed on a yearly basis.
C They are the functional unit for absorption.
D They are increased in number in celiac disease.

5 Diseases of the terminal ileum would most likely result in a deficiency in which of the following substances?

A Iron
B Vitamin B_{12}
C Folate
D Magnesium

6 The enteric nervous system is best characterized by which of the following statements?

A It contains fewer neurons than the spinal cord.
B It must have input from the CNS to control complex functions.
C It may contain neurons that may have many different neuro-transmitters.
D It has most of the cell bodies located extrinsic to the GI organs.

References

Gastroenterology and Hepatology (MKSAPXII). Philadelphia, PA: American College of Physicians, 2000.

Johnson LR: *Gastrointestinal Physiology*. St. Louis, MO: Elsevier Science, 2001.

U.S. Dept. of Health and Human Services: *Digestive Diseases Statistics*. Washington, DC: National Institutes of Health, 1995, NIH publication no. 95-3873.

Yamada T (ed): *Textbook of Gastroenterology*. Philadelphia, PA: J. B. Lippincott, Williams & Wilkins, 2003.

Zakim D, Boyer T: *Hepatology: A Textbook of Liver Disease*. Philadelphia, PA: W. B. Saunders, 1990.

2

Regulation of the Digestive System

■ CHAPTER OUTLINE ■

■ LEARNING OBJECTIVES ■

At the completion of this chapter, the reader should be able to:
- List the types of regulatory systems that control the digestive system.
- Explain why the digestive system requires such complex control mechanisms.
- Describe the major differences in the five categories of neural control systems involved in the regulation of the digestive system.
- Explain how the enteric endocrine system differs from the classic endocrine system.
- Describe the major characteristics of regulatory peptides.
- List the physiologic events that are regulated by the major transmitters or hormones in the digestive tract.

R.T., a 56-year-old homemaker and mother of three children, presented with diarrhea and epigastric pain. Ten years ago she first developed epigastric pain. An upper GI radiograph was unremarkable. Seven years later, pain developed in her epigastrium 2 months after her son moved away, which was a stressful time for her. After several weeks of inadequate pain relief from escalating doses of antacids, she sought the advice of her primary care physician, who placed the patient on cimetidine, an antagonist to histamine type 2 receptors (H_2-receptor antagonist), twice daily and scheduled a follow-up visit in 6 weeks.

Five days later the patient presented to a local emergency room with black stools and weakness. Her blood pressure was 135/65 mm Hg when lying down but fell to 95/40 mm Hg when sitting. Nasogastric lavage revealed bright-red blood that only partially cleared with 5 gallons of lavage. Endoscopy showed a visible vessel in a 1.5×1.0 cm ulcer in the duodenal bulb and several additional ulcers in the postbulbar region. Injection of the site with a solution of epinephrine stopped the bleeding. Three days later the patient was discharged on the proton pump inhibitor omeprazole. She had continued to take one or two pills daily and was unable to discontinue them because of recurrent abdominal pain, despite many letters from her HMO administrator urging her to do so.

Over the past year she noted more frequent episodes of pain and progressively severe diarrhea. She had taken two pills nearly every day for months. She also reported a 12-lb weight loss despite a good appetite.

Her laboratory values were all normal, except a complete blood count that revealed her hemoglobin to be 8.9 (low) and her mean corpuscular volume to be 72 (low).

The patient was sent for a 2-hour analysis of her blood and for a computerized tomographic (CT) scan. These findings confirmed the presumptive diagnosis, and she was referred to a genetics counselor and a surgeon.

Introduction

In 1902, Bayless and Starling reported their discovery of the first hormone, the GI hormone secretin. This seminal work established the concept that chemical substances can be transported in the blood to regulate physiologic events. In this same work they coined the term *hormone* and emphasized the important interaction of such hormones with neural reflexes. A decade later these same investigators demonstrated that complex reflexive behavior of the small intestine occurred even when a loop of small intestine was isolated from extrinsic neural input. Many decades later, the importance of these discoveries was appreciated when it became apparent that the GI tract had the capacity to regulate digestive functions through extraordinarily complex intrinsic neural and endocrine systems—the enteric nervous system and the enteroendocrine system, respectively. Digestive system functions are closely regulated by both extracellular and intracellular control mechanisms. This chapter provides a broad overview of the mechanisms that regulate digestive functions. These regulatory systems are frequently mentioned in the discussion of normal physiology and pathophysiology of specific organs in subsequent chapters of this book.

The first part of this chapter covers how digestive functions are influenced by extracellular control mechanisms, and the final sections briefly outline the functions of several key transmitters, including nitric oxide and regulatory peptides. It must be remembered, however, that although each of the control mechanisms are discussed separately for the sake of clarity, the cells of the digestive system in vivo are constantly influenced by a variety of chemical signals simultaneously.

Cell–Cell Communications

Organs of the digestive system are constantly influenced by a complex array of extracellular chemical signals. Chemical transmitters originating from nerves, hormone-secreting cells, and inflammatory cells modulate cell functions within all the organs of the digestive system. An very complex array of receptors on the surface of the cell receives a variety of chemical signals simultaneously; secondary messengers interact through signal transduction pathways within the cell to integrate these communications and stimulate a response.

The complex regulatory control functions of the digestive system coordinate the six specific functions performed by the organs of the digestive system. As illustrated in Figure 2-1, these cell–cell transmitters act by one of four mechanisms. *Neural transmitters* are released by neurons into a narrow synaptic cleft to reach target receptors on the adjacent tissues. *Endocrine cells* release hormones into the adjacent capillaries, which distribute them via systemic circulation to receptors on both local and distant target cells. *Paracrine communication* is achieved by the release of chemical transmitters into the interstitial space surrounding nearby cells. *Autocrine secretion* is a special type of paracrine communication that provides feedback inhibition to reduce further secretion of the same hormone. Thus, GI functions are influenced by an array of extracellular communications: by extrinsic neural input originating in the CNS, by neural fibers residing in the intrinsic nervous system, and from a variety of local and system hormones that are released from cells distributed throughout the digestive tract. Although most cells within each organ tend to share a primary function, interspersed within the predominant cell type are cells that perform other, often quite distinct functions at the same

Specific Functions of Digestive Organs
Absorption
Secretion
Motility
Metabolism
Defense
Regulation

Transmission of visceral afferent information involves participation of most of the neurons in both the sympathetic and parasympathetic pathways.

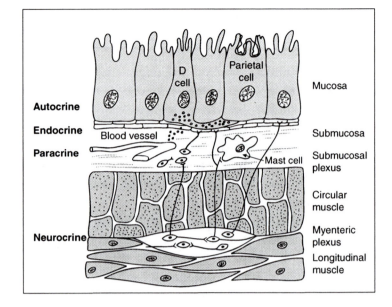

Fig. 2-1.

Four types of cell–cell communications occur throughout the GI tract: autocrine, endocrine, paracrine, and neurocrine. The layers of the luminal organs are labeled on the right. Chemical messengers are released by mucosal enteroendocrine cells, submucosal inflammatory cells, and neurons in the submucosal and myenteric plexus.

time. The coordination of these diverse types of activities is necessary to maximize the efficiency of the digestive processes and of the digestive system's defense against the harsh intraluminal contents.

The extrinsic neurons innervating the digestive system are collectively known as the autonomic nervous system. Classically, the autonomic nervous system has been described as having two subdivisions: the *parasympathetic nervous system* and the *sympathetic nervous system*. The greatest source of neural influence on digestive functions is derived from neurons that have their cell of origin within the wall of the digestive tract. Collectively, this highly complex, ubiquitous intrinsic nervous system of the GI tract is known as the *enteric nervous system (ENS)*.

Similarly, hormones that regulate digestive functions originate both from outside the digestive tract and from cells intrinsic to it. Hormonal communications that originate from sites outside the digestive tract, which make up the endocrine system proper, have important influences on the digestive system. The most important endocrinologic influences on the digestive system, however, originate from hormones secreted by intrinsic endocrine cells. These digestive hormones originate from islet cells in the pancreas and from a huge number of hormone-secreting cells distributed diffusely throughout the mucosa of most tubular organs of the digestive system, the *enteroendocrine cells*. Enteroendocrine cells secrete a surprisingly large number of digestive hormones, nearly all of which are peptides.

COMPLEX COMMUNICATION SYSTEMS

Before discussing each of these regulatory systems specifically, it is important to consider why such complex cell–cell communication systems are needed.

Massive Size of the Digestive System

First, the digestive system is massive in size compared to all other organ systems. It includes seven distinct organs: esophagus, stomach, small intestine, large intestine, gallbladder, liver, and pancreas. Each of these organs is relatively large and therefore presents considerable challenges to regulation and distribution. Not only are there seven distinct organs, but one of the seven, the liver, is the largest (second only to the skin): Its normal weight is 1400–1600 g. For proper digestion to occur, it is important for the mucosa of the distal small intestine to be able to influence the movement of materials through the stomach and proximal intestine, 800 cm upstream. For example, peptide YY (PYY), released from mucosal endocrine cells in the ileum in response to an increase in intraluminal fat and other nutrients, causes slowing of upper intestinal motility. Thus the sheer size of the digestive tract requires that complex regulatory systems be available to orchestrate functions in this physically large array of organs.

Functions of the Digestive System

Second, complex control mechanisms are needed because of the *variety of functions* performed by these seven organs. The major functions of the digestive system are: absorption, secretion and digestion, motility, metabolism, mucosal defense, and regulation. The impact of disease on the digestive system can be most fully appreciated by considering how it impacts each of these functions of the system.

Absorption.   It is intuitively clear that the primary function of the digestive tract is absorption. Interestingly, although there are seven organs in the digestive tract, nearly all absorption is achieved by just one, the small intestine. It alone accounts for absorption of 85% of the fluid taken in and nearly all ingested nutrients. The colon is involved in the absorption of the remaining 1–1.5 L of water and the electrolytes it contains. Because less than 200–250 ml of semisolid excreta remain from the 1.5–2 L of ingested food and over 7 L of daily secretions, this is an extraordinarily efficient (98%) system. Absorption of nutrients occurs through several distinct mechanisms, including active transport, cotransport, pores, and diffusion. Although nearly all absorption occurs in the small bowel, other luminal organs have a capacity for absorption. Nonnutrient absorption of electrolytes and fluid by the gallbladder concentrates bile, leading to the more efficient storage of bile salts until their release is stimulated by a meal. As mentioned, the colon also absorbs fluid and electrolytes, leading to the solidification of stool. Small amounts of nutrients are absorbed by organs other than the small intestine. The gastric mucosa has been shown

to absorb ethanol. The colon absorbs vitamin K and short-chain fatty acids in normal individuals. Fatty acids are a major nutrient source for colonic epithelial cells. In disorders characterized by fat malabsorption, as in patients with Crohn's disease who have had a long segment of terminal ileum resected, the colon absorbs excess oxalate. This may lead to the formation of calcium oxalate kidney stones.

Secretion.   The digestive system secretes 7 L of fluid a day to assist with digestion, transit, and absorption. To optimize the efficiency of the digestive process, secretion must be regulated to correlate with intraluminal demand. Although this secretion is most commonly associated with the luminal organs, it is important to remember that the digestive system's solid organs (the liver and pancreas) are also major secretory bodies. Secretions produced by cells of the digestive tract are complex but can be divided into two types for simplification. Most secretions are preformed substances that are found in serum, such as water, electrolytes, and bilirubin. Other specialized secretory cells are involved in the secretion of substances that have been synthesized by the cell. These include enzymes, mucus, neurotransmitters, hormones, bile salts, and transport proteins.

Motility.   Motility of the gut serves three distinct functions: storage, mucosal protection, and nutrient delivery. In some organs, contractions are organized to lead to the storage and timely release of intraluminal contents. Storage is a key motility function of the gallbladder, stomach, and colon. Motility serves to protect the mucosa by limiting contact time and enhancing the mixing of intraluminal contents with digestive and immunologically active secretions. Finally, motility serves to deliver nutrients to the mucosal surfaces for absorption in a timely fashion. When considering the regulation of a given organ's motility, it is useful to consider how the contractile events that characterize the motility patterns of that organ change throughout the day. In general, this is best seen as changes that occur in response to fasting and eating. Other, less apparent but important types of motility are the contractions of the muscularis mucosa and villi that alter the adjacent unstirred water layer.

Metabolism.   Metabolism for the rest of the organism is greatly influenced by the digestive system. The liver contains the primary metabolic machinery of the body, performing many complex biochemical transformations and storing a key energy source, glycogen. It is also responsible for the removal of fat-soluble, protein-bound toxins and waste products. Pancreatic endocrine cells regulate fat and glucose metabolism throughout the body. The small bowel plays a major role in the metabolism of fat through the resynthesis of triglycerides and the synthesis of apolipoproteins.

Defense Mechanisms and Immunity.   The intraluminal contents of the digestive tract pose a constant and considerable risk to the rest of the organism because of the caustic chemical character and microorganism content of intraluminal fluids. In fact, some have argued that the lumen of the GI tract is not actually part of the body but simply a tube within a tube. Thus it is essential to maintain differentiation of the polarity of the epithelial cells that line the tube and to maintain mechanisms to protect the integrity of the lining of the tube against a potentially injurious environment. The digestive system is protected by immunologic and nonimmunologic defense mechanisms. Immune defenses consist of the intra-epithelial lymphocytes, lamina propria leukocytes, M cells, Peyer's patches, gut-associated lymphoid tissue (GALT), and Kupffer's cells of the liver. Together with Peyer's patches and intestinal lymph nodes, the inflammatory cells of the small intestine make up nearly 25% of its total weight. Nonimmune mechanisms play an equally important role defending the organism through the protective effects of mucus, motility, acid secretion, and the integrity of cell–cell tight junctions.

Heterogeneity of Cells of the Digestive System

Complex regulatory mechanisms are needed because of the heterogeneous nature of cell types within each organ. To fully appreciate the complexity of the digestive system, it must be understood that within a given organ adjacent cells may be involved with the performance of each of these functions within millimeters of each other. It is important to note that another function that is closely regulated by these systems is *cell growth*. Several regulatory peptides have a trophic effect on cells of the same or other organs of the digestive system. Thus, in addition to activating acid-secreting (parietal) cells of the stomach, the hormone gastrin has a trophic effect on these cells that increases their number. An example of this type of organ-to-organ communication is the effect of enteroglucagon, released from the distal ileum and colon, on the number and height of absorptive cells in the duodenum and jejunum.

EXTRINSIC NEURAL CONTROL OF THE DIGESTIVE SYSTEM

For most of the twentieth century, GI functions were thought to be regulated by nerves from the CNS that were modulated by gut hormones. We now know from patients and animals that have undergone multivisceral organ transplants (stomach, pancreas, liver, small intestine, and colon) that much of the gut can function almost normally even when devoid of all extrinsic neural input. Nevertheless, the CNS plays a key role in normal gut function. The importance of this interaction is known as the brain–gut axis.

Voluntary Influence by the CNS

Voluntary neurons of the CNS influence digestive function by mediating control of swallowing and the muscles of the pelvic floor (primarily the puborectalis muscle) and the external anal sphincter. Indirect voluntary CNS control occurs through conditioned responses and emotion and stress associations. The CNS also modifies digestive function by the interpretation of sensory function.

Mediation of the Brain–Gut Axis
Four types of nerves mediate the brain–gut axis: voluntary motor neurons from the CNS, involuntary motor neurons from the sympathetic and the parasympathetic nervous systems, and visceral afferent neurons.

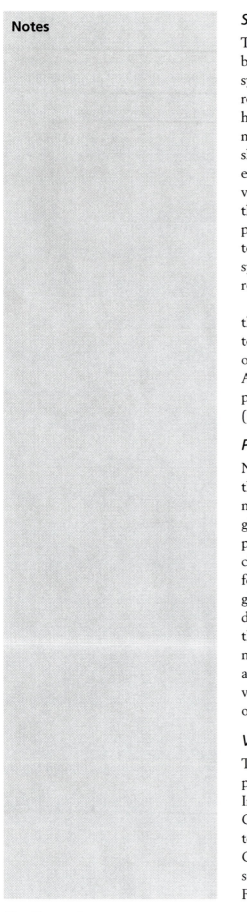

Sympathetic Nervous System

The CNS modulates digestive functions through the two involuntary branches of the autonomic nervous system, the sympathetic nervous system and the parasympathetic nervous system. The fight-or-flight response of the sympathetic nervous system primarily provides an inhibitory tone to digestive functions. This results in an inhibition of motility and secretion and a reduction of mesenteric blood flow to shunt blood to the muscles involved with fight and flight. The notable exception to the widespread inhibitory effect of the sympathetic nervous system is its excitatory effect on enteric sphincters. This reduces the flow of luminal contents from one organ to another. Efferent, postganglionic sympathetic neurons contain the adrenergic transmitters norepinephrine and, to a lesser extent, dopamine. Perivascular sympathetic neurons also often contain the peptide transmitter neuropeptide Y (NPY).

Sympathetic communications reach the digestive system through the splanchnic nerve and the paravertebral, celiac, superior mesenteric, and inferior mesenteric ganglia. Spinal visceral afferent neurons originate in the dorsal root ganglia along several levels of the cord. As will be discussed, nearly one-third of these neurons contain the peptide transmitters substance P or calcitonin gene-related peptide (CGRP) or both.

Parasympathetic Nervous System

Neurons in the parasympathetic nervous system project fibers into the digestive tract via the vagus and pelvic nerves. Nearly all efferent nerves in the parasympathetic nervous system are pre- and postganglionic cholinergic fibers. Peptidergic transmitters are also involved in parasympathetic communications, particularly the neurotransmitter cholecystokinin (CCK). Approximately 80% of all vagal fibers are afferent neurons carrying information to the CNS via the nodose ganglion. Parasympathetic nerves generally have a stimulatory effect on digestive system functions. Input from the vagal nerves is extensive throughout the esophagus and stomach but decreases throughout the more distal GI tract. In fact, neurons that innervate the oropharynx and esophagus are specifically organized in a viscerotropic order from ventral to caudal in the vagal neural complex. No other digestive organ has a specific viscerotropic organization in the CNS.

Visceral Afferent Neurons

The CNS receives nociception and sensory input from neurons in the parasympathetic and sympathetic (spinal afferent) nervous pathways. Information about painful abdominal conditions also reaches the CNS through the spinothalamic pathways carrying input from mesenteric neurons. Sensory information from the digestive system to the CNS is much less precise and less accurate than that received from somatic sensory pathways. The explanation for this is multifaceted. First, although most extrinsic nerves reaching the digestive system are afferent, the density of afferent nerves per square centimeter is less than that in the somatic system. Second, the visceral sensory nerves from each of the GI organs enter the spinal afferent pathways through several spinal levels. This reduces the accuracy of localization and is partly responsible for the phenomenon of referred pain. Third, fibers carrying visceral pain information are unmyelinated C-fibers. These fibers transmit information more slowly and less precisely than myelinated somatic sensory fibers. Finally, the majority of receptors in the digestive tract that carry information to the CNS are relatively nonspecific and respond to a variety of stimuli. These nonspecific receptors are known as "naked free" nerve endings. Extrinsic neural reflexes that depend on afferent reflex pathways have been demonstrated to influence both secretory and motor events. Afferent fibers containing CGRP are also involved in gastric reflexes that help mediate mucosal protection. Afferent CGRP fibers reflexively stimulate bicarbonate secretion and increased mucosal blood flow. Thus, afferent innervation to the GI tract is not only involved with nociception.

Intrinsic Neural Control by the Enteric Nervous System

Though extrinsic nerves provide important modulating effects on digestive function, specific events of the digestive system are mediated by intrinsic neurons under the control of reflex responses of the ENS. There are about 10 million nerves in the ENS. Not only is this an order of magnitude greater than that of all sympathetic and parasympathetic nerves, it is more than the number of nerves in the spinal cord. Since the experiments of Bayless and Starling over a century ago, it has been known that even complicated GI motility events (such as small intestinal peristalsis) can occur in the absence of extrinsic neural innervation. Likewise, secretory responses to local physical or chemical stimulation, sphincter contraction or relaxation in response to the distention of distal or proximal adjacent bowel loops, respectively, and esophageal peristalsis have all been demonstrated in vitro. These and other experimental data derived from direct recordings in the ganglia of the gut indicate that complex neural pathways exist in the local neurons that make up the ENS. Although important input can be demonstrated to occur through reflexes through paraspinal ganglia and from the CNS, the ENS is the site where most digestive tract functions are regulated.

Anatomy of the ENS

Cell bodies of the ENS are located in the myenteric (Auerbach's) plexus and submucosal (Meissner's) plexus. Electrophysiologic and ablation studies have demonstrated that the myenteric plexus is the dominant nerve center that regulates both mucosal function and contractions of the muscularis propria. Meissner's plexus receives information from local sensory nerves and modifies epithelial cell function and submucosal blood flow.

The **ENS** serves as an intrinsic, semiautonomous network of nerves constituting the hard wiring of the gut.

Neural circuitry in the myenteric plexus has been described as an intrinsic computer that, when triggered, initiates patterned programmed responses. The ENS's responses are thought to be primarily reflexively controlled. These hard-wired reflex pathways are then modulated by sympathetic postganglionic and parasympathetic preganglionic fibers and by intestinal hormones. A model of this neural circuitry that has been proposed for the peristaltic reflex is summarized in Chapter 4.

Detailed analysis of the nerves in the ENS has shown that they vary widely in shape, content of neurotransmitters, and electrophysiologic characteristics. Dogiel characterized three shapes of enteric neurons: Dogiel type I neurons are monopolar neurons with a single dendritic process that is much longer than types II or III neurons. Unlike somatic nerves, however, which carry signals over considerable distances, Dogiel type I neurons are typically less than 1 cm long and rarely extend over 1–2 cm. Dogiel types II and III neurons have multiple axons and dendritic processes that provide a mechanism for multiple neural inputs. Nearly all of these neurons are less than 1 cm long. These neurons are well suited to function as local neural reflexes and as motor neurons.

Electrophysiologic Characteristics of the ENS

Enteric neurons can be distinguished by the electric characteristics of the nerves, determined by recording the responses to stimulation of neural processes. This classification is based on the length and shape of the action potential and by the characteristic of the resting membrane potential. A summary of these characteristics is shown in Table 2-1. These characteristics, first determined in recordings from the myenteric neurons in the guinea pig small intestine, have provided a framework for describing enteric neurons elsewhere in the

Table 2-1. Neuron Type

NEURON TYPE ELECTROPHYSIOLOGIC	DOGIEL	RMP/ AMPLITUDE	TTX SENSITIVE [SODIUM CHANNEL]	IH FINDINGS	MYENTERIC PLEXUS FAST EPSP[a] (4–40 ms)	SLOW EPSP (15–120 s)	IPSP
AH-II After-hyperpolarization Ca^{2+}-dependent K$^+$ channel	II ? sensory	59/83 Higher/high	No Ca^{2+} and Na$^+$	Calbindin	Less often have fast EPSP	40% Noncholinergic serotonin	Rare
S-I Repetitive spike discharges after depolarization	I, III, IV Uniaxonal	54/68 Less/low	Yes	VIP, ENK, Dyn	Prominent inhibition by hexamethonium; ? sympathetic	75% muscarinic and some second ? substance P	Rare

Note. RMP = resting membrane potential; TTX = tetrodotoxin; IH = immunohistochemical; EPSP = excitatory postsynaptic potential; IPSP = inhibitory postsynaptic potential; VIP = vasoactive intestinal peptide; ENK = enkephalin; Dyn = dynorphin.
[a]Fast EPSPs are the major synaptic input in the enteric nervous system; they are seen in 70% of myenteric and 90% of submucosal neurons.

gut and for understanding reflex circuitry. Two primary nerve types have been described, AH (after-hyperpolarization) and S neurons.

Neurotransmitters in the ENS

The complexity of the ENS is demonstrated by its size, its functional variability, and the remarkable number of neurotransmitters it contains. Nerves in the ENS contain most (if not all) of the same transmitters present in the CNS. In fact, many of the neurotransmitters now known to be critical to CNS communications were first discovered in the ENS. Dozens of transmitters can be identified in every few millimeters of the length of the digestive tract. Even within organs like the esophagus and gallbladder, which have relatively limited function and repertoire of responses, the complex array of neurotransmitters is similar to that found in other luminal organs of the GI tract. Characterization of transmitters by location or by their specific functions is not practical, because each type of nerve and each type of transmitter can be found throughout the GI tract and is involved in a variety of functions. Acknowledging this risk of oversimplification, several of the better understood transmitters and their functions are listed in Table 2-2.

In several recent studies, it has been shown that most neurons in the ENS contain more than one transmitter. In fact, many ENS neurons contain four or more transmitters. When stimulated, a neuron in the ENS may release a single transmitter or several different transmitters simultaneously. Many transmitters in the ENS bind to several subtypes of receptors with variable affinity. Regulatory peptides, serotonin γ-aminobutyric acid (GABA), and acetylcholine have multiple receptor subtypes. In fact, there are more than five specific receptor subtypes to the transmitter serotonin (5-hydroxytryptamine, or 5-HT). Thus the response to the stimulation of a nerve varies by the type and number of transmitters released and by the types and numbers of ligand receptors present on the target organ.

All of the classic neurotransmitters—including norepinephrine, epinephrine, dopamine, serotonin, acetylcholine, and GABA—are found throughout the GI tract. The adrenergic amines, epinephrine and norepinephrine, are located only in extrinsic sympathetic pathways, but acetylcholine, serotonin, and GABA are found in nerves of the ENS. In addition to these transmitters, over the past few decades over 30 different peptide transmitters and hormones have been identified in the GI tract.

Perhaps the most important transmitter discovered over the past two decades, however, is nitric oxide (NO). For many years, stimulation of the wall of the luminal organs of the GI tract has been shown to cause reflexive relaxation. The inhibitory reflex was shown to be critical to the normal functioning of GI sphincters and to the reflexes that mediate peristalsis. Studies of these reflexes with a variety of specific antagonists to sympathetic transmitters, acetylcholine, and many neuropeptides failed to identify the chemical transmitter that mediated

NO is a profoundly important inhibitory transmitter.

Table 2-2. Regulatory Peptides and Primary Function

REGULATORY PEPTIDE	AMINO ACID CHAIN LENGTH	PRIMARY FUNCTION
Cholecystokinin	33–58	Events associated with lipid and protein digestion (pancreatic enzyme secretion, gallbladder contraction, delayed gastric emptying); trophic to pancreas; controls satiety
Enteroglucagon	37	Trophic to small intestine; released in malabsorptive states
Gastric inhibitory peptide	42	Glucose-dependent insulin release; inhibits gastric secretion and stimulates small bowel secretion
Gastrin	17	Acid secretion; trophic to stomach and pancreas
Gastrin-releasing peptide	27	Stimulates secretion by mucosal cells, neurons, and mammalian bombesin-hormone–secreting cells
Motilin	22	Initiates phase III of the migrating myoelectric complex (MMC) in the proximal GI tract
Neurotensin	13	Vasodilation, stimulates secretion
Pancreatic polypeptide	36	Regulates pancreatic secretion
Peptide YY	36	Related from ileum; inhibits motility and secretion of the upper GI tract (the ileal brake)
Secretin	27	Stimulates pancreatic fluid and bicarbonate secretion
Somatostatin	28	Important inhibitory transmitter; inhibits secretion by neurons, hormone-secreting cells, and epithelial cells
Substance P	11	Regulates vasodilation, muscle contraction and secretion; sensory transmitter in sympathetic neurons
Vasoactive intestinal polypeptide	28	Stimulates secretion of fluid and electrolytes; inhibits muscle contraction

these reflexes. This elusive transmitter became known as the non-adrenergic, noncholinergic (NANC) inhibitory transmitter. Most authorities feel that NO is the transmitter responsible for sphincter relaxation throughout the digestive tract and in other essential NANC inhibitory reflexes. Although many of the specific functions of this key neurotransmitter remain incompletely understood, reflexes that involve NO include esophageal and intestinal peristalsis, inhibition of mucosal secretion, and relaxation of all GI sphincters.

Endocrine System of the GI Tract

The hormonal control system of the GI tract differs from hormones in the endocrine system in several ways. Most notably, GI hormones are not secreted by discrete endocrine organs but by specialized mucosal endocrine cells that are interspersed between other types of cells in the stomach, pancreas, and small and large intestines. GI hormone-secreting cells are found in the islets of the pancreas and interspersed between the mucosal cells throughout the columnar cell–lined epithelium. These specialized mucosal cells are known as *enterochromaffin* cells because of their histologic staining characteristics. By far the greatest number of hormone-secreting cells of the digestive system are the enteric endocrine cells found in the mucosa. Hormones released by the digestive system circulate in levels that are typically 1000-fold less than that of other hormones, such as insulin. Most digestive hormones have a very brief circulation time. Most are unbranched, relatively short peptides that are rapidly degraded by enzymes in tissues and in blood. The kidney plays an important role in the metabolism of several peptides, including gastrin.

Enteric endocrine cells may contain a variety of different types of chemical messengers, including histamine, dopamine, and regulatory peptides. These hormones can be released as classic hormones into the vascular system or into the interstitial space in a paracrine fashion. Hormonal messengers have the advantage of being able to simultaneously affect regions of the digestive tract that are physically separated by considerable distance. CCK, one of the more extensively studied hormones, mediates the response to fat. Intraluminal carbohydrates and proteins have little effect on its release. In the circulation it exerts an effect on the stomach (delayed emptying), pyloric sphincter (contraction), gallbladder (contraction and secretion), sphincter of Oddi (sphincter relaxation), small intestine (contractility), and pancreas (secretion of enzymes and electrolyte solution). Furthermore, this hormone influences the CNS satiety centers. Thus a single hormone can influence complex responses, complementary responses, and responses that are distant from one another.

Similarly, but on a much smaller scale, hormones released into the interstitial space in a *paracrine* fashion can simultaneously influence the variety of different cell types within a local region. Thus the interstitial release of histamine by enterochromaffin-like (ECL) cells in the gastric mucosa influences the secretion of acid by parietal cells, the release of gastrin by mucosal endocrine cells, blood flow, and immunologic functions. Paracrine release may occur from the base of the cell or from specialized extensions that come into direct contact with the target cells, thus simulating neurocrine release.

Many of the islet cells in the pancreas secrete regulatory peptides that have an important influence on GI functions. These cells characteristically surround the insulin-secretory beta cells of the islets.

Some can be found interspersed between pancreatic secretory cells. Glucagon, pancreatic polypeptide, and somatostatin are examples of GI peptides released from islets.

The largest number of GI hormone-secreting cells and the greatest variety of hormones are released by *specialized mucosal endocrine cells.* They are found in surprisingly large numbers interspersed among the predominant type of epithelial cell in the mucosa from the stomach to the colon. Some of these enteric endocrine cells release their transmitters in an endocrine fashion (e.g., gastrin, CCK, PYY, enteroglucagon, motilin), others in a paracrine manner (e.g., histamine), and others as both (e.g., somatostatin).

Mucosal endocrine cells have a specialized structure that provides a means of detecting them by standard hematoxylin-eosin-stained histologic sections, if they are well oriented. The use of specialized histochemical stains (immunohistochemistry) for neuron-specific enolase, chromogranin, or for specific peptides permits their definitive recognition. They have a pyramidal shape that appears triangular in crosssection. Most are "open type," with numerous microvilli that extend into the lumen at their apex. These microvilli appear to sample the chemical nature of the luminal contents. Others appear to have a closed apical end, without contact with the lumen. The cell contains an abundance of mitochondria, rough endoplasmic reticulum (RER), and Golgi apparatus suitable for its function as a secretory cell. Just above the basal aspect of the cell are numerous secretory granules filled with synthesized messengers, poised for release. Regulatory peptides are released by the process of exocytosis.

Although mucosal endocrine cells can be found throughout the columnar cell–lined mucosa of the digestive tract, the hormones they contain show a functionally distinct distribution (Table 2-3). For

Table 2-3. Origins and Locations of Major Digestive System Hormones

GUT HORMONE	CELL OF ORIGIN	PRINCIPAL LOCATION
Somatostatin	D cells[a]	Throughout gut and pancreas
Glucagon	Alpha cells	Pancreas (body and tail)
Pancreatic polypeptide (PP)	. . .	Pancreas (head and uncinate process)
Gastrin	G cells	Gastric antrum
Cholecystokinin	. . .[a]	Duodenum
Secretin	S cells	Duodenum (less so in jejunum)
Gastric inhibitory polypeptide	K cells	Duodenum and jejunum
Motilin	M cells	Duodenum and jejunum
Neurotensin	N cells[a]	Ileum (less so in jejunum)
Enteroglucagons	L cells	Ileum and colon
Peptide YY	L cells	Ileum and colon

[a]Indicates peptides that are often found extensively in neurons.

example, gastrin, which regulates acid secretion from the stomach, is located in gastric hormone-secreting cells. CCK is located primarily in duodenal mucosa, where it is poised to regulate the digestion of fats as they are emptied from the stomach. Motilin, a hormone that regulates fasting motility, is located in the upper small intestine, where it can respond to a prolonged absence of nutrients. In contrast, PYY, which delays motility of the stomach and upper small intestine when nutrients enter the distal intestine because of incomplete absorption, is located in endocrine cells of the ileal mucosa. In contrast, somatostatin, which has a key inhibitory paracrine effect, is evenly distributed throughout the digestive tract.

Regulatory Peptides

GENERAL CHARACTERISTICS

Regulatory peptides are the most abundant type of chemical transmitters in the GI tract. Most are also found in the CNS, hence the name *brain–gut peptides*. They are all nonbranching chains of 3 to 69 amino acids that are initially synthesized as inactive proteins (prohormones). These peptides may be released as hormones, parahormones, or neurotransmitters. Several of these peptides are released by more than one type of cell. Somatostatin is released by all three mechanisms. Before discussing specific peptides and their known functions, it is important to review some of the special characteristics of this family of chemical transmitters.

Regulatory peptides are most commonly known by acronyms made up of the first letter in each word of the particular peptide's name or indicating a special structural aspect. Unfortunately, the original name given to a peptide often provides little information about the function of the peptide as we understand it today. When the earliest peptides were discovered, such as secretin, gastrin, and CCK, they were isolated from extracts of mucosa by scientists in search of a peptide that controlled a given function. Their names provide information about their physiologic significance. More commonly these days, however, this is not the case. It may be because the original function of the peptide was unknown or was described incorrectly. Examples include substance P (SP), gastric inhibitory peptide (GIP), and vasoactive intestinal polypeptide (VIP). More recently, biologically active peptides were isolated before their function was known. Many of these peptides are named because of a unique aspect of their structure. For example, PYY was given its name because it has a tyrosine molecule on both the amino and carboxyl terminals (Y being the one-letter abbreviation for tyrosine). PHI, peptide histidine isoleucine, is the peptide with amino-terminal histidine and carboxyl-terminal isoleucine (H and I being the one-letter abbreviations for histidine and isoleucine, respectively). Therefore, regulatory peptides are usually referred to by their two- to four-letter acronym, despite the fact that the full name that those letters represent may have little or no biologic significance.

Table 2-4. Peptide Families

SECRETIN–VIP	NEUROMEDIN
Secretin	Substance P
Vasoactive intestinal peptide (VIP)	Neuromedin A
Peptide histidine methionine (PHM)	Neuromedin B
Peptide histidine isoleucine (PHI)	
Gastric inhibitory peptide (GIP)	**PANCREATIC POLYPEPTIDE**
Glucagon	Peptide YY (PYY)
Glycetin	Neuropeptide (NPY)
Enteroglucagon	Pancreatic peptide (PP)
Oxyntomodulin	
Glucagon-like peptides (GLP-1 and GLP-2)	**OPIOID PEPTIDE**
	Enkephalin
CHOLECYSTOKININ (CCK)–GASTRIN	Dynorphin
CCK 8	
CCK 16	
CCK 33	
Gastrin	

Many regulatory peptides show considerable homology in their amino acid sequence, particularly in the carboxyl terminus that determines receptor specificity. Grouping by structural families does not relate to the type of cell in which the peptide is found or to its function. Examples of regulatory peptide families are discussed later and are listed in Table 2-4. In some circumstances, structurally similar peptides may be coreleased by the same cell. This is true for VIP and peptide histidine methionine (PHM), two neuropeptides. More commonly, the inclusion of two peptides in a family indicates little about their function or the type of cell in which they reside. For example, peptides of the pancreatic polypeptide (PP) family show greater than 50% amino acid homology and even greater homology at the active carboxyl terminal, yet each is secreted by different types of cells: NPY from neurons, PP from islet cells, and PYY from the enteroendocrine cells of the ileum.

Regulatory peptides are often transcribed from the same *prepropeptide gene*. This is particularly true of regulatory peptides that coexist in the same cell (e.g., PHI, VIP). On the other hand, some peptides within the same family can generate different regulatory peptides from the same gene. The gene that encodes the synthesis of calcitonin in the C cells of the thyroid gland also encodes for CGRP, a neurotransmitter. The preprohormone gene that encodes the prohormone for glucagon in pancreatic cells encodes the sequences for enteroglucagons in the ileum, including oxyntomodulin and glucagon-like peptides 1 and 2 (GLP-1, GLP-2).

The effect of the release of a regulatory peptide is determined by the amount released and by its biologic activity. Regulatory peptides are characterized by the various modifications they undergo after they are synthesized known as *posttranslational processing*, which markedly alters their biologic activity. After a peptide sequence is translated from its respective mRNA, it may be shortened to variable lengths that differ considerably in their biologic activity. Gastrin and CCK are two important examples of this type of posttranslational processing. Biologically active forms of CCK may exist in lengths of 33, 8, and 7 amino acids. All share the identical terminal heptapeptide. Lengthening the heptapeptide of CCK by a single amino acid to CCK-8 increases its potency 100-fold. A second type of posttranslational processing is sulfation. Sulfation further increases CCK's receptor affinity another 3- to 10-fold.

Another characteristic of regulatory peptides shared by many other types of neurotransmitters is that a single peptide may serve as a ligand to several distinct receptor subtypes. Peptide sequences may activate a variety of distinct receptor subtypes. For example, the opioid family of peptides has at least three receptor subtypes, and each specific subtype may produce opposite effects at different sites. For instance, delta opioid receptors stimulate pyloric contractions while inhibiting contractions in the adjacent duodenum.

MECHANISMS OF CELLULAR REGULATION

The influence of regulatory peptides and other transmitters on cellular functions is highly regulated at three levels: (1) within the neuron or endocrine cell releasing the transmitter, (2) during diffusion and circulation to the target organ, and (3) within the target organ. Within the regulatory cell, the ultimate effect of a transmitter is determined by its rate of synthesis, posttranslational processing, rate of packaging, the types of transmitters with which it is packaged, and its rate of release. As mentioned, both NO and regulatory peptides have rapid rates of degradation. The pathway a transmitter takes to reach the target cell therefore influences its potency. Thus the concentration of a neuropeptide released into a synaptic space is likely to be considerably greater than that of a hormone released into the interstitial space by paracrine mechanisms, and concentrations of both will be considerably less than that of a hormone released into the circulation. These are important considerations when the potential effects of a given transmitter are being studied by application to a target organ. Furthermore, the effect of the transmitter on a target organ is determined by the number of receptors present on the membrane of the target cell, the magnitude of secondary messenger response following peptide–receptor binding, and the interplay between secondary messengers within the target cell. Advances in cell biology are beginning to clarify just how highly regulated each of these individual steps is.

There are several key mechanisms through which these cellular events are regulated. Activation of the endocrine cell or neuron results in stimulation of the nucleus to synthesize a transmitter. Nucleic acids contain the information that directs all cellular functions by directing the conversion of information from DNA into RNA through the process of transcription. RNA polymerase explores DNA in the nucleus for specific sequences that serve as promoters. Through the action of accessory proteins (sigma factors), the primary RNA sequences produced are then modified. Sequences that are not transcribed (introns) are removed, and the remaining exons are spliced together to produce carrier RNA, called messenger RNA or mRNA. Transcription always progresses from the 5-end to the 3-end. The DNA sequence provides the information specifying the RNA codons, which in turn determine the amino acid sequence of the regulatory peptide. Other segments of the gene direct the transcription process. The promoter sequence specifies the starting site for transcription. Enhancers increase the number of sequences transcribed. They may be adjacent to the gene or at some distance from the transcription sequence.

The information encoded in the mRNA directs the synthesis of the regulatory peptide through translation. After mRNAs are translated into specific polypeptides, further processing occurs. Key to the proper processing of the newly synthesized prohormone is correct intracellular trafficking. The leading edge of most secreted peptides begins with a hydrophobic leader or "signal sequence" that enhances its movement through the lipid bilayer of the endoplasmic reticulum (ER)–Golgi apparatus. The long chains of linear polypeptides are transformed into three-dimensional structures by their exposure to specific pH and ionic conditions, as well as by alterations of the three-dimensional structure by the formation of disulfide bonds, protease cleavage, phosphorylation, methylation, glycosylation, and covalent linkage to other peptides. Reduction in peptide length influences the duration of biologic activity of a peptide. Nearly all regulatory peptides require amidation of the carboxyl-terminal sequence. Sulfation increases the activity of several peptides and is critical to the activity of several, including serotonin. Posttranslational processing plays a major role in determining the biologic activity of the initial coded sequence of amino acids and provides a number of steps through which a diversity of peptides are produced.

Synthesized and processed prohormones are then packaged and concentrated into secretory granules. When activated, these granules are extruded from the cell through the process of exocytosis. The membrane of the secretory granule fuses with the cell membrane and the contents of the granule are emptied into the extracellular space. In the case of neurocrine and paracrine release, the peptide diffuses only a short distance to the target cell receptors. In the case of hormones, the peptide diffuses into the capillary via fenestrations in the adjacent capillary wall, circulates in the blood, then reaches the target organ by rediffusing through the fenestrations of the capillaries to the target organ.

Receptors are specific complex glycoprotein molecules residing in cellular membranes, which activate biologic responses when occupied by specific ligands known as agonists. The ligand can bind the receptor when three-dimensional configuration and electrophilic interactions between them are complementary. Once a specific fit occurs between ligand and receptor, the receptor undergoes a conformational change, resulting in the activation of subunits of the molecule. This in turn results in the initiation of a cascade of intracellular events that eventually results in the desired effect, such as secretion or contraction.

Once activated, the cell responds through an increasingly better understood series of events that communicate the activated state to the cell organelles. Most regulatory peptides activate the target cell by binding to G protein–coupled receptors. These receptors have seven membrane-spanning regions, including one that binds to guanylate cyclase and can activate signal transduction pathways or channels to effect cell activation. A typical example of this type of activation is the binding of VIP to a stimulatory G protein (Gs), which in turn increases the intracellular concentration of cyclic adenosine monophosphate (cAMP) through the activation of adenylate cyclase. In the same cell, another receptor may be bound to an inhibitory G protein (G_i), such as NPY or somatostatin, which decreases adenylate cyclase activity. Activated adenylate cyclase results in the production of increased concentrations of cAMP from ATP, which in turn activates cAMP-dependant protein kinases, such as protein kinase A. Protein kinases in turn activate other intracellular kinase events. This cascade of events provides multiple steps for further regulation and checks and balances within the cell.

Activated receptors may also activate cellular functions by altering the intracellular concentration of calcium (Ca^{2+}). Activation of G proteins stimulates the release of Ca^{2+} from intracellular organelles, such as the ER. This occurs as a result of the effect of G protein on inositol-1,4,5-triphosphate (IP_3). In some cells, the resting membrane potential can be altered, resulting in the opening of Ca^{2+} channels, which are closed in the resting state, and the inward flow of Ca^{2+}. Small flushes of Ca^{2+} from the extracellular space can stimulate a further increase in the concentration of unbound intracellular Ca^{2+} by the release of intracellular stores. Intracellular Ca^{2+} binds to calmodulin to form a Ca^{2+}–calmodulin complex, which in turn increases the phosphorylation of important proteins and enzymes within the cell.

Many cells besides enteric neurons become activated by an alteration of the resting membrane potential, permitting the transport of a specific ion, including all smooth muscle cells, endocrine cells, and secretory cells. The resting membrane potential is established by the relative permeability of the plasma membrane to selected ions, such as Ca^{2+}, potassium (K^+), sodium (Na^+), and chloride (Cl^-). Changes in the rate of opening and closing of these channels result from conformational changes of the channels. This process is known as *gating*. For most of these cells there is a background permeability, primarily to K^+, which establishes the resting membrane potential. *Depolarization* of the cells occurs when inward Na^+ (neurons) or Ca^{2+} (smooth muscle cells) channels open sufficiently to reach threshold potential.

Specific regulatory peptides of known clinical significance are summarized next. An outline of these and other peptides is found in Table 2-2.

Secretin-VIP Family

The largest family of regulatory peptides is the secretin-VIP family. This family includes secretin, VIP, PHM, PHI, glucose-dependent insulinotropic peptide (GIP, previously known as gastric inhibitory peptide), glucagon, the enteroglucagons glycetin and oxyntomodulin, and GLP-1 and GLP-2. As already mentioned, the first hormone to be identified was secretin. Bayless and Starling coined the name after they demonstrated that a substance released from extracts of the duodenum could influence pancreatic secretion of bicarbonate (HCO_3^-). They also correctly demonstrated that secretin release was determined by duodenal acidification. Ingested nutrients, bile, oleate, and alcohol are less potent stimulants. Secretin remains the most important mediator of pancreatic HCO_3^- secretion, an effect that is potentiated by CCK. It also stimulates the secretion of HCO_3^- from Brunner's glands in the duodenum. Secretin is released from endocrine cells in the duodenal mucosa. It is metabolized primarily by the kidney.

VIP shares considerable homology with secretin, but in contrast, VIP is a neurotransmitter, not a hormone. For nearly a decade, VIP was the leading candidate for the NANC inhibitory transmitters that are now thought to be mediated by NO. Nevertheless, VIP appears to play a crucial role in many NANC inhibitory reflexes, perhaps by interacting directly with NO. PHM is structurally very similar to VIP and is translated from the same gene. It is released from the same neurons as VIP and shares several similar effects. VIP release from neuroendocrine tumors of the pancreas or duodenum causes life-threatening diarrhea.

Glucagon, glycentin, oxyntomodulin, GLP-1, and GLP-2 are all synthesized from the same preproglucagon gene. Glucagon is released from the pancreas, predominantly from cells in the body and tail. It opposes many of the metabolic effects of insulin by regulating the rates of glycogenolysis, lipolysis, gluconeogenesis, and ketogenesis. Glycentin, the predominant form of glucagon released from enteroglucagon cells in the ileum and colon, contains the entire glucagon sequence with amino and carboxyl extensions. Enteroglucagon is released in response to nutrients, primarily fats, in the ileal lumen. It has a trophic effect on proximal intestinal epithelial cells and is released in disorders characterized by steatorrhea in a compensatory response to malabsorption. Like glucagon, it slows gastric emptying and inhibits gastric acid secretion.

CCK-Gastrin Family

CCK and gastrin are the leading peptides in the CCK family of regulatory peptides. In 1905, gastrin became the second peptide discovered. It was one of the first peptides to be chemically characterized and also one of the first to be sequenced. It is found primarily in the gastric antrum. Less than 15% of circulating gastrin is derived from enteroendocrine cells in the duodenum. Its primary function is to regulate the secretion of acid from gastric parietal cells. Gastrin stimulates the release of acid directly and by enhancing the release of histamine from ECL cells in the lamina propria of the stomach. Its release is stimulated by gastrin-releasing peptide (GRP) released from neurons that originate in the myenteric plexus in the presence of protein and low-acid contents in the stomach. Its release is inhibited in the presence of intraluminal acid by a number of mediators, all or most of which are mediated by somatostatin. Gastrin hypersecretion occurs in neuroendocrine tumors and in conditions in which acid secretion from the stomach is impaired by atrophy of the gastric parietal cells or by medications. For reasons that are not completely understood, neuroendocrine tumors that secrete gastrin almost never arise from the stomach but from neoplasms in the pancreas and duodenum.

CCK stimulates a variety of functions associated with fat ingestion, including pancreatic secretion of enzymes, contraction of the gallbladder, relaxation of the sphincter of Oddi, the induction of satiety, contraction of the pylorus, and delayed gastric emptying. It is found primarily in endocrine cells in the duodenum and upper jejunum but can also be seen in enteric nerves in the colon.

PANCREATIC POLYPEPTIDE FAMILY

The pancreatic polypeptide family is composed of three peptides that share considerable sequence homology, but each is secreted by different types of regulatory peptidesecreting cells. PP is released from endocrine cells in the body and the uncinate process of the pancreas. PYY is released from enteroglucagon-containing endocrine cells in the ileum and proximal colon. In contrast, NPY is released from neurons. NPY is located in two types of neurons. Most are intrinsic neurons that originate in the ENS and can be found distributed in all layers of the gut wall. A smaller subset of fibers that contain NPY are extrinsic neurons that also contain norepinephrine and originate from cells in the sympathetic nervous system. Most of these fibers are localized in a perivascular distribution. Studies performed to evaluate the significance of colocalized transmitters have shown that NPY can potentiate the effect of norepinephrine on the lower esophageal sphincter and blood vessels.

The physiologic importance of PP is unknown. It is released in response to vagal stimulation. Levels increase not only when food enters the stomach but in response to the sight or smell of food. This characteristic of PP has been used to measure the integrity of vagal input to the gut in disorders associated with gut neuropathies such as diabetes. PYY appears to be an important mediator of the reflex slowing of upper GI motility and secretions that occurs when nutrients, particularly fat, reach the distal small intestine. This response is known as the ileal brake. Enteroglucagon and neurotensin may also be mediators of this response.

ORPHAN PEPTIDES

Several peptides that have clinically important effects on digestive system function have not been found to be related in structure to other peptides. These peptides therefore do not belong to any peptide family and have been categorized as orphan peptides. Two clinically important ones are somatostatin and motilin.

Somatostatin is found in the pancreas, in mucosal endocrine cells, and in neurons throughout the digestive tract. It acts as a neurocrine, endocrine, paracrine, and autocrine transmitter. Nearly all nerves that contain somatostatin are located in the myenteric plexus. It has been said that a more appropriate name for this peptide would be inhibin, because its effects as a neurotransmitter, paracrine transmitter, and hormone are almost always inhibitory. It mediates the inhibitory effects of VIP, CGRP, and secretin on acid secretion from gastric parietal cells. The potent inhibitory effects of somatostatin have been mimicked by an 8-amino-acid synthetic analog of this important peptide, sandostatin. A disulfide bond in the structure of this analog gives it a longer circulating half-life, which has led to its use as an inhibitor of hormone secretion from neuroendocrine tumors, to treat diarrhea in patients with AIDS, and lower mesenteric blood pressure in patients with variceal bleeding.

Motilin is localized in ECL cells in the small intestine, predominantly in the duodenum. In contrast to most enteric hormones, the circulating levels of motilin decrease in response to a meal. Peak levels are observed in a cyclical pattern during fasting. Eating and the infusion of several enteric hormones, including gastrin and CCK, stop this cycling pattern and decrease motilin levels. The rise in motilin levels correlates well with the onset of phase III motor activity of the interdigestive cycle in the duodenum. Although the precise correlation of the timing of these two events has been the subject of much controversy, most data suggest that motilin is responsible for initiating this phase of forceful contractions in the upper but not the lower digestive system. These forceful contractions normally traverse from the stomach to the terminal ileum, sweeping undigested food and sloughed epithelial cells in front of it. For this reason, the migrating motor complex (MMC) is known as the intestinal housekeeper. Selectively structured macrolidelike molecules, including erythromycin, mimic the response of motilin, perhaps by acting on receptors. This has led to the development of several macrolidelike agents to be used as promotility substances.

Summary

Complex regulatory systems direct and modulate the intricate cascade of diverse activities that make up the functions of the digestive system. These include absorption, secretion, digestion, motility, metabolism, and mucosal defense. Selected enteric hormones also regulate cell growth. Two notable enteric hormones involved in this trophic regulatory role are gastrin and enteroglucagon. Important interactions between the CNS and digestive system are mediated by brain–gut interactions. These extrinsic nerves primarily modulate digestive functions, except in the esophagus, where vagal nerves are important mediators of peristalsis, the stomach, and the external anal sphincter. Most extrinsic fibers in both parasympathetic and sympathetic pathways are afferents. Nearly all complex motor and secretory reflexes in the gut are mediated by the intrinsic ENS, mainly by nerve pathways that have their cell bodies located in the myenteric plexus. The complexity of the ENS is remarkable and appears increasingly so with the discovery of new transmitters and new ways that transmitters interact with each other and with target cells, from transcription to the secondary messengers they stimulate in the target cells. Transmitters in the ENS mirror the diversity of those found in the CNS, such that the largest number of transmitters are known as brain–gut peptides. Over 30 such peptides have been discovered in enteric neurons or hormone-secreting cells. Perhaps the most important neurotransmitter discovered, however, is not a peptide but a combination of nitrogen and oxygen. This molecule, NO, is the leading candidate transmitter to mediate many NANC inhibitory reflexes. Many of these transmitters have been shown to have clinical and pathophysiological significance.

CASE STUDY: *RESOLUTION*

Progressive resistance to acid suppression therapy associated with recurrent duodenal ulcers and diarrhea should raise suspicion for the presence of a gastrinoma. This neoplasm is usually benign but may be malignant. Elevation of the fasting level of the hormone gastrin above 100 pg/dl strongly supports the diagnosis. A paradoxical increase in gastrin levels 30, 60, or 120 minutes following a secretin infusion (secretin stimulation test) is pathognomonic. A CT scan revealed a mass in the tail of the pancreas, which was resected.

An elevation in gastrin levels in hypochlorhydria (reduced acid secretion) is commonly due to inhibition of acid secretion by proton pump inhibitors or H_2-receptor antagonists. Hypochlorhydria is also seen in patients with chronic gastritis, pernicious anemia, or prior gastrectomy or vagotomy.

---

*R*EVIEW *Q*UESTIONS

Directions: For each of the following questions, choose the one best answer.

1 Several highly complex regulatory systems of the digestive system control the widely diverse events that occur during fasting and in

response to eating. Which control mechanism is correctly matched with the physiologic response?

Control Mechanism	Physiologic Event
A Endocrine	Response of the stomach, pancreas, and gallbladder to a meal
B Paracrine	Secretory response to mucosal injury
C Autocrine	Recognition of distention of the vermiform appendix
D Neurocrine	Proximal contraction and distal relaxation in response to distention

2 Which physiologic event is correctly matched with the location of the neurons involved?

Physiologic Event	Control Mechanism
A Rectal distention	Superior mesenteric ganglion
B Lower esophageal sphincter relaxation	Nitric oxide (NO) neurons in the submucosal plexus
C Ulcer-induced noxious stimulation	Calcitonin gene-related peptide (CGRP) neurons in the dorsal root ganglia
D Relaxation of the sphincter of Oddi	Vagal motor complex

3 Which of the following describes a pathway by which sensory information about the digestive tract reaches the CNS?

A Vagal afferent nerves passing through the spinothalamic tract
B Spinal afferent CGRP nerves passing through the dorsal root ganglia to the spinal cord lamellae
C NO-containing nerve originating in the myenteric plexus
D Neurons in the spinothalamic tract carrying information from the femoral nerve

4 Hormone release is an important mechanism for the regulation of cell growth. Which of the following is a major trophic hormone?

A Motilin
B Secretin
C Enteroglucagon
D Somatostatin

5 Which of the following events is mediated by somatostatin?

A Feedback inhibition of gastrin release
B Stimulation of amylase secretion
C Cycles of motor activity during fasting in the small intestine
D Regulation of upper digestive motility in response to nutrients in the ileum

6 Which of the following physiologic events is mediated by NO?

A Relaxation of the lower esophageal sphincter

B Inhibition of gastrin release

C Contraction of circular muscle fibers downstream from a distention

D Relaxation of the pelvic floor muscles (e.g., puborectalis) during defecation

7 Which of the following statements best describes regulatory peptides?

A There is diversity in the number of amino acids among different peptides in this class.

B Posttranslational processing is uncommon.

C The complex three-dimensional structure is the result of branching side chains.

D They are categorized into families by the types of cells involved and their function.

8 Cells of the digestive system are under a constant tone of inhibition from various regulatory pathways. Which of the following inhibitory events is a correct description of normal physiology?

A In the presence of high concentrations of acid in the antrum, somatostatin inhibits the secretion of gastrin.

B Norepinephrine inhibits intestinal motility during digestion of a meal.

C VIP inhibits bile secretion during fasting.

D NPY inhibits pancreatic secretion and intestinal motility in response to excess food in the ileum.

References

Furness JB, Young HM, Pompolo S, et al: Plurichemical transmission and chemical coding of neurons in the digestive tract. *Gastroenterology* 108:554–563, 1995.

Geoghegan J, Pappas TN: Clinical uses of gut peptides. *Ann Surg* 225:145–154, 1997.

Holst JJ, Fahrenkrug J, Stadil F, et al: Gastrointestinal endocrinology. *Scand J Gastroenterol* 216:27–38, 1996.

Johnson LR: *Gastrointestinal Physiology*. St. Louis, Mo.: Elsevier Science, Mosby, 2001.

Pearson RK, Anderson B, Dixon JE: Molecular biology of the peptide hormone families. *Endocrinol Metab Clin North Am* 22:753–774, 1993.

Schultz SG, Wood JD, Raunder BB (eds): *The Gastrointestinal System*, vols 1 and 2. Bethesda, Md.: American Physiological Society, 1989.

Watson JD, Gilman M, Witkowski J, et al (eds): *Recombinant DNA*, 2nd ed. New York: W. H. Freeman, 1992.

3

Anatomy, Histology, and Embryology of the GI Tract

▪ CHAPTER OUTLINE ▪

▪ LEARNING OBJECTIVES ▪

At the completion of this chapter, the reader should be able to:
- Evaluate the mature consequences of the embryologic development of the gastrointestinal (GI) tract.
- Outline the general anatomy of the GI system.
- Outline the general organization of the GI tract into four layers: mucosa, submucosa, muscularis externa, and serosa.
- Correlate structural specializations to specific functions with attention to propulsion, protection, secretion, digestion, mixing, absorption, lubrication, and defense.
- Recognize the normal histologic appearance of the esophagus, stomach, and intestines in the light microscope.
- Differentiate the specific ultrastructural functions of specialized GI cells: chief cells, parietal cells, enteroendocrine cells, Paneth cells, enterocytes, and goblet cells.

A newborn presented with jaundice, dark urine, and acholic stools. Physical examination revealed jaundice and hepatomegaly. The serum bilirubin was elevated to 10 mg/dl. The prothrombin time was 2 seconds prolonged. Evaluation revealed extrahepatic biliary atresia.

Atretic lesions of the extrahepatic bile ducts are the most common malformation of the biliary passages. The incidence is 5–10 cases per 100,000 live births. The occlusion may result from persistence of the solid stage of duct development, perhaps secondary to a noxious agent or infection during late fetal development. Biliary cirrhosis ensues, with ascites, portal hypertension, and vitamin deficiencies.

Introduction

Congenital anomalies involving the GI tract are not uncommon. The development of the fetus is an intricately timed process for the growth and differentiation of organ systems and cell types. This chapter presents anatomy and histology and reviews the embryologic development of the digestive system.

Embryology

The primitive gut tube is created by embryonic folding during the 4th week of development. Initially, this endodermal tube consists of a blind-ending cranial foregut, a blind-ending caudal hindgut, and a midgut open to the yolk sac via the vitelline duct (Figure 3-1). The abdominal portion of the tube is suspended by a dorsal mesentery; ventral mesenteries also attach to the abdominal esophagus, stomach, and superior part of the duodenum. The ectodermal oral and anal extremities of the canal fuse to the endodermal gut tube to produce a patent lumen. The adult derivatives of the primitive gut are discussed in Table 3-1.

Brief details of the embryology of each major GI organ are discussed.

ESOPHAGUS

At week 4 of development, a small diverticulum appears at the ventral wall of the foregut. This eventually is partitioned by the esophageal tracheal septum, which splits the foregut into a ventral respiratory primordium and a dorsal esophagus. Initially, the esophagus is quite short; however, it lengthens with the descent of the heart.

STOMACH

Also at week 4 of development, a fusiform dilation of the foregut appears, with the dorsal side growing faster than the ventral side.

Notes

The GI tract forms from a foregut, midgut, and hindgut. Each of these regions develops in association with specific blood vessels.

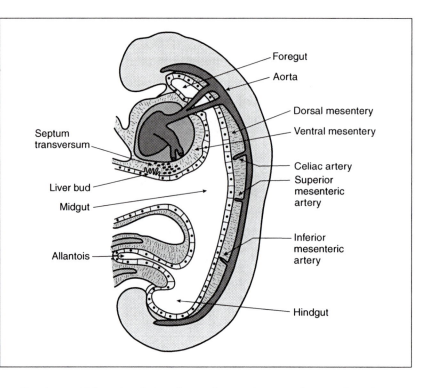

Fig. 3-1. Midsagittal Section of a 25-Day Embryo Showing Foregut, Midgut, and Hindgut

Table 3-1. Adult Derivatives of the Primitive Gut

FOREGUT DERIVATIVES[a]

- The oral cavity, pharynx, tongue, tonsils, and salivary glands
- The upper and lower respiratory system
- The esophagus and stomach
- The duodenum, proximal to the opening of the common bile duct
- The liver, gallbladder, bile duct, and pancreas

MIDGUT DERIVATIVES[b]

- The small intestine, including the duodenum distal to the opening of the common bile duct
- The cecum, appendix, ascending colon, and the right half to two-thirds of the transverse colon

HINDGUT DERIVATIVES[c]

- The left, distal portion of the transverse colon, the descending colon, sigmoid colon, rectum, and superior portion of the anal canal
- The epithelium of the urinary bladder and most of the urethra

[a]The blood supply to the thoracic foregut is five branches from the aorta. The blood supply to the abdominal foregut is the celiac artery.
[b]The blood supply of the midgut is the superior mesenteric artery.
[c]The blood supply of the hindgut is the inferior mesenteric artery. The distal (ectodermal) anal canal is supplied by rectal arteries, which branch from the internal pudendal arteries.

This creates the greater and lesser curvatures of the stomach. During the seventh week, the stomach also rotates 90° clockwise so that the greater curve is displaced to the left. This rotation explains why the left vagus nerve supplies the anterior stomach wall and the right vagus supplies the posterior wall. This movement also drags along the ventral mesentery of the stomach, creating the lesser sac.

DUODENUM

This portion of the intestine is formed from the terminal foregut and the cephalic midgut, which are joined at the site of the hepatic diverticulum. As the stomach rotates, the duodenum begins to take on its adult C-looped shape and is forced retroperitoneal. During month 2, when the accessory digestive glands are actively proliferating, the lumen of the duodenum may be temporarily obliterated as a result of endodermal mitoses.

LIVER AND BILIARY APPARATUS

The liver, biliary tree, and gallbladder arise at week 4 from an outpouch of the distal foregut. This hepatic diverticulum expands in the ventral mesentery toward the septum transversum, between the pericardial cavity and the yolk sac. Note that the penetration of the liver divides the ventral mesentery into the falciform ligament (connecting the liver to the ventral body wall) and the lesser omentum (connecting the liver to the stomach and duodenum). Hepatoblasts at the cranial end of the liver bud differentiate into cords of liver cells and the biliary epithelium. The hepatic sinusoids arise from the interlacing of liver cords with septal remnants of the umbilical and vitelline veins. Liver growth pushes into the septum transversum to create the bare area of the liver that protrudes through the diaphragm and is therefore not covered with peritoneum. A second diverticulum, caudal to the liver bud, forms the cystic duct and the gallbladder. Finally, the connection between the liver bud and the foregut narrows and fuses with the cystic duct to give rise to the common bile duct.

Functionally, the liver becomes hematopoietic at week 6. Bile formation begins at week 12. Fetal bile is what colors the meconium. At this point, the liver makes up 10% of the total fetal weight. At birth, the bile acid pool is less than half its relative size in adults and is recycled enterohepatically to maintain the critical micellar concentration of bile acids.

PANCREAS

On day 26, another duodenal bud begins to grow into the dorsal mesentery, the dorsal pancreatic bud. A few days later a ventral pancreatic bud pushes into the ventral mesentery just caudal to the cystic duct. As the duodenum rotates to form its C-loop, the ventral bud passes behind the duodenum to lie just below the dorsal bud in the dorsal mesentery. Late in week 6 the two buds fuse to form the definitive pancreas. The dorsal bud gives rise to the head, body, and tail of the pancreas, and the ventral bud gives rise to the uncinate process. The duct of the ventral bud becomes the main pancreatic duct, which empties into the duodenum via the common bile duct; however, the duct of the dorsal bud may persist as an accessory pancreatic duct with an independent entry site into the duodenum. Like the duodenum, the pancreas fuses with the posterior body wall to become secondarily retroperitoneal.

The exocrine cells of the pancreas (digestive enzymes and bicarbonate secretions) differentiate from the endodermal pancreatic buds. The source of the endocrine cells of the islets of Langerhans (insulin and glucagon secretions) is uncertain.

SPLEEN

At the end of the fourth week a mesenchymal thickening develops in the dorsal mesentery. This condensation differentiates into the spleen. Note that the spleen is of mesodermal origin and is not a diverticulum of the gut endoderm. The rotation of the stomach displaces the spleen toward the left. The remaining mesenteric connections form the splenorenal ligament (to the left kidney) and the gastrosplenic ligament (to the greater curve of the stomach).

SMALL INTESTINE AND COLON

In the fifth and sixth weeks of development, the rapid growth of the liver and the continuing elongation of the midgut force a primary intestinal loop to herniate into the umbilicus. At its apex, this loop is connected to the yolk sac via the vitelline duct. The cephalic limb of this loop becomes part of the duodenum, the jejunum, and part of the ileum; the caudal limb becomes the remainder of the ileum, the cecum, the appendix, the ascending colon, and part of the transverse colon. As it herniates, the loop rotates 90° counterclockwise around the superior mesenteric artery, which forms the central axis of the primary intestinal loop. At the end of the 10th week, the intestinal loop begins to retract into the abdominal cavity and rotates an additional 180°. By the 11th week, the intestinal loop is completely retracted, and the ascending and descending colons become fixed to the right and left posterior abdominal walls, respectively, to become secondarily retroperitoneal organs.

COLON, RECTUM, AND ANUS

The terminal hindgut, the cloaca, is an endodermal cavity without direct contact to the surface ectoderm. As development proceeds, a transverse ridge, the urorectal septum, forms and divides the cloaca into the anterior primitive urogenital sinus and the posterior anorectal canal. At week 7, this septum reaches the cloacal membrane, and the perineal floor is formed. At the same time, the anal pit forms from an ectodermal depression and eventually ruptures into the rectum. Thus, hindgut endoderm gives rise to the distal portion of the transverse colon, the descending colon, and the rectum, with the inferior mesenteric artery as its blood supply; the ectoderm gives rise to the lower anal canal, with the rectal arteries as its blood supply. The junction of the rectum and anus is demarcated by mucosal folds called the pectinate line, where columnar epithelium meets stratified squamous epithelium.

Overview of GI Histology

The tubular portion of the GI tract is organized into four general layers: the mucosa, the submucosa, the muscularis externa, and a serosa or adventitia. Figure 3-2 summarizes the organization of the GI tract and illustrates the various specializations that occur along its length. This basic design is present from the oral cavity to the anus.

MUCOSA

The mucosa lines the inner luminal surface of the gut tube. The mucosa is composed of three parts: epithelium, lamina propria, and muscularis mucosae.

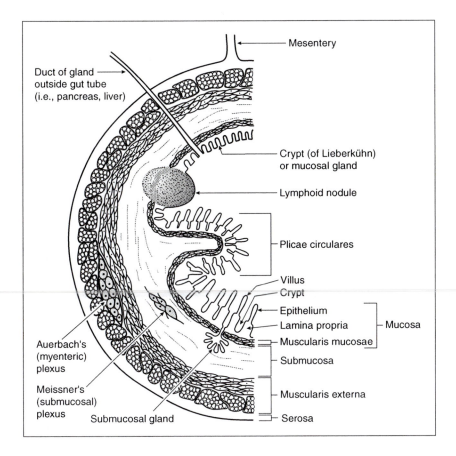

Fig. 3-2. General Organization of Gastrointestinal Tract into Four Layers

The lower two-thirds of the diagram illustrates the villi and crypt structure of the small intestine; the upper third illustrates the large intestinal mucosa with only crypts.

Epithelium

The structure of the epithelium varies according to function. A quick glance at the types of epithelium and specialized cells present gives an understanding of the function of that GI segment:

- **Protection:** The stratified squamous epithelia in the esophagus and anus provide protection from friction.
- **Secretion:** The surface mucous cells and enzyme-producing pits in the stomach release specific secretions.
- **Absorption:** Villi and microvilli augment the surface area of the simple columnar small-intestinal epithelium for absorption.

Lamina Propria

This connective tissue layer supports the epithelium both physically and biochemically and attaches it to the underlying muscle layer. The lamina propria projects into the villi and contains fenestrated capillaries and lymphatic capillaries to facilitate absorption. Frequent lymphocytes and lymphatic nodules act as a defensive barrier against organisms that may penetrate the epithelium.

Muscularis Mucosae

This smooth muscle layer is usually circumferential, peripheral to the lamina propria. However, individual smooth muscle cells are found in the lamina propria all the way to the tips of the villi. Contraction of the muscularis mucosae results in the independent movement and folding of the mucosa and therefore aids in the processes of digestion and absorption.

SUBMUCOSA

The submucosa is a loose connective tissue layer with blood vessels, collagen, and elastin. It is sandwiched between the muscularis mucosae and the muscularis externa. Submucosa also extends into the core of the *plicae circulares*, which are folds of the entire mucosa found in the small intestine, and *rugae*, comparable mucosal folds in the stomach. Two segments of the GI tract that secrete large amounts of mucus (the esophagus and duodenum) have glands that penetrate into the submucosa. The *submucosal (Meissner's) plexus* of autonomic nerves and ganglia is usually found in the submucosa, adjacent to the muscularis externa. The submucosal plexus regulates the function of the mucosal and submucosal blood vessels and smooth muscles. The submucosal plexus consists of unmyelinated sympathetic postganglionic fibers, which originate from the prevertebral group of ganglia, and parasympathetic ganglion cell bodies, which synapse with preganglionic fibers from the vagus nerve.

MUSCULARIS EXTERNA

The muscularis externa consists of two layers of perpendicularly oriented smooth muscle, an inner circular and an outer longitudinal one.

The smooth muscle of these layers is innervated by the *Auerbach's plexus*. This is also called the myenteric ("within muscle") plexus because it lies at the junction of the circular and longitudinal muscle layers. Again, parasympathetic preganglionic fibers from the vagus nerve terminate on ganglia cells, and sympathetic postganglionic fibers from the prevertebral ganglia contribute to this plexus. Interstitial cells of Cajal, type I (ICC-I), interact with the cells of the myenteric plexus and may be the origin of myogenic slow waves in the GI tract. When examined with an electron microscope, smooth muscle cells of the muscularis externa are connected by gap junctions. Numbers of these low-resistance open channels permit the spread of depolarization waves, which result in the baseline contractions of slow waves.

Contraction of mainly the circular layer of smooth muscle produces the local mixing of luminal contents called segmentation. Peristaltic contractions move the GI contents distally and mostly involve the longitudinal muscle layer of the muscularis externa.

Serosa or Adventitia

Much of the GI tract is suspended by mesentery. The thin layer of connective tissue that envelopes these segments is called the *serosa*. There is a small amount of loose connective tissue through which blood vessels and nerves travel. On the outer surface is a simple squamous epithelium called the mesothelium. However, some portions of the GI tract are embedded in other tissue, such as the esophagus in the mediastinum or retroperitoneal portions of the small and large intestines. The outer layer of these tubes is an *adventitia*, which blends into surrounding connective tissue.

Esophagus

Anatomy

The esophagus is a 25-cm-long tube that extends from the epiglottis to the cardiac orifice of the stomach. It enters the mediastinum posterior to the trachea at the level of the 6th cervical vertebra and passes through the diaphragm to enter the stomach at the 10th thoracic vertebra. The two vagus nerves travel with the thoracic esophagus—the left vagus anteriorly and the right vagus posteriorly. These nerves accompany the esophagus, lymphatic vessels, and branches of the left gastric blood vessels through the diaphragm. The esophagus is a conduit for swallowed food and is not involved in storage or significant digestion of food.

As a result of its location in the neck, thorax, and abdomen, there are three different blood supply loops for the esophagus: The upper third is supplied by the inferior thyroid artery and veins; the middle third is supplied by branches of the descending thoracic aorta and azygous veins; the lower third is supplied by branches of the left gastric artery and veins.

Notes

The esophagus is characterized by stratified squamous epithelium with rete pegs, submucosal glands, and the gradual substitution of smooth muscle for skeletal muscle within the muscularis externa.

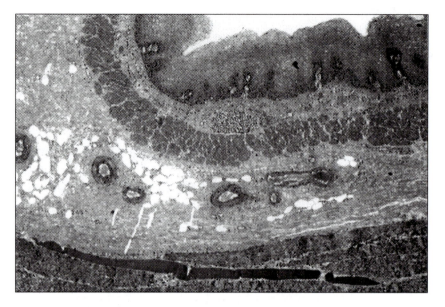

Fig. 3-3. Layers of the Esophageal Wall (Human)

The esophageal mucosa contains stratified squamous epithelium with rete pegs and lymphocytes in the lamina propria; the submucosa contains mucus-secreting glands; the muscularis externa contains smooth muscle with a few fibers of skeletal muscle (hematoxylin-eosin; 70×).

HISTOLOGY

Mucosa

The mucosa of the esophagus displays stratified squamous nonkeratinized *epithelium*. The stratification protects against the friction of swallowed food and insulates against extremes of hot and cold. Folds of lamina propria push the epithelium into rete pegs; this interdigitation of lamina propria and epithelium is another structural reinforcement against friction (Figure 3-3).

In the *lamina propria*, mucous glands can be found in the lower third and occasionally the upper third of the esophagus. These are relatively small glands, named cardiac glands because they secrete a neutral mucus similar to the glands of the cardiac portion of the stomach. Isolated lymphocytes as well as lymphatic nodules are frequently observed in the esophageal lamina propria. This layer of connective tissue borders epithelium contiguous with the external body surface. Exposure to outside pathogens is potentially greater here; therefore, there is a need for lymphocyte defenders.

A prominent *muscularis mucosae* is composed of longitudinally oriented smooth muscle fibers. The combination of stratified squamous epithelium with rete pegs and longitudinally oriented muscularis mucosae readily identifies a tissue section as esophagus.

Submucosa

Mucus production by the esophageal (submucosal) glands facilitates swallowing. These large glands are present throughout the length of the esophagus, although most of the liquid in the esophagus actually originates as saliva.

Muscularis Externa

The mechanisms of swallowing and the propulsion of food down the length of the esophagus are coordinated by both skeletal muscle and smooth muscle. The muscularis externa in the top third of the esophagus is composed of skeletal muscle and is under voluntary control. The middle third displays a mixture of skeletal and smooth muscle. In the final third, the muscularis externa is composed entirely of smooth muscle. At all levels, the muscularis externa is formed by two layers, an inner circular and an outer longitudinal one. Swallowing is involuntary past the upper third of the esophagus and is controlled by the deglutination (swallowing) reflex centers in the medulla and lower pons.

Adventitia

The esophagus descends through the thorax in the central mediastinum. Its outermost layer is therefore an adventitia. There is no serosa in the esophagus.

Stomach

The stomach serves a variety of functions. First, it provides *storage* for ingested food; the organ is a large expansion along the GI tube and is restricted by a tight pyloric (exiting) sphincter. Second, the stomach is the site for *proteolytic digestion*. The degradative enzymes pepsin (proteins), rennin (milk), lipase (fats), and a highly acidic environment facilitate digestion. Third, the stomach *mixes* its contents using thick smooth muscle layers. Fourth, *absorption* of water, salts, alcohol, and some drugs takes place across the stomach wall. Fifth, *secretion* of vitamin B_{12} intrinsic factor, which binds and preserves dietary vitamin B_{12} for later absorption in the ileum, takes place in the stomach. These general functions should be kept in mind when the structure of the tissues and specialized cells of the stomach are examined.

ANATOMY

The stomach is a dilated storage pouch along the upper abdominal portion of the GI tract (Figure 3-4). Much of the stomach lies just under the lower ribs. The organ has a greater curve (convex, left) and a lesser curve (concave, right) because of its asymmetric expansion. The lesser curve is attached to the underside of the liver by two layers of peritoneum, the lesser omentum. These peritoneal layers then expand to surround the anterior and posterior aspects of the stomach as serosa, rejoining at the greater curve to form the greater omentum. The stomach is divided into the following parts: the *cardiac orifice* at the junction with the lower esophagus; the *fundus*, a dome-shaped projection upward and to the left of the cardia; the *body*, from the level of the cardia to the bend of the lesser curve; the *antrum*,

The stomach is characterized by epithelial pits and glands and by rugae, large submucosal folds.

Gastric pits are all lined with surface mucous cells. Gastric glands of the fundus, body, and antrum are composed of mucous neck cells (acidic mucus), parietal cells (HCl and vitamin B_{12} intrinsic factor), chief cells (pepsinogen, rennin, and lipase), and a variety of enteroendocrine cells.

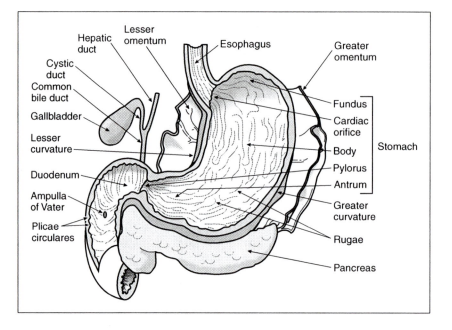

Fig. 3-4. Longitudinal Section of the Stomach Showing Anatomical Relationships to Neighboring Organs and General Wall Structure

descending deepest into the abdomen, from the bend of the lesser curve to the pylorus; and the *pylorus*, a tubular portion with a thick muscular wall, which forms the pyloric sphincter. The entrance to the stomach at the cardiac orifice and the exit of the stomach at the pylorus are relatively fixed compared to the mobile middle.

The nerves of the stomach are derived from the celiac plexus of the sympathetic nervous system and from both the right and left vagus nerves. Due to the rotation of the stomach as it enters the abdomen, the left vagus nerve innervates the anterior wall, whereas the right vagus nerve innervates the posterior wall.

HISTOLOGY

The stomach is organized into the same four general layers as the rest of the GI tract. The unique stomach mucosa is characterized by pits and glands. Figure 3-5 summarizes the structure and cell types of the gastric pits and glands. The simple columnar epithelium is composed of a homogeneous population of surface mucous cells. The apical ends of the cells are filled with secretory vesicles of mucus, which is a neutral carbohydrate-rich glycoprotein. Surface mucous cells act as a buffer zone to protect the mucosa from the caustic environment in the stomach lumen. Gastric pits descend from the surface into the lamina propria. These pits are also lined by surface mucous cells. Two or three gastric glands empty into the base of each pit. The gastric glands are different in each anatomic region of the stomach (cardia, fundus and body, pylorus). The lamina propria is filled with invaginating gastric pits and glands and is only seen as small amounts of intervening connective tissue. Directly under the

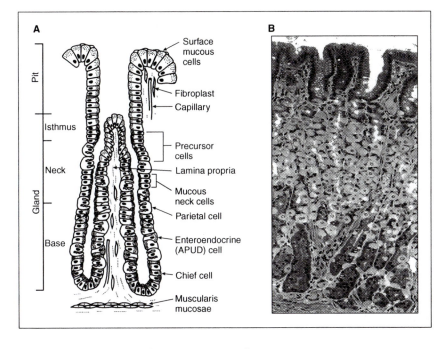

Fig. 3-5. Stomach Mucosa

The stomach mucosa is organized into pits lined by surface mucous cells, into which empty gastric glands composed of mucous neck cells, parietal cells, chief cells, and enteroendocrine cells. (A) Drawing. (B) Micrograph (human) (hematoxylin-eosin; 350×).

base of the gastric glands is a thin muscularis mucosae composed of circularly oriented smooth muscle. The stomach wall has large, visible mucosal folds with a central core of submucosal tissue called rugae. Together, the pits, glands, and rugae serve to increase the surface area of the mucosal layer available for the secretion of digestive enzymes and acid.

The muscularis externa expands to include three layers of smooth muscle: inner oblique, middle circular, and outer longitudinal. In most histologic preparations, this is difficult to appreciate because of variation in section orientation. However, the thickness of the overall muscle is notable.

Cardia

The cardiac glands are composed primarily of small, pale-staining mucous cells. There are, however, a few bright pink, eosinophilic, acid-producing parietal cells. The cardiac pits are irregular and shallow; the cardiac glands are highly coiled. The ratio of the length of pits to glands is approximately 1:1. The transition from the esophagus to the cardiac stomach is sharp and dramatic, from stratified squamous epithelium with esophageal glands to simple columnar epithelium invaginated into pits and glands. This rapid shift in tissue structure is indicative of the immediate change in function from conduit to digestion.

Fundus, Body, and Antrum. The glands of these regions are referred to by a variety of names: *gastric glands* (major secretors of stomach), *zymogen glands* (contain stored secretory or "zymogen" granules), or *fundic glands* (location). These glands secrete the digestive enzymes and acid into the stomach. They are characterized by chief cells and parietal cells (see Figure 3-5A). Although these regions of the stomach serve different physiologic functions, they all display similar histologic structure and are therefore grouped together here.

The mucosa of the fundus, body, and antrum displays deep, straight pits and long glands that coil only at the base. The ratio of the length of pits to glands is approximately 1:4. The gastric glands have an isthmus, neck, and base. The *isthmus* drains into the base of the pit. Mucous neck cells found here secrete an acidic glycoprotein; they display cytoplasmic basophilia resulting from increased amounts of rough endoplasmic reticulum (RER) and contain larger secretion granules than surface mucous cells. The *neck* (middle) of the gastric gland contains mucous neck cells and acid-producing parietal cells. The *base* of the gastric gland is made up of chief cells (digestive enzymes), parietal cells, and a variety of enteroendocrine cells.

Parietal (oxyntic) cells secrete 0.1 N hydrochloric acid (HCl) and vitamin B_{12} intrinsic factor. In hematoxylin-eosin–stained light micrographs (see Figure 3-5B), parietal cells appear as plump, round acidophilic cells with a homogeneous pink cytoplasm and a central nucleus. Visualization with the electron microscope reveals cytoplasmic specializations that permit secretion of the strong solution of HCl. The apical plasma membrane folds into a deep, trenchlike invagination with numerous microvilli called an *intracellular canaliculi*. The surrounding area of the cytoplasm is filled with smooth-surfaced vesicles, the *tubulovesicular system*. These vesicles fuse with the canaliculi when acid secretion is stimulated. Together, the intracellular canaliculi and the tubulovesicular system augment the surface area for H^+-K^+-ATPase pumps and Cl^--ATPase pumps, which release hydrogen ions (H^+) or chloride ions (Cl^-), respectively, into the stomach lumen. The cytoplasm is also densely packed with mitochondria. The mitochondria provide ATP for active transport occurring at the canalicular surface. The basolateral plasma membrane of the parietal cell contains receptors for histamine, gastrin, and acetylcholine, all of which stimulate acid secretion. The hormones somatostatin, prostaglandin, and gastric inhibitory peptide inhibit parietal cell HCl secretion.

Figure 3-6 summarizes the reactions that result in the secretion of HCl:

1. H^+ is pumped into the lumen of the gland in exchange for potassium ion (K^+) by H^+-K^+-ATPase. This energy-requiring reaction pulls all the others behind it.
2. Water is hydrolyzed into H^+ and OH^-. This provides a constant source of H^+ for export.

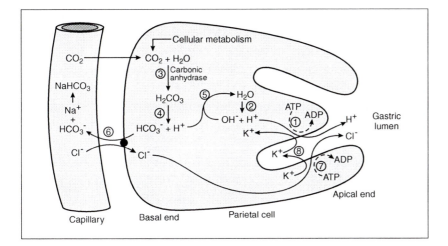

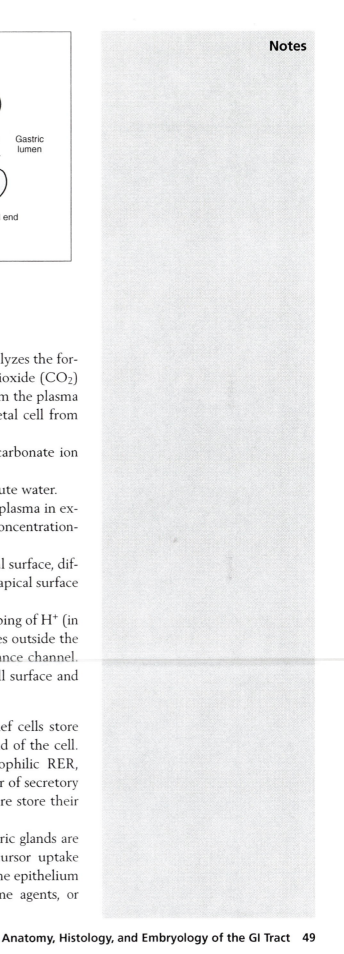

Fig. 3-6. Gastric Parietal Cell

Schematic mechanism of acid secretion.

3. The cytoplasmic enzyme carbonic anhydrase catalyzes the formation of carbonic acid (H_2CO_3) from carbon dioxide (CO_2) and water (H_2O). The CO_2 either diffused in from the plasma and interstitial fluids or was present in the parietal cell from ambient metabolism.

4. Carbonic acid immediately ionizes to form a bicarbonate ion (HCO_3^-) and an H^+.

5. The H^+ combines with the free OH^- to reconstitute water.

6. The HCO_3^- diffuses out of the cell and into the plasma in exchange for a Cl^-. This exchange is facilitated by a concentration-driven antiporter.

7. The Cl^-, which enters the parietal cell at the basal surface, diffuses across the cell and is transported out at the apical surface by a conductance channel.

8. The transport of Cl^- (in step 7) exceeds the pumping of H^+ (in step 1). Therefore, the buildup of negative charges outside the cell causes K^+ to diffuse out through a conductance channel. K^+ continually cycles in and out of the apical cell surface and provides an elegant means for the export of H^+.

Chief cells secrete pepsinogen, rennin, and lipase. Chief cells store abundant basophilic secretory granules in the apical end of the cell. In contrast, the basal cytoplasm is packed with basophilic RER, understandable for a cell that is a very active synthesizer of secretory proteins. Chief cells are regulated secretors and therefore store their secretory products in condensed zymogen granules.

The third type of cells found in the base of the gastric glands are enteroendocrine cells. Enteroendocrine or amine precursor uptake and decarboxylase (APUD) cells are single cells within the epithelium that secrete substances that act as hormones, paracrine agents, or neurotransmitters. These cells are found throughout the stomach, small intestine, and to some extent in the colon. Enteroendocrine cells can be distinguished in electron micrographs because of their basal concentration of secretory granules. These secretions are released at the basal end of the cell and move by diffusion through the interstitial fluid of the lamina propria or via the bloodstream. Table 3-2 offers a summary of the major types, secretions, and actions of enteroendocrine cells in the GI tract.

Because of the extreme conditions within the lumen of the stomach, the renewal rate of the gastric surface mucous cells is rapid, every 2–6 days. On the other hand, the cells deep within the gastric gland turn over at the much slower rate of approximately once a year. The isthmus of the gastric gland serves as a source of stem cells for both the surface mucous cells, as well as the cell types deep in the base of the gland. This renewal process can be damaged by aspirin, bile salts, and alcohol. However, when the epithelium is damaged and cells are

Table 3-2. GI Enteroendocrine Cell Secretions

CELL	LOCATION	HORMONE	ACTION
A	Stomach and small intestine	Glucagon	Stimulates hepatic glycogenolysis
D	Stomach and small and large intestines	Somatostatin	Inhibits release of other GI hormones
EC	Stomach and small and large intestines	Serotonin	Increases gut motility
ECL	Stomach	Histamine	Stimulates HCl secretion
G	Stomach and small intestine	Gastrin	Stimulates HCl secretion and pyloric motility
I	Small intestine	Cholecystokinin	Stimulates secretion of pancreatic enzymes and gallbladder contraction
K	Small intestine	Gastric inhibitory peptide	Inhibits HCl secretion
Mo	Small intestine	Motilin	Stimulates intestinal peristalsis
N	Small intestine	Neurotensin	Increases blood flow to ileum and decreases peristalsis of intestines
S	Small intestine	Secretin	Stimulates secretion of bicarbonate and water from pancreas
VIP	Stomach and small and large intestines	Vasoactive intestinal peptide	Stimulates ion and water secretion and increases intestinal peristalsis

lost, re-epithelialization begins within minutes as long as the basement membrane remains intact. Adjacent cells thin and extend lamellipodia via microfilament action to cover the exposed areas.

Pyloric Region

This area is notable for mucus-secreting glands. The pyloric region is characterized by deep pits (equal to those in the body) but short glands. The pit-to-gland ratio is close to 1:1. The glands are also coiled, unlike the straighter glands of the body. The pyloric glands contain mucus-secreting cells and enteroendocrine cells but few parietal or chief cells. G cells (gastrin-secreting) are primarily found in the pylorus. The rate of renewal of surface mucous cells is slower in the pylorus, with life spans up to 2 months. It is interesting to note that the pylorus is a frequent site of peptic ulcers; with pyloric resection, many of the G cells are removed, which aids the patient by decreasing parietal cell acid secretion.

A pyloric sphincter is formed by a thickening of the middle circular layer of the muscularis externa. This is a substantial constriction, which prevents leakage of the stored stomach chyme.

Small Intestine

ANATOMY

The small intestine is approximately 6 m in length. It is divided into three sections: the duodenum, the jejunum, and the ileum. The major functions of the small intestine are further digestion, absorption, production of GI hormones, and immunologic defense.

Duodenum

The duodenum is only 25 cm long. It curves around the head of the pancreas, where the ampulla of Vater receives the fused common bile duct (bile from the liver and gallbladder) and pancreatic duct (pancreatic digestive enzymes). These two ducts usually join together and are surrounded by circular muscle fibers called the sphincter of Oddi. The first few centimeters of the duodenum are suspended by a mesentery, but the duodenum rapidly becomes retroperitoneal. The arterial supply of the upper third of the duodenum is the superior pancreaticoduodenal artery, the second branch of the celiac artery. The lower two-thirds is supplied by the inferior pancreaticoduodenal artery, a branch of the superior mesenteric artery.

Jejunum and Ileum

The jejunum measures 2.5 m; the ileum measures 3.5 m. Both are attached to the posterior abdominal wall by a fold of peritoneum, which creates a suspending mesentery. The attachment of the mesentery provides access for the superior mesenteric artery and vein, lymphatic vessels, and for autonomic nerves of the superior mesenteric plexus. The jejunal mesentery is attached above and to the left of the

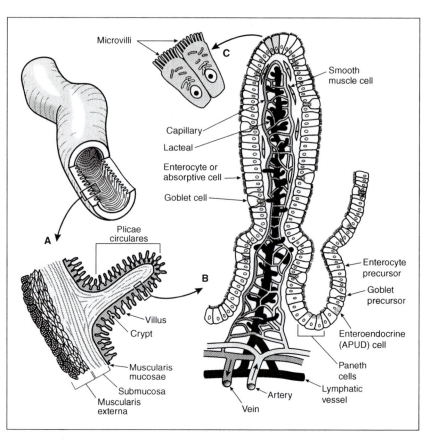

Fig. 3-7. Structural Specializations of the Small Intestine

(A) Plicae circulares. (B) Villi and crypts with capillary loops and lacteals.
(C) Enterocytes with microvilli.

abdominal aorta and passes diagonally below and to the right of the
aorta to provide attachment for the ileum.

HISTOLOGY

Understanding the functions of the small intestine is facilitated by
knowledge of the structural specializations of its tissues and cells
(Figure 3-7).

General Concepts

Plicae circulares. These are visible folds, circularly arranged
around the lumen of the small intenstine. Plicae circulares (also
called valves of Kerckring) are folds of the mucosa that contain a
central core of submucosal tissue. Therefore, the muscularis mucosae also extend into the plicae circulares. Plicae circulares increase
the surface area of the organ, but because of the muscle are also important as mechanical mixers. These folds are the most extensive in
the jejunum.

Villi. Villi are projections of the epithelium with a core of lamina
propria. The muscularis mucosae do not follow the connective tissue

into the villi. Villi can be leaf- or finger-shaped (tallest in jejunum, shortest in the ileum). The lamina propria core contains diverse connective tissue structures: white blood cells (WBCs), lymphocytes, plasma cells, eosinophils, lacteals (blind-ending lymphatic capillaries), arterioles from the submucosal artery, a rich fenestrated capillary network (permeable to macromolecules), unmyelinated nerves, and smooth muscle cells, which are scattered from the muscularis mucosae out to the tip of the villus. Contraction of these scattered muscle cells forces lymph from lacteals into larger lymphatic vessels.

The villus epithelium is composed of two cell types, enterocytes and goblet cells. *Enterocytes*, the columnar absorptive cells of the small intestine, display an apical striated border of microvilli. *Goblet cells* secrete mucin for protection of surface enzymes and for lubrication. Indeed, as more food is absorbed from the intestinal lumen, the need for lubrication rises, and the goblet cells increase from only a few in the epithelium of the upper small intestine to being more prominent in the large intestine surface epithelium.

Microvilli. These are folds in the apical plasma membrane of each individual enterocyte. Microvilli greatly increase the surface area for nutrient digestion and absorption. Extending from the microvilli is a thick glycoprotein coat called the *glycocalyx*. The glycocalyx contains hydrolytic enzymes, such as enterokinases (enteropeptidases), dipeptidases, and disaccharidases. These are intrinsic membrane proteins, which span the bilayer and expose their enzymatic active sites toward the small intestine lumen.

The digestive process that began in the stomach is continued in the small intestine lumen via the pancreatic enzymes. Glycocalyx enterokinase enzymatically converts pancreatic trypsinogen to its active form, typsin, which in turn activates the remaining pancreatic enzymes. These pancreatic enzymes then reduce most protein and carbohydrates to di- or tripeptide and disaccharide forms. Enzymes of the glycocalyx complete the protein and carbohydrate digestion to individual amino acids and monosaccharides.

The second major class of intrinsic proteins of the microvillus plasma membrane is the nutrient symporters. These carriers cotransport amino acids or monosaccharides with sodium ion (Na^+). These are passive processes that use an existing Na^+ electrochemical gradient generated within the enterocyte by basolateral Na^+-K^+-ATPase active transporters. Together, the microvilli and glycocalyx are responsible for the absorption of sugars, amino acids, and lipids.

Crypts. Crypts are invaginations of the epithelium that extend down into the lamina propria between projecting villi. Structurally, they are analogous to the pits of the stomach. Many of the cells in the crypt serve as precurosrs for enterocytes or goblet cells of the villi. However, at the base of the crypts are *Paneth cells*. These large cells have abundant basal RER and large, apical, acidophilic storage granules. Paneth

Specialized cells of the small intestine are the enterocytes, goblet cells, Paneth cells, enteroendocrine cells, and M cells.

Notes

Together, **M cells, lymphocytes, plasma cells, and secretory IgA** presensitize the GI tract to luminal antigens.

cell granules contain lysozyme, an antibacterial substance that degrades bacterial cell walls. Therefore, Paneth cells may be involved in population control of gut bacteria. Enteroendocrine cells are also scattered through the small-intestinal crypts. See Table 3-2 for a summary of the enteroendocrine cells of the small intestine.

Gut-Associated Lymphoid Tissue (GALT). Although lymphoid cells are transient, they are always found throughout the GI tract lamina propria, submucosa, and even the epithelium itself. The GI tract, being continuous with the outside of the body, is potentially exposed to many foreign antigens. Diffuse lymphocytes, clustered lymphocytes, and solitary nodules are not unusual in any portion of the GI tract. Aggregated nodules, a cluster of nodules, many with pale secondary centers, are found in the ileum (called Peyer's patches) and in the appendix.

At the site of Peyer's patches, the overlying villi are frequently absent. The epithelium covering a patch contains specialized epithelial cells called *M cells*. M cells take up a representative sampling of intraluminal antigens by pinocytosis at their apical surface. Vesicle contents are transferred by transcytosis only to be released at the basolateral surface. M cells are cup-shaped, with the flat "base" facing the intestinal lumen. The "cup" portion is filled with intraepithelial lymphocytes that express major histocompatibility complex (MHC) class II and are capable of antigen presentation. These cells then migrate from the surface of the nodule into the center and stimulate the maturation of B lymphocytes into a clone of plasma cells. The plasma cells, in turn, produce large quantities of immunoglobulin A (IgA), a dimeric form of antibody, which is released into the lamina propria. Enterocyte basolateral plasma membranes contain a glycoprotein receptor for IgA called the secretory component (SC). Once IgA binds to SC, the complex is taken up by endocytosis. The secretory component remains with the IgA and is transported to the apical surface of the enterocyte. Eventually the transport vesicle fuses with the apical plasma membrane and releases secretory IgA into the intestinal lumen. Other plasma cells migrate to lymph nodes, where they continue to proliferate. These plasma cell clones also secrete IgA, which is taken up by a SC receptor in the liver. The SC-IgA is released into bile canaliculi and finds its way into the lumen of the duodenum with the flow of bile. Secretory IgA binds antigens and enterotoxins, decreases the adherence of microbes to the epithelial surface, and neutralizes viruses and bacterial toxins. Clearly, M cells and IgA help clear unwanted antigens before they even have the opportunity to broach the wall of the GI tract.

Bordering the patches are high endothelial venules, which express unique integrins to recognize T and B lymphocytes. These high venules have endothelial walls that are slightly thicker than most simple squamous endothelia. They are typical of venules where lymphocytes

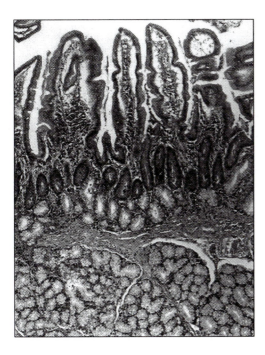

Fig. 3-8 . Duodenum (Human)

Long villi with few goblet cells and dense
Brunner's glands cross the muscularis mucosae
to empty into the base of the intestinal crypts
(hematoxylin-eosin; 150×).

Notes

Histologic identification of small
intestine segments depends on
the presence of specific (although
sometimes minor) features.

adhere and undergo diapedesis (passage of lymphocytes through
endothelia), thus allowing lymphocytes to exit the circulation and
enter the interstitial fluid of the connective tissue.

Regions of the Small Intestine

Duodenum. The duodenum is approximately 25 cm long and
curves around the head of the pancreas. Duodenal villi are leaflike in
shape (broad, flat); this appearance is varied in microscopic specimens, depending on the plane of sectioning (Figure 3-8). There are
very few goblet cells in the epithelium, because there is little need for
lubrication yet. The most distinguishing feature of the duodenum are
Brunner's glands in the submucosa. (The only other portion of the GI
tract that has glands in the submucosa is the esophagus.) Brunner's
glands are branched tubuloalveolar glands that produce a neutral or
slightly alkaline mucous secretion to neutralize the acidic chyme
arriving from the stomach.

Jejunum. The jejunum is 2.5 m long. It displays the best-developed
plicae circulares and numerous, long, fingerlike villi (Figure 3-9). There
are a moderate number of goblet cells, more than in the duodenum.
The jejunum is the major area for final digestion and absorption in the
small intestine.

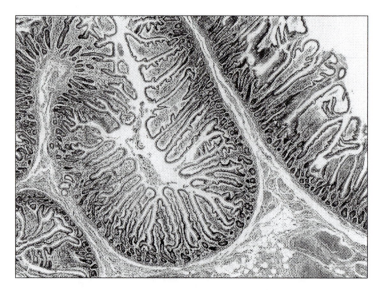

Fig. 3-9. Jejunum (Human), Longitudinal Section

Typical elaborate plicae circulares and long villi with an intermediate number of goblet cells (hematoxylin-eosin; 25×).

Ileum. The ileum is the longest portion of the small intestine (3.5 m). The ileum is characterized by Peyer's patches and short, club-like villi (Figure 3-10). There are only shallow crypts and low plicae circulares. The epithelium of the ileum contains a large percentage of goblet cells. Absorption of the vitamin B_{12}–intrinsic factor complex and bile acids takes place in the ileum.

A   B

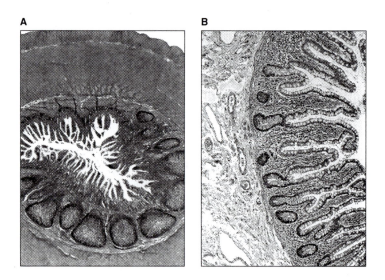

Fig. 3-10. Ileum

(A) Cat. Peyer's patches aggregate on the antimesenteric aspect of the lumen of the ileum (hematoxylin-eosin; 25×). (B) Human. Villi of the ileum are short and clublike with a high density of goblet cells; the base of the crypts contain eosinophilic Paneth cells (hematoxylin-eosin; 120×).

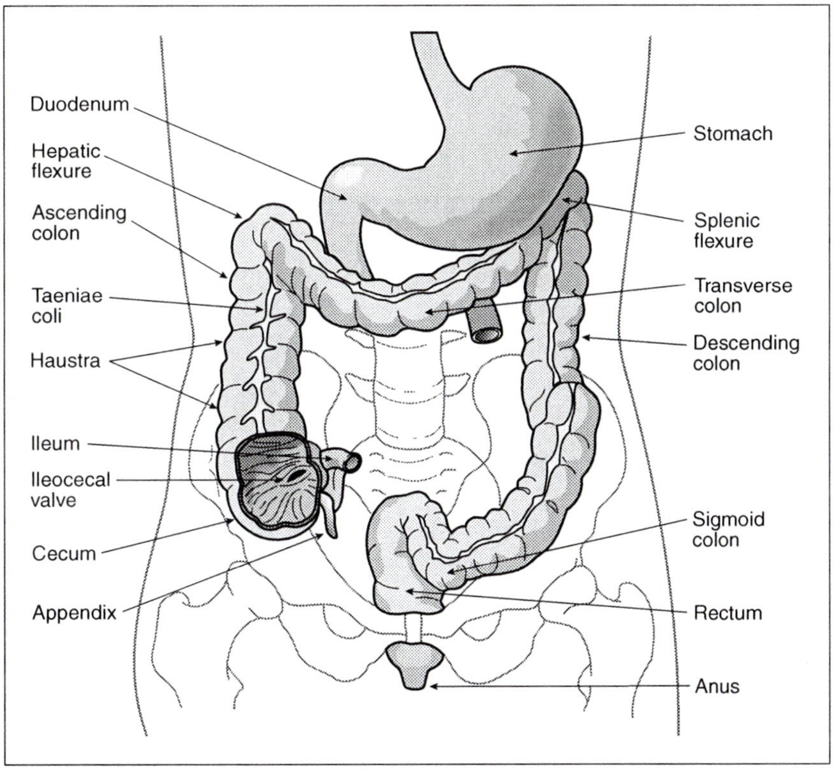

Fig. 3-11. Anatomic Regions of the Large Intestine: Ileocecal Valve to Anus

Large Intestine

The large intestine extends from the ileocecal valve to the anus and is divided into the cecum; the vermiform appendix; the ascending, transverse, descending, and pelvic colon; the rectum; and the anus (Figure 3-11). The major functions of the large intestine are the reabsorption of water and salts and the elimination of undigested feces.

Anatomy

Cecum and Appendix

The cecum of the large intestine lies in the right iliac fossa, below the level of entry of the ileum. Extending downward from the cecum is the vermiform appendix, a narrow, blind tube. The appendix is situated one-third of the way along a line between the anterior superior iliac spine and the umbilicus. Within the abdominal cavity, the appendix is located by following the taeniae coli longitudinal muscular bands from the cecum all the way to the base of the appendix.

Ascending, Transverse, and Descending Colon

The ascending colon extends upward from the cecum to the inferior surface of the right lobe of the liver, where it turns sharply left, forming the right colic or hepatic flexure. The transverse colon continues across the abdominal cavity, suspended within the transverse mesocolon, to the left colic or splenic flexure. The left colic flexure is

Notes

The large intestine is characterized by crypts containing many goblet cells and large submucosal blood vessels.

considerably higher than the right colic flexure and is suspended from the diaphragm by the phrenocolic ligament. The descending colon curves to the midline at the pelvic inlet and continues as the sigmoid colon. It is suspended by the pelvic mesocolon and becomes continuous with the rectum at the level of the third sacral vertebra.

The front and sides of the ascending and descending colon are covered by peritoneum, yet the posterior aspects fuse with the posterior abdominal wall, rendering them retroperitoneal structures.

Rectum and Anus

The rectum is 13 cm in length. It follows the curve of the sacral and coccygeal vertebrae. Then it bends downward and backward as the rectum pierces the levator ani muscle of the pelvic floor to continue as the anus. The upper half of the rectum is covered by peritoneum on its anterior and lateral aspects; the lower rectum is retroperitoneal and is embedded in the pelvic fascia. In women, the peritoneum reflects over the superior aspect of the uterus, lines the floor of the abdominal cavity above the cervix, and then reflects over the anterior aspect of the midrectum. Abdominal bleeding settles into this low point, the rectouterine pouch (of Douglas), and can be easily detected by a needle aspiration through the upper posterior wall of the vagina. The mucosa, submucosa, and circular muscularis externa of the rectum form three permanent crescent-shaped folds called the plicae transversales recti.

The anal canal is approximately 4 cm long. The mucosa is thrown into a series of longitudinal folds called the anal columns. Large veins within the columns can enlarge to produce hemorrhoids. The lumen of the anal canal is constricted by the internal and external anal sphincter muscles. The internal sphincter is a thickening of the circular layer of the muscularis externa and consists of smooth muscle. The external sphincter, on the other hand, is composed of skeletal muscle and is under voluntary control.

HISTOLOGY

Colon

The mucosa of the colon appears smooth when viewed in a gross specimen; neither plicae circulares nor villi are present. Throughout the large intestine, the muscosa is composed of only crypts with no villi. The epithelium consists of simple columnar absorptive cells, goblet cells, and a few enteroendocrine cells (Figure 3-12). Paneth cells are absent. Although hematoxylin-eosin-stained sections illustrate many goblet cells, enterocytes predominate in the proximal colon at a 4:1 ratio. A glycocalyx is present, but it does not contain hydrolytic enzymes as it does in the small intestine. The basolateral surface of the absorptive cells contains Na^+-K^+-ATPase used to power the retention of salts at the apical surface. The lamina propria contains numerous fenestrated capillaries and large veins for the assimilation of

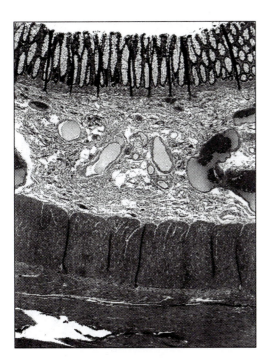

Fig. 3-12. Colon (Human)

The section, taken through a taeniae coli of
the muscularis externa, shows crypts with a
large number of goblet cells and submucosal
blood vessels (hematoxylin-eosin E; 80×).

reabsorbed fluids and ions. The lamina propria of the colon is unique,
however, in its lack of lymphatic capillaries. This deficit contributes to
the slow rate of metastasis of certain colon cancers. Lymphatic circulation only extends as far in as muscularis mucosae. GALT of the
colon includes multiple (and frequently large) solitary lymphatic nodules and isolated lymphocytes, plasma cells, and eosinophils.

The outer logitudinal layer of the muscularis externa of the colon
is clustered into three bands called taeniae coli. These logitudinal
bands of muscle are easily recognized at the gross anatomic level;
puckering between taeniae creates the protruding haustra of the
colon. The outer serosa of the transverse colon frequently contains
pendulous projections of fat.

Appendix

The appendix epithelium is identical to that of the colon—crypts
only, with numerous goblet cells (Figure 3-13). However, the appendix has a very small lumen diameter. There are lymphatic nodules
aggregated around the entire lumen (unlike the ileum, where the
Peyer's patches cluster on the antimesenteric side of the lumen). Frequently, debris remains preserved in the lumen.

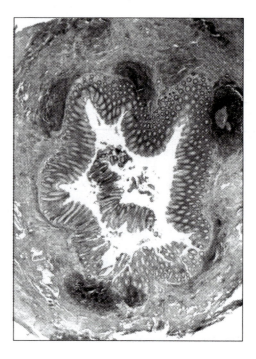

Fig. 3-13. Appendix (Human)

Aggregated lymphoid nodules surround a
small, debris-filled lumen lined by crypts
with goblet cells (hematoxylin-eosin; 30×).

Rectum

The rectal lumen is lined by three large semilunar folds with cores of
submucosal tissue called plicae transversales recti. The epithelial ratio
of absorptive cells to goblet cells shifts closer to 1:1. The crypts are
usually deeper than in the upper large intestine, and solitary lymphatic
nodules are common. The submucosa is characterized by veins with
large lumens, which aid in the reabsorption of water. The muscularis
externa contains a continuous sheet of logitudinal smooth muscle,
with no taeniae coli, and is bordered by an adventitia, as the rectum is
embedded in retroperitoneal connective tissue.

Anus

The anal mucosa folds longitudinally into anal columns or anal valves.
The epithelium changes to stratified squamous (Figure 3-14). This
change alone implies the lack of absorption and the increase in friction in the anus. The submucosa is well vascularized with terminal
branches of the superior rectal artery and rectal venous plexus. Enlargement of these submucosal veins produces internal hemorrhoids.
The submucosa also contains nerves and Pacinian corpuscles for
deep-pressure sensation. The muscularis mucosae disappears in the
anus, but the circular layer of the muscularis externa thickens to form
the internal anal sphincter. The external anal sphincter is formed by
skeletal muscle of the perineal floor.

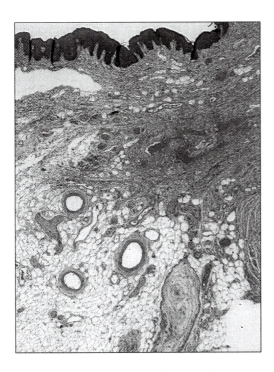

Fig. 3-14. Anus (Human)

Stratified squamous epithelium lines the anal lumen; a broad submucosa includes large blood vessels, fat, and a Pacinian corpuscle (hematoxylin-eosin; 60×).

REVIEW QUESTIONS

Directions: For each of the following questions, choose the one best answer.

1 Nontropical sprue involves malabsorption resulting from an intolerance to wheat gluten. Based on your knowledge of the structure and function of the normal GI tract, which of the following defects would be seen early in this condition?

A Enzyme defects in enteroendocrine cells
B Blockage of main pancreatic ducts
C Destruction of enterocyte microvilli
D Decline in endogenous bacterial population of the colon
E Spastic contraction of the muscularis externa

2 In a patient with vitamin B_{12}-deficient anemia, which of the following is the *least* probable cause?

A Surgical resection for carcinoma, removing most of the distal ileum
B Hiatal hernia with reflux of stomach contents

C Atrophy of the gastric glands in the fundus and body of the stomach

D Colonization of the small intestine by masses of bacteria

E Aspirin-induced gastric ulcers

3 Which of the following statements concerning acid secretion by gastric parietal cells is *true*?

A It results in a decrease in blood pH.

B It produces carbon dioxide and water from carbonic acid (H_2CO_3).

C It is accomplished via an H^+-Cl^--ATPase.

D It requires H^+-K^+-ATPase stored in the tubulovesicular system to be inserted into the canalicular membrane.

E It requires the basolateral import of K^+.

4 A unique histologic feature most helpful in identifying the duodenum is the presence of

A Brunner's glands.

B Peyer's patches.

C surface mucous cells.

D Paneth cells.

E goblet cells.

References

Fitzgerald MJT, Fitzgerald M: *Human Embryology.* London: Bailliere Tindall, 1994.

Gartner LP, Hiatt JL: Digestive system II: alimentary canal. In *Color Textbook of Histology.* Philadelphia, PA: Saunders, 1997, pp 312–37.

Johnson LR: *Gastrointestinal Physiology.* St. Louis, MO: Elsevier Science, Mosby, 2001.

Moore KL, Persaud TVN: *The Developing Human,* 5th ed. Philadelphia, PA: Saunders, 1993.

Neutra MR: The gastrointestinal tract. In *Cell and Tissue Biology,* 6th ed. Edited by Weiss L. Baltimore, MD: Urban and Schwarzenberg, 1988, pp 641–84.

4

Overview of Gastrointestinal Motility

▦ CHAPTER OUTLINE ▦

▦ LEARNING OBJECTIVES ▦

At the completion of this chapter, the reader should be able to:
- List the sequential cellular events that lead to contraction of intestinal circular muscle.
- Describe the importance of tone in the GI tract.
- Contrast segmenting contractions, peristalsis, and tonic contractions.
- Describe the mechanisms involved and importance of the intestinal housekeeper function of the migrating myoelectric or motor complex (MMC) recorded in the interdigestive period.

CASE STUDY: *INTRODUCTION*

Y.S. was a 70-year-old woman who presented with a 3-year history of progressively worsening bloating, nausea, and vomiting. She first presented with diarrhea 3 years prior to admission. A colonoscopy was negative, and she was given the diagnosis of irritable bowel syndrome. Over the next year, her symptoms worsened, and she noted progressive abdominal distention despite a 15-lb weight loss. Two years prior to admission she was admitted to another hospital for evaluation of her progressive weight loss and a radiograph that was interpreted as showing a small intestinal obstruction. All laboratory studies were normal except for a decreased albumin level and mild normocytic anemia. Electrophoresis of the serum immunoglobulins and urine was normal. A CT scan of the abdomen and pelvis was normal except for multiple dilated loops of small and large intestine. A gastric emptying test (nuclear study) showed severely delayed emptying at 2 hours. A repeat colonoscopy, including deep mucosal biopsies from the rectum, was normal. She was prescribed antibiotics that were to be taken for the first week of each month on a rotational basis.

Introduction

Contents of the digestive system vary, and include life-sustaining nutrients, highly caustic organic and inorganic acids, and dense concentrations of potentially injurious bacteria in the colon. To sustain health, luminal contents must move through the digestive tract in an oral-to-anal direction at a rate that allows time for mixing, digestion, and absorption. In fact, the movement of material through the lumen of the digestive system is precisely regulated and varies with the caloric content, type of nutrients, and osmolality of the material. Furthermore, esophageal, gastric, and intestinal contractions must limit the retrograde movement of luminal contents from distal to proximal organs. Luminal contents move down the digestive system as the result of contractions regulated by a complex interaction of electrical, neural, and hormonal control mechanisms. The release of chemical transmitters by immune cells also has a major effect on digestive contractions, particularly in the presence of inflammation. The contractile and regulatory events that mix and transport luminal contents through the digestive system are collectively referred to as GI motility.

The movement of luminal contents is measured in terms of rates of transit. Normal transit times through digestive organs vary greatly, from a few seconds in the esophagus to 2–3 days in the colon. These highly varied transit rates result from equally variable patterns of GI motility. To fully understand the normal motility patterns of each of the tubular organs, it is necessary to appreciate how these patterns vary between fasting and feeding. Each of these highly varied patterns, however, ultimately results from similar fundamental cellular electrical and contractile physiologic mechanisms.

Patterns of contractions propel luminal contents at a rate that optimizes digestion and absorption. GI motility delivers nutrients to the small intestine in a timely manner to optimize digestion and absorption. Motility also provides for storage, mixture, and delivery of nutrients for absorption; storage of waste products; reservoir functions to limit energy use during fasting; limitation of the exposure of the mucosa to luminal contents; propulsion of waste products and bacteria from the small intestine; and a variety of other important functions that enhance the efficiency of the digestive system. Disorders causing impaired GI motility can adversely influence any or all of these functions.

The specific characteristics of the motility of each organ are discussed in more detail in the chapters that follow. This chapter provides an overview of the physiology of motility by describing the mechanisms of excitation–contraction coupling that are shared by the luminal organs and discusses their physiologic importance. Understanding these physiologic principles provides a foundation to understand the pathophysiology of each organ and the potential treatment options to restore the patient to health.

GI Contractions

MECHANISMS OF CONTRACTION

Smooth muscle in the GI tract is primarily located in three layers of muscles found in most luminal organs: muscularis mucosae, circular muscle, and longitudinal muscle. The lamina muscularis mucosae is a thin layer of muscle that lies just inside the basal lamina of the epithelial cells. It is thought to be involved primarily in mixing fluid at the surface of the lumen. The circular and longitudinal muscle layers constitute the overwhelming majority of muscle in the gut wall. Together they are known as the muscularis propria. The two layers are oriented perpendicular to each other and, as their names imply, are oriented around or down the longitudinal axis of the gut lumen. In the esophagus, the two layers have a more spiral orientation. When patients have spasms of the esophagus, this spiral orientation creates a corkscrew appearance that can be seen on x-ray.

Two types of muscles are found in the digestive system. Striated muscles are found in the pharynx, upper esophageal sphincter, proximal esophagus, and external anal sphincter. All other GI muscles are smooth muscles; thus, most GI muscles are smooth. Striated muscles are sometimes designated as voluntary and smooth muscles as involuntary. Although conceptually useful, this convention can be misleading. Smooth muscle contractions also mediate esophageal peristalsis, vomiting, belching, defecation, and fecal retention; yet each of these events can be initiated voluntarily.

GI muscles are smooth muscle except for those of the pharynx, upper esophageal and external anal sphincters, and proximal esophagus.

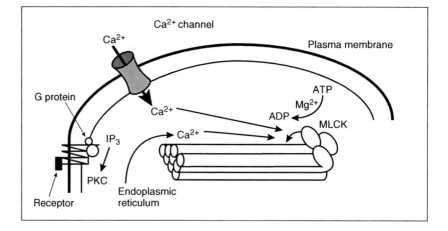

Fig. 4-1. Calcium (Ca²⁺) Channel

Final activation of smooth muscle contraction is mediated by an increase in the cytoplasmic concentration of Ca^{2+}. In the presence of Ca^{2+} and ATP, myosin light-chain kinase activates the conformational interaction between actin and myosin to cause contraction. Intracellular Ca^{2+} released from the endoplasmic reticulum is mediated by protein kinase C. Concentrations of protein kinase C are increased through the release of inositol triphosphate (IP₃) after the activation of seven transmembrane-crossing receptors that are associated with the heterodimer G proteins. Extracellular Ca^{2+} enters the cell through Ca^{2+} channels through the gating process. PKC = protein kinase C; Mg^{2+} = magnesium; ADP = adenosine diphosphate; MLCK = myosin light-chain kinase.

All muscles share similar basic mechanisms of excitation–contraction coupling. The specific cellular mechanisms for smooth muscle contraction are less well understood than for striated muscle, but presumably they are very similar. Ultimately, all muscle contractions depend on cross-bridge movement between actin (light-chain) and myosin (heavy-chain) fibers (Figure 4-1). Actin–myosin cross-bridge cycling is initiated in the presence of increased cytosolic calcium (Ca^{2+}). The concentration of intracellular Ca^{2+} is altered by two closely related mechanisms that provide Ca^{2+} from both intra- and extracellular sources.

Extracellular Ca^{2+} enters the cell as the result of changes in the resting membrane potential of the cell, leading to the opening of Ca^{2+} channels. Like many other types of cells within the digestive system, muscles become activated by alteration of the resting membrane potential. Enteric neurons, endocrine cells, and secretory cells all exhibit membrane excitability and specific permeability characteristics for selected ions. The resting membrane potential is established by the relative permeability of the plasma membrane to selected ions such as Ca^{2+}, K^+, and Na^+. The membrane potential changes when a chemical alteration influences membrane permeability. Thus, biologic membranes set up specific charges within the cell by activating selected ion pumps, such as the Na^+-K^+-ATPase and the Ca^{2+} pumps. Each pump will require ATP and, therefore, cellular oxygen.

The membrane potential influences the rate of opening and closing of Na$^+$, chloride (Cl$^-$), K$^+$, and Ca^{2+} channels through conformational changes of the channels. This process is known as *gating*. For most of these cells there is background permeability, primarily to K$^+$, which establishes the resting membrane potential. Depolarization of the cells occurs when inward Na$^+$ (neurons) or Ca^{2+} (smooth muscle cells) channels open.

Ion channels are pores through the cell membrane that are just narrow enough to permit the movement of a single ion. Each channel has the ability to distinguish between specific anions and cations. When these channels undergo conformational change, the channel itself becomes closed or sequentially opened to permit the transport of specific ions. The development of specific ion channel antagonists, such as the Ca^{2+} channel antagonist, has provided a clinically effective treatment of hypertension, angina, and smooth muscle spastic disorders, including diffuse esophageal spasm, and has provided an important class of agents to evaluate channel physiology.

Intracellular Ca^{2+} is stored in the smooth endoplasmic reticulum (ER) or in specialized organelles known as calciosomes. Stored Ca^{2+} is released in response to the activation of signal transduction pathways that activate specific protein kinases. This may occur as a result of inositol 1,4,5-triphosphate (IP$_3$), a by-product of phosphatidylcholine under the influence of phospholipase C and G protein activation. In turn, increased release of intracellular Ca^{2+} results in the formation of Ca^{2+}–calmodulin complex, which in turn increases the phosphorylation of myosin light-chain kinase.

Actin–myosin cross-bridge cycling is also dependent on the presence of ATP. Activated phosphate bonds serve as the source of energy to drive this reaction. As cytosolic Ca^{2+} concentrations return to normal, actin–myosin cross-bridging recycles and the muscle relaxes.

Smooth muscle contractions may occur in a tonic or phasic pattern. In general, tonic contractions require less energy, involve fewer cross-bridge cyclings, and may occur independent of the depolarization of the cell membrane. Phasic contractions result when the cell membrane depolarizes, resulting in the inward flux of extracellular Ca^{2+}. The cell is later repolarized by the outward flow of K$^+$. Changes in smooth muscle membrane potential depend primarily on potentials generated by the transmembrane movement of Ca^{2+} and K$^+$. Smooth muscle contractions occur independently of Na$^+$ channels and are therefore resistant to Na$^+$ channel antagonists, such as tetrodotoxin.

Recent studies of esophageal muscles suggest that the flux of Cl$^-$ is what determines the resting membrane potential in this muscle. Experimental evidence suggests that Cl$^-$ channels are critical to esophageal peristalsis. Peristaltic sequences persist when Na$^+$ channels are completely blocked by agents that eliminate nearly all neural functions. In contrast, peristalsis is completely abolished by Cl$^-$ channel antagonists.

Slow waves, the basal electric rhythm of intestinal motility, are measurable, repetitive depolarization-repolarization patterns.

Each GI organ has a characteristic **slow-wave frequency.**

REGULATION OF GI CONTRACTIONS

Contractions of the GI tract occur in complex, often repetitive patterns that are modified by input from complex regulatory mechanisms. Contractions are regulated by the intrinsic properties of muscle, extrinsic hormones, extrinsic nerves, and intrinsic neurons and by electrical pacemaker potentials. It is important to appreciate that the final contractile event is the result of the summation of stimulatory and inhibitory neural, hormonal, and immune influences.

Electrical Properties of Smooth Muscles

Two fundamental types of electrical control activity can be recorded from intestinal smooth muscle: controls of timing and of rhythm. The pacemaking potentials of the gut control the timing of phasic contractions. Also known as basal electric rhythm, the potentials are important in determining the rhythm of contractions. More commonly, however, these controls are known descriptively as slow waves. Slow waves are precisely timed, rhythmic depolarization and repolarization of the muscularis propria of the stomach and intestine, independent of the presence or absence of a stimulus or contraction. This repetitive depolarization–repolarization moves in an oral-to-anal (aborad) direction. Thus, when slow waves are evaluated from multiple cells using extracellular electrodes, multiphasic potentials are recorded that appear similar to the QRS complex of an electrocardiogram (ECG) (Figure 4-2). Unlike the ECG signal, however, slow waves are the result of pacemaker potentials, not contractions, as is the case for the QRS complex of the ECG.

Slow-wave potentials occur with a highly precise rhythmicity that is specific for the organ from which they are recorded. The presence of such rhythmic depolarizations enhances the probability of contractile events occurring at the peak of cell depolarization, thus creating a mechanism for coordinating the timing of rhythmic smooth muscle contractions. This coordination of contractions by the electrical control activity is important not only to facilitate the aboral movement of waves of contraction down the digestive tract but to ensure that these contractions occur at the same time in a plane of circular muscles to create a moving ring of contraction.

Slow waves of the GI tract occur in a characteristic frequency specific to each organ (Table 4-1). Slow-wave activity has been

Table 4-1. Slow-Wave Frequencies

ORGAN	FREQUENCY (CONTRACTIONS/MIN)
Esophagus	. . .
Fundus	. . .
Antrum	3
Duodenum	14–15
Ileum	11–13
Colon	Mixed: 3, 6, and others

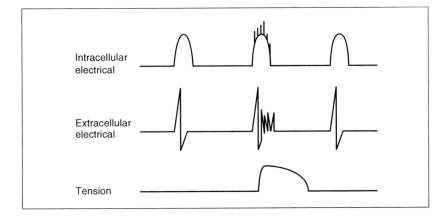

Fig. 4-2. Schematic Representation of the Changes in Electric Potential and Force Transducer Recordings from GI Muscles over the Period of 30–60 Seconds

The upper tracing shows the periodic depolarization and repolarization of a single smooth muscle cell. Smooth muscle cells develop this characteristic periodic change from the resting membrane potential of 50–70 mV to create what is known as electrical control activity or, more commonly, slow waves. Recording the same event from bipolar electrodes placed over the intracellular electrode generates a tracing similar to the second tracing. Note the consistent interval that occurs between slow waves, whether or not there is associated electrical response activity or spike potentials. Note that in the first and third slow waves, no spike activity is seen, and hence no contraction is recorded. In contrast, the second slow wave has apparently reached threshold potential, resulting in the opening and closing of multiple channels, which are recorded as tiny spikes on the top of the slow wave in the cellular recording and as spikes after the slow wave on the extracellular recording. These rapid changes in membrane potential reflect the opening of calcium channels, which in turn resulted in the contraction recorded on the tension tracing.

recorded inconsistently in the esophagus and gastric fundus. In contrast, rhythmic, high-amplitude, very precisely timed pacemaker potentials are generated in the upper portion of the gastric corpus 3 times per minute. These waves of depolarization–repolarization travel down the stomach in a ringlike fashion toward the pyloric sphincter. Slow-wave potentials in the gastric antrum can be recorded by a study called an electrogastrogram by placing electrodes on the abdominal wall over the stomach and recording activity. These pacemaker potentials appear critical to the normal functioning of the stomach. Disorders of slow-wave rhythms have been associated with abnormalities of gastric emptying and nausea. In the small intestine, slow waves also occur with precise rhythm but at a much faster rate than in the stomach. In the colon, slow-wave frequencies are less distinct and may represent a composite of several pacemaker potential frequencies.

These electrical control signals are generated by specialized cells in the area of the muscularis propria known as the *interstitial cells of Cajal* (ICC). In the small intestine, these cells are located on

the luminal side of the circular muscle layer. Signals generated by these cells travel quickly around the circumference of the lumen and more slowly in an aboral direction. The speed of transmission is a function of the density of specialized cellular organelles known as *gap junctions*. Electrical communications between the cells are the result of cell-to-cell cross-communication through gap junctions. This results in a syncytial network of cells that rapidly transmit electrical signals, permitting the organization for the electrical propagation of peristalsis.

Patterns of GI Contractions

TONIC CONTRACTIONS

Smooth muscle contractions can be viewed as either tonic or phasic. Either type of contraction may impede or accelerate the transit of intraluminal contents. Tonic contractions show relatively little change over time. Tonic contractions of the gastric fundus, gallbladder, and colon promote the movement of intraluminal contents down the GI tract by exerting a relatively low pressure (5–15 mm Hg) for prolonged periods. Although these organs are anatomically and physiologically different in many ways, they share the characteristic of being storage organs. The colon stores fecal material. The fundus stores ingested food so that it can enter the digestive process in a timely fashion that will maximize the efficiency of digestion and absorption. The gallbladder stores bile secreted by the liver. Bile is then emptied in response to a meal if the food contains fat or selected amino acids. This reduces the flow of these structurally complex bile salt molecules during fasting, thus reducing their exposure to the lumen and reducing the expenditure of energy that would be needed to reabsorb them from the small intestine. The fundus fills through the process known as receptive relaxation. It then propels liquids through the stomach by exerting a tonic pressure at the top (proximal) end of the stomach. The gallbladder relaxes during fasting to permit the filling of bile under the influence of a closed sphincter of Oddi at the end of the common bile duct. In response to eating, the sphincter opens, and the gallbladder tonically contracts to expel its contents gradually over 1–2 hours.

GI Sphincters

In contrast to the low-pressure tonic contractions of the large organs, sphincters are narrow zones of tonically contracted muscles that impede the transit of luminal contents between organs of the digestive tract. The resting pressures of sphincters vary from 10 to 70 mm Hg. Most sphincters also have superimposed phasic contractions. In the pyloric sphincter and the lower esophageal sphincter (LES), these phasic contractions often exceed 100 mm Hg. Sphincteric control of flow is an essential component of normal motility. A list of GI sphincters is shown in Table 4-2. Most sphincters can be recognized as a

Table 4-2. GI Sphincters and Disorders Associated with Sphincter Dysfunction

SPHINCTER	ASSOCIATED DISORDERS
Upper esophageal sphincter (UES)	Cricopharyngeal achalasia
	Zenker's diverticuli
Lower esophageal sphincter (LES)	Achalasia
	Gastroesophageal reflux disease
Pylorus	Gastric ulcers
	Hypertrophic pyloric stenosis
Sphincter of Oddi	Biliary dyskinesia
Ileocecal valve	Bacterial overgrowth
Anal sphincters	Hirschsprung's disease
	Fecal leakage

Notes

Sphincteric muscle is characterized by higher-pressure tonic contractions and superimposed phasic contractions.

thickening of the circular muscle layer at the junction of two luminal organs. Others, such as the LES, cannot be appreciated by gross inspection but can be precisely defined as a zone of increased pressure by using physiologic pressure-recording devices. Furthermore, strips of sphincteric muscle examined in vitro can be distinguished from adjacent strips of nonsphincteric muscle by their increased active resting tone, increased resistance to stretch (passive tone), and (in smooth muscle sphincters) contraction in response to norepinephrine. Sphincter muscles maintain a tonic contraction between luminal organs to slow retrograde flow and regulate the forward flow of materials. This tonic contraction is maintained as a result of myogenic properties of the muscle and in response to tonic neural input. A small amount of retrograde flow occurs normally across the LES and pylorus. Retrograde flow in normal individuals occurs across the LES as a result of intermittent transient relaxations (TLESRs). No retrograde flow of fluid or air occurs in healthy individuals across the sphincter of Oddi or the anal sphincters.

Forward flow across the sphincter occurs when these specialized zones of muscle relax. A number of clinical disorders of motility are characterized by an inability of sphincters to maintain adequate tone or to relax normally. Examples of disorders associated with sphincteric dysfunction are shown in Table 4-2. Relaxation must be both complete and, in most circumstances, well coordinated with contractile waves that are propelling luminal contents forward. Because of the clinical importance of sphincters, scientists have long sought to understand the mechanisms responsible for maintaining sphincter tone and relaxation. Characteristically, proximal distention leads to sphincter relaxation, whereas distention of the lumen distal to the sphincter leads to contraction. This intermittent relaxation is under neurologic control. The two striated muscle sphincters, the upper esophageal sphincter and external anal sphincter, are under voluntary control by neurons in the CNS. All other sphincters are composed of smooth muscle and relax reflexively under the influence of neurons that have their cell bodies in the myenteric plexus

NO is the neurotransmitter responsible for relaxation of sphincter smooth muscle.

Segmentary contractions churn and mix luminal contents for maximum exposure to mucosal epithelium, promoting digestion and absorption.

between the longitudinal and circular muscle layers. For many years, the neurotransmitter responsible for this relaxation was unknown. Although it was repeatedly shown that this relaxation was neurally mediated, it was also clear that it was not due to neurons in the sympathetic (adrenergic) or parasympathetic (cholinergic) pathways. Nitric oxide (NO) has been shown to be responsible for the relaxation of GI sphincters by these nonadrenergic, noncholinergic (NANC) neurons. A peptide neurotransmitter, vasoactive intestinal polypeptide (VIP), is colocalized in these neurons and interacts with NO.

PHASIC CONTRACTIONS

Phasic contractions may either impair or accelerate intestinal transit. Peristaltic contractions, segmenting contractions, contractions occurring during the intestinal housekeeper, contractions during fasting, and spasms are examples of phasic contractions. The most common contractions recorded during fasting or feeding in both the small and large intestines are phasic contractions, which occur randomly and are known as segmenting contractions. The random nonpropagating nature of segmenting contractions results in the mixing of luminal contents and an increased exposure of contents with the surface epithelium. This in turn increases the effect of the mucosal digestive and absorptive functions. An increase in the frequency of segmental contractions impedes the transit of material through the GI tract. Likewise, phasic contractions that occur in a retrograde fashion (anal-to-oral direction) will impair transit. Retrograde contractions are known to be important in the vomiting reflex and in the back-and-forth movement of intraluminal contents in the large intestine.

Peristalsis

Peristalsis is the orderly movement of a circular ring of contraction down (aboral direction) the GI tract. It is the only normal pattern of phasic contraction seen in the esophagus and gastric antrum, and it can also be recorded in the intestine. Mechanisms responsible for this orderly movement of phasic contractions are incompletely understood. Complex patterned behaviors, such as peristalsis, require the development of an upstream contraction and distal relaxation. As the wave moves in an anal direction, the adjacent muscles must first relax, then contract. This pattern of muscle relaxation and contraction is mediated by the sequential activation of adjacent program circuits so that specific motor neurons are activated and deactivated in a timely fashion. Afferent stimuli from the mucosa that can stimulate a peristaltic sequence are detected by neurons that have their cells of origin in the submucosal plexus or paraspinal nuclei, such as the inferior or superior mesenteric ganglia. The neurons involved in the peristaltic reflex are localized to the myenteric plexus and are of two morphologies. The propagation of these programmed events is controlled by a "switch" or "gate" that commands neurons. Most of these driver network neurons are thought to be of a Dogiel type I morphology, with long axons and short, stubby dendrites. Long, Dogiel type I neurons also encircle the lumen circumferentially to activate groups of motor neurons. Excitatory and inhibitory motor or effector neurons that synapse with smooth muscles have more extensive dendrites and shorter axons. These are described as Dogiel type II–III motor neurons. It is likely that serotonin (5-hydroxytryptamine) plays a key role as a transmitter in the Dogiel type I neurons. Contraction is mediated by acetylcholine-containing neurons. Substance P may also contribute to contraction. NO mediates distal relaxation, perhaps through an interaction with VIP. Thus, through the interplay of motor neurons that have a primarily inhibitory effect and other similarly shaped cells containing excitatory transmitters, complex patterns can be generated through the appropriate sequential activation of inhibition followed by excitation of enteric neurons.

COMPLEX MULTIORGAN PATTERNS OF CONTRACTION

In addition to isolated phasic patterns of contractions occurring in a single organ, several contractile events can traverse from one organ to another. Thus, although peristalsis of the esophagus terminates at the LES and "colonic mass action" does not occur in other organs, there are several complicated contractile events that are multiorgan in nature.

Interdigestive Migrating Motor Complex (IMMC)

During fasting, the digestive system is not entirely dormant. Cyclical patterns of inactivity mix with easily recognized patterns of contractile activity. These patterns develop in the proximal stomach and the LES, then traverse the entire small intestine to the ileocecal sphincter. These repetitive patterns of contraction do not propagate into the colon. The gallbladder and sphincter of Oddi are also involved. The cyclical pattern of relaxation, followed by two patterns of contractile activity, is known as the IMMC and is characterized by three phases of contractile activity. Depending on the size and caloric content of a meal, the fed pattern of contraction gradually ends after 2–4 hours, to be replaced by the first phase of the IMMC. During phase I, the bowel is at rest, as if in a recovery phase from the considerable expenditure of energy during the digestive cycle. After 30–60 minutes of minimal contractile activity, intermittent, apparently random segmenting phasic contractions can be seen in a pattern that is very similar to that seen during a fed phase of digestion. The duration of phase II is highly variable but generally lasts about 1 hour. After the period of mixing contractile activity, phase III begins.

Phase III is the most easily recognized pattern of contraction. It is also known as the intestinal housekeeper. It is a very forceful contractile event lasting 8–12 minutes over 3–6 cm of the GI tract. These forceful contractions move down the tract from the proximal stomach and LES to the distal ileum. These contractile events propel all intraluminal contents toward and eventually into the colon. The wave of contraction can cleanse the stomach and small intestine of residual undigested material and dying luminal cells. Artifacts larger than 4 mm that were retained in the stomach through the effects of the pyloric sphincter and so kept from interfering with the digestion of nutrients are propelled to the colon. Thus, phase III serves to cleanse the bowel of its intestinal waste, an important function that has led to the name of the intestinal housekeeper. Patients with small intestine bacterial overgrowth are known to have impairment or absence of phase III activity.

Mechanisms responsible for phase III of the IMMC are incompletely understood. The initiation of phase III activity in the duodenum is very closely associated with the release of the GI hormone motilin. The further progression of the IMMC involves intrinsic opioidlike neurotransmitters distally. The potent smell of food, eating, and the infusion of food into the duodenum produce immediate termination of IMMC cycling by the hormone gastrin, regardless of where the activity front (phase III) is at that time. Phase IV is a short transition period between the constant activity of phase III and the quiescence of phase I (see also Chapter 28 and Figure 28-5).

Vomiting

Vomiting is a complex, multisystem reflex initiated by the central vomiting center located in the medulla. When vomiting occurs, the epiglottis closes, and there is a massive sympathetic discharge and very forceful antiperistaltic contractions. These retrograde contractions begin in the duodenum, progress upward through the stomach, and eventually result in relaxation of the LES and movement of the material through the esophagus. Vomiting can be initiated by gastric receptors, cortical input from learned or aversive responses, vestibular irritation, or by the activation of chemoreceptors in the chemoreceptor trigger zone of the medulla.

CASE STUDY: *RESOLUTION*

Over the next 2 years, Y.S. lost an additional 40 lbs. She attributed this to the fact that all foods made her feel bloated after the first few bites. She denied dysphagia. The abdominal distention was worse, and the diarrhea persisted. The antibiotics had been discontinued. She denied arthralgias of the extremities. There was no history of diabetes, Raynaud's phenomenon, or atherosclerotic disorders. On physical examination, the patient appeared cachectic and weak, with mild dyspnea and a protuberant abdomen. Her blood pressure was 90/60 mm Hg, her pulse was 60 beats/min, and her respiratory rate was 22 breaths/min. The breath sounds were decreased bilaterally, and percussion revealed dullness at both bases. The bowel sounds were hypoactive. A succussion splash was elicited. The abdomen was severely distended and tympanitic. There were no masses or tenderness, and no evidence of a fluid wave or shifting dullness. There was no peripheral edema, and the skin was normal on the extremities. The rectal examination was normal; stool in the rectal vault was negative for occult blood. She was severely anemic. The albumin was 2.6 g/dl, and the cholesterol was 110 mg/dl. Liver chemistries and renal function were normal. A chest radiograph revealed bilateral pleural effusions. Paracentesis showed that the fluid was a transudate bilaterally, and the cytology examination was negative. A repeat CT was unchanged. The patient was discharged to a skilled nursing facility to receive total parenteral nutrition.

REVIEW QUESTIONS

Directions: For each of the following questions, choose the one best answer.

1 Which of the following statements most accurately describes striated muscles?

   A Only striated muscles can be influenced voluntarily.
   B Striated muscles are found in the upper (UES) and lower esophageal sphincters (LES).
   C Striated muscles are found in the lower digestive tract.
   D Striated muscle contractions do not depend on calcium.

2 Which of the following statements best describes the characteristics of slow waves?

   A Slow waves occur more frequently when contractions occur.
   B Slow waves are generated by cells in the submucosal plexus.
   C Slow waves occur more frequently than contractions.
   D Esophageal slow waves occur at a frequency of 5 contractions per minute.

3 Which of the following statements best describes GI sphincters?

   A Most sphincters contain some striated muscles.
   B All sphincters are composed of a thickening of the longitudinal muscle.
   C Sphincters contract in response to adrenergic (sympathetic) stimulation.
   D Sphincters prevent the retrograde flow of air and fluid.

4 Which of the following statements best describes the interdigestive migrating motor complex (IMMC)?

A Motilin, a neurotransmitter, mediates the propagation of the IMMC through the jejunum and ileum.

B Loss of phase III may be associated with an overgrowth of intestinal bacteria.

C Undigested solids leave the stomach during phase I of the IMMC.

D Phase III can be distinguished from the fed pattern by the frequency of retrograde contractions.

E The amplitude of phase III is increased in the colon.

References

Anand N, Patterson WG: Role of nitric oxide in esophageal peristalsis. *Am J Physiol* 266:G123–31, 1994.

Hartshor DJ, Kawamura T: Regulation of contraction-relaxation in smooth muscles. *News Physiol Sci* 7:59–64, 1992.

Johnson LR: *Gastrointestinal Physiology*. St. Louis, MO: Elsevier Science, Mosby, 2001.

Makhlouf GM: Smooth Muscle of the Gut. In *Textbook of Gastroenterology*, 4th ed., Edited by Yamada T. Philadelphia, PA: Lippincott, Williams & Wilkins, 2003.

5

GI Electrolyte and Fluid Secretion

■ CHAPTER OUTLINE ■

■ LEARNING OBJECTIVES ■

At the completion of this chapter, the reader should be able to:
- Evaluate the mechanisms through which saliva is secreted and the physiologic functions of saliva.
- Assess the secretory effects of secretin, gastrin, 5'-adenosine monophosphate (5'-AMP), histamine, cholecystokinin (CCK), and acetylcholine (ACh).
- Describe the secretion of hydrochloric acid (HCl) and recognize the cellular regulatory pathways.
- Analyze the primary regulatory mechanisms of pancreatic fluid secretion.
- Identify what cystic fibrosis transmembrane conductance regulator (CFTR) is and explain how it is regulated in GI epithelial cells.

CASE STUDY: *INTRODUCTION*

The patient was a 43-year-old man with a 2-month history of intermittent epigastric abdominal pain and watery diarrhea that resulted in dehydration and required resuscitation with intravenous fluids. Although the patient did not have obvious blood in his feces, occult blood was detected, and he was anemic. Physical examination was unremarkable. Stool studies for ova and parasites were negative. An upper endoscopic evaluation showed a hiatal hernia, distal esophagitis, and antral gastritis. Antral biopsies showed dense infiltration with eosinophils. A peripheral blood smear showed no elevation in the white blood cell (WBC) count or the number of eosinophils. The patient was diagnosed as having eosinophilic gastroenteritis, was briefly treated with prednisone, and received long-term treatment with oral cromolyn and omeprazole. His abdominal pain and diarrhea resolved within a couple days of treatment.

Introduction

Secretion, motility, and absorption are the essential functions of the GI tract. Therefore, alterations in fluid secretion may create a variety of pathophysiologic conditions. This chapter provides an overview of the cellular and tissue elements important in the regulation of GI fluid secretion and examines mechanisms by which altered regulation of secretion results in disease. Because of the emerging appreciation of the important role of ion channels in GI electrolyte secretion, ion channel effects are emphasized. To avoid overlap with another segment of this book, hepatocyte secretion (see Chapter 9) is not covered. In addition, secretion is only half the equation of GI fluid balance; the other half is absorption (see Chapters 6 and 7).

FUNCTIONS OF GI SECRETIONS

There are three dominant functions of GI secretions: transport, defense, and lubrication.

Transport

Beginning with the addition of saliva, all food is transported through the GI tract with the assistance of fluid. In addition, a variety of digestive enzymes flow to their appropriate alimentary zone after being released into specialized secretory ducts.

Defense

Specialized immunoglobulins secreted into the GI tract aid in mucosal defense. In addition, secreted fluids that possess antimicrobial enzymes and detergents dilute the concentration of pathogens, possibly destroy them (e.g., acid in the stomach), and transport them out of the body. Last, secreted mucus establishes a protective barrier, impairing attachment of pathogens to the epithelium.

Lubrication

Secreted fluids and mucus lubricate and protect the mucosal surface of the GI epithelium from injury. In addition, the mucous layer provides an essentially normal microenvironment for cells in an extreme location, such as the stomach.

MOVEMENT OF ELECTROLYTES

There are three basic cellular units responsible for movement of electrolytes: carriers, pumps, and channels.

Carriers

Carriers are either *symporters* (cotransporters) or *antiporters* (exchange carriers). In symporters, the carrier protein simply binds and transfers ions from one surface of the cell to the other. In antiporters, one ion is transported across the membrane in exchange for another. In general, carriers facilitate the transfer of electrolytes through the cell at a rate greater than would take place by simple diffusion.

Pumps

Pumps require energy (typically ATP) to move ions in a set direction, generally against the concentration gradient. Carriers and pumps transport relatively low volumes of ions through cell membranes; vastly more move through ion channels ($>10^6$ ions/s).

Channels

Ion channels are transmembranous proteins inserted in the lipid membrane of cells. Channels characteristically show a preference for one kind of ion over another; this is known as selectivity. Examples include cation channels, which are more permeable to positively charged ions than negatively charged ions (e.g., K^+ and $Na^+ \gg$ than Cl^-). There are particular cation channels that may also be selective for certain cations (e.g., K^+ channel is permeable to K^+ but not to Ca^{2+}). Although the regulation of the open or closed positions requires energy, the flow of ions through a channel is passive down electrochemical gradients. This capacity to allow prodigious quantities of ions to move quickly makes ion channels a key regulatory site of epithelial ion transport.

It is essential to keep in mind the effective architectural arrangement of GI epithelia. Like other epithelia, these cells are polarized, having apical and basolateral surfaces. An essential function of an intact gut epithelium is to maintain the polarity of the cell so that ions may move in predetermined directions; such movement is known as *vectoral flow*. Loss of polarity and disrupted vectoral flow is thought to be pathogenic in a variety of epithelial disorders.

Notes

Duct delivery systems and direct secretion are the basic modes of secretion in the GI tract.

SECRETORY SYSTEMS

Typically, approximately 7 L of fluid a day are secreted by the GI tract. This is accomplished through two basic modes of secretion: duct delivery systems and direct secretion.

Duct Delivery Systems

Salivary ducts (1.5 L), the pancreatic duct (1.5 L), and the bile duct (about 20% of the 0.5 L/day of bile secreted is from ducts, about 80% is from hepatocytes) each secrete fluids into the GI tract.

Direct Secretion

Fluid and electrolytes are secreted directly into the lumen of the alimentary canal from individual cells lining the alimentary tract (e.g., intestine, 1 L; HCl in stomach, 2.5 L).

Classical Secretory Units

ORAL CAVITY

Saliva is produced by the parotid, sublingual, and submandibular glands and delivered to the mouth through ducts. Cuboidal epithelial cells lining these ducts regulate and modify the amount of potassium (K^+), sodium (Na^+), bicarbonate (HCO_3^-), and chloride (Cl^-) released into saliva. Ion secretion is initiated in the acinus, stimulated through parasympathetic innervation coupled to intracellular calcium (Ca^{2+}) signaling systems, and modulated by various hormones. The regulation of electrolyte concentration is coordinated by effects on several systems, including various ion channels (K^+, Cl^-) and transporters (Na^+-K^+ pump, a Na^+-hydrogen ion [H^+] antiporter, and a Na^+-K^+-Cl^- cotransporter) (Figure 5-1). In turn, the amount of water secreted depends on the concentration of these ions, and the amount of mucus secreted depends on the gland type. The cumulative effect is the secretion of a slightly hypertonic fluid from the gland, which is subsequently modified by the salivary epithelial cells to a hypotonic solution when delivered to the mouth. Because a primary job of this duct epithelium is to reclaim electrolytes, when saliva flow is increased, there is less time for reuptake of ions. *Although K^+ concentration has a slightly inverse relationship to salivary flow rate, concentrations of Na^+, Cl^-, and HCO_3^- are increased.* Consequently, the higher the flow rate, the higher the osmolality, and the higher the alkalization of saliva.

Alkaline saliva is useful in maintaining a neutral oral pH as well as in neutralizing gastric acid refluxed into the esophagus. Saliva also enhances taste; lubricates food to aid in swallowing; contains secretory immunoglobulin A (IgA) and antimicrobial enzymes (e.g., lysozyme) that retard bacterial, viral, and fungal growth in the proximal gut; and contains digestive enzymes (e.g., amylase, lipase) to initiate digestion. Xerostomia (dry mouth) is found in a variety of disorders (e.g., Sjögren's disease, systemic amyloidosis, radiation injury following treatment of head and neck cancer) that frequently present

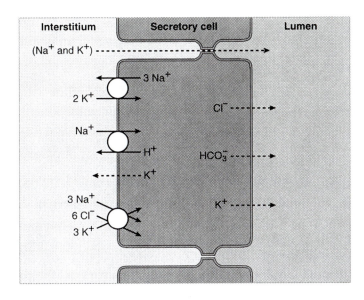

Fig. 5-1. Salivary Secretion

This figure illustrates a salivary gland acinar secretory cell and its fluid and salt transport properties. Along the basolateral surface there is an ATP-dependent Na^+-K^+ pump that provides the electrical chemical gradient for subsequent ion secretion. By taking 2 K^+ from the interstitium and secreting 3 Na^+, an electrochemical driving force is created that powers the activation of the Na^+-K^+-$2Cl^-$ cotransporter, which brings fresh ions into the cell. Carbonic acid that accumulates as a by-product of HCO_3^- formation is removed from the cell into the interstitium through a Na^+-H^+ antiporter. HCO_3^-, K^+, and Cl^- move into the lumen (depicted by arrows that slope downward) driven by their electrochemical gradients, in part through ion channels. Cations, Na^+ and K^+, are pulled into the lumen through cation selective intercellular pathways driven by the lumen's negative potential established by HCO_3^- and Cl^- secretion.

as complaints of dysphagia, altered taste, increased problems with dental caries, and heartburn. Heartburn is a frequent complaint of patients with the common medical problem of gastroesophageal reflux disease (GERD), often resulting in reflux esophagitis.

STOMACH

The stomach secretes a variety of compounds into the GI tract, with each cell type specializing in the secretion of a particular product. The secretory cells of the stomach line the oxyntic glands, forming gastric pits. Neck and surface cells secrete mucus and HCO_3^-; parietal cells secrete HCl and intrinsic factor; chief cells secrete pepsinogen; and endocrine cells secrete gastrin, histamine, and somatostatin. Although HCl is secreted into the lumen of the stomach, the mucosal cells of the stomach are buffered from this acid bath by the concomitant production of a mucus layer rich in HCO_3^-, which maintains the pH of the cellular membrane at about 7. Factors that alter the balance between the mucosal barrier and acid secretion can have important implications for ulcer formation and GI bleeding (see Chapter 11).

HCl Secretion

Beginning in the cephalic phase of digestion, vagal release of gastrin-releasing peptide initiates release of gastrin from antral G cells. Once food enters the stomach (gastric phase), there is a marked increase in gastrin release, which plays a significant role in stimulating parietal cells to secrete HCl.

Understanding the cellular basis of gastric acid secretion has been the foundation of an exciting and fruitful area of research and drug development. As with other forms of fluid secretion, the cellular elements involved are ion channels and pumps. On the apical surface of parietal cells, H^+ is secreted from a H^+-K^+-ATPase. However, the secretion and uptake of Na^+, K^+, Cl^-, and HCO_3^- from a host of channels and transporters at the apical and basolateral surfaces are required to keep the electrolytes in balance and help drive H^+ secretion into the lumen. The rate of secretion is regulated by histamine (from endocrine and mast cells), gastrin (from G cells), and acetylcholine (Ach) (from the vagus nerve), binding to their respective receptors on parietal cells (Figure 5-2). Histamine's actions dominantly increase

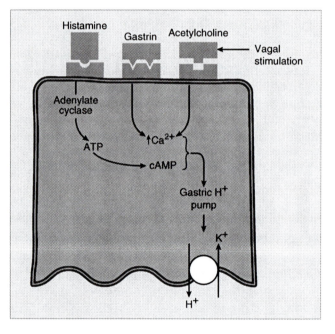

Fig. 5-2. Gastric Acid Secretion

H^+ secretion is driven by an ATP-dependent H^+-K^+ pump inserted into the apical membrane of parietal cells. Histamine, gastrin, and ACh bind to receptors expressed on the basolateral membranes of parietal cells, which results in other an increase in cAMP (histamine) or an increase in Ca^{2+} (gastrin, ACh). The increased activity of these intracellular signaling systems, in turn, increases the activity of the H^+-K^+ pump, resulting in H^+ secretion and HCl formation. *Source:* Modified from Rhoades and Tanner 1995, p. 538.

intracellular cyclic (cAMP) concentration, whereas gastrin and ACh work through effects on intracellular Ca^{2+}. Both pathways converge on the H^+-K^+-ATPases to increase their activity and increase acid output. First-generation antisecretory drugs known as H_2 blockers (i.e., cimetidine, famotidine, nizatidine, ranitidine) bind to the histamine receptor, block its interaction with its natural ligand, and result in partial inhibition of acid production. Proton pump inhibitors (e.g., omeprazole, lansoprazole) work by irreversibly binding H^+-K^+-ATPases. Rather than only blocking one pathway, proton pump inhibitors block acid production at the final cellular step and thus have proven to be extremely potent antisecretory drugs. They offer a greater magnitude of antisecretory benefits and have now become commonly used drugs in the treatment of severe esophagitis, ulcers, and hypersecretory disorders (e.g., gastrinomas).

CASE STUDY: *CONTINUED*

Omeprazole was an excellent choice to treat the patient's esophagitis and gastritis (resulting from excess acid secretion). Cromolyn was used to decrease release of histamine and other inflammatory mediators (e.g., leukotrienes) from mast cells.

Nonacid Secretion

Lining the gastric pits are chief cells, which secrete proenzyme pepsinogens. Their conversion to active pepsins is facilitated by gastric acid. Pepsins are particularly effective at proteolysis of collagens, a major protein in many foods. Mucous cells, also lining the pits, secrete mucins, which are mixed with HCO_3^-, phospholipids, and water to form a mucous barrier to acid, pepsin, bile salts, and other irritants. In part by the actions of an apical Cl^-–HCO_3^- exchanger, HCO_3^- is also secreted from mucous cells. Production of mucus is stimulated by both the vagus nerve and HCl. Other possible mediators and causes of impaired mucus production are actively under investigation and may be important in the pathogenesis of peptic ulcer and ulcers induced by the use of nonsteroidal anti-inflammatory drugs (NSAIDs). Independent of acid production, intrinsic factor is also secreted by parietal cells; it is necessary for vitamin B_{12} (cobalamin) absorption downstream in the distal ileum. Deficiencies in vitamin B_{12} may result in pernicious anemia and are a signal of possible gastric epithelial cell injury.

DUODENAL CLUSTER UNIT

The duodenal cluster is a grouping of the proximal duodenum, pancreas, and biliary tree into one system united by their integrated regulation. Although a significant percentage of pancreatic secretion is produced by cephalic stimuli, the most important phase of pancreatobiliary secretion is the intestinal phase. Secretion is initiated at the level of the duodenum where luminal pH, osmolality, and nutrient mix are sensed by specialized endocrine cells. In response to decreased pH, increased protein, or increased osmolality, these cells secrete secretin and cholecystokinin (CCK) and also stimulate vagal impulses. In turn, this stimulates pancreatic and biliary secretion into the duodenum.

Exocrine Secretions of the Pancreas

As in saliva, water enters into pancreatic juice through passive movement in response to altered ion concentrations in the lumen of the pancreatic duct. Regulation of luminal ion concentration dictates the amount of fluid secreted. Again, as with saliva, the dominant physiologic ions are Na^+, K^+, Cl^-, and HCO_3^-. Unlike saliva, increased flow of pancreatic juice increases only Na^+ and HCO_3^- concentrations, while the concentration of Cl^- falls, and K^+ is unaffected. A recent discovery has been the recognition that a cAMP-dependent Cl^- channel gene, cystic fibrosis transmembrane conductance regulator (CFTR), is expressed and its protein product delivered to the apical surface of pancreatic (and biliary) epithelial cells, through which Cl^- enters the lumen. Once there, it activates Cl^-–HCO_3^- exchangers to increase reuptake of Cl^- and allow efflux of HCO_3^-, resulting in the alkalization of pancreatic (and biliary) secretions. Defects in this gene result in malfunctioning or absent CFTR channels and ultimately the devastating pancreatic (and biliary) complications ensue as seen in patients with cystic fibrosis.

Secretin, released by duodenal cells into the blood in response to decreased intraluminal pH, predominantly controls alkaline delivery. Circulating secretin then binds to receptors on pancreatic (and biliary) duct cells, causing an increase in cAMP and subsequent activation of CFTR (Figure 5-3). In contrast to the elaborate control of anion secretion, Na^+ and K^+ enter the lumen through unregulated paracellular movement.

In response to duodenal release of CCK and the release of a variety of vagal neurotransmitters (e.g., vasoactive intestinal polypeptide [VIP], ACh, gastrin-releasing peptide), a number of enzymes (mostly proteases) are secreted into the pancreatic fluid. These enzymes are variably effective at digesting starches, fats, and proteins (see Chapter 6). Without effective pancreatic transport, about 50% of nutrient digestion would be lost. Pancreatic fluid release is also important for regulating intraduodenal pH, which must be nearly neutral for the enzymes to be effective.

Biliary Duct Cell Secretion

Biliary duct cell secretion has many similarities to that of pancreatic duct cells. Important exceptions may be that biliary duct cells have greater control over Na^+ and water transcellular transport and that there is significant hepatobiliary signaling (see Figure 5-3).

Inhibition of Secretion

Inhibitory pathways are also important for regulating secretion. *Glucagon* inhibits the volume and enzymatic content of pancreatic

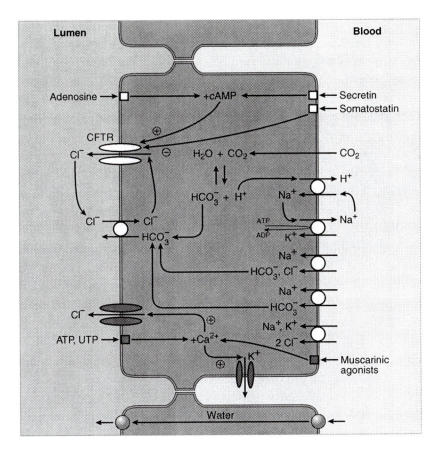

Fig. 5-3. Ion Transport in Biliary Epithelial Cells

The dominant secretory pathways are the Cl^- channels and the $Cl^- - HCO_3^-$ exchangers located on the apical surface. Additional transporters located on the basolateral surface provide electrical and chemical balance to the cell and allow for accumulation of ions for secretion. In addition to other transporters and channels described in GI epithelial cells, biliary cells also have a channel, aquaporin, through which water is secreted transcellularly. Nonselective cation channels and K^+ channels have unknown cellular locations and are shown between cells. Binding of select autocrine, paracrine, and endocrine factors to their receptors are also shown along with the second messenger systems being activated by these factors.

juice and raises its pH. *Somatostatin* has similar effects, and its analog, octreotide, is used clinically to reduce pancreatic flow in settings of pancreatic fistulas or duct disruption. *Pancreatic polypeptide (PP)* is another intrinsic pancreatic hormone, and it causes feedback inhibition of pancreatic (and biliary) secretion. There is an emerging body of knowledge regarding intraluminal (intestinal lumen) feedback of pancreatic secretion. This model, based mostly on rat studies, is currently being incorporated into the treatment plan of chronic pancreatitis.

INTESTINE

With respect to volume, intestinal secretion of fluid and electrolytes appears to play a minor role in physiologic GI secretion. However, the capacity of the intestine to secrete fluid is important in a variety of

pathologic processes, typically resulting in diarrhea. Thus, most data are on pathologic intestinal fluid secretion from which an understanding of normal physiology has been deduced. The average adult (male) intestinal tract measures 660 cm (500 cm of small intestine, 160 cm of colon), and with the microvilli, the surface area contained within that length is amplified many times. In this way, the surface area over which electrolytes may be transported is augmented from 3300 cm^2 to 2 million cm^2. Consequently, aberrant intestinal secretion can rapidly result in life-threatening loss of fluid and electrolytes.

The Cl$^-$ channel is the essential unit regulating secretion in the intestine. The cooperative activities of Na$^+$-K$^+$-2Cl$^-$ cotransporters and Na$^+$-K$^+$-ATPases result in enhanced intracellular Cl$^-$ concentrations. The regulated opening of a variety of Cl$^-$ channels results in rapid movement of Cl$^-$ from the cell interior into the lumen. This movement creates a driving force for the paracellular movement of water (osmosis). By regulating Cl$^-$ movement, the volume and rate of intestinal secretion are controlled. The best-studied Cl$^-$ channel involved with intestinal fluid secretion is the CFTR channel. Defects in this protein have been found to be the cause of cystic fibrosis, which often results in impaired fluid secretion of the intestine as well as of the pancreatic and biliary ducts. Although Cl$^-$ is the predominant ion secreted by the intestine, K$^+$ and HCO$_3^-$ are also secreted and can be clinically important in diarrhea-induced metabolic acidosis and hypokalemia.

A variety of substances, both intrinsic and extrinsic to the gut, can stimulate intestinal secretions of fluid. Among the endogenous compounds are histamine, prostaglandins, and atrial natriuretic factor. Among the exogenous compounds are bile salts, laxatives, and bacterial toxins (*Vibrio cholerae*). In general, these factors bind to selective receptors expressed on epithelial cells that initiate subsequent signaling cascades, which ultimately regulate an ion channel or other transporter. Often more than one messenger system is involved, and there is frequently overlap between stimulatory and inhibitory pathways. Some of the more common messenger systems are cAMP, intracellular Ca^{2+} (e.g., Ca^{2+}-calmodulin-dependent kinase II, protein kinase C), lipid mediators (inositol phosphates), and cyclic guanosine monophosphate (cGMP). Variable numbers of receptors expressed on the membrane, variability in the concentration of the ligand interacting with the receptor, or the presence and concentration of other competing ligands or inhibitors make possible an innumerable array of responses that may alter the balance of fluid and electrolyte secretion.

V. cholerae *and* Escherichia coli

Cholera is the quintessential disorder of intestinal fluid secretion. Although rarely seen in contemporary industrialized countries, cholera remains an important health problem in developing areas and serves as a model for elucidating the mechanism of a disease that plagues tourists, that is, travelers' diarrhea. Rather than destroying (ulcerating) the mucosa, these disorders are classified as enterotoxigenic diarrheas; the pathogens involved secrete toxins that bind selectively to enterocytes to stimulate Cl⁻ secretion. Both *V. cholerae* and *E. coli* (enterotoxigenic) toxins activate cAMP-dependent Cl⁻ channels, which can drive intestinal secretions up to many liters a day and, with cholera, result in death (85%) if untreated.

Microenvironmental Regulation of Secretion

As already mentioned, a large number of neural, endocrine, and paracrine factors have been recognized as altering GI secretion. Work over the past several years has elucidated novel paracrine factors that may enter the microenvironment of the epithelial cell and transiently (rather than constitutively) alter its secretion. The identification of these substances may offer insights into the pathogenesis of diseases not previously understood.

Although myriad initiating mechanisms and diverse sources of autacoids exist (e.g., vascular endothelial cells; neurons; intestinal epithelial cells; mast cells, which play a pivotal role; lymphocytes; and granulocytes, such as neutrophils, eosinophils, and basophils), in general, a primary event "activates" one or more of these cell types. This activation changes the behavior of cells and results in the release of other signaling molecules. An integrated model representing this cascade is presented in Figure 5-4. For simplicity, two select mediators are discussed separately. In vivo, however, they are interdependent. The paracrine factors discussed are nitric oxide and 5'-AMP.

Nitric Oxide (NO)

NO is a lipophilic compound synthesized by NO synthase (NOS) from L-arginine. There are both constitutive and inducible forms of

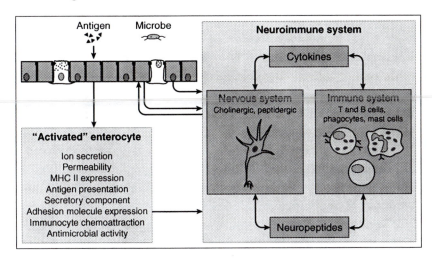

Fig. 5-4. Immunophysiology of the Intestine

This figure is an illustration of the neuroimmunologic effects on GI epithelial cells. A prerequisite step in neuroimmunologically mediated intestinal injury is the activation of the enterocytes. MHC II = major histocompatibility complex II. *Source:* Modified after Perdue and McKay 1994, p. G160.

NOS that appear to be important in GI function. In general, the constitutive form (cNOS) is important for physiologic functions, whereas the inducible form (iNOS) appears to be important in inflammation.

In general, a decrease in NO formation leads to the activation of mast cells. These activated mast cells then release a variety of autacoids, including histamine (increasing HCl production in the stomach), numerous cytokines, and platelet-activating factor (PAF). PAF, in turn, may stimulate "filtration secretion." In essence, filtration secretion occurs through increased paracellular permeability of fluid and is independent of Cl⁻ secretion. PAF also stimulates prostaglandins and enteric neurons to activate ion channel secretions of anions. The sum effect of this secretion is diarrhea. It is possible that NO may itself stimulate Cl⁻ channels, thereby increasing secretion. NO activates CFTR in lymphocytes; the direct effect of NO on GI epithelial cell secretion has not been clarified.

5'-AMP

PAF and interleukin-5 also serve as eosinophil recruiting factors and promote migration of eosinophils into the intestinal epithelium. Neutrophils are also recruited into the epithelium. Both cell types secrete 5'-AMP, which is converted to adenosine by an intestinal ecto-5'-nucleotidase. In turn, adenosine binds to its receptors on intestinal cells, resulting in increased cAMP. Subsequently, this rise in cAMP results in activation of cAMP-dependent Cl⁻ channels, thereby promoting secretion of Cl⁻ and fluid. Arachidonic acid and cytokines released by eosinophils may themselves amplify this secretion by also activating cAMP-dependent Cl⁻ channels.

CASE STUDY: *RESOLUTION*

Eosinophilic gastroenteritis is a disorder of unknown etiology with varied clinical manifestations, depending on the site and layer of the stomach or intestine involved. The most commonly involved organs are the stomach and small intestine. The layer of involvement can typically be deduced by the patient's symptoms: (1) mucosa: diarrhea, vomiting, cramping, and occult blood; (2) muscularis: symptoms of intestinal obstruction (e.g., abdominal pain, distention, nausea, vomiting); and (3) serosa: eosinophilic ascites or pleural effusions.

Thus the case presented at the beginning of the chapter appears to involve the mucosal layer. Although the exact mechanisms by which eosinophilic gastroenteritis causes symptoms are not clear and an optimum treatment strategy is unknown, increased understanding of epithelial physiology and ion transport makes it possible to intervene rationally. In the case described, glucocorticoids were used to destroy eosinophils, cromolyn was used to stabilize mast cells (decreased release of mast cell molecules prevents continued migration of eosinophils), and omeprazole was used to decrease proton secretion (i.e., acid) of the stomach. With these agents, the patient's symptoms abated, his diarrhea resolved, and he had no further episodes of dehydration. As the factors regulating the balance between GI epithelial cells and their environment become better understood, it may be possible to control or cure the illnesses that afflict them.

REVIEW QUESTIONS

Directions: For each of the following questions, choose the one best answer.

1 Which statement best characterizes the secretion of acid from stomach cells?

A Gastrin and histamine mediate a rise in intracellular cAMP, which results in activation of a Na^+-H^+ pump to secrete acid.

B ACh (from the vagus nerve) and histamine mediate a rise in intracellular Ca^{2+} to open Cl^- channels to secrete HCl.

C Histamine works primarily to increase cAMP, which stimulates a H^+-K^+-ATPase to secrete acid.

D Somatostatin increases acid output.

E In normal conditions, stomach acid secretion results in a pH of less than or equal to 2 at the apical surface of the stomach epithelium.

2 Which of the following statements regarding the effect of secretion on GI secretion is *true*?

A Secretin inhibits pancreatic fluid secretion.

B Secretin promotes bile flow by increasing the formation of bile acids.

C Secretin promotes pancreatic duct cell secretion by stimulating an increase in intracellular Ca^{2+}, which results in the opening of Na^+ channels and an increase in Na^+ and water secretion.

D Secretin opens HCO_3^- channels in pancreatic and biliary duct cells and releases HCO_3^- and water into the digestive tract.

E Secretin modulates Cl^- channels and Cl^-–HCO_3^- exchangers to increase secretion and alkaline concentration of bile and pancreatic fluid.

3 Which of the following statements concerning GI cellular transport proteins is *true*?

A Symporters and antiporters require ATP to move electrolytes up their electrochemical gradient.

B Cotransporters and exchange carriers are proteins that facilitate transfer of ions without the need for ATP.

C Pumps passively move ions from greater to lesser concentrations.

D Ion channels require energy to transport large numbers of ions against their electrochemical gradients.

4 With increased saliva flow rates, what ionic combination is most likely to result?

A There is an increased concentration of Cl^- and HCO_3^- but a decreased concentration of K^+.

B There is an increased concentration of K^+ and HCO_3^- but a decreased concentration of Cl^-.

C There is an increased concentration of Na^+ and Cl^- but a decreased concentration of K^+ and HCO_3^-.

D There is an increased concentration of K^+ and Na^+ but a decreased concentration of Cl^- and Mg^{2+}.

5 CFTR protein is best described as a

A protein that is heavily secreted in sweat and saliva but is reduced in these areas of patients with cystic fibrosis.

B mammalian lipid in which Cl^-–HCO_3^- exchangers are inserted and which is responsible for secretion of Cl^- and HCO_3^- in the pancreas, airway, and intestines but is not present in liver or biliary tissues.

C unique pancreatic duct cell secretory protein essential for protein digestion.

D cAMP-dependent anion pump.

E cAMP-dependent anion channel.

6 Which of the following statements regarding the effects of NO is *true*?

A Decreased NO release results in activation of mast cells.

B Increased NO release causes an increase in filtration secretion; therefore, a decrease in NO release works to decrease diarrhea.

C Increased NO release results in increased release of PAF, which activates ion channels to secrete more fluid.

D Only circulating mast cells require activation before they release their factors; mucosal mast cells can release their contents in the absence of activation.

7 Which of the following statements concerning 5′-AMP and its effects on GI epithelium is *true*?

A 5′-AMP is the neutrophil-derived secretagogue and is only released by neutrophils and basophils.

B 5'-AMP is converted to adenosine, which binds to adenosine receptors present on GI epithelial cells, and activates Ca^{2+}-dependent Cl^- secretion.

C 5'-AMP is converted to cAMP-dependent Cl^- channel secretion.

D 5'-AMP is broken down by ecto-5'-nucleotidase, and its metabolite activates cAMP-dependent Cl^- channel secretion.

References

Alican I, Kubes P: A critical role for nitric oxide in intestinal barrier function and dysfunction. *Am J Physiol Gastrointest Liver Physiol* 270:G225–G237, 1996.

Johnson LR: *Gastrointestinal Physiology.* St. Louis, MO: Elsevier Science, Mosby, 2001.

Kwiatkowski AP, McGill JM: Electrolyte transport in biliary epithelium. *J Lab Clin Med* 130:8–13, 1997.

Montrose MH, Keely SJ, Barrett KE: Electrolyte secretion and absorption: small intestine and colon. In *Textbook of Gastroenterology*, 4th ed. Edited by Yamada T. Philadelphia, PA: Lippincott Williams & Wilkins, 2003.

Perdue MH, McKay DM: Integrative immunophysiology in the intestinal mucosa. *Am J Physiol Gastrointest Liver Physiol* 267:G151–G165, 1994.

Resnick MB, Colgan SP, Patapoff TW, et al: Activated eosinophils evoke chloride secretion in model intestinal epithelia primarily via regulated release of 5'-AMP. *J Immunol* 151:5716–5723, 1993.

Rhoades RA, Tanner GA (eds): *Medical Physiology.* Boston, MA: Little, Brown, 1995.

Sartor RB: Cytokines in intestinal inflammation: pathophysiological and clinical considerations. *Gastroenterology* 106:533–539, 1994.

Yamada T, Alpers DH, Owyang C, et al (eds): *Textbook of Gastroenterology*, 2nd ed. Philadelphia, PA: J. B. Lippincott, 1995.

6

Digestion and Absorption

■ CHAPTER OUTLINE ■

■ LEARNING OBJECTIVES ■

At the completion of this chapter, the reader should be able to:
- Evaluate the role of each of the organs of the digestive system in digestion and absorption.
- Identify the signs and symptoms of maldigestion.
- Develop a differential diagnosis of major diseases causing altered digestion and absorption.
- Predict the region of the GI tract affected by a disease based on the deficiencies of specific vitamins and nutrients.

CASE STUDY: *INTRODUCTION*

A 26-year-old woman was seen in the clinic complaining of diarrhea, fatigue, and a 22-lb (10-kg) unintentional weight loss. Her medical history was unremarkable, but she did remember having similar problems with diarrhea during childhood and adolescence, though it was never this severe. She noted that for the past 6–8 months she has experienced multiple large, bulky, foul-smelling daily stools but never watery diarrhea or blood. She denied pain other than some abdominal cramping. This cramping was associated with abdominal distention, borborygmi, and increased flatus. Despite her weight loss, she had a good appetite and was actually eating more than ever. This fact was confirmed by her husband. She denied vomiting, fever, or chills and had not traveled outside her hometown. She also noted that she had missed her period for the past 4 months but that she had excluded pregnancy with a home pregnancy test.

On the basis of this history, the patient's medical problem was suspected to be one of maldigestion or malabsorption. A careful physical examination was performed, which helped guide the physician to the correct diagnosis.

Introduction

One of the fundamental problems faced by every living thing is how to assimilate environmental nutrients for the growth and maintenance of its own body. This problem can be illustrated by a person's consumption of a hamburger (Figure 6-1). The biochemical components of a hamburger are exactly the nutrients needed for growth and body maintenance. However, there are two major hurdles in using

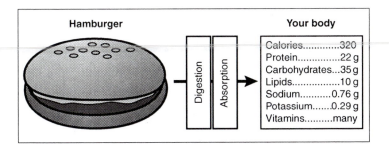

Fig. 6-1. Assimilation of a Hamburger into the Human Body

The digestive tract of a healthy human is capable of digesting almost all of the complex biochemicals in the meats, grains, vegetables, and dairy products that make up the basic elements of a hamburger. Once digested, each element is absorbed by one or another mechanism for utilization by the body while leaving the useless waste behind.

Notes

At each level of the GI tract, various coordinating mechanisms optimize digestion and absorption.

hamburgers to build healthy bodies. The first is that the burger must be broken down into its components. The mechanism used by living animals to meet this challenge is called *digestion*. The second issue is that the nutrients must be moved from the environment to the organism. The mechanism used by living animals to overcome this problem is called *absorption*. The primary purpose of the digestive system and GI tract is to facilitate digestion and absorption. Digestion and absorption are accomplished by means of a number of specific mechanisms at specific locations throughout the GI tract.

Through the work of many physicians and scientists over many years, we now know both the site and mechanism of each component of the digestive and absorptive processes for every important nutrient. Using this information, we can learn about the location and extent of many GI diseases resulting from the disruption of specific digestive or absorptive mechanisms. This chapter is designed to explain some of the most important mechanisms used by the human body to break down proteins, carbohydrates, and fats into their components and move these components from the intestinal lumen into the bloodstream.

Organization

The digestive system is designed to break down complex nutrients sequentially into smaller and smaller components (digestion) until they are reduced to a molecular size that can be transported from the intestinal lumen to the body (absorption). However, a meal cannot be digested and absorbed at the rate of consumption. Therefore, a number of coordinating mechanisms are employed by the body to optimize the digestion and absorption processes at each level of the GI system and to propel the meal through the stomach and intestines at rates consistent with the meal size, consistency, and nutritional content. This process begins in the mouth and ends in the colon (Table 6-1).

Table 6-1. Overview of the GI System

ORGAN	DIGESTION	ABSORPTION
Mouth	**Mechanical** Biochemical	None
Stomach	**Mechanical** Biochemical	Minimal
Duodenum	**Coordination** Mechanical Biochemical	Important
Liver	**Biochemical**	None
Pancreas	**Biochemical**	None
Jejunum and ileum	**Mechanical** **Biochemical**	**Very important**
Colon	Minimal	Important

Note. Bold indicates primary functions.

MOUTH

The process of breaking down food into absorbable molecules begins in the mouth. The function of the mouth is primarily mechanical (teeth and saliva) and secondarily biochemical (specific components of saliva).

Teeth

The teeth play an important role in crushing, shredding, and grinding large, complex nutrients into small pieces. The importance of the mechanical function of teeth is illustrated by patients with poor dentition. Indeed, many of the signs and symptoms of maldigestion in these patients resolve with correction of this problem.

Saliva

While in the mouth, food is mixed with saliva. Saliva, which is secreted through the ducts of the parotid, submandibular, and sublingual glands, consists of a hypotonic electrolyte solution, mucins, salivary amylases, and some antimicrobial and other proteins. The sublingual glands also produce lingual lipase (see Lipids). The volume, toxicity, and electrolyte composition of saliva is under autonomic nervous system control. Salivary flow increases with the sight and smell of food and with chewing. Like pancreatic juice, saliva is high in sodium bicarbonate ($NaHCO_3$), which helps maintain a neutral oral pH, thereby protecting the dental enamel from acid-producing bacteria. The mucus in saliva acts as a mechanical lubricant as the food bolus begins its descent through the esophagus and into the stomach.

In addition to lubricating the food bolus, saliva serves an important biochemical digestive purpose through salivary amylase. Salivary amylase initiates the digestion of complex carbohydrates by attacking the carbohydrate branch points (see later discussion). This greatly reduces the size of starch molecules, thereby reducing the viscosity of the food bolus. Digestion of carbohydrates by salivary amylase and lipids by lingual lipase continues in the stomach until the pH is reduced below 4 by gastric acid. The final digestion stages of the carbohydrates and lipids are completed in the small intestine by the action of pancreatic amylase and lipase.

CASE STUDY: CONTINUED

Physical examination revealed a thin, white woman sitting comfortably on the examination table. Her temperature and blood pressure were normal, and she had a pulse of 60 beats/minute. Examination of her head and neck revealed normal eyes, good dentition, and moist mucous membranes.

This stage of the physical examination is important because some autoimmune diseases (e.g., Sjögren's syndrome) affect the salivary glands, resulting in diminished salivary secretion. In addition, common prescription drugs, such as antidepressants and antihypertensives, may inhibit salivation. Diminished salivary secretion results in a dry mouth with dental caries, difficulty in chewing and swallowing, and altered taste. This may lead to diminished food intake and weight loss.

This patient's history, including prescription drug use, and the determination by physical examination of moist mucous membranes and normal teeth made a problem with the oral cavity unlikely.

A dry mouth usually results in weight loss from diminished food intake, whereas poor dentition interferes with the initial stages of digestion.

STOMACH

After the chewed food is transferred through the esophagus, which has no digestive or absorptive function, it enters the stomach. In the stomach, the food is mechanically stored and liquefied while the biochemical digestion of proteins is initiated. The stomach has limited absorptive capacity (see Table 6-1).

Functionally, the stomach may be divided into two components: (1) the proximal stomach, which includes the fundus and the corpus, or body; and (2) the distal stomach, which includes the antrum and the pylorus.

Proximal Stomach

Mechanically, the proximal stomach serves as a reservoir and enlarges with food intake through a process controlled by the vagus nerve called receptive relaxation. The tonic contraction of the fundus in the postprandial period plays an important role in enhancing gastric emptying, especially of liquids. The rate of gastric emptying is controlled by many factors through enteric and autonomic nervous system reflexes and hormones originating in the duodenum, small intestines, colon, and pancreas.

Biochemically, the proximal stomach makes several major contributions to digestion and absorption. Gastric juice is secreted by ductless oxyntic glands in the gastric mucosal layer of the proximal stomach. Gastric juice primarily contains (1) pepsinogen, secreted by the chief cells in the base of the oxyntic glands; (2) hydrochloric acid, produced by the parietal cells in the oxyntic gland neck; (3) mucus, secreted by mucous cells in the oxyntic gland neck and surface mucous cells; and (4) intrinsic factor, which is secreted by the parietal cells and is essential for the protection and later absorption of cobalamin (vitamin B_{12}).

Pepsinogen. Pepsinogen is a proenzyme that autoactivates into pepsin in an acid environment. Pepsin hydrolyzes proteins at aspartic amino acids and therefore plays an important role in early digestion of collagen in meats. These hydrolyzed proteins play an important role in stimulating the release of gastrin from the gastric antrum and cholecystokinin (CCK) from the duodenum. Pepsin activity terminates when the gastric contents mix with alkaline pancreatic juice in the small bowel.

Hydrochloric Acid (HCl).   HCl appears to play several roles in the stomach, including acting with pepsin to denature and digest proteins and to kill bacteria.

Mucus.   The mucus protects the inner lining of the stomach from the digestive juices.

Distal Stomach.   The gastric antrum and pylorus serve as a coordinated unit to triturate the gastric contents into liquefied chyme. Peristaltic waves begin at the gastric pacemaker along the greater curvature of the stomach and increase in strength as they sweep through the antrum toward the pylorus. The food and chyme are thereby trapped in a high-pressure area at the distal end of the stomach. Most of the contents are squirted back into the stomach, and a small amount of chyme containing particles smaller than 1 mm in diameter passes through the pylorus and into the duodenum. In this way food is mechanically liquefied and mixed with biochemically important gastric juice.

Notes

The stomach liquefies food, stores it, and slowly releases it into the small intestine at rates that allow the small intestine to accommodate volume and osmolarity.

CASE STUDY: *CONTINUED*

The physical examination was continued. The patient's abdomen was slightly distended but nontender. Specifically, there were no scars over her upper abdomen, and no succussion splash was heard with a stethoscope; the upper abdomen was nontender.

Surprisingly, many people have lived a relatively normal life without their stomach, as long as they receive vitamin B_{12} injections. However, malabsorption syndromes are occasionally related to the stomach (Table 6-2). Peptic ulcer disease, which may cause pain with eating may result in edema, spasms, or stenosis of the pylorus and subsequent gastric outlet obstruction. Gastric outlet obstruction or gastric emptying delay is suggested on physical examination by moving the patient from side to side and listening over the stomach for a succussion splash several hours after the last meal. However, the symptoms of gastric outlet obstruction are nausea and vomiting with limited food intake rather than maldigestion, as suggested by this patient's history.

Prior to the introduction of histamine- (H_2-)receptor antagonists in the late 1970s (e.g., cimetidine, ranitidine), many individuals with refractory peptic ulcer disease underwent partial gastric resections. These surgeries eliminated the pylorus and often resulted in rapid "dumping" of a hyperosmolar meal into the intestine, causing intestinal distention, osmotic fluid shifts, release

The duodenum is a sensory organ stimulating bile and pancreatic secretion through hormones and changing motility patterns of the stomach and GI tract through neural reflexes.

Table 6-2. Site-Specific Causes for Maldigestion and Malabsorption

STOMACH

Postgastrectomy
Zollinger-Ellison syndrome
Achlorhydria

LIVER: CHRONIC BILE SALT DEFICIENCY

Primary biliary cirrhosis and
    primary sclerosing cholangitis
Depleted bile salt pool as a result
    of ileal disease or resection
Unconjugated bile salts as a result
    of bacterial overgrowth

PANCREAS: PANCREATIC EXOCRINE INSUFFICIENCY

Chronic pancreatitis
Cystic fibrosis
Neoplasm

SMALL INTESTINE

Celiac disease
Crohn's disease
Whipple's disease
Lactase deficiency
Eosinophilic gastroenteritis
Tropical sprue
Short bowel syndrome
Bacterial overgrowth
AIDS
Lymphangiectasia
Diabetes mellitus
Motility disorders
Infectious causes
Lymphoma

Source: Modified from Uhl M, Cooke AR: Malabsorption syndromes. In *Consultations in Gastroenterology.* Philadelphia, PA: W. B. Saunders, 1996, p. 77.

of counterregulatory and vasoactive hormones, and rapid absorption of carbohydrates, with hyperglycemia followed by hypoglycemia. These symptoms could be avoided by small meals with restricted liquids.

Finally, gastric acid hypersecretion, as seen in Zollinger-Ellison syndrome (a gastrin-secreting tumor), can cause maldigestion and diarrhea by changing the pH of the small intestine and destroying pancreatic enzymes. This rare tumor can be identified by measuring elevated gastrin levels in the serum after administration of intravenous secretin or by measuring basal gastric acid output.

This patient had no history or signs of peptic ulcer disease and no surgical scars; thus, a disease of the stomach was an unlikely cause of her symptoms.

DUODENUM

The duodenum is the initial portion of the small intestine, and much of the discussion of the small intestine that follows applies to the duodenum. However, the duodenum is considered separately here because it is central in coordinating digestion and absorption.

The duodenum is an ideally located sensory organ because it receives the partially digested gastric contents, and it is where bile and pancreatic juices enter the digestive tract. From this important location, the duodenum influences the magnitude and rate of gastric emptying, the volume of pancreatic and biliary secretions, and the pattern of small intestine motility. The control signals include activation of sensory nerves in the duodenum and release of peptide hormones from the duodenum.

The sensory nerves in the duodenum are sensitive to stretch, acid, various lipids, glucose, amino acids, pH, and other luminal factors. It has recently been discovered that sensory nerves are also stimulated by duodenal hormones (e.g., CCK, secretin). Vagal afferent fibers relay information to the brainstem on the type of nutrients, the volume, and the osmolarity of the chyme in the duodenum. Sensory fibers also relay information to enteric ganglia and other nerves. Sensory nerve relays are involved in the regulation of gastric motility, small intestine motility, pancreatic secretion, and hormone release.

The duodenum is also rich in regulatory peptides, including the GI gut hormones. Duodenal peptide hormones are primarily stimulatory in nature, causing secretion of digestive enzymes from the pancreas and increasing bile flow from the liver and gallbladder. They also increase digestion by delaying gastric emptying, thus lengthening the time available for digestion. The most important regulatory peptides in the duodenum are secretin and CCK. Conversely, peptide hormones from the hindgut are usually inhibitory, slowing down the transit of nutrients.

PANCREAS

The pancreas is a large retroperitoneal gland with a main duct and, occasionally, an accessory one that empty pancreatic juices into the duodenum. The pancreatic juice contains a bicarbonate (HCO_3^-)-rich fluid derived from ductal cells and digestive enzymes derived from acinar cells. The pancreas also contains endocrine cells that control the utilization of nutrients after absorption. Only the exocrine function of the pancreas is considered here because it plays a central role in the biochemical digestion of chyme and because exocrine pancreatic failure can lead to severe maldigestion.

The acinar cells, located at the terminal end of the pancreatic ducts, secrete a large number of digestive proenzymes, including proteases (trypsinogen I, II, and III; chymotrypsinogen A and B; several proelastases and procarboxypeptidases), prophospholipases, ribonucleases, and deoxyribonucleases. In addition, the pancreas secretes amylase and lipase in the active form. When pancreatic secretion is stimulated by a meal, the proenzymes amylase and lipase are secreted into the duodenum. When trypsinogen encounters the intestinal brush-border enzyme enterokinase, an N-terminal octapeptide is cleaved, transforming trypsinogen into active trypsin. Trypsin initiates a proenzyme activation cascade, resulting in immediate availability of all pancreatic digestive enzymes within the duodenum. In general, pancreatic enzymes digest large, complex molecules into less complex molecules, whereas small-intestinal enzymes break the simpler molecules into their primary elements for absorption.

The duct cells secrete a HCO_3^--rich fluid that serves to buffer the acidic fluid entering the small intestine from the stomach. The

When pancreatic enzymes enter the duodenum, the duodenal enzyme enterokinase activates trypsin, which in turn initiates a proenzyme activation cascade, resulting in immediate availability of all digestive enzymes within the small intestine.

Interruption of the enterohepatic circulation of bile salts at any point may result in fat maldigestion.

buffering action is important for the protection of the small intestine mucosa and to optimize pancreatic and small intestine enzyme activity. The duodenum also has the capacity to secrete HCO_3^-, thereby complementing the role of pancreatic HCO_3^- secretion.

CASE STUDY: *CONTINUED*

The patient's bowel sounds were active, with frequent borborygmi but no high-pitched sounds suggestive of a bowel obstruction. The rectal examination was normal, with normally brown stools that had no evidence of blood on guaiac testing.

Pancreatic insufficiency may result in all of the signs and symptoms noted in this case. Although the patient had no history of alcohol use, cystic fibrosis, or chronic abdominal pain, the possibility of pancreatic insufficiency required additional testing.

LIVER

The liver plays an important role in the digestion and absorption of intestinal lipids through the biliary tree. Bile is a complex fluid, in part because it serves as a vehicle for the secretion of bile acids (or bile salts) that are essential for lipid digestion and excretion of xenobiotics and endogenous toxins. Bile acids are synthesized from cholesterol in the liver. The bile acid pool, however, consists of primary bile acids and secondary bile acids produced by the action of intestinal bacteria on the primary bile salt.

The amount of bile salts needed each day for proper digestion of lipids far exceeds the amount synthesized. Therefore, up to 95% of the bile acids that are secreted during a meal are reabsorbed in the terminal ileum, transported through the portal vein to the liver, and resecreted into the biliary system, where they are either resecreted or stored in the gallbladder. Interruption of the "enterohepatic circulation" of bile acids by disease of the liver, biliary tree, or loss of the terminal ileum may result in the loss of bile salts during a meal, causing maldigestion of fats, resulting in steatorrhea.

CASE STUDY: *CONTINUED*

On examination the patient had no signs of liver disease (e.g., jaundice), impaired secretion of bile salts (e.g., light-colored stools, suggesting an inability to secrete bilirubin metabolites through the biliary system), or reabsorption (e.g., resection of the terminal ileum).

The bile salts play an important role in the digestion of lipids, especially complex long-chain fatty acids. However, the clinical features of liver disease are evident before significant maldigestion of lipids becomes clinically recognized.

SMALL INTESTINE

The small intestine is both the anatomic and physiologic center of the alimentary tract and is essential to life. The small intestine—including the duodenum, jejunum, and ileum—plays an important role in digestion through enzymes located on the enterocyte brush borders. In general, small intestine digestion reduces small, partially digested nutrients into absorbable elements. Thus the small intestine, in concert with the mouth, stomach, pancreas, and hepatobiliary system, participates in the mechanical and biochemical digestion of nutrients to prepare them for eventual absorption. The critical role of absorption occurs almost exclusively in the small intestine.

Small-Intestinal Digestion

Further nutrient breakdown of chyme occurs in the small intestine through the action of several enzymes. *Enterokinase* activates trypsinogen, which activates other digestive enzymes secreted by the pancreas. *Disaccharidases*, such as maltase, which catalyzes the hydrolysis of maltose into glucose; sucrase, which hydrolyzes sucrose into one glucose and one fructose; lactase, which hydrolyzes lactose into one glucose and one galactose; trehalase; and isomaltase complete the digestive breakdown of the carbohydrates. *Peptidases*, such as amino-oligopeptidase and dipeptidase, further break down proteins. The small intestine's mixing of chyme promotes lipid emulsification but adds little to lipid digestion. After digestion at the brush border, the nutrients are ready to be absorbed into the body through the intestinal mucosa.

Small-Intestinal Absorption

Absorption is dependent on active and passive transport systems and requires a large surface area. This is accomplished by exposing the digested nutrients to a small-intestinal luminal surface area of 2 million cm^2. This massive absorptive area is compressed into a tube measuring 6 meters and containing countless villi and microvilli that project into the lumen. Nutrients enter the small intestine through the duodenum and are thoroughly mixed and slowly propelled through its length by the coordinated action of the smooth muscle layers that make up a major portion of the intestinal wall. These contractions are orchestrated by the enteric nervous system, which is influenced in turn by neural input from the autonomic nervous system and by the milieu of circulating regulatory hormones.

The nature of the small intestine changes between the duodenum and terminal ileum. Iron, fat-soluble vitamins, zinc, and—to a large degree—calcium (Ca^{2+}) are absorbed predominantly in the duodenum and jejunum. Folate is absorbed *only* in the jejunum, and vitamin B_{12} and bile acids are absorbed *only* in the terminal ileum. Thus deficiencies of specific vitamins or minerals can give clues to the location of small intestine pathologic conditions.

The upper small intestine absorbs fat-soluble vitamins, folate, iron, zinc, and Ca^{2+}. **The lower small intestine** absorbs bile salts and vitamin B_{12}.

CASE STUDY: *CONTINUED*

Active bowel sounds with borborygmi but without high-pitched bowel sounds were noted. The patient's skin was dry, and she had symmetric vesicular eruptions on her neck, elbows, wrists, and knees that appeared to have been scratched.

A number of diseases that affect the small intestine are associated with maldigestion and malabsorption syndromes (see Table 6-2). Maldigestion usually reflects a loss of function of specific enzymes, as illustrated by lactase deficiency. Malabsorption syndromes arise from site-specific damage to the small-intestinal mucosa. Celiac disease (gluten-sensitive enteropathy) results from an upper small intestine reaction to the gluten in wheat, rye, barley, and oats. Biopsies of the duodenum or jejunum may be striking because of the loss of villi. Loss of villi results in a markedly diminished surface area and malabsorption. Involvement of the duodenum and jejunum results in the malabsorption of iron, folic acid, Ca^{2+}, and vitamins D and E. Celiac disease is sometimes associated with a skin disorder, dermatitis herpetiformis, as described on the patient's physical examination. The diagnosis is usually made by small-bowel biopsy and supported with serologic tests (e.g., antigliadin or antiendomysial antibodies); clinical improvement comes with a gluten-free diet. Small intestine biopsies in tropical sprue are similar to celiac disease, but tropical sprue occurs primarily in endemic areas and responds to antibiotics rather than diet. Other diseases that cause chronic inflammation in the small intestine, including Whipple's disease and eosinophilic gastroenteritis, also must be considered.

Crohn's disease is an idiopathic inflammatory bowel disease most commonly located in the terminal ileum. Malabsorption occurs with extensive small intestine involvement or extensive surgical resection. Resection of the distal small intestine because of Crohn's disease, infarction, multiple-obstructing adhesions, or injury results in bile salt malabsorption, steatorrhea, and vitamin B_{12} deficiency.

Malabsorption syndromes occur from small-intestinal dysmotility (e.g., from diabetes, scleroderma, autonomic neuropathies) and the resulting bacterial overgrowth. Excessive bacteria in the upper small intestine deconjugate bile salts, leading to fat maldigestion, and they metabolize carbohydrates, resulting in gas, acid production, and diarrhea.

Obstruction of the lymphatics by congenital malformation, lymphoma, or other causes results in steatorrhea and hypoalbuminemia. The diagnosis is made by observing dilated lacteals on small-bowel biopsy.

The diagnosis of small-bowel disease is made by radiographic studies and multiple small-bowel biopsies (because some diseases have a patchy distribution). Small intestine mucosal function tests, such as the ability to absorb D-xylose from the intestine and excrete it in the urine, are also useful.

Because this patient had a history of a similar problem in the past, evidence of significant malabsorption with weight loss and skin lesions suggestive of dermatitis herpetiformis, celiac disease was suspected. Serum transglutaminase antibody test was ordered, along with a complete blood count, iron studies, routine chemistries including albumin, and a prothrombin time. An upper GI endoscopy with intestinal biopsies was scheduled. Endoscopy with biopsies was chosen over radiographic studies in this case because adequate biopsy specimens are usually diagnostic of celiac disease, whereas radiographic tests would likely show nonspecific mucosal changes. In addition to these tests, the patient was started on a gluten-free diet.

COLON

The colon primarily serves as a waste container until the appropriate time for emptying. Although the role of the colon in digestion is minimal, it continues to play an important role in the absorption of water.

Biochemical Digestion and Absorption of Specific Nutrients

CARBOHYDRATES

The average American consumes approximately 300 g of carbohydrates a day in the form of starch (50%), sucrose (30%), lactose (6%), maltose (2%), and other sugars (i.e., trehalose, glucose, fructose, sorbitol, cellulose, hemicellulose, and pectins). The basic chemical structure of carbohydrates is shown in Figure 6-2.

Salivary amylase and pancreatic amylase are most efficient in digesting the internal bonds connecting chains of sugar molecules in starches and glycogen. Specifically, salivary amylase favors the 1:6 branches, whereas the pancreatic amylase hydrolyzes internal 1:4 bonds, resulting in the formation of di- and trisaccharides. The small intestine brush border contains a variety of specific disaccharidases, including maltase, isomaltase, sucrase, lactase, and trehalase. On hydrolysis, the resulting monosaccharides are ready for absorption.

Most of the absorption of monosaccharides is by specific carrier systems. *Glucose* absorption from the intestine occurs by passive as well as active transport, primarily in the jejunum. Aqueous channels between the enterocytes and pores in the brush border allow for some passive diffusion. For the most part, however, dietary *hexoses* are too large to be absorbed in the necessary quantities through this means. *Fructose* is transported by facilitated diffusion. In addition, the sodium gradient drives active transport carrier systems. *Glucose* and

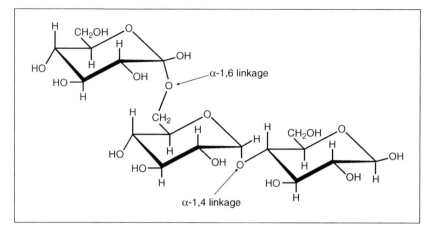

Fig. 6-2. Carbohydrate Digestion

Complex polysaccharides are hydrolyzed by salivary amylase, which cleaves at α-1,6 linkages and some α-1,4 linkages. Pancreatic amylase digests primarily at interior α-1,4 linkages, producing mono-, di-, and trisaccharides. Further digestion occurs through small intestine disaccharidases. Although cellulose, the chief component of wood and plant fibers, consists of chains of glucose molecules, none of the enzymes produced in humans digest the β linkage, making cellulose "indigestible."

galactose are the prototypic examples for active monosaccharide absorption. The absorptive process as driven by sodium (Na^+) is illustrated in Figure 6-3.

Recognition of the Na^+-dependent glucose and galactose transporter has very important clinical implications. For example, children with severe dehydration and volume depletion cannot be given oral saline solution for rehydration because the saline solution causes an osmotic diarrhea. Therefore, giving salt water worsens the problem of dehydration and volume depletion. The addition of glucose to the electrolyte rehydration solution results in the transport of glucose, Na^+, chloride (Cl^-), and water across the intestinal wall. This simple application of intestinal physiology has saved hundreds of thousands of lives!

Maldigestion of carbohydrates results in well-recognized symptoms of bloating, intestinal gas formation, and diarrhea. For example, consider the common condition of lactase deficiency (commonly called lactose intolerance)(Figure 6-4). Lactase is a brush-border enzyme that hydrolyzes lactose, a disaccharidase present in dairy products, into glucose and galactose. Expression of this enzyme diminishes with aging. By adulthood, about 15% of whites and nearly 90% of African Americans and Asians have a lactase deficiency, with symptoms developing after the consumption of one or more glasses of milk. Failure to hydrolyze lactose results in excess luminal fluid produced by osmotic forces and related effects. Bacterial fermentation results in the formation of organic acids, gases, and other by-products that further increase the osmotic load. The results vary among

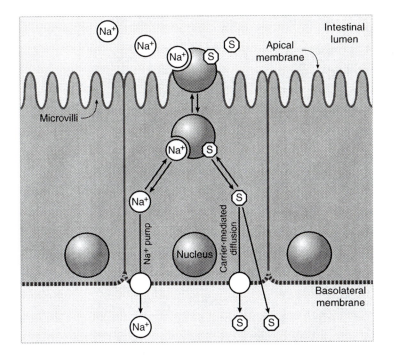

Fig. 6-3. Na⁺-Dependent Carrier System for Glucose and Galactose

Transport of sugars (S) into the body is driven by the high Na^+ electrochemical gradient using an apical carrier molecule. Once the sugar is inside the cell, transport across the basolateral membrane is mediated by another carrier system. The process is driven by the ATP-dependent Na^+ pump, which maintains the high Na^+ electrochemical gradient.

individuals, but abdominal distention, bloating, flatulence, and osmotic diarrhea are common.

PROTEINS

The average American consumes 70–100 g of protein a day. These proteins are broken down into 21 common amino acids. As proteins, the amino acids are linked by peptide bonds that couple the α-carboxyl group of one amino acid with the amino acid residue of the next (Figure 6-5). The structural and functional nature of the protein is dependent on the nature of the amino acid side chain (R).

Because of the variety of side chains, a number of different specific peptidases are required to digest dietary proteins. Thus, gastric pepsin I and II, the pancreatic endonucleases (i.e., trypsin, chymotrypsin, elastase), and carboxypeptidases are necessary to hydrolyze proteins at specific amino acids. The intestinal brush border also contains a number of endopeptidases and exopeptidases that digest at specific amino acids or at peptide sequences. The final products of these peptidases are free amino acids and di- and tripeptides.

The L-isomers of amino acids are absorbed through Na⁺-dependent active transport systems in much the same manner as the

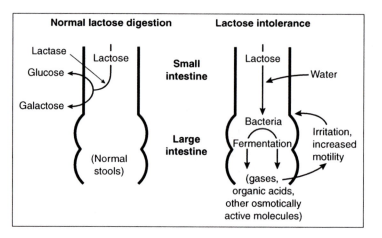

Fig. 6-4. Lactase and Lactase Insufficiency

The stylized small intestine and colon demonstrate the effects of adequate lactase expression (*left*) and inadequate lactase expression (*right*). When adequate lactase is expressed to digest dietary lactose, the disaccharide is hydrolyzed into glucose and galactose and absorbed in the small intestine (*left*). When dietary lactose exceeds the digestive capacity of expressed lactase, undigested lactose draws fluids into the small and large intestine by osmosis. Bacteria ferment the lactose, creating gases, organic acids, and other osmotically active molecules. This results in additional fluid shifts into the intestinal lumen and intestinal irritation with increased motility, borborygmi, diarrhea, and flatulence.

monosaccharides (see Figure 6-3) and by passive amino acid transport systems. Separate carrier systems for neutral, basic, acidic, and imino amino acids have been demonstrated, but carriers for di- and tripeptides also exist, providing redundancy to the absorption process. Once di- and tripeptides are transported into the enterocytes, they are finally broken down into free amino acids. The free amino acids cross the basolateral membrane of the enterocytes by another passive transport system, thereby entering the body.

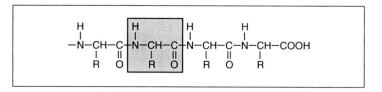

Fig. 6-5. Basic Structure of Proteins

The shaded box encloses the amino nitrogen, α-carbon, and carboxyl carbon from one amino acid in linkage with other amino acids, which form the basic backbone structure of proteins. The *R* group represents the side chain that distinguishes the 21 common amino acids from one another. The digestive system produces a variety of specific peptidases that selectively hydrolyze proteins at specific amino acids.

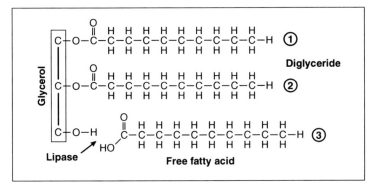

Fig. 6-6. Hydrolysis of a Triglyceride by Lipase

Lingual, gastric, and pancreatic lipases hydrolyze triglycerides in the 1 and 3 position, leaving two free fatty acid molecules and a monoglyceride. Pancreatic cholesterolesterase is capable of completing the digestion to free fatty acids and glycerol.

LIPIDS

The average American consumes 120–150 g of lipids a day. The main forms of dietary lipids are long-chain (more than 14 carbons) triglycerides (Figure 6-6). In addition, the diet contains phospholipids, cholesterol, and fat-soluble vitamins.

Because digestion and absorption occur in an aqueous environment, several coordinated processes are necessary for lipids to be digested and absorbed. These include secretion of bile and lipases, emulsification of the lipid in an aqueous environment, ester hydrolysis, and solubilization of lipolytic products within bile salt micelles.

Bile salts play a critical role in efficient fat digestion. Bile salts contain a flat, cholesterol-derived core, with a hydrophobic surface on one side and a hydrophilic surface on the other. When the concentration of bile salt monomers reaches a critical concentration, the bile salts form a water-soluble micelle with a hydrophobic center. The formation of micelles is important because emulsified fat particles are 200–500 nm in diameter, whereas micelles are only 3–10 nm in diameter. This markedly increases the solubility and surface area of the lipid–aqueous interface, enhancing the exposure of lipids to lipolytic enzymes.

The initial phases of lipid digestion occur with *lingual lipase*. Lingual lipase differs from pancreatic lipase because of its preference for position 3 of triglycerides (as in Figure 6-6), its preferential hydrolysis of medium-chain and polyunsaturated fatty acids, and the fact that its activity is not significantly affected by bile salts or colipase. In the absence of pancreatic lipase, between 40% and 70% of dietary fats are absorbed, in part because of lingual and gastric lipases.

The most important enzyme for the digestion of triglycerides is *pancreatic lipase*. Pancreatic lipase is secreted by the pancreas in an active form, but this form is reversibly inhibited by bile salts. The activity of pancreatic lipase is increased 40–50% by *colipase*, a pancreatic protein secreted with lipase in a 1:1 ratio that is activated in

Pancreatic lipase is the most important enzyme for triglyceride digestion.

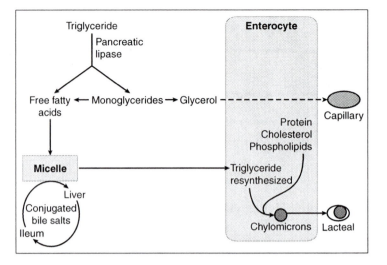

Fig. 6-7. Digestion, Absorption, and Resynthesization of Triglycerides

Formation of micelles by bile salts is a central process in the digestion and absorption of triglycerides. Once the micelles enter the enterocytes, the triglycerides are resynthesized and packaged into chylomicrons for transport through the body.

the intestinal lumen by trypsin. Colipase enhances triglyceride digestion by associating with bile salts on the surface of lipid micelles to form a docking site for pancreatic lipase. The active site of lipase is then positioned for rapid hydrolysis of the 1 and 3 fatty acids from the triglyceride backbone. The pancreas also secretes pancreatic phospholipase A_2, which digests phospholipids, and *pancreatic cholesterolesterase*, which digests a variety of lipids, including triglycerides, sterols, and vitamin esters.

Once triglycerides are broken down into monoglycerides and free fatty acids and incorporated into micelles, they are quickly absorbed in the upper small intestine cells (Figure 6-7). Short-chain and medium-chain fatty acids are absorbed into the cells directly. In addition, long-chain fatty acids may have a specific transporter. Once the monoglycerides and long-chain fatty acids enter the enterocytes, they are resynthesized into triglycerides and packaged with proteins (e.g., apoproteins), cholesterol, and phospholipids to form chylomicrons. The chylomicrons are transported to the lymphatic lacteals and through the lymphatic system to eventually join the cardiovascular system. The bile acids are reabsorbed in the terminal ileum and recycled through the liver.

VITAMINS

Vitamins are organic compounds that are vital for metabolism but cannot be synthesized by the body. Vitamins are characterized by their relative solubility in water or fat. Examples of two vitamins, thiamine (vitamin B_1) and vitamin A, illustrate the chemical nature of

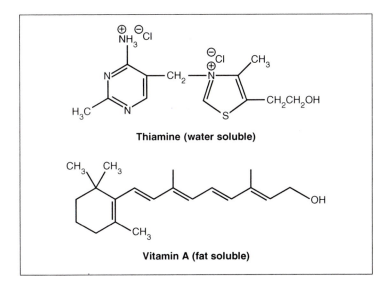

Thiamine (water soluble)

Vitamin A (fat soluble)

Fig. 6-8. Water-Soluble and Fat-Soluble Vitamins

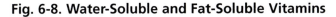

The chemical nature that renders vitamins soluble in water or fat is illustrated. Several water-soluble vitamins require special transport systems for absorption. Fat-soluble vitamins are absorbed with other lipids in micelles.

these vitamins as a basis for their solubility (Figure 6-8). The water-soluble vitamins are absorbed by passive diffusion and carrier-mediated mechanisms. Thiamine, folic acid, vitamin C, and vitamin B_{12} have specific carrier systems. Absorption of vitamin B_{12} in the terminal ileum also requires the secretion of intrinsic factor from the stomach. The fat-soluble vitamins (i.e., vitamins A, D, E, and K) are absorbed with other fats in bile-salt micelles as already described.

SITE-SPECIFIC CAUSES FOR MALDIGESTION AND MALABSORPTION

The process of digestion and absorption is critical to the functioning of the human body. This chapter has defined the role of each part of the GI tract in these functions and has focused on digestion and absorption of different nutrients. In subsequent chapters, the pathophysiology and diseases will be discussed when something interferes with the normal process either through developmental or genetic processes or acquired diseases. Table 6-2 demonstrates examples of site-specific causes of maldigestion and malabsorption.

CASE STUDY: *RESOLUTION*

The first laboratory tests to return included a white blood count of 4.3×10^9/L (normal: $4.5–11 \times 10^9$/L), hemoglobin of 8.6 g/dl (normal: 12–15 g/dl), hematocrit 27.5 ml/dl (normal: 35–47 ml/dl), mean corpuscular volume of 58.4 fl (normal: 80–100 fl) with iron 50 μg/dl (normal: 65–165 μg/dl), total iron-binding capacity

of 388 μg/dl (normal: 250–420 μg/dl), and iron saturation of 13% (normal: 25–50%). These tests, combined with a hemoccult-negative stool and amenorrhea, suggested iron-deficiency anemia from poor iron absorption in the duodenum and jejunum. Other laboratory tests included an albumin of 3.2 g/dl (normal: 3.5–5.0 g/dl), suggesting protein malabsorption, and transglutaminase antibody test was positive, suggesting celiac disease.

Biopsy of the small intestine showed total villus atrophy, hyperplastic crypts, and mixed plasmacytic and lymphocytic infiltration of the lamina propria, which demonstrated the site of malabsorption and confirmed the suspicion of celiac disease. The patient responded to a gluten-free diet with resolution of the diarrhea, appropriate weight gain, and eventual resumption of normal periods.

REVIEW QUESTIONS

Directions: For each of the following questions, choose the one best answer.

1 A 51-year-old woman is brought to the clinic by her husband because of fatigue and 30-lb weight loss (from 125 lbs down to 95 lbs) over the past 8 months; however, her weight has remained stable at 95 lbs for the past 2 months. She denies any abdominal pain, bloating, or diarrhea and has only one small bowel movement per week. She has had no previous surgery and is now postmenopausal. She had lost 20 lbs previously but gained it back. Her only medications are an antidepressant and multiple vitamins. On physical examination her pupils were moderately dilated, her sclera were nonicteric, her mouth was dry, and she had no lymphadenopathy. Her abdomen was scaphoid with occasional bowel sounds, and on rectal examination, there was brown, guaiac-negative stool. Her complete blood count revealed a mild, normocytic anemia. A recent CT scan of the abdomen was reported as normal. Based on this information, the physician should order which of the following tests?

A Antigliadin and antiendomysial antibody tests
B A small-bowel biopsy
C A pancreatic function test to exclude chronic pancreatitis
D A colonoscopy
E Gynecology and psychiatry consultations

2 A woman brings her sick grandchild to the clinic. The child is 1 year old and has been sick for the past 3 days. The illness began with a runny nose, fussiness, and a low-grade fever. On the second day, the child began vomiting, followed by diarrhea at a rate of 8–10 green, watery stools a day. There was no blood, mucus, or worms in the diaper, but the volume was large enough to overwhelm the absorbance capacity of the diaper and further the distress of the caretakers. Today the vomiting only occurred after the child drank a large amount of apple juice, but the diarrhea has continued. On examination, the child appears mildly dehydrated, has not stopped urinating, and appears to have a viral syndrome. The physician advises the woman to give the child frequent small volumes of liquid. The liquid suggested by the physician is most likely to be

A distilled water.
B 0.9% sodium chloride solution.
C 0.9% sodium chloride with 10% sucrose.
D honey water.
E over-the-counter electrolyte solution from the grocery store.

3 A 45-year-old woman with a history of Crohn's disease and a 50-cm resection of her terminal ileum is concerned about fat absorption. The physician should inform her that the loss of this section of small intestine may result in

A loss of the fatty acid–absorbing portion of her small intestine.
B loss of part of the bile salt-absorbing portion of her small intestine.
C the inability to absorb fat-soluble vitamins.
D the loss of lipase absorption.
E folate deficiency.

4 Which of the following statements concerning colipase is *true*?

A It is useless without trypsin.
B It is secreted with gastric lipase.
C It is absolutely necessary for pancreatic lipase activity.
D It is secreted in the active form.
E It is required for activation of every type of human lipase.

5 What is the most important portion of the GI tract for survival?

A Stomach
B Pancreas
C Biliary system
D Small intestine
E Colon

References

Castro GA: Digestion and absorption. In *Gastrointestinal Physiology*, 4th ed. Edited by Johnson LR. St. Louis, MO: Mosby Year Book, 1991.

Notes

Ciclitira PJ, Ellis HJ: Celiac disease. In *Textbook of Gastroenterology.* Edited by Yamada T. Philadelphia, PA: Lippincott, Williams & Wilkins, 2003.

Despopoulos A, Silbernagl S: *Color Atlas of Physiology,* 4th ed. New York, NY: Thieme Medical, 1991, pp 200–216.

Halsted CH, Lōnnerdal BL: Vitamin and mineral absorption. In *Textbook of Gastroenterology.* Edited by Yamada T. Philadelphia, PA: Lippincott, Williams & Wilkins, 2003.

Johnson LR: *Gastrointestinal Physiology.* St. Louis, MO: Elsevier Science, Mosby, 2001.

Montrose MH, Keely SJ, Barrett KE: Electrolyte secretion and absorption: small intestine and colon. In *Textbook of Gastroenterology.* Edited by Yamada T. Philadelphia, PA: Lippincott Williams & Wilkins, 2003.

Uhl M, Cooke AR: Malabsorption syndromes. In *Consultations in Gastroenterology.* Edited by Snape WJ. Philadelphia, PA: W. B. Saunders, 1996, pp 75–83.

7

Management of Water and Electrolytes

■ **LEARNING OBJECTIVES** ■

At the completion of this chapter, the reader should be able to:

- Describe the basic pathways and mechanisms involved in intestinal fluid and electrolyte transport.
- List the specific transport mechanisms for the sodium (Na^+), potassium (K^+), chloride (Cl^-), and bicarbonate (HCO_3^-) ions and various solutes.
- Identify the complex intracellular and extracellular regulatory systems involved in control of intestinal transport.
- Define the pathophysiology and treatments of specific diseases that alter intestinal transport.
- Appreciate the clinical importance of understanding intestinal transport through specific clinical examples.

Water transport is a passive process indirectly regulated by the active transport of electrolytes and solutes.

Case Study: *Introduction*

A 62-year-old woman was admitted to the hospital with severe diarrhea, dehydration, and hypokalemia (low potassium). Diarrhea initially occurred several times per week but progressed and now occurred on a daily basis. It was described as large in volume, watery, and associated with mild, crampy abdominal pain. Prior outpatient evaluation included stool cultures, which failed to demonstrate an infectious cause. Barium studies and endoscopy revealed normal mucosa without evidence of an inflammatory or malabsorptive process.

Introduction

Each day the intestinal tract is met with the formidable task of converting a highly variable intake of nutrients into a usable pool from which it must extract water, electrolytes, and nutrients and excrete waste. This remarkable feat is accomplished through elaborated pathways in the small and large intestines under regulatory control from several sources. In health, these pathways run flawlessly. However, a host of diseases can alter these pathways and can cause, in some cases, life-threatening conditions. As demonstrated in the case study, an understanding of normal intestinal function and the pathophysiology of various disease states is crucial for clinicians to be able to develop specific therapeutic strategies for their patients with intestinal disease.

Fluid Management

The presence of water in the lumen of the intestine is critical to maintain fluidity of the luminal contents. This allows digestive enzymes to contact food particles and digested nutrients to diffuse to the epithelial surface. Under normal physiologic conditions, the amount of water is closely regulated so that digestion and absorption are optimized.

The daily fluid load varies with the composition of meals ingested but typically approximates 9 L (see Chapter 5). It characteristically comprises approximately 1.5 L of oral intake and 7 L of endogenous intestinal secretions, including 1.5 L of saliva, 2.5 L of gastric juice, 0.5 L of bile, 1.5 L of pancreatic juice, and 1 L of small intestine secretions (Figure 7-1). Most of this fluid is absorbed by the small intestine along with digested nutrients and electrolytes. Only approximately 1.5–2 L of fluid reach the colon each day. The colon absorbs most of the remaining fluid, allowing typically only 100 ml to be excreted in the stool under normal circumstances.

The active transport of electrolytes generates an osmotic gradient between the lumen of the intestine and the tissue compartment. Water moves between these two compartments so that contents are maintained in an iso-osmotic state.

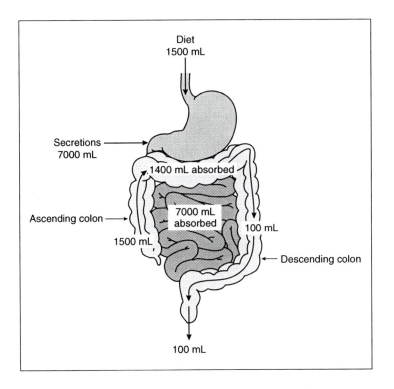

Diet
1500 mL

Secretions
7000 mL

1400 mL absorbed

7000 mL
absorbed

Ascending colon

100 mL

1500 mL

Descending colon

100 mL

Fig. 7-1. Normal Function of the Intestinal Tract

The intestinal tract secretes and absorbs a large volume of fluid on a daily basis. The volumes shown are typical of a normally functioning intestinal tract. Diarrhea results when either the small bowel delivers a volume that exceeds the colon's absorptive capacity (approximately 5 L) or when the colon's absorptive capacity is impaired and it cannot absorb the normal ileocecal volume.

The gut has a tremendous capacity to absorb water and solutes. This is due in part to its amplified surface area, achieved by the many folds, villi, and microvilli. Together, the folds, villi, and microvilli amplify the surface area of the intestine approximately 600-fold. The colon alone has the capacity to absorb up to 5 L water per day. As will be discussed later, the amount of fluid secreted or absorbed can be altered by different endogenous and exogenous compounds. Diarrhea occurs when either an abnormally large volume of fluid enters the colon, exceeding its maximal absorptive capacity, or when the absorptive capacity of the colon is reduced.

The most dramatic example of a secretory diarrhea is produced by the enterotoxin of *Vibrio cholerae*. The toxin causes the small intestine mucosa to secrete an enormous volume of isotonic fluid while leaving absorption intact. This volume overwhelms the absorptive capacity of the colon, leading to as much as 10–20 L of stool water per day excreted along with electrolytes.

Despite delivery of a normal volume to the colon, diarrhea can also occur if the absorptive capacity of the colon is altered. A simple example of this is the osmotic diarrhea that follows the ingestion of magnesium sulfate, a poorly absorbable osmotically active substance.

The **osmolar gap** is the difference between the expected stool osmolality of 290 mOsm/kg and calculated stool osmolality of $2(Na^+ + K^+)$.

Polarity of the epithelial cell derives from the functional differences between the luminal and serosal surfaces.

Table 7-1. Causes of Diarrhea

OSMOTIC (OSMOTIC GAP > 50 mOsm/L)	SECRETORY (OSMOTIC GAP > 50 mOsm/L)
Lactose intolerance	Hormone-induced VIPoma,
Magnesium-containing antacids	gastrinoma, and carcinoid tumor
Sorbitol	Bile salt malabsorption
	Vibrio cholerae toxin

Note: VIP = vasoactive intestinal peptide.

Normally, as stool leaves the colon, its osmolality is equal to that of the serum (approximately 290 mOsm/kg). Under ordinary circumstances, the electrolytes Na^+, K^+, Cl^-, and HCO_3^- constitute the major osmoles in feces. However, the presence of a nonabsorbable, osmotically active substance such as magnesium sulfate increases the osmolality of the stool, leading to increased stool water volume and thus diarrhea.

Clinically, differentiating between a secretory and osmotic diarrhea can be helpful when evaluating patients with diarrhea (Table 7-1). Stool osmolality (S Osm) can be estimated by the formula: S Osm = $2(Na^+ + K^+)$. Under normal physiologic conditions, this value is less than 50 mOsm/kg. An osmolar gap greater than 50 mOsm/kg suggests the presence of a nonabsorbable solute causing the diarrhea. An osmolar gap less than 50 mOsm/kg suggests the presence of a secretory stimulant.

Overview of Intestinal Structure and Transport

A basic understanding of the intestinal epithelial cell and its components is critical to the understanding of fluid and electrolyte transport in the gut. The epithelia of the small and large intestines consist of a single layer of columnar cells joined together close to the luminal surface by tight junctions. The epithelial cell has *polarity*, in that the apical (luminal) surface contains different elements from those of the basolateral (serosal) membrane, and these therefore serve different functions. In general, this difference typically consists of active transport mechanisms at one surface and passive transport at the other, which leads to a specialized transcellular movement of electrolytes and solutes. The characteristics of the tight junctions and the specific transport proteins contained within the apical and basolateral membranes determine the distinct functional characteristics of an intestinal segment.

The transport properties of the epithelium vary from one intestinal segment to the next. The functional differences between the small intestine and colon have been well established. Functional differences also exist within a given segment of intestine. For example, the less permeable tight junctions in the distal colon allow for Na^+ absorption against a steep gradient as compared to the relatively "leaky" tight junctions found in the proximal colon.

Segmental differences have been noted along the crypt–villus axis as well. Evidence suggests that crypt and villus cells have distinct transport properties. Crypt cells exhibit predominately secretory features, whereas villus cells function primarily as absorptive cells. It seems that epithelial cells acquire different membrane transport proteins as they migrate from the crypt to the villus surface. This concept that absorption and secretion occur separately is further supported by the separate regulatory mechanisms of these cells. This feature has important clinical implications, in that a pathologic process can affect one function while leaving another intact.

Electrolytes and solutes move across the epithelium through either *active* or *passive* transport mechanisms. The passive transport of uncharged solutes requires no energy and is dependent solely on the solute's transmembrane concentration gradient. Passive transport of a charged substance, however, is dependent on both the concentration gradient and the *electrochemical gradient,* or potential difference, for the given substance. Because epithelial cells typically have a net negative intracellular charge, intracellular movement of cations and extracellular movement of anions are favored.

Active transport refers to the net movement of solute or ion against or in the absence of a concentration or electrochemical gradient. This is often referred to as uphill movement. As a result, active transport can create an electrochemical gradient across the cell membrane. This process requires energy, usually derived from the hydrolysis of ATP. Because of this energy requirement, active transport is always *transcellular,* or across the cell membrane. Passive transport can be transcellular or *paracellular,* occurring between epithelial cells through their tight junctions.

As in other cells, the membrane of the epithelial cell consists of a lipid bilayer with a hydrophilic exterior and a hydrophobic interior. Specialized membrane proteins called channels, carriers, and pumps are required for solutes and electrolytes to traverse this lipid bilayer. Together these regulatory proteins control the transmembrane transport of solutes and electrolytes into and out of the cell.

Channels are essentially selective "protein pores" within the epithelial cell membrane. They allow for movement of a specific solute or electrolyte across the membrane. Channels have the ability to open and close quickly. Their opening and closing is regulated by several factors, including intracellular mediators, ionic concentrations, and voltage. *Carriers* are specialized membrane proteins capable of transporting either solute or multiple ions across the membrane. In general, carrier-mediated transport occurs at a much slower rate than that through channels. Like enzymes, carriers exhibit structural specificity for their ligands and are subject to competitive inhibition and saturation kinetics. *Pumps* are carriers that require energy to transport a solute against an electrochemical gradient. The classic example is the Na^+-K^+-ATPase pump located in the basolateral membrane. This pump uses energy from the hydrolysis of ATP to exchange intracellular Na^+ for extracellular K^+. Three Na^+ ions are exchanged for two K^+ ions with each cycle of the pump. This results in the electrically

The unique transport properties of a particular intestinal segment are determined by the specific transport proteins within the epithelial membrane and the characteristics of the adjoining tight junctions.

negative, low Na⁺, high K⁺ content characteristic of the intracellular space.

SPECIFIC ION TRANSPORT

With these basic principles of transport defined, let us now discuss the specific transport mechanisms for various ions.

Na⁺ Absorption

Na⁺ absorption occurs through two distinct mechanisms known as (1) electrogenic absorption and (2) electroneutral absorption. As depicted in Figure 7-2A, the Na⁺-K⁺-ATPase pump located in the basolateral membrane creates an electrochemical gradient, which drives the movement of Na⁺ from the intestinal lumen into the intracellular space. This process is facilitated by Na⁺-specific channels located in the apical membrane. Because there is no counterflow of charge coupled with the apical transport of Na⁺, an apical transmembrane potential is generated—thus the term *electrogenic Na⁺ absorption*.

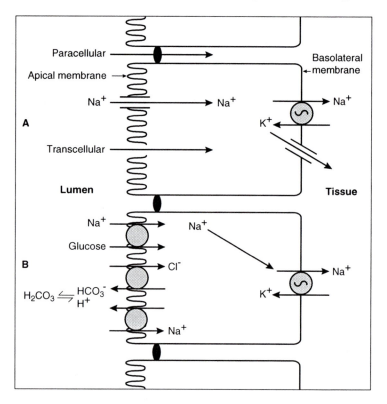

Fig. 7-2. Electrogenic Na⁺ Absorption and Electroneutral NaCl Absorption

(A) Electrogenic Na⁺ absorption. These apical Na⁺ channels, found largely in the distal colon, are inhibited by amiloride. The mineralocorticoid aldosterone enhances this mechanism by increasing the number of apical Na⁺ channels and stimulating the Na⁺-K⁺-ATPase pump. (B) Electroneutral NaCl absorption. This system is found throughout the small intestine and is facilitated by glucocorticoids. The routes of transcellular and paracellular absorption and an example of Na⁺-coupled nutrient transport (using glucose) are also shown.

Electrogenic Na$^+$ absorption occurs in the ileum, cecum, and distal colon. The fact that the apical Na$^+$ channels in the distal colon are inhibited by the diuretic amiloride whereas those in the ileum and cecum are not suggests that a different class of channels exist in these segments. The mineralocorticoid aldosterone facilitates Na$^+$ absorption in the distal colon by increasing the number of Na$^+$ channels present in the apical membrane and by increasing the activity of the Na$^+$-K$^+$-ATPase pump. This results in water conservation and suggests that the distal colon contributes to overall fluid homeostasis.

A significant portion of total Na$^+$ absorption in the intestine is coupled to Cl$^-$ movement in *electroneutral sodium chloride (NaCl) transport*. This process, illustrated in Figure 7-2B, involves two separate apical membrane carriers. One carrier exchanges extracellular Na$^+$ for intracellular H$^+$, and the other exchanges extracellular Cl$^-$ for intracellular HCO$_3^-$. Because both carriers operate at the same rate, no net charge is generated—thus the term electroneutral NaCl transport. As with electrogenic Na$^+$ absorption, the Na$^+$-K$^+$-ATPase pump creates an electrochemical gradient that drives the apical absorption of luminal Na$^+$. The export of H$^+$ maintains electrical neutrality. This in turn facilitates the extracellular movement of HCO$_3^-$, which itself drives the intracellular movement of Cl$^-$ to maintain neutrality. The end result is NaCl absorption coupled with water and carbon dioxide secretion with maintenance of intracellular pH.

Cl$^-$ Transport

The absorption of Cl$^-$ probably occurs by both passive and active transport mediated through Na$^+$-dependent and -independent mechanisms. Electrogenic Na$^+$ absorption creates an electrical gradient that favors Cl$^-$ absorption. Electroneutral Na$^+$ absorption likely accounts for a significant portion of Cl$^-$ absorption, and an active Na$^+$-independent mechanism appears to involve an electroneutral Cl$^-$–HCO$_3^-$ exchanger located at the apical surface.

Secretion of Cl$^-$ occurs through an electrogenic transport mechanism driven by the Na$^+$-K$^+$-ATPase pump. As illustrated in Figure 7-3, a single carrier located in the basolateral membrane binds Na$^+$, K$^+$, and Cl$^-$ and transports them from the circulation into the epithelial cell in the ratio 2 Cl$^-$:1 K$^+$:1 Na$^+$. Cl$^-$ accumulates intracellularly until it exceeds its electrochemical equilibrium with the intestinal lumen. When the Cl$^-$ channels located in the apical membrane open, Cl$^-$ moves down its electrochemical gradient into the intestinal lumen. K$^+$ exits the basolateral membrane through K$^+$-specific channels, thus balancing the large Cl$^-$ flux across the apical membrane.

K$^+$ Transport

Little is known about the intestinal absorption of K$^+$ in humans. Until recently it was believed (wrongly) that K$^+$ transport was passive and occurred by the paracellular route. However, evidence now supports the existence of active transcellular transport mechanisms for K$^+$

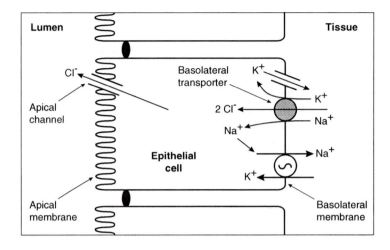

Fig. 7-3. Cl⁻ Secretion

The basolateral transporter carries two Cl⁻ anions with one Na⁺ and one K⁺ cation. This process is driven by the Na⁺ electrochemical gradient generated by the Na⁺-K⁺-ATPase pump. K⁺ ions exit through channels at the basolateral membrane.

absorption and secretion. On the basis of animal studies, investigators believe that an electroneutral H⁺-K⁺-ATPase pump located in the apical membrane is responsible for K⁺ secretion. These transporters, found mainly in the colon and regulated by aldosterone, may play a significant role in K⁺ homeostasis.

K⁺ secretion appears to be passive in the small intestine. In the colon, K⁺ secretion occurs concurrently with Cl⁻ secretion. Evidence suggests that the Na⁺-K⁺-ATPase pump and the Na⁺-K⁺–2 Cl⁻ cotransporter are involved the same way they are in Cl⁻ secretion. K⁺ then exits the cell through apical K⁺ channels in an electrogenic manner. The overall movement of K⁺ is then determined by the conductances of the apical and basolateral membranes. Glucocorticoids and aldosterone enhance active K⁺ secretion, whereas this is inhibited by the prostaglandin inhibitor indomethacin.

HCO₃⁻ Transport

HCO₃⁻ anion secretion is important not only in the pancreas and bile ducts but in the proximal gut as well. HCO₃⁻ secreted in the proximal duodenum is used to create the mucus–bicarbonate layer that overlies the epithelial cells of the duodenum. HCO₃⁻ performs an important protective function, preventing mucosal ulceration by neutralizing gastric acid secretion. HCO₃⁻ also helps create the ideal pH environment for optimal digestive enzyme function. HCO₃⁻ secretion occurs to a lesser degree in the ileum and colon. The physiologic role of HCO₃⁻ secretion in the distal gut is not clear, but it may function in Cl⁻ conservation through the Cl⁻–HCO₃⁻ exchange.

Evidence supports the existence of two separate mechanisms for HCO₃⁻ secretion. In both systems, the Na⁺-K⁺-ATPase pump provides

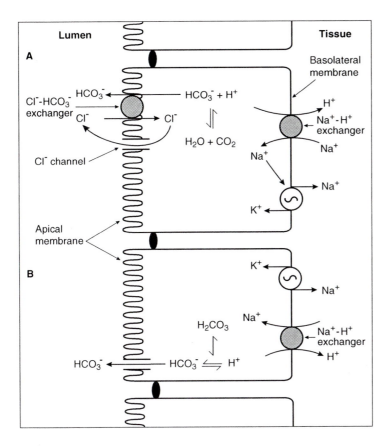

Fig. 7-4. Two Mechanisms Believed to Exist for HCO_3^- Secretion

(A) HCO_3^- secretion coupled with Cl^- recycling at the apical membrane. The intracellular H^+ that are generated exit the basolateral membrane via the Na^+–H^+ exchanger driven by the Na^+-K^+-ATPase pump. (B) The Cl^--independent secretion of HCO_3^-. In this system, HCO_3^- exits the cell through a specific channel in the apical membrane.

the electrochemical gradient that drives a Na^+-H^+ exchanger located in the basolateral membrane. Intracellular HCO_3^- is derived from the action of carbonic anhydrase on water and carbon dioxide. In one mechanism (Figure 7-4A), a Cl^-–HCO_3^- exchanger and a Cl^- channel located in the apical membrane work together to yield a net HCO_3^- secretion while recycling Cl^-. In the second system (Figure 7-4B), a HCO_3^--specific channel located in the apical membrane allows HCO_3^- efflux into the intestinal lumen.

REGULATION OF TRANSPORT

The elaborate array of transport channels, carriers, and pumps is kept running smoothly by an equally elaborate regulatory system. For simplicity, this system can be divided into two classes: (1) *extracellular mediators*, including luminal, neural, hormonal, and inflammatory components; and (2) *intracellular mediators*, such as second messengers that respond to extracellular stimuli. However, it is important to

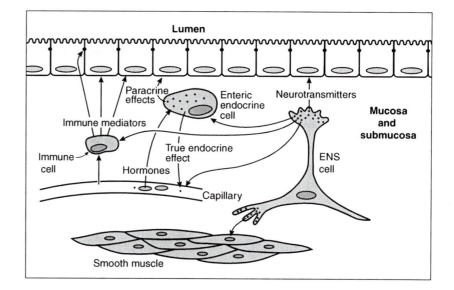

Fig. 7-5. The Complex Regulatory System Governing Intestinal Transport

Each component regulates the epithelial cells as well as other regulatory systems. The immune cell shown is located in the lamina propria and is meant to represent the entire spectrum of immunologic effector cells.

realize that these components interact with one another to form this complex regulatory system (Figure 7-5).

Extracellular Regulation

The intestinal epithelium is exposed to a vast array of extracellular mediators. Luminal factors, such as ingested nutrients, bacterial toxins, inflammatory mediators, neurotransmitters, and hormones, alter intestinal transport.

Hormonal regulation in the gut can occur through the classic endocrine effects from distant glands. However, the intestinal tract is also governed by its own intrinsic endocrine cells, which reside in the crypts and exert local (or paracrine) effects. In response to luminal contents, local endocrine cells release hormones that interact with epithelial cell receptors and lead to an alteration in transport. Other extraintestinal regulatory signals, such as neural input, also regulate these intrinsic endocrine cells.

Hormones such as mineralocorticoids, glucocorticoids, and insulin appear to have regulatory effects at physiologic levels. Some hormones—for example, serotonin and vasoactive intestinal peptide (VIP)—exert their effects only when present in excess quantities, typically as a result of endocrine tumors (e.g., VIPoma). An abbreviated list of transport regulatory hormones is provided in Table 7-2.

Neural Regulation

Neural input plays an important role in fluid and electrolyte transport. Tonic sympathetic and parasympathetic input influences

Table 7-2. Intestinal Secretagogues

STIMULANT	INTRACELLULAR MEDIATOR
Endogenous	
Neural	
Acetylcholine	Calcium
Substance *P*	Calcium
Calcitonin	Calcium
VIP	cAMP
Paracrine	
Secretin	cAMP
Glucagon	cAMP
Gastrin	Unknown
Immune	
Prostaglandins	cAMP
Arachidonic acid	cAMP
Histamine	Calcium
Lipoxygenase metabolites	Unknown
Miscellaneous	
Atrial natriuretic factor	cGMP
Motilin	Unknown
Luminal	
Bacterial endotoxins	
Vibrio cholerae	cAMP
Escherichia coli (heat-labile)	cAMP
Escherichia coli (heat-stable)	cGMP
Yersinia	cGMP
Bile salts	cAMP + ?calcium
Fatty acids	cAMP + ?calcium
Laxatives	Unknown

Note. cAMP = cyclic adenosine monophosphate; cGMP = cyclic guanosine monophosphate; VIP = vasoactive intestinal peptide.

intestinal transport. Alteration in the balance of these neural pathways can have deleterious clinical effects. For example, patients with long-standing diabetes may develop autonomic neuropathy with loss of sympathetic stimulation. This may explain the diarrhea seen in diabetic patients and the effectiveness of α_2-adrenergic agonists, such as clonidine, used to treat the disorder.

As with the enteric endocrine cells, the gut contains its own intrinsic neuronal network known as the *enteric nervous system (ENS)*. The ENS is complex and independently integrates the neural activity of the epithelium, smooth muscle, and blood vessels of the gut with input from the central nervous system. The ENS consists of two ganglion plexuses known as Meissner's and Auerbach's plexuses. Meissner's plexus is located in the submucosa, and Auerbach's plexus is found in the smooth muscle layer of the intestine. It is the latter that plays the major role in regulating transport.

Sensory input from the ENS probably comes from changes in the luminal content or volume. As in other neural systems, interneurons relay information from sensory neurons to motor neurons through cholinergic mediators. The motor neurons influence the epithelial cell as well as paracrine, endocrine, smooth muscle, and inflammatory cells in the submucosa (see Figure 7-5).

Immunologic Regulation

The role of immune cells located in the lamina propria of the intestine in regulating ion and water transport has been recognized. The entire spectrum of immune cells, including B and T lymphocytes, plasma cells, macrophages, mast cells, and polymorphonuclear cells (PMNs), normally occupy the lamina propria. These cells release various mediators that alter transport through direct influences on local epithelial cells and other regulatory systems. Diseases that incite an inflammatory reaction in the gut lead to the release of inflammatory mediators. For example, histamine, serotonin, and adenosine all are potent secretagogues that when released from mast cells, affect the ENS and epithelial cells while promoting prostaglandin release. Bacterial enteric infections lead to an increase in the number of PMNs, which release potent secretagogues, such as superoxides, hydrogen peroxide, and the cytokines interleukin-1 and -3. The eicosanoids, especially prostaglandins, play a key role in the secretory response to inflammation. Inflammatory mediators can also affect fluid transport by altering the permeability of tight junctions. The exact role of these inflammatory mediators in the idiopathic inflammatory diseases ulcerative colitis and Crohn's disease, however, is still unclear.

Luminal Factors

The osmotic load of the intraluminal contents generates a significant regulatory force for intestinal transport. Because the intestinal epithelium is unable to generate an osmotic gradient, the intake of relatively hypertonic nutrients leads to rapid movement of water into the lumen to maintain osmotic equilibrium. As nutrients are absorbed along the intestinal tract, the secreted fluid is reabsorbed so that this osmotic equilibrium is maintained. As previously mentioned, the presence of a nonabsorbable substance within the lumen prevents fluid reabsorption, resulting in diarrhea.

A common cause of osmotic diarrhea is lactose intolerance. Lactose, the disaccharide glucose-galactose, is not readily absorbed by the intestinal mucosa. The brush border enzyme lactase breaks down the disaccharide into its readily absorbable monosaccharide constituents. People who suffer from a relative deficiency of lactase develop diarrhea associated with lactose ingestion as a result of the osmotic load created by the nonabsorbable disaccharide.

Systemic Factors

Intestinal transport is also regulated by systemic factors, such as pH, volume status, and blood flow. Electroneutral NaCl absorption is stimulated in the presence of metabolic acidosis and inhibited by metabolic alkalosis. Hypovolemia results in a net increase in intestinal fluid absorption in an effort to conserve intravascular volume. Several factors, including cardiopulmonary mechanoreceptors, carotid barore-ceptors, angiotensin II, and sympathetic stimulation of the ENS, mediate this response. Finally, an increase in intestinal blood flow results in stimulation of both secretion and absorption.

Intracellular Mediators

Many diverse and heterogeneous agents stimulate intestinal fluid and electrolyte transport. This barrage of external stimuli is translated into intracellular *second messengers* that ultimately alter the membrane transport machinery. Most of the cellular events that link these stimulants to changes in transport are not known. Table 7-2 lists the second messengers associated with the different secretagogues.

Many endogenous and exogenous secretagogues mediate their effects through intracellular cyclic AMP (cAMP). In general, these ligands bind to the receptor portion of the membrane-bound adenylate cyclase complex as depicted in Figure 7-6. Binding of the secretagogue activates the G protein within the complex, which in turn activates the adenylate cyclase subunit. This then converts intracellular ATP to cAMP. Increased intracellular cAMP activates protein kinases, which phosphorylate a specific target protein, such as an ion channel or carrier. Phosphorylation changes the activity of these transport proteins, thereby altering fluid and electrolyte transport. A similar cascade

Notes

Three Messenger Systems. Three distinct second messenger systems (of possibly many) have been well described: (1) cAMP, (2) cGMP, and (3) intracellular Ca²⁺.

Endogenous substances such as VIP and prostaglandins and exogenous agents such as the bacterial toxin of *V. cholerae* act through the second messenger system.

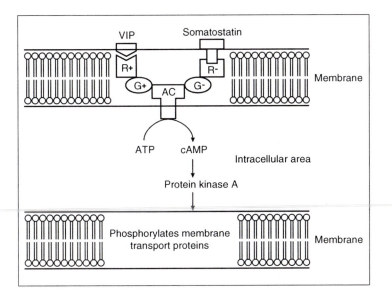

Fig. 7-6. Intracellular cAMP Second Messenger System

Secretagogues such as VIP bind to a stimulatory membrane receptor (R+), which activates its associated G protein (G+). This in turn activates the membrane-bound adenylate cyclase (AC) subunit. Increased intracellular cAMP levels lead to activation of protein kinases, which phosphorylates membrane transport proteins. Phosphorylation results in a structural change that results in a functional change. The binding inhibitory ligands, such as somatostatin, have the opposite effect.

Drug Effects. The antidiarrheal effects of drugs such as phenothiazines and loperamide are in part due to their inhibition of the intracellular Ca²⁺-mediated cascade.

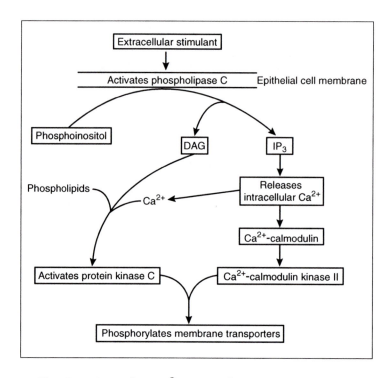

Fig. 7-7. Complex Ca²⁺ Second Messenger System

As with cAMP, the ligand binds to the membrane receptor, which, through a G protein subunit, alters the activity of membrane bound phospholipase C. Activated phospholipase C converts phosphoinositol to IP₃ and DAG. Rising intracellular IP₃ levels lead to the release of Ca²⁺ from intracellular stores. Together DAG, Ca²⁺, and phospholipids activate protein kinase C, which alters transport protein structure and function. Also, the increase in intracellular Ca²⁺ permits the Ca²⁺-calmodulin complex to form, which activates Ca²⁺-calmodulin kinase II. This complex also alters transport protein structure and function.

exists for cyclic guanosine monophosphate (cGMP)-mediated intracellular regulation.

Intracellular Ca²⁺ also plays an important role as a second messenger (Figure 7-7). In the absence of regulatory factors, intracellular Ca²⁺ is maintained at a low concentration relative to the extracellular space. A transient rise in intracellular Ca²⁺ concentration leads to activation of the Ca²⁺–calmodulin complex. This complex activates various protein kinases, which ultimately results in secretion. One mechanism for increasing intracellular Ca²⁺ is the release of intracellular Ca²⁺ stores. This is caused by receptor-mediated release of phosphoinositol metabolites, such as inositol triphosphate (IP₃) and diacylglycerol (DAG) from the cell membrane.

SPECIFIC ABSORPTIVE STIMULI

Table 7-3 summarizes intestinal absorptive stimuli. A few are discussed next. Both glucocorticoids and mineralocorticoids function as endogenous absorptive stimuli. The mineralocorticoid aldosterone and its analogs stimulate amiloride-sensitive electrogenic Na⁺ absorption

Table 7-3. Intestinal Absorptive Stimuli

ENDOGENOUS	PHARMACOLOGIC
Angiotensin II	Clonidine
α-Adrenergic agonists	Colchicine
Aldosterone	Codeine
Glucocorticoids	Lithium
Opioids	Phenothiazines
Somatostatin	Propranolol
Peptide XY	Steroids
Prolactin	Verapamil

and K^+ secretion in the distal colon. The effect of this mechanism on overall transport is limited, however, because these receptors are restricted to the distal colon. Glucocorticoids, on the other hand, have a much more significant overall effect on Na^+ absorption. They stimulate Na^+ absorption throughout the small bowel and colon, independent of amiloride-sensitive Na^+ conductance channels. Because glucocorticoids stimulate Na^+ absorption over a larger area, they are more potent stimulators of Na^+ absorption. In addition to their anti-inflammatory effects, this profound effect on Na^+ absorption may account for the potent antidiarrheal effects of glucocorticoids in inflammatory bowel disease.

Catecholamines, such as epinephrine, stimulate electroneutral NaCl absorption and inhibit HCO_3^- secretion in the ileum. These effects are mediated through stimulation of α_2-receptors. Opiates (such as codeine, morphine, and loperamide) are the most effective pharmacologic class of antidiarrheal medications. Opiates and opioid peptides such as enkephalins exert their constipating effects through various mechanisms, all of which are mediated by opioid receptors in the gut. Stimulation of the μ-, δ-, and κ-receptors affect smooth muscle tone. Stimulation of the δ-receptors results in fluid and electrolyte absorption in the small intestine. It seems that the constipating effect of opioids is largely due to their antimotility actions on smooth muscle rather than their absorptive effects.

Somatostatin, a tetradecapeptide hormone, is ubiquitous in the body, including the GI tract. In the gut it is synthesized by a class of enteric endocrine cells known as delta, or D, cells. Among the many effects of somatostatin are a slowing of gastric and intestinal motility, inhibition of gastric acid secretion, and stimulation of both NaCl and water absorption in the ileum and colon. Although somatostatin does not appear to have an effect on basal water secretion, it does inhibit the activity of several secretagogues, including VIP and serotonin. these antisecretory properties of somatostatin led to the development and clinical use of the long-acting synthetic somatostatin analog octreotide. Other peptide hormones, such as peptide XY, angiotensin II, and insulin, function as absorptive stimuli. The physiologic significance of this activity is not known.

Increased intestinal levels of prostaglandins and leukotrienes are found in idiopathic inflammatory bowel disease (e.g., ulcerative colitis, Crohn's disease) and are likely play a role in the pathogenesis of the diarrhea characteristic of this disorder.

SPECIFIC SECRETAGOGUES

As a general class, secretagogues can be divided into exogenous mediators, such as bacterial endotoxins, and endogenous stimuli, including neurotransmitters, hormones, and inflammatory mediators. Although many secretagogues have been identified, they all appear to exert their effects through one of the three intracellular mechanisms previously discussed (see Table 7-2).

A major cause of morbidity and mortality worldwide, infectious diarrhea is often caused by bacteria producing and releasing a toxin that stimulates secretion. The secretory diarrhea of *V. cholerae* is caused by cholera toxin. This enterotoxin irreversibly stimulates adenylate cyclase activity, thereby producing an unregulated increase in intracellular cAMP levels. This in turn leads to an inhibition of electroneutral NaCl absorption by the villus epithelial cells and stimulation of Cl^- secretion in crypt epithelial cells. Voluminous life-threatening diarrhea and hypokalemia result. Supportive therapy for this condition takes advantage of intact absorptive mechanisms. The oral rehydration solution used in cholera contains Na^+, glucose, and amino acids and hence uses the intact Na^+-coupled nutrient absorptive pathways, which are unaffected by the enterotoxin. This allows water and nutrient absorption to take place in lieu of massive secretory secretory stimulation. Other enterotoxins, such as the heat-labile enterotoxin of *Campylobacter* and *Escherichia coli*, act in a similar fashion.

The heat-stable enterotoxin of *E. coli* stimulates the intracellular production of cGMP. This leads to a series of consequences similar to that with cAMP. Therefore, electroneutral NaCl absorption is inhibited and Cl^- secretion enhanced. Other enterotoxins from bacteria such as *Klebsiella* and *Yersinia enterocolitica* also mediate their effects through cGMP.

Other luminally active endogenous secretagogues include bile salts and long-chain fatty acids. Both of these substances are normally absorbed in the small intestine. However, with malabsorption, bile acids and long-chain fatty acids enter the colon and cause diarrhea. In the case of bile acids, it seems that only the dihydroxy bile acids such as chenodeoxycholic acid with the hydroxyl group in the α (not β) position produce diarrhea. The exact mechanisms leading to diarrhea are not clear but are likely to be multifactorial. Chenodeoxycholic acid may produce diarrhea by solubilizing the surface membranes of the epithelial cells, thereby increasing their permeability. Also, Cl^- secretion may be amplified through second messenger systems. Long-chain fatty acids are believed to exert a similar effect.

There is an emerging appreciation for the role of arachidonic acid metabolites, particularly prostaglandins, in the endogenous regulation of intestinal secretion. Most gut prostaglandins arise from the inflammatory cells in the submucosa. Prostaglandins exert their secretory effects by stimulating adenylate cyclase activity.

Substances such as VIP and serotonin alter transport when produced in excess quantities, but their role in normal physiologic intestinal transport remains unclear. VIP is secreted by neurons in the intestinal mucosa. When produced in excess, usually by a tumor (e.g., VIPoma), VIP causes an increase in adenylate cyclase activity and net secretion. Serotonin, normally found in enteric neurons and enterochromaffin cells, causes a secretory diarrhea when produced in excess by carcinoid tumors. The intracellular effects of serotonin are mediated through intracellular Ca^{2+}.

Summary

The mechanisms of intestinal water and electrolyte transport and their regulatory systems are intricate and complex. Recent advances in physiology have uncovered some of these transport mechanisms and their respective roles in the pathogenesis of many diarrheal disorders. This has led to the development of pharmacologic agents designed to target these specific mechanisms and thereby treat patients with a variety of intestinal diseases. The basic knowledge of Na^+–nutrient cotransport led to the development of a simple yet life-saving oral rehydration solution used in the treatment of cholera worldwide. Discovering the effects of abnormally high VIP levels in patients with VIPoma and the antagonistic effects of somatostatin paved the way for the development of a highly effective synthetic somatostatin preparation for clinical use.

As our understanding of intestinal transport mechanisms increases, new therapies will undoubtedly be developed to combat clinical disease further. From the foregoing examples, it should be obvious that all practicing clinicians need a basic understanding of intestinal transport in health and disease to facilitate the best care for their patients.

CASE STUDY: *RESOLUTION*

In the hospital, the patient experienced up to 5 L diarrhea per day, which persisted despite fasting. Analysis of stool electrolytes and osmolarity suggested the presence of a secretory diarrhea. Serum gastrin levels were normal, but serum VIP level was markedly elevated. Thus, the diagnosis of VIPoma was suspected. An abdominal CT scan revealed a mass in the tail of the pancreas with evidence of liver metastases. A biopsy of the lesion showed microscopic features of an endocrine tumor. Special marker studies confirmed the diagnosis of VIPoma.

The patient was started on subcutaneous somatostatin, with marked improvement in the diarrhea. Because of metastatic disease, the patient was not considered an operative candidate and therefore was treated with chemotherapy. As a result of the somatostatin, the patient experienced improvement of the diarrhea and maintained good quality of life.

REVIEW QUESTIONS

Directions: For each of the following questions, choose the one best answer.

1 A patient with Crohn's disease (regional enteritis) required surgical resection of 50 cm of terminal ileum. Which of the following statements would characterize the expected diarrhea?

A Secretory diarrhea (stool osmolar gap > 50 mOsm/L)
B Secretory diarrhea (stool osmolar gap < 50 mOsm/L)
C Osmotic diarrhea (stool osmolar gap > 50 mOsm/L)
D Osmotic diarrhea (stool osmolar gap < 50 mOsm/L)

2 Which one of the following statements is *true* of intestinal epithelial cells?

A They are characterized by the absence of tight junctions.
B They allow ions to move freely across the apical membrane.
C They demonstrate functional polarity.
D They show similar transport properties throughout the intestinal tract.

3 A patient underwent a urinary bladder resection for a primary bladder cancer. To maintain some urinary control, the surgeons joined the ureters to the sigmoid colon. The patient subsequently developed a hyperchloremic, hypokalemic metabolic acidosis. Which of the following statements explains this finding?

A Excess urinary Na^+ entering the colon leads to excess NaCl absorption.
B Excess urinary Cl^- entering the colon leads to excessive HCO_3^- secretion.
C Excess urinary HCO_3^- leads to net colonic H^+ secretion.

4 A patient with long-standing diabetes mellitus presents with diarrhea. Extensive evaluation fails to uncover a specific cause. The physician suggests that the diarrhea may be related to the patient's diabetes. Which of the following medications should be considered in trying to treat this disorder?

A Somatostatin   **C** Steroids
B Magnesium sulfate **D** Clonidine

5 Which of the following substances stimulates fluid and electrolyte absorption?

A Vasoactive intestinal polypeptide (VIP)
B Prostaglandins
C Somatostatin
D Enterotoxin of *V. cholerae*

6 A patient with ulcerative colitis is admitted to the hospital with severe diarrhea and dehydration. As part of therapy, the physician prescribes glucocorticoids. The following day the patient notes a marked decrease in the diarrhea. Although this may be in part due to the anti-inflammatory effects of the glucocorticoids, some of this effect is likely to be due to

A rehydration with NaCl.
B glucocorticoid inhibition of HCO_3^- secretion.
C stimulation of amiloride-sensitive electrogenic Na^+ absorption in the distal colon.
D stimulation of Na^+ absorption throughout the intestinal tract.

References

Johnson LR: *Gastrointestinal Physiology.* St. Louis, MO: Elsevier Science, Mosby, 2001.

Montrose MH, Keely SJ, Barrett KE: Electrolyte secretion and absorption: small intestine and colon. In *Textbook of Gastroenterology*, 4th ed. Edited by Yamada T, et al. Philadelphia, PA: Lippincott, Williams & Wilkins, 2003, p 308.

Powell DW: Ion and water transport in the intestine. In *Physiology of Membrane Disorders.* Edited by Andreoli TE, Hoffman JF, Fanestil DB, et al. New York, NY: Plenum Press, 1986, p 559.

8

Liver Anatomy and Physiology

▓ CHAPTER OUTLINE ▓

▓ LEARNING OBJECTIVES ▓

At the completion of this chapter, the reader should be able to:

- Describe important gross anatomic features of the liver, gallbladder, and biliary drainage system.
- Describe the blood flow of the liver, including unique differences with respect to other organs.
- Outline the normal histology of the liver in terms of physiologic units.
- Relate damage to liver histology in common types of hepatic injury.
- Describe the effect of cirrhosis on the normal histology of the liver.
- Describe the embryologic development of the liver.
- Discuss the unique cell types that compose the liver and outline their major functions.

CASE STUDY: *INTRODUCTION*

A 70-year-old man with a history of atherosclerotic cardiovascular disease suffered a myocardial infarction associated with a significant period of profound hypoxia lasting approximately 1 hour. In the recovery period following effective treatment of heart disease, a variety of systemic alterations were noted, including neurologic deficits, renal failure, and hepatic dysfunction. The latter was especially severe, and workup led to a liver biopsy performed 6 days after myocardial infarction (Figure 8-1). Supportive measures including careful dietary guidelines led to recovery of hepatic function.

This patient with severe coronary artery disease had a myocardial infarction with hypoxia suffered ischemic injury to the liver as seen in Figure 8-1. Supportive measures aimed at maintaining blood pressure and good oxygenation and avoiding hepatotoxins led to complete recovery of hepatic function and normalization of liver tests.

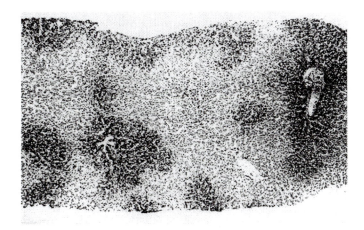

Fig. 8-1. Marked Recent Centrilobular and Midzonal Hepatocellular Necrosis with Preservation of Periportal Liver Parenchyma

The appearance is consistent with marked recent ischemic necrosis.

Introduction

The liver is the largest organ of the body, weighing 1200–1500 g and accounting for 1/50 of total body weight. Its relative size is even greater in infancy, amounting to 1/18 of body weight. The liver is situated in the right upper quadrant and is guarded on all sides by the rib cage, except for a small portion of the anterior surface of the left lobe that occupies part of the epigastrium. The liver often responds to

disease processes by an increase or decrease in size. Assessment of liver size is therefore a useful clinical maneuver in the physical examination; size may be reasonably estimated at bedside by a combination of palpation and percussion. As bedside ultrasound becomes a more ubiquitous tool, it will undoubtedly be used to evaluate the liver. In the normal state, the lower edge is felt on abdominal palpation just beneath the costal ridge in the midclavicular line. The span in the same vertical direction, using percussion of the chest, does not usually exceed 15 cm. Liver volume may be accurately determined by CT scan or magnetic resonance imaging (MRI).

The vascular supply of the liver is unique because of the presence of dual input, consisting of (1) high-pressure, oxygen-rich arterial flow via the hepatic artery and (2) low-pressure, oxygen-poor venous flow from the intestinal tract via the portal vein. Total hepatic blood flow fluctuates during the day according to splanchnic blood flow, with two-thirds derived from the portal circulation and the remainder from the hepatic artery. Separation of blood flow from these two sources is maintained through successive branching of the vascular tree within the liver; the blood flows only mix just prior to contact with individual hepatocytes at the level of the hepatic sinusoids. Elegant three-dimensional reconstructions of hepatic blood flow, using detailed methods to outline the vascular tree, have confirmed the absence of shunts between the hepatic artery and portal vein channels in the normal state. Venous blood from the liver is collected in tributaries of the hepatic veins, which unite to empty into the inferior vena cava.

The liver is responsible for production of bile. Bile is a complex, highly saturated fluid, initially produced by hepatocytes and then modified by selective absorption and secretion by bile duct epithelium, accessory peribiliary glands, and the gallbladder. The resultant bile, rich in cholesterol, phospholipids, and bile salts, enters the duodenum by way of the common bile duct through the ampulla of Vater to mix with intestinal contents, optimizing food absorption in the small bowel.

These anatomic considerations lay the basis for the essential physiologic functions of the liver. This organ has a major synthetic role, producing many proteins vital for use throughout the body. The liver synthesizes bile, which is delivered to the small intestine by an independent pathway of biliary drainage to assist nutrient uptake. It receives intestinal absorption via a low-pressure portal venous system and proceeds to actively modify and detoxify incoming fats, proteins, carbohydrates, minerals, and chemical compounds. To accomplish all of these tasks, it is highly dependent on maintaining the structural integrity of both its microscopic anatomy and cellular organelles and keeping molecular pathways operative within individual hepatocytes. The structure and function of the liver can be adversely affected by a great many disease processes commonly encountered in clinical practice. For these reasons, better understanding of the biologic basis of liver injury remains a central part of the practice of modern medicine.

Basic Embryology

The liver first appears at 3 weeks gestation as a cellular outgrowth of the hepatic diverticulum sprouting from the developing foregut. The histogenesis of the liver originates from three tissue elements: (1) foregut endoderm, producing epithelial-derived parenchymal cells, including hepatocytes and bile ducts; (2) mesenchyme from the septum transversum, contributing vascular and supporting elements, including portal tracts; and (3) mesenchyme of coelom, creating structural support for positioning the organ in the abdominal cavity. The primordial liver begins as budlike cellular clusters from the hepatic diverticulum surrounded by mesenchyme. At 4 weeks gestation, through rapid growth and coalescence of the enlarging buds, there is a thick, anastomotic cellular sheet of hepatocytes organized into rudimentary sinusoids. This rudimentary organization of the liver is referred to as *hepatic muralium*. Progressive remodeling of the liver parenchyma ensues, reducing the masslike growth to two-cell-thick plates at the time of birth. The adult pattern of uniform single-cell plates throughout the entire organ is not reached until 4 years of age.

Vascular flow undergoes extensive change during the transition from fetal development to birth. Blood flow to the liver during gestation is mainly from the oxygen- and nutrient-rich umbilical vein through a major branch, therefrom joining the portal vein. Most umbilical vein blood is diverted through the liver via the ductus venosus and enters the inferior vena cava. During fetal life, hepatic artery and splanchnic blood flow is relatively nutrient- and oxygen-poor and correspondingly small in volume. To achieve the adult pattern, umbilical blood flow ceases, leading to involution of the portal vein component, which becomes the *ligamentum teres* in parallel with involution of the ductus venosus as the *ligamentum venosum* (Figures 8-2 and 8-3).

Notes

Elements in Histogenesis of the Liver
Foregut endoderm
Mesenchyme from septum transversum
Mesenchyme of the coeloma

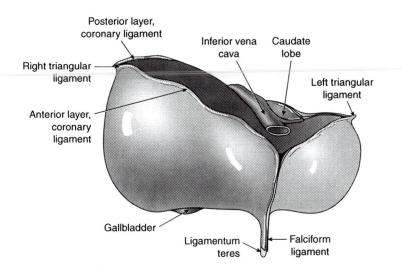

Fig. 8-2. Diaphragmatic Surface of the Liver Showing the Relationships of the Hepatic Ligaments.

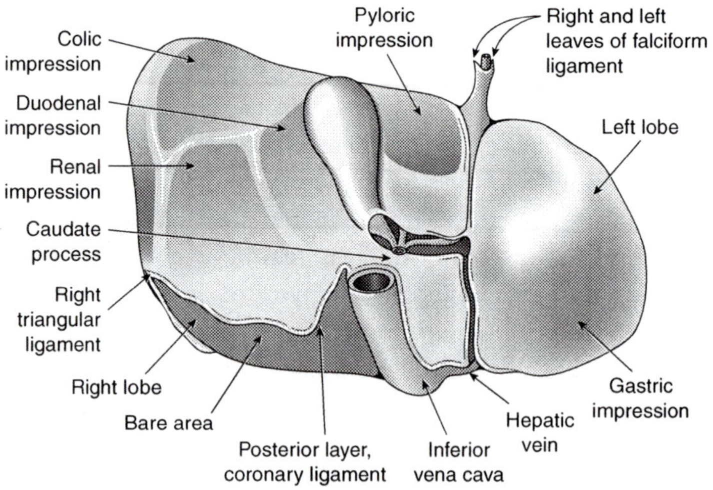

Fig. 8-3. Diagram of the Visceral Surface of the Liver

Notice the *H* pattern made up of the gallbladder, inferior vena cava, lesser omentum and porta, ligamentum teres, and ligamentum venosum

At the same time, hepatic artery and portal vein blood flow via the splanchnic veins dramatically increases.

The liver has important hematopoietic function during fetal development that is first evident at 6 weeks gestation. At 12 weeks, the liver is the major site of hematopoiesis, taking over that function from the yolk sac. After 12 weeks, there is a progressive decline in hematopoietic activity as the bone marrow takes on the function. Nevertheless, hematopoiesis—confined mainly to erythroid production—is present at birth and may still be seen for several weeks thereafter. Bile synthesis by hepatocytes can be demonstrated at 6 weeks gestation; however, bile flow into the small intestine requires an additional 6 weeks before it is achieved. During this time, connections between the hepatocytes and the developing intrahepatic and extrahepatic biliary tree are actively being formed. Production of adult-type bile requires the participation of cellular elements throughout the biliary tree and is not reached until near full term, continuing to develop well after birth. Thus it can be seen that although much liver development occurs early in gestation, many essential aspects of liver function are not attained until after birth.

Gross Anatomic Divisions of the Liver

When examined grossly, the liver demonstrates two major lobes, right and left, accompanied by two lesser segments protruding from the undersurface, designated the caudate and quadrate lobes. These lesser segments appear to arise from the right, contributing to the greater size of the right lobe, which is approximately six times larger in volume than the left lobe. This grossly observed separation of right and

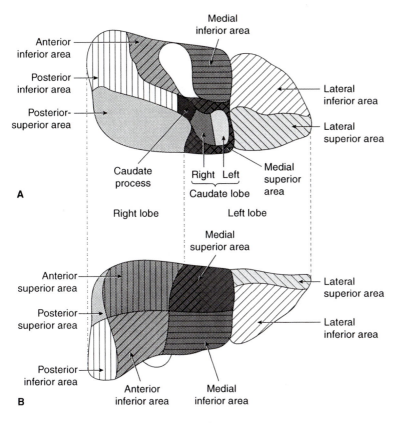

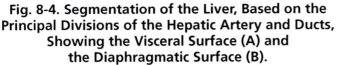

Medial
inferior area

Anterior
inferior area

Posterior
inferior area

Posterior-
superior area

Lateral
inferior area

Lateral
superior area

Caudate
process

Right   Left

Caudate lobe

Medial
superior
area

Right lobe

Left lobe

Medial
superior area

Anterior
superior area

Lateral
superior area

Posterior
superior area

Lateral
inferior area

Posterior
inferior area

Anterior
inferior area

Medial
inferior area

A

B

**Fig. 8-4. Segmentation of the Liver, Based on the
Principal Divisions of the Hepatic Artery and Ducts,
Showing the Visceral Surface (A) and
the Diaphragmatic Surface (B).**

left lobes is demarcated by (1) the falciform ligament, a fold of peritoneum, on the anterior surface; (2) the ligamentum venosum on the posterior surface; and (3) the fissure of the ligamentum teres inferiorly (see Figures 8-2 and 8-3). The division of liver into demarcated lobes is, however, artificial and not in keeping with the branching hierarchy of vascular supply and biliary drainage of the organ.

A more functional division of liver anatomy, consistent with vascular perfusion and bile drainage, recognizes two more equally sized lobes divided in the midline vertical plane (Figure 8-4). Using gross landmarks to demarcate this functional subdivision, the line between the right and left lobes is seen to run from the inferior vena cava posteriorly to the gallbladder anteriorly. Both caudate and quadrate lobes now become part of the left lobe of liver, leading to a more equal division of the total liver mass. Each lobe may be subdivided first into medial and lateral sectors and each sector then further subdivided into anterior and posterior subsectors. Although this topographic sectioning of the liver correlates better with vascular and biliary flow, it should be recognized that no connective tissue demarcations exist to mark territorial boundaries. Nevertheless, this approach is useful in the surgical resection of individual segments of the liver.

Notes

Functions of Hepatocytes
Molecular synthesis
Carbohydrate and fat metabolism
Blood detoxification
Initial bile formation

The anatomic variations that may affect the basic gross appearance of the liver should also be noted. A *Riedel's lobe*, which consists of a downward, tonguelike projection of liver tissue from the right lobe, may be encountered. This finding is not uncommon and is more frequently seen in women. It is important to recognize a Riedel's lobe so that it is not construed as a tumor mass or ectopic kidney. *Accessory lobes* represent connective tissue–demarcated individual liver segments present as part of an otherwise normal liver or separate from a main organ. Accessory lobes, which are uncommon, may be aberrantly placed and possess an independent blood supply and bile duct.

Liver Histology

CELLULAR ELEMENTS

The liver is constituted from five basic cell types that interact both anatomically and physiologically to perform the diverse functions of this organ. Although the bulk of liver is composed of hepatocytes, participation by and communication among all cells by paracrine signaling mechanisms are fundamental to normal function of the organ.

Hepatocytes

Hepatocytes account for 60% of total adult liver mass and are primarily responsible for molecular synthesis, carbohydrate and fat metabolism, blood detoxification, and initial bile formation. They are arranged in single-cell-thick plates and lack basement membranes, enabling them to be in intimate contact with the circulation. Hepatocytes have a polygonal shape, being 30–40 μm in greatest dimension. In most cells there is a single round nucleus in the center with a prominent nucleolus. Occasional binucleated cells may be found. The hepatocyte cytoplasm is slightly basophilic in color and granular in texture when viewed with standard hematoxylin-eosin staining after formaldehyde fixation. The polygonal cell shape with central round nucleus and prominent nucleous imparts a liverlike quality that is characteristic of this type of cell.

Hepatocytes are spacially polarized, with three functional surfaces. The largest surface, occupying 70% of total hepatocyte surface area, is the *basolateral region*, which is positioned to interact with sinusoidal fluid. The basolateral surface manifests abundant basal plasma cell infoldings associated with numerous secretory vacuoles, consistent with strong absorptive and secretory activity. Synthesized proteins and repackaged lipids are directed into the circulation by the basolateral surface. The second polarized surface is the *canalicular surface* located directly opposite the basolateral region. Bile produced in the hepatocyte cytoplasm is actively secreted into canaliculi, which are spaces created by the apposition of adjacent hepatocytes. The canaliculi manifest plasma surface microvilli and are supported by tight junctions, which define points of attachment between adjacent hepatocytes. The third surface is the *lateral surface*. Its hallmark is prominent intercellular junctions of various types, including gap junctions, tight junctions, and desmosomes, designed to facilitate intercellular communication between hepatocytes.

In keeping with their strong synthetic function, hepatocytes possess abundant smooth and rough endoplasmic reticulum (RER), free ribosomes, and Golgi organs. The RER and free ribosomes are primary centers for production of proteins, which include albumin, α_1-antitrypsin, lipid-associated proteins, and coagulation pathway factors, to name just a few. Hepatocytes possess large quantities of glycogen, which are stored as an immediate source of glucose and potential energy. The cytoplasm contains numerous membrane-bound vesicles, reflecting both absorptive and secretory activity. As part of the detoxification function, hepatocytes possess numerous lysosomal vesicles, including hydrogen peroxide–containing *peroxisomes* used to mediate intracellular organelle breakdown and chemical detoxification. Also, lipid droplets are frequently present and may coalesce to sufficient size to be visible on light microscopy as pale vacuoles of varying size. Final, a variety of intracellular filaments and microtubules are present within hepatocytes. The most prominent are situated beneath the canalicular membrane and possess contractile properties designed to massage bile down the canaliculi in the direction of biliary excretion. To support this large array of metabolic and subcellular organelle activity, the hepatocytes contain abundant mitochondria for energy production.

Bile Duct Cells

Bile duct cells line the full length of the intrahepatic and extrahepatic biliary tree. They not only serve as a channel lining to conduct bile but actively modulate the composition of bile and physically propel it in the direction of the small intestine. Numerous microvilli and secretory vesicles at the apical surface in contact with the bile stream attest to the intimate interaction between bile duct epithelium and biliary fluid. Tight junctions between adjacent cells, supported by intermediate filaments, provide the basis for a strong cellular tube system for conducting bile. The smallest branches of the biliary tree receive the drainage of the bile canaliculi and are referred to by a variety of names, including ductule, cholangiole, and *canals of Hering*. Ductular bile cells are cuboid in shape and relatively small. As bile drains into progressively larger bile duct branches, the biliary epithelial cells become columnar and progressively larger in size. Bile duct cells are primarily responsible for the addition of mucin to the bile.

Endothelial Cells

Hepatocytes are arranged in a broad array of one-cell-thick plates covered by endothelial cells. More specifically, endothelial cells are interposed between flowing blood and hepatocytes in such a way as to create a space referred to as the space of Disse. Thus, hepatocytes do not directly contact blood but instead interact with a filtrate of

Kupffer's cells are fixed tissue macrophages in the liver and constitute an important element of the reticuloendothelial system.

blood created by the liver endothelial cells. Certain cellular features distinguish hepatic endothelial cells from those in the rest of the body. Liver endothelial cells possess more holes, known as fenestrae, and manifest prominent endocytotic vacuoles. Also, liver endothelial cells lack basement membranes in many areas. These features permit a greater capacity for contact between hepatocyte and noncellular elements of blood. Additionally, endothelial cells possess an immunological function. They may function as antigen-presenting cells (APCs) in the context of both MHC-I and MHC-II restriction, resulting in the development of antigen-specific T cell tolerance. They secrete cytokines, eicosanoids (such as prostanoid and leukotrienes), endothelin-1, nitric oxide, and some components of the extracellular matrix.

Perisinusoidal Cells

Perisinusoidal cells in the normal state are indistinct, being scattered between the endothelial cells and hepatocytes in the spaces of Disse. They have been referred to by a variety of terms including Ito cells, stellate cells, and fat-storing cells. They are better seen using sections 1 μm thick or by electron microscopy, where they are seen to contain lipid vacuoles. Cell processes extend around endothelial cells in a fashion that suggests they may control capillary size and cross-sectional diameter. Much remains to be learned of their biologic functions; however, studies support a role in lipid and vitamin A metabolism, control of vascular flow and permeability, production of extracellular membrane proteins, and liver regeneration. They are key players in the development of hepatic fibrosis, the precursor of cirrhosis. Acute hepatocellular damage leads to transformation of quiescent stellate cells into myofibroblastlike cells that play a critical role in the development of the inflammatory fibrotic response.

Kupffer's Cells

Kupffer's cells occupy a position within the liver sinusoids, being situated internal to the endothelial cells. Their location in direct contact with hepatic blood flow renders them ideally positioned for phagocytic activity of bloodborne products delivered to the liver. Normally small and inconspicuous in the resting liver, they undergo enlargement and proliferation in response to an insult to the organ mediated through the bloodstream, such as viral hepatitis. Kupffer's cells are fixed tissue macrophages residing in the liver and constituting an important element of the host reticuloendothelial system. They modulate immune responses via antigen presentation, suppression of T cell activation by antigen-presenting sinusoidal endothelial cells, and participate in the development of oral tolerance to bacterial superantigens. In addition to their role in immune response, Kupffer's cells have been shown to release and respond to paracrine signaling molecules and play an important role in maintaining overall liver size.

Additional Cellular Elements

In addition to the cells just described, the liver contains other cellular elements. Liver-associated lymphocytes represent a resident population of lymphocytes contributing to the hepatic immune response. Nerve cells, primarily arising from the celiac sympathetic ganglion, distribute fibers through the liver.

Extracellular Matrix of the Liver

The extracellular matrix of the liver is relatively small compared to that of other organs. In the normal state, it accounts for only 5%–10% of total hepatic weight. The extracellular matrix assumes greater importance in disease states, when it is responsible for production of excessive connective tissue, resulting in the gross appearance of cirrhosis. The greatest amount of extracellular material in the normal state is found in the capsule of the liver, referred to as *Glisson's capsule*. The next largest concentration of extracellular matrix is in the portal tracts, where it surrounds vascular, biliary, and lymphatic channels. A variety of extracellular matrix proteins may be found in the liver. Collagens represent the largest groups of protein, with types I and III collagens accounting for over 95% of all proteins. Glycoproteins, including laminin and fibronectin, as well as proteoglycans (such as heparan sulfate) contribute to the normal extracellular matrix of the liver. In addition to its essential structural role, the extracellular matrix participates in intercellular communication and growth homeostasis.

CELLULAR ORGANIZATION

Hepatic Sinusoids and the Spaces of Disse

As discussed, hepatocytes do not directly contact blood flowing through the liver. Instead, a loose barrier of endothelial cells exists, creating narrow spaces between the external surface of the endothelial cells and the basolateral region of the hepatocytes. These spaces are referred to as the *spaces of Disse* and normally contain a transudate high in plasma proteins and similar in composition to that of plasma as a result of the high porosity of liver endothelial cells. From the spaces of Disse hepatocytes remove absorbed food material, such as proteins, amino acids, lipids, sugars, and other biomolecules, and into the same spaces synthetic molecules (such as proteins and lipids) are released. The size of the spaces can be controlled by perisinusoidal cells. Obliteration of the spaces of Disse occurs in several disease processes, including alcoholic liver disease and sickle-cell anemia.

Portal Tracts

The *portal tracts*, also known as *portal triads*, are distinguishing microscopic features of liver consisting of branches of the portal vein, bile duct, and hepatic artery, supported by a small amount of loose connective tissue. They are bounded by hepatocytes at their periphery, which exist in a well-defined single row referred to as the *limiting*

Hepatic triads consist of branches of the portal vein, bile duct, and hepatic artery.

plate. Also running in the portal tracts are branches of nerve fibers and lymphatics. There exists a close size relationship between each of the elements within the portal tracts so that the larger portal tracts contain more proximal branches of the portal vein, hepatic artery, and bile duct, whereas smaller tracts carry smaller, more peripheral branches of these entities. Portal tracts are primarily responsible for bringing blood to the liver and carrying bile away from it.

Portal tracts undergo a complex embryologic development during the stage of hepatic muralium. The presence of mesenchyme surrounding vascular channels, destined to become the portal venous and hepatic arterial system, induces the conversion of limiting plate hepatocytes in the muralium to become a two-cell layer of bile duct epithelial cells. Over time, the bilayered biliary epithelium organizes into bile duct–like structures containing lumina. Some of these "ductular hepatocytes" remain as the canals of Hering, receiving the drainage directly from the bile canaliculi. Other ductular hepatocytes evolve into bile ducts and invade the mesenchyme surrounding the vascular structures of the developing portal tracts. Through a process of involution, many of the primordial bile ducts atrophy and disappear, leaving behind a tubular structure destined to become the single bile duct of that portal tract. This process of ductal plate remodeling occurs actively during mid- to late gestation and may even continue after birth. Disorders that lead to failed remodeling, referred to as ductal plate malformations, may produce a range of biliary alterations including disease states known as congenital hepatic fibrosis and polycystic liver disease.

The liver possesses a rich lymphatic drainage designed to remove excess fluid collected in the spaces of Disse. At the periphery of the portal tracts, small lymphatics take up the excess fluid in the spaces of Disse and channel it into progressively larger lymphatics, running primarily in the portal tracts. Hepatic lymph is very high in protein, reflecting the plasma filtrate normally found in the spaces of Disse. Hepatic lymph also contains abundant cells, including perisinusoidal cells and liver-associated lymphocytes, which travel in the thoracic duct. Hepatic lymph accounts for 15%–20% of total lymph and constitutes most of the lymph flowing in the thoracic duct.

Liver Lobule

In 1933, Kiernan defined the spatial organization of liver cells in relationship to blood flow in the form of a classic *liver lobule.* In the center of the lobule was the smallest branch of the hepatic vein, collecting blood that had traversed through the sinusoids. The portal tracts were situated at the periphery of the lobule. Hepatic vein and portal vascular supply were envisioned as extensive tunnels distributed throughout the liver, oriented perpendicular to one another and never directly connected. Between these vascular systems were liver cells distributed in one-cell-thick plates, receiving blood in one direction and moving bile in the other. The liver lobule with its centrally placed hepatic vein

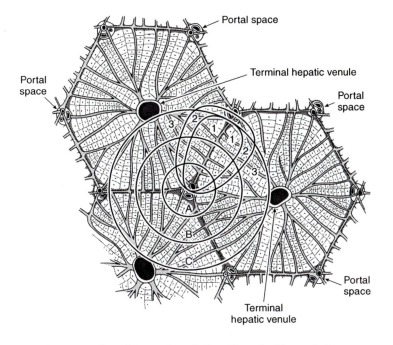

Portal space

Portal space

Terminal hepatic venule

Portal space

Portal space

Terminal hepatic venule

Fig. 8-5. Blood Supply of the Simple Liver Acinus

The oxygen tension and the nutrient level of the blood in the sinusoids decrease from zone 1 through zone 3. Zones 1', 2', and 3' indicate corresponding volumes in a portion of an adjacent acinar unit. Circle A encloses the area commonly designated as periportal; B and C represent the areas more peripheral to the portal space.

Notes

The **acinus,** now thought to be the basic liver unit, consists of parenchymal liver cells grouped into three zones surrounding terminal vessels.

branch was thus defined as the fundamental functioning unit of the liver, organized to carry out all physiologic activity.

Liver Acinus

In 1954, Rappaport reexamined the structural organization of the liver with an emphasis on disease-related tissue alterations (Figure 8-5). In this initial article and through a series of supplementary reports, he redefined the basic structural functionality of the liver in terms of the *liver acinus.* The liver acinus is centered on the portal tract, reflecting the directionality of blood flow into the liver. The liver acinus then defines hepatic parenchyma in a topographic distribution around the portal tract. Three zones of hepatic parenchyma are recognized, reflecting relative oxygenation. Zone 1 is oxygen-rich because of its proximity to the portal blood supply. Zone 3, in contrast, is oxygen-poor because it is farther away from distribution of the portal blood flow. Zone 2 is intermediate in position. This microcirculatory acinus concept proved a better model in correlation with disease processes, predicting greater relative sensitivity in zone 3 as a result of a comparatively more vulnerable blood supply. The validity of the Rappaport model is supported by the pattern of liver damage in ischemia, viral hepatitis, and toxic injury, which is mainly zone 3 in distribution.

Since the pioneering work of Rappaport, the microcirculatory acinus model has been refined by Latimer and others to provide even better correlation with histologic patterns of injury. The present concept of a metabolic acinus has emerged, and it appears to serve best as the basic functioning unit of the liver—that is, the smallest amount of tissue subserving organ functions whose blood supply is provided by terminal vessels. Rappaport's refined model recognizes three zones of liver parenchyma: (1) a periportal zone that is relatively rich in oxygen and closest in position to vascular inflow, (2) a midzone situated equidistant from portal tract and terminal hepatic venule, and (3) a centrilobular zone that is relatively oxygen-poor and especially vulnerable to a variety of disease processes.

CASE STUDY: *CONTINUED*

The clinical case highlights the utility of the acinus concept. The patient suffered an episode of ischemic injury sufficient to cause liver failure. The liver biopsy revealed extensive centrilobular and midzonal hepatic necrosis consistent with vulnerability of these regions to a decline in tissue oxygenation. Only periportal hepatocytes were preserved, consistent with the acinus concept. It is interesting that despite extensive necrosis, the preserved periportal hepatocytes were capable of dramatic regeneration.

Functional Heterogeneity of the Liver

There is evidence that zonal distributions of hepatocytes are morphologically, physiologically, and biochemically distinct. The differences are sharpest between periportal and centrilobular hepatocytes and are outlined in Table 8-1. It is recognized that zone designation across the

Table 8-1. Zonal Differences in Hepatocytes

DISTINCTIONS	PERIPORTAL	CENTRILOBULAR
Morphologic	Smaller cell size and branching hepatic plates	Larger cell size and nonbranching parallel plates
Physiologic	Drug detoxification and urea formation from amino acids	Ammonia detoxification, urea formation from ammonia, bile formation, and glucose using (glycogenolysis)
Biochemical	Glucose forming (gluconeogenesis), fatty acid oxidation, citric acid cycle, and respiratory chain	
Pathologic	Immunologic injury—chronic active hepatitis	Ischemic injury, drug toxicity, alcoholic injury, and viral hepatitis

hepatic sinusoids is in reality a gradient and that differences are only relative in degree. Nevertheless, the value of the acinar concept is that it has done much to explain the distribution of many disease processes, which may in turn be used to infer the etiologic nature of liver injury in patients presenting with hepatic dysfunction of unknown origin.

Liver Regeneration

The liver is an organ of *conditional renewal*. Hepatocytes are relatively long-lived, with an average life span of about 120 days but a capability of survival for many months and possibly years. Under normal conditions, only a small fraction of hepatocytes traverse the cell cycle in active proliferation. Notwithstanding this low rate of cell turnover, hepatocytes can undergo dramatic proliferation in response to injury and cell loss. The same holds true for bile duct epithelial cells. Hence the designation of the liver as an organ of conditional renewal.

Liver cells manifest both adaptive hyperplasia and hypertrophy. The latter refers to an increase in individual cell size resulting from an increase in cytoplasmic organelles. This change is best seen in the context of drug toxification, where prominent enlargement of hepatocytes reflects proliferation of smooth endoplasmic reticulum designed to increase chemical biotransformation. Adaptive hyperplasia may be seen when there is an increase in functional demand, as occurs in a variety of metabolic alterations involving carbohydrate and lipid metabolism. The mechanisms to stimulate liver cell hypertrophy and proliferation are unclear but are known to involve growth regulatory genes including c-*fos*, c-*jun*, c-*myc*, and inducible nitric oxide synthase, as well as cytokines such as epidermal growth factor, tumor necrosis factor, interleukin-6, and TGF-α and -β. Although cell proliferation in the liver can be dramatic, it should be noted that proliferating cells cannot reconstitute the normal architecture of the liver that may have been lost as a result of tissue damage. This fundamental fact explains the nodular pattern of cirrhosis, which reflects cell proliferation without proper cellular alignment and architectural integrity.

Cell death in the liver is characterized by cell shrinking, cytoplasmic condensation, nuclear loss, and eventual disappearance of individual hepatocytes as they fall into the hepatic sinusoids and are carried away by flowing blood. This process of cellular degeneration is referred to as *apoptosis*. Apoptosis is not a passive process but is in fact quite active under the control of a variety of growth regulatory genes. Furthermore, the topographic pattern of apoptosis is not random but likely occurs more frequently in the centrilobular zone 3 hepatocytes, which are relatively more vulnerable because of their poorer blood supply. This has given rise to a theory of "streaming liver cells," in which hepatocytes proliferating in the periportal regions are caused to slide down the hepatic plate toward the centrilobular regions, where they ultimately die and are carried away. Although the streaming liver cells concept is spatially attractive, full proof awaits further documentation and scientific support.

The Aging Liver

The total mass of the liver is seen to vary inversely with age so that by age 90, approximately two-thirds of hepatic mass is lost. The aging liver also becomes darker in color, which can be attributed to the cytoplasmic accumulation of lipofuscin pigment. Lipofuscin represents a wear-and-tear product within the cell derived from effete cell membranes that are no longer capable of being broken down within lysosomes. In certain lysosomal enzyme disorders, lipofuscin accumulation is enhanced, with prominent accumulation at younger ages. A variety of other cellular alterations have been associated with advancing age, including fat accumulation, cell shrinkage, and nuclear shape alterations.

Extrahepatic Biliary Tree and Gallbladder

Biliary drainage begins at the hepatocyte with movement across the canalicular membrane of the cell into the bile canaliculus. Movement of bile toward portal tracts is first along bile canaliculi and then via canals of Hering into interlobular bile ducts. The latter are situated in a central position in the portal tract. Proceeding in a centripetal direction toward the hilum of the liver, bile is collected into progressively larger bile ducts until drainage into the major right and left hepatic bile ducts takes place. As a rough guide, interlobular bile ducts less than 100 μm in diameter are known as small; those approximately 100 μm in diameter are designated medium-sized; and those larger than 100 μm are called large bile ducts.

The right and left hepatic ducts usually join to form the common bile duct at a position outside the liver. The common duct proceeds toward the duodenum, giving rise to a major branch called the cystic duct, which connects to the gallbladder. The common duct enters the pancreas obliquely, where it unites with the main pancreatic duct to form the ampulla of Vater. In approximately 10%–15% of people, the common duct and main pancreatic duct exist as independent conduits and fail to unite, an anatomic variation referred to as pancreas divisum. The mucosa of the ampulla of Vater protrudes into the duodenum as the duodenal papilla. The latter serves as an easily recognizable landmark for endoscopic cannulation of the pancreaticobiliary tree.

The gallbladder is a pear-shaped sac with an approximate capacity of 50 ml. It usually is loosely attached to the undersurface of the liver; however, this may vary from individual to individual. There may be virtually no connection, resulting in a freely mobile gallbladder that may extend into the right lower quadrant. Alternatively, the gallbladder may be entirely buried within the substance of the liver. The gallbladder may be divided into three zones. The zone closest to the cystic duct is referred to as Hartmann's pouch, which may join the cystic duct in a tortuous manner at the neck of the gallbladder. The narrowing and tortuosity of drainage of the gallbladder accounts for the impaction of gallstones in Hartmann's pouch. The middle zone is referred to as the body of the gallbladder. The distal region is called the fundus of the gallbladder.

The extrahepatic biliary tree and gallbladder share a similar microscopic anatomy, consisting of a fibromuscular wall lined by mucin-producing columnar epithelium similar to that seen in the intrahepatic bile ducts. Present beneath the surface epithelial layer and organized into small acinar units are peribiliary glands with connecting ducts. The peribiliary glands provide additional mucin to the bile, supplementing that derived from the bile duct lining cells. The mucosa of the gallbladder is noted for outpouchings of surface mucosa, which extend into and through the muscular fibers constituting the wall. These outpouchings are called Rokitansky-Aschoff sinuses.

Liver Biopsy

Obtaining a piece of liver tissue and examining it by microscopic analysis represents one of the most useful methods for identifying the cause of liver disease, assessing severity of injury, and predicting the effectiveness of specific treatments. In clinical practice, this is commonly done by inserting a needle through the abdominal wall into the liver and removing a representative core of tissue for histologic analysis. The procedure is not without attendant risks; however, the information obtained greatly outweighs the small hazards of the biopsy. The tissue is fixed in formaldehyde, sectioned at 3–4 μm, and subjected to a series of histologic stains including hematoxylin-eosin, periodic acid–Schiff (with and without diastase), reticulin, and trichrome stains. There are other methods for obtaining a liver biopsy with laparoscopic assistance; in some cases where bleeding may be of higher concern, a biopsy of the liver may be obtained by the interventional radiologist via the jugular vein.

Using hematoxylin-eosin as a routine screening stain, the liver tissue is examined for architectural integrity. Portal tracts, hepatic sinusoids, and hepatic vein branches are examined and their spatial relationship to each other evaluated. In the process, the liver acinus is evaluated for its presence, size, shape, and cellular content. Following this, a more detailed examination of the liver is done, still using the routine hematoxylin-eosin stain. The portal tracts are evaluated for the presence and number of portal vein, hepatic artery, and bile duct branches. The liver plates are assessed for number-of-cells thickness, and the hepatic vein branches are assessed for patency and structural alterations. Individual hepatocytes are carefully examined for their morphologic preservation, color, and histologic characteristics. Routine stain analysis is completed by searching for excessive numbers of Kupffer's cells and other inflammatory cells, the presence of cancer cells arising in the liver or seeded into the liver by metastasis, and the presence of any foreign material.

Special stains may then be reviewed. The reticulin stain, outlining the delicate extracellular material associated with endothelial cells,

Microscopic anatomy of the extrahepatic biliary tree and gallbladder is similar and resembles that of intrahepatic ducts.

provides a sensitive means to detect collapse of parenchyma, which may arise from tissue loss or changes in architectural orientation of the liver cells. The trichrome stain positively highlights collagen, which may support the presence of cirrhotic changes. The periodic acid–Schiff (with and without diastase) is an excellent way to pick up early hepatocyte degeneration, highlighted by the positive staining of collapsed and dying liver cells. These stains may in turn be supported by more specialized histologic stains designed to show positively specific cellular alterations. These include (1) Prussian blue to show excessive iron accumulation, (2) rhodamine to show excessive copper accumulation, and (3) orcein to detect the surface coat protein accumulation of hepatitis B virus, to name just a few. Even in cases where disease etiology remains unclear after microscopic examination, the changes present in the liver biopsy tissue may serve as a baseline to assess histologic progression seen in future liver biopsy specimens.

CASE STUDY: *RESOLUTION*

The clinical case highlights the utility of the acinus concept. The mechanism of liver injury was ischemia, which preferentially damages the centrilobular zones of the hepatic parenchyma related to relatively poorer oxygenation. As can be seen in the biopsy, the brunt of the ischemic necrosis is evident in the centrilobular regions. In fact, the degree of ischemic injury involved the midzonal portions of the liver parenchyma as well. Only the periportal hepatocytes were preserved fully, which is consistent with the acinus concept. Despite the extensive degree of hepatocellular injury, the patient made a full recovery largely because of the abundant regenerative capacity of the remaining periportal hepatocytes. Although functional recovery was complete, it is quite reasonable that the liver was left with varying degrees of scarring affecting areas that underwent necrosis of the entire acinus. It is fortunate that the liver has a large functional reserve, enabling the patient to suffer little or no permanent functional deficit.

REVIEW QUESTIONS

Directions: For each of the following questions, choose the one best answer.

1 Under normal circumstances, the direction of bile flow is *best* described by which one of the following pathways?

   A Hepatic artery via endothelial cells into the spaces of Disse

   B Hepatocytes via canaliculi toward portal tracts

C Kupffer's cells via bile ducts to ligamentum teres
D Enterochromaffin cells via crypts of Lieberkühn to gallbladder

2 Which one of the following subcellular organelles is primarily responsible for drug detoxification?

A Nucleus   **C** Mitochondria
B Golgi apparatus   **D** Peroxisomes

3 How many cells thick are liver cell plates in the normal adult?

A 1–2   **D** 10–20
B 3–4   **E** approximately 100
C 5–6

4 Which one of the following statements concerning hepatic artery blood flow and portal vein blood flow is *true*?

A Intravascular pressure is approximately equal.
B Oxygen saturation is approximately equivalent.
C Both enter the hepatic parenchyma via portal tracts.
D Only hepatic artery blood flow proceeds to bile formation.

5 Which one of the following statements is *true*?

A The concept of a liver acinus as outlined by Rappaport, though useful conceptually, is theoretical and unrelated to physiologic activities of the liver.
B All blood supplying the liver is venous in type with low oxygen saturation.
C In cirrhosis, the normal anatomy and histology of the liver are preserved.
D Hepatocytes, bile duct epithelial cells, and Kupffer's cells are all capable of regeneration.

6 Liver damage resulting from hypoxia most commonly affects which one of the following sites?

A Hepatocytes situated adjacent to the portal tract (limiting plate)
B Bile duct epithelial cells positioned next to the central vein branch
C Kupffer's cells in the midzone between central vein and portal tract
D Hepatocytes situated around the central vein branch
E Hepatocytes present in a subcapsular location

7 Which one of the following statements about the gallbladder is *true*?

A Its blood is supplied via branches from the portal vein.
B It is the main site where free water is added to bile.

C It is the most common site for stone formation.
D It is designed to trap debris emanating from the liver.

8 Which of the following is found in the center of the linear acinus?

A Common bile duct
B Ampulla of Vater
C Portal tract
D Ligamentum teres

References

Jones AL: Anatomy of the normal liver. In *Hepatology: A Textbook of Liver Disease*, 3rd ed. Edited by Zakim D, Boyer TD. Philadelphia, PA: W. B. Saunders, 1996, pp 3–31.

Jones AL, Labreque DR: Morphology of the liver. In *Diseases of the Liver and Biliary Tract*. Edited by Gitnick G, Labreque DR, Moody FG. St. Louis, MO: Mosby Year Book, 1992, pp 7–24.

Klatskin G: *Histopathology of the Liver.* New York: Oxford University Press, 1993, pp 3–18.

Kmiec Z. Cooperation of liver cells in health and disease. *Adv Anat Embryol Cell Biol.* 2001;161:III–XIII,1–151.

Koniaris LG, McKillop IH, Zimmers TA. Liver regeneration. *J Am Col Surg.* 2003; 197(4),634–657.

Rappaport AM, Borowy ZI, Lotto WN: *Anat Rec* 119:11, 1954.

Rappaport AM, Wanless IR: Physioanatomic considerations. In *Diseases of the Liver*, 7th ed. Edited by Schiff L. Philadelphia, PA: J. B. Lippincott, 1993, pp 1–41.

Sherlock S: Clinical examination of the liver and biliary system. In *A Colour Atlas of Liver Disease*, 2nd ed. St. Louis, MO: Mosby Year Book, 1991, pp 9–34.

9

Liver Metabolism, Physiology of Bile Formation, and Gallstones

▧ CHAPTER OUTLINE ▧

▧ LEARNING OBJECTIVES ▧

At the completion of this chapter, the reader should be able to:
- Review pathways of carbohydrate, amino acid, and ammonia (NH_3) metabolism.
- Review fat and cholesterol metabolism.
- Discuss the role of the liver in protein synthesis and degradation.
- Outline detoxification mechanisms of the liver.
- Review the role of the liver in hormone metabolism.
- Review pathways of fat, cholesterol, and bile acid metabolism.
- Describe the origins, major components, and functions of bile.
- Outline mechanisms of bile secretion.
- Discuss the role of the enterohepatic circulation.
- Describe briefly the anatomy and physiology of the biliary tract.
- Define factors involved in gallstone formation.

Metabolism, interconversion, and disposal of biologic substances are critical functions of the liver.

Amino acids are the major fuel for the liver.

CASE STUDY: *INTRODUCTION*

Mr. W., a healthy 45-year-old engineer, made an appointment for a complete physical, because he had not had a physical examination in several years. The physician's office requested that he have a routine blood analysis prior to his visit. His blood work showed nothing unusual except for elevations in alanine aminotransferase (ALT, 135 U/L, which is more than 3 times normal) and in serum aspartate aminotransferase (AST, 85 U/L, which is more than 2.5 times normal). Physical examination was unremarkable except for a body weight 20% above normal recommendations. He claimed that he was very busy and in a high-pressure situation at work and did not always have time to eat anything other than fast food. Because of his work situation, he did not have the time or energy to participate in regular exercise. He felt well, except for being tired a lot, and had not had any unexplained illness. He denied risk factors for hepatitis and admitted to drinking alcohol socially. His hepatitis screen was negative. Further testing showed normal levels for fasting glucose, albumin, alkaline phosphatase, bilirubin, serum iron, ceruloplasmin, α_1-antitrypsin, and thyroid hormone, but no change in his ALT and AST values after 6 months. His fasting triglyceride level was 350 mg/dl, and his cholestrol was 195 mg/dl. Antinuclear antibodies were absent.

Mechanisms of Normal Hepatic Metabolism

The liver plays a central role in the metabolism and interconversion of biologic substances. After digestion, the liver has exposure to all nutrients delivered from the intestines. It may use, store, repackage, and/or deliver theses nutrients to peripheral tissues. Because of the sensitivity of hepatic metabolic pathways to hormones, the liver can respond quickly to provide energy-producing biochemicals as needed. The liver also plays a crucial role in detoxifying xenobiotics and waste products resulting from normal metabolism. Furthermore, biliary excretion plays a unique and critical role in eliminating lipophilic substances, such as drugs, bilirubin, and cholesterol, from the body.

CARBOHYDRATE METABOLISM

When considering hepatic carbohydrate metabolism, think *glucose!* The liver plays a central role in glucose homeostasis, as outlined in Figure 9-1. The hepatocyte has glucokinase, which traps glucose in the cell by phosphorylation. Energy needs in the fed or fasted state and the insulin:glucagon ratio are key factors in the regulation of glucose storage and release.

AMINO ACID AND NH₃ METABOLISM

The liver uses amino acids as fuel to a great extent, as shown in Figure 9-2. To metabolize amino acids for energy, the liver must remove

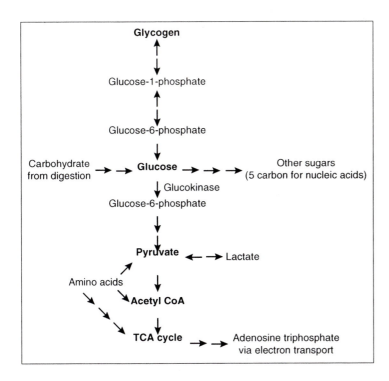

**Fig. 9-1. Overview of Hepatic Carbohydrate
Metabolism**

Hepatic glycogen provides a critical store of glucose for the whole body. The insulin:glucagon ratio regulates glucose storage and release for energy generation. CoA = coenzyme A; TCA cycle = tricarboxylic acid or Krebs cycle.

the amino group by *transamination* reactions in which the amino group is transferred to α-ketoglutarate to create *glutamate*. Two transaminases, ALT (also called serum glutamate pyruvate transaminase or SGPT) and AST (also called serum glutamate oxaloacetate transaminase or SGOT) have particular diagnostic value when appearing in the

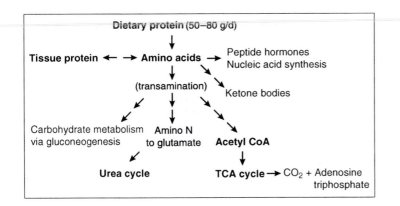

**Fig. 9-2. Overview of Amino Acid Metabolism
in the Liver**

CoA = coenzyme A; TCA cycle = tricarboxylic acid or Krebs cycle.

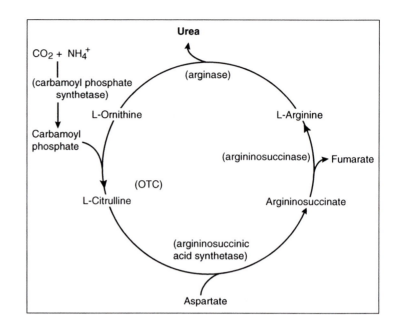

Fig. 9-3. Outline of Hepatic Urea Cycle

NH_4^+ = ammonium ion; OTC = ornithine transcarbamoylase.

serum as a result of hepatocellular damage. A rise in both enzymes suggests liver damage.

Urea Cycle

The use of amino acids as fuel and removal of their amino groups necessitate a mechanism to metabolize or inactivate this potential source of toxic ammonia. The urea cycle, outlined in Figure 9-3, is unique to the liver, because only the liver has arginase. The urea cycle disposes of ammonia and amino groups, which enter the liver as free ammonia in portal blood from the intestine or from glutamate and glutamine. Urea cycle activity accounts for up to 90% of nitrogenous waste in urine. Hyperammonemia may be a result of inborn errors of metabolism or of liver disease.

ROLE OF THE LIVER IN PROTEIN SYNTHESIS AND DEGRADATION

The liver is the site of synthesis of all serum proteins except immunoglobulins, as shown in Table 9-1. These proteins include serum albumin, a major protein for transport and maintenance of osmotic pressure; other proteins are important in transport and defense. The liver also removes most serum proteins and glycoproteins that have been targeted for degradation; removal from the blood is by means of a highly specific cell surface receptor. The liver then transports the protein to the lysosome, where the protein is degraded, and then the liver recycles or metabolizes the liberated amino acids.

ENZYMATIC DETOXIFICATION MECHANISMS OF LIVER

The liver detoxifies many substances, including drugs, environmental pollutants, plant chemicals, and food additives, through a number

Table 9-1. Important Blood Proteins Made by the Liver

Albumin (the major blood protein, about 50%)	Transports fatty acids, steroid hormones, fat-soluble vitamins and drugs, Ca^{2+} ions, and lipophilic substances
Glycoprotein transport proteins	Transcortin (corticosteroid-binding globulin)
	Thyroid-binding globulin
	Sex hormone (testosterone-estradiol)-binding globulin
	Transferrin (iron transport)
Acute phase proteins (acute phase of inflammatory response)	Ceruloplasmin
	α_1-Antitrypsin
	α_1-Acid glycoprotein
	α_2-Macroglobulin
Blood coagulation proteins	Factors I (fibrinogen), II (prothrombin), V, VII, IX, X, XII, XIII

of metabolic strategies. The first step in metabolism of such substances is usually by a so-called phase 1 reaction, in which mixed-function oxidation, reduction, or deacetylase reactions are catalyzed by P-450 enzymes. The polar intermediates formed by the phase 1 reactions are then conjugated to other compounds by the so-called phase 2 reactions, which include sulfation, glucuronidation, acylation, and conjugation with the tripeptide glutathione (Glu-Cys-Gly).

One source of drug toxicity may be metabolites from phase 1 reactions that are possibly highly reactive or toxic intermediates that may not be conjugated immediately. These intermediates may bind to cellular proteins or may oxidize cell components, causing cell injury or death. One important example of such toxicity occurs during the metabolism of acetaminophen. In chronic alcoholics or in normal individuals who are fasting, even normal doses of acetaminophen can be hepatotoxic. Hepatotoxicity of drugs and other chemicals may be intrinsic, dose-related, or idiosyncratic. Idiosyncratic reactions may be due to alternate metabolism of the compound in some individuals or to hypersensitivity reactions caused by the immunogenicity of proteins altered by reactive toxins.

Many factors influence the rate and route of xenobiotic metabolism. Phase 1 reactions are often diminished with age, hypoxia, smoking, acute alcohol ingestion, use of oral contraceptives, and presence of liver disease. Chronic alcohol ingestion appears to increase certain phase 1 reactions, as does the use of a variety of drugs. Phase 2 reactions are less susceptible to such factors. However, fasting may reduce the amount of available glucose for glucuronidation, and several congenital enzymopathies may result in reduced or absent phase 2 enzyme activity.

ROLE OF LIVER IN HORMONE METABOLISM

The liver clears hormones from the circulation, thus permitting the regulation of the amount of available hormone. In severe liver disease, the ability of the liver to clear hormones may be compromised, thus altering the availability and actions of these biologic mediators. *Steroid hormones* are normally metabolized to a more water-soluble and less biologically active form. Reactions are mostly hydroxylations via P-450 enzymes; these hydroxylations are site-specific for the various carbons of the steroid ring. Some enzymes perform reductive functions, that is, reduction of unsaturated steroids. Steroids may also be conjugated to sulfates or glucuronic acid. In several species, metabolism is gender-specific. The liver is also a major site of clearance of a number of *peptide hormones*, such as growth hormone, insulin, glucagon, and so on. Peptide hormones are cleared by a mechanism of protein uptake and then degraded in the lysosome, as noted for other proteins.

PATHWAYS OF LIPID METABOLISM: FATTY ACIDS, TRIGLYCERIDES, CHOLESTEROL, AND BILE ACID SYNTHESIS

The liver regulates the metabolism and interconversion of acetyl coenzyme A (CoA) units to synthesize and degrade fatty acids and synthesize cholesterol and bile acids, as outlined in Figure 9-4. The acetyl CoA units may also be used for energy in situations of glucose depletion. Fat retention in the liver (fatty liver or steatosis) occurs in a number of circumstances, such as with heavy alcohol use, after ingestion of certain drugs (e.g., estrogens) and with obesity. A fatty liver is usually reversible if the cause is removed.

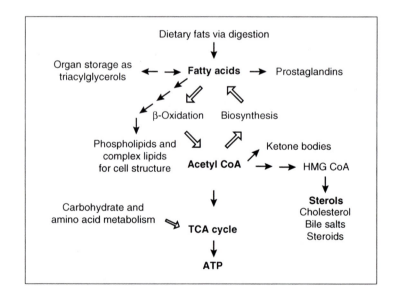

Fig. 9-4. Overview of Fat Metabolism

Open arrows depict complex multistep pathways. CoA = coenzyme A; HMG = 3-hydroxy-3-methylglutaryl; TCA cycle = tricarboxylic acid or Krebs cycle.

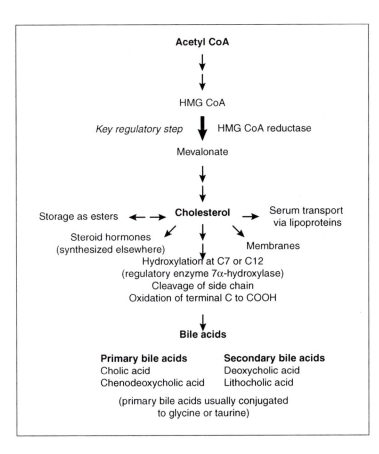

Fig. 9-5. Overview of Cholesterol Metabolism and Bile Acid Synthesis

CoA = coenzyme A; HMG = 3-hydroxy-3-methylglutaryl.

Notes

The reaction catalyzed by HMG CoA reductase is the rate-limiting step in cholesterol synthesis, thus providing a site of action for certain cholesterol-lowering therapeutic agents.

Cholesterol and Bile Acid Synthesis

Acetyl CoA units from fat metabolism are used to synthesize cholesterol and bile acids in the liver. Cholesterol has several fates in the liver: esterification and storage, exportation bound to lipoproteins, and conversion to bile acids, as shown in Figure 9-5. The rate-limiting step in cholesterol synthesis is that which is catalyzed by 3-hydroxy-3-methylglutaryl coenzyme A reductase (HMG CoA reductase). Bile acid synthesis is unique to the liver, and this pathway uses a significant portion of the cholesterol in the liver; this pathway is regulated by the rate-limiting enzyme 7α-hydroxylase. The liver produces primary bile acids and conjugates them to either taurine or glycine. Secondary bile acids are formed by gut bacteria prior to their reuptake by the enterohepatic circulation.

Biliary System

ORIGINS OF BILE

Bile components are synthesized or assembled by the hepatocytes and transported across the hepatocyte to the canalicular membranes,

Notes

Contraction of the gallbladder is regulated by meal-induced release of CCK.

Bilirubin is the most important and prevalent of the bile pigments.

where some are secreted by energy-requiring processes. Because the components of bile are often hydrophobic, they use specialized carriers within the hepatocyte. When the bile acids and the bilirubin enter the hepatocyte from the blood, they bind to specific transport proteins (bile acid–binding proteins and ligandin, respectively) and are individually transported to the endoplasmic reticulum, where each substance undergoes conjugation and bile components are assembled. Bilirubin, because of its toxicity and insolubility, undergoes conjugation with glucuronic acid to form mono- and diglucuronides by the enzyme *bilirubin uridine diphosphate-glucuronosyltransferase* (UDPGT). The diglucuronide form predominates (> 80%) in normal bile.

Bile flow into the canaliculus is promoted by bile acids (*bile acid–dependent flow*) carrying along organic anions in bilirubin and promoting secretion of water as a response to the osmolality of the bile acids. This flow is enhanced by secretin. *Bile acid–independent flow* (so called because a plot of bile salt versus bile flow shows additional bile flow when the bile acid concentration equals zero) is poorly understood but accounts for 30%–50% of flow. Ductular flow is unidirectional because of secretory pressure. As ducts within the biliary tree become larger, flow is enhanced by secretin. In the ducts, water is removed along with sodium chloride (NaCl) (thus concentrating the bile), and bicarbonate (HCO_3^-) is added. Once bile reaches the gallbladder, further concentration occurs. Contraction of the gallbladder is regulated by meal-induced release of cholecystokinin (CCK).

MAJOR COMPONENTS OF BILE

Approximately 500 ml of bile are secreted into the digestive tract each day. Bile is composed of carefully balanced proportions of *bile acids*, *phospholipids*, and *cholesterol*, as noted in Table 9-2. Water makes up about 82% of bile by wet weight. Cholesterol is an extremely hydrophobic molecule, whereas both bile acids and phospholipids are

Table 9-2. Solute Composition of Bile

SUBSTANCE	COMPOSITION (%) BY DRY WEIGHT (TOTAL)
Bile salts	67
Chenodeoxycholates	27
Cholates	23
Deoxycholates	10
Lithocholates	5
Ursodeoxycholates	2
Phospholipids (mainly lecithins)	22
Proteins, glycoproteins	5
Cholesterol	4
Bilirubin	<1
Other substances: electrolytes, amino acids, and peptides	<1

amphipathic molecules, containing both hydrophobic and hydrophilic ends. Thus the combination of these three molecules permits micellar formation, which allows all components to remain in solution. Disruption of this delicate balance may contribute to gallstone formation.

The major primary bile acids in bile, *cholic acid* and *chenodeoxycholic acid*, are synthesized by the liver and secreted directly into bile. The major secondary bile acids, *deoxycholic acid* and *lithocholic acid*, are formed from the primary bile acids by bacterial action in the gut and returned via the enterohepatic circulation to the liver for re-excretion in the bile. Bile acids may also be conjugated to taurine or glycine (e.g., taurocholic acid, glycochenodeoxycholic acid). The predominant phospholipid in bile is *lecithin* (phosphatidylcholine).

Secondary components of bile are *bile pigments* ($< 2\%$ of total solids), with *bilirubin* being the most important and the most prevalent. Bilirubin, a product of heme catabolism, is excreted conjugated to one—or, more often, two—glucuronide molecules to enhance its limited solubility. Bile also contains *inorganic ions* (sodium [Na^+] > potassium [K^+], and calcium [Ca^{2+}]), chloride (Cl^-), and HCO_3^-, with cations more numerous than anions. The "extra" cations are found surrounding the charged bile acid carboxyl (COO^-) groups. Bile also contains a number of hydrophobic compounds, which may be conjugated to glucuronide or sulfate molecules (steroid hormones and metabolites, drugs). Proteins in the bile include *biliary glycoproteins* (mucins), serum proteins including albumin, immunoglobulins, and an array of enzymes.

Hepatic bile and gallbladder bile differ somewhat in composition in normal patients. In general, hepatic bile has a somewhat higher concentration of cholesterol and somewhat lower concentration of bile acid than gallbladder bile. However, the major difference is the concentration of all components, with gallbladder bile more concentrated as a result of action of the gallbladder mucosa in removing water and other solutes. Bile in the gallbladder is also more acidic. Composition of bile is influenced by diurnal variation, length of fasting periods, sex, and hormones, especially estrogens. Alterations in dietary lipids have a significant or modest effect, depending on the species. However, a high-fiber diet may influence the composition by altering the gut metabolism of bile acids and the enterohepatic return of bile acids to the liver.

FUNCTIONS OF BILE

Emulsification of lipids during digestion is a critical role of bile. Enzymes (lipases) digesting triglycerides, the major dietary lipid, are much more active in the presence of bile components, especially the bile acids, as a result of increased solubility, surface area, and accessibility of the substrates. The solubilities of lipophilic products of digestion are also enhanced by bile salts and phospholipids. *Disposal of hydrophobic materials* is another function of bile. Cholesterol is excreted as both the free form and as lithocholic acid. Other substances include bilirubin, hormones and their metabolites, pigments, drugs and their metabolites, and fat-soluble vitamins. Thus the biliary route of excretion is critical, because the hydrophobic natures of these substances prevent their disposal by the urinary route.

ROLE OF THE ENTEROHEPATIC CIRCULATION

Bile acids that have added to and mixed with the digestion products pass through the small intestine, and in the terminal ileum there is a high-affinity uptake system that captures the bile acids and returns them to the liver via the portal vein. The bile acids so returned include the secondary bile acids, which are a product of bacterial deconjugation (removal of taurine and glycine) and dehydroxylation at carbon 7 (C7) of the steroid ring. This process of recapture is called the *enterohepatic circulation*. It is highly efficient, returning 99% of the bile acids to the liver. Only about 1% of bile acids are excreted in the feces.

The basis for treatment of hypercholesteremia with cholestyramine and similar anion-binding resins is that these resins bind bile acids tightly and prevent their reuptake in the enterohepatic circulation. This loss of bile acids forces the liver to convert more cholesterol to bile acids and thus helps rid the body of excess cholesterol. This strategy works best when coupled with a HMG-CoA reductase inhibitor, such as lovastatin.

ANATOMY AND PHYSIOLOGY OF THE BILIARY TRACT

Gross Anatomy

The biliary tract begins with the hepatic canaliculi, progressing to ductules, larger ductules, and interlobular ducts, which turn into two hepatic ducts from the right and left lobes of the liver. These ducts join to become the common hepatic duct. After the cystic duct, which connects the gallbladder, joins the common hepatic duct, the structure is known as the common bile duct. The latter empties into the duodenum and is regulated by the sphincter of Oddi. The most important arterial supply is from the cystic artery, left hepatic artery, and occasionally the right hepatic artery. It should be noted that both the ductular system and the arterial supply are characterized by frequent individual variations between subjects. The innervation of the gallbladder and the biliary ducts is supplied by both parasympathetic (vagal) and sympathetic fibers (from the celiac plexus). Both afferent and efferent fibers are present. Adrenergic neurons supply the smooth muscle of the gallbladder. The afferent fibers giving rise to pain from the biliary tract travel in the sympathetic nerves to the celiac ganglia.

Microscopic Anatomy

The mucosa of the gallbladder is characterized by folds with cores of connective tissue (as in the intestinal villi). There is a thin layer of epithelial cells lining the gallbladder. Between adjacent cells are long, narrow, convoluted channels, which are closed by tight junctions at the luminal surface but open at the serosal surface; these channels are active in fluid resorption. Goblet cells are not present in the gallbladder but are present in the common bile duct. In the gallbladder, the epithelial cells contribute glycoproteins to the bile. The muscularis consists of smooth muscle, longitudinal and circular, with the latter more active in in vitro preparations. CCK acts directly on the smooth muscle of the gallbladder.

Functions of the Gallbladder

A major function of the gallbladder is *storage of bile during interdigestive periods*. Bile flows from canaliculi toward the small intestine because of secretory pressure generated by hepatocytes and ductular epithelium. Bile enters the gallbladder as a result of closure of the sphincter of Oddi and the resistance of flow through the terminal bile duct during the interdigestive period. During the fasting period, some bile is secreted in synchrony with the migrating motor complex (MMC, or "housekeeping wave") of the GI tract, especially during intense duodenal contractions associated with this wave.

The gallbladder also affects the *concentration of bile*. The gallbladder can hold up to 50 ml of fluid. During fasting, the liver output far exceeds this volume. While in the gallbladder, the bile is concentrated by the active transport of electrolytes, namely, Na^+, which is coupled with either Cl^- or HCO_3^-. Absorption of water molecules depends on the active absorption of these ions and is itself passive. The loss of ions and water serves to concentrate the remaining ions and other solutes of bile, sometimes up to 20-fold. Despite such a concentration, the contents remain isotonic because of the presence of lipid micelles.

Contractions of the gallbladder also result in *delivery of bile during digestion*. During a meal, the gallbladder musculature contracts and empties the gallbladder in a gradual manner. This contraction is triggered mainly by CCK, which is released as a result of stimulation of the duodenal mucosa by digestion products, especially lipids. Flow of bile from the gallbladder through the common bile duct and into the duodenum is the net result of the *contraction* of the gallbladder and the *relaxation* of the sphincter of Oddi (the smooth muscle sphincter that is located at the ampulla), both influenced by the release of CCK. There may be minor contributions from the musculature of the cystic and common bile ducts.

Regulation of Biliary Tract Motility

During the interdigestive period, about 20% of the emptying of the gallbladder occurs as a result of the periodic MMC. During relaxation between MMCs, hepatic bile flows into the gallbladder with a concomitant dilution of gallbladder bile. During the resting phase, the gallbladder concentrates the bile as already noted. This periodic contraction of the gallbladder during the interdigestive period may prevent or minimize the accumulation of microcrystals, which may in turn inhibit the formation of gallstones.

During the digestive period, gallbladder emptying occurs as a result of delivery of food to the duodenum or, experimentally, by the administration of CCK. A large number of studies have been performed to assess the degree and rate of gallbladder emptying. It appears that administration of a fatty meal to subjects produces a 55%–75% emptying of the gallbladder over a 30–45-minute time period. Similar values were obtained by continuous infusion of CCK, using two noninvasive techniques, radionucleotide cholescintigraphy and real-time ultrasonography.

During digestion, hormonal regulation is a critical part of the process. CCK, a key player, was isolated in 1928 by Ivy and Oldberg, who extracted a substance from upper small intestine mucosa that when injected intravenously caused the emptying of the gallbladder. They named this substance cholecystokinin ("that which excites or moves the gallbladder"). Since then, many studies have shown that CCK is released when a fatty meal is eaten or introduced into the duodenum or when bombesin is administered. The released CCK has several molecular forms, the most prevalent being CCK-33 and CCK-8, the latter being the carboxy-terminal octapeptide of the larger form. These forms seem to be equipotent in their stimulation of the gallbladder to contract, and they exhibit similar binding affinities to the CCK receptor on gallbladder smooth muscle.

Many studies of the relationship between CCK and gallbladder emptying have been performed. After a fatty meal, plasma CCK rises markedly within 2–6 minutes and reaches a maximum level within 16 minutes. The increase in CCK is closely followed by a significant decrease in gallbladder volume, and maximum gallbladder emptying occurs 2 minutes after the peak of CCK. It should be noted that these studies do not factor out the individual contributions of the *contraction* of gallbladder smooth muscle and the *relaxation* of the sphincter of Oddi to gallbladder emptying as a result of CCK stimulation.

A hormone that is also notable for its effect on decreasing gallbladder contractility is progesterone. In pregnant women, there is a direct correlation between rising serum progesterone levels and increased fasting and residual gallbladder volumes. Experiments have shown that the gallbladder contains progesterone receptors and that progesterone reduces the responsiveness of the gallbladder to such stimuli as CCK, acetylcholine, and histamine. In spite of these influences, pregnant women rarely develop gallstones. Minor influences on gallbladder contractility include secretin, vasointestinal peptide (VIP), polypeptide YY (PYY), and pancreatic polypeptide (PP).

The neural control of the gallbladder is both parasympathetic and sympathetic. With respect to parasympathetic control, in spite of documented vagal and cholinergic stimulation of gallbladder smooth muscle, the question of the physiologic significance of vagal input to the gallbladder remains unanswered. Theories include involvement during gastric and intestinal phases of digestion, maintenance of muscle tone, and possible modulation of hormonal stimulation. Furthermore, vagotomy is associated with the development of gallbladder stasis. The stimulation of the sympathetic nerves (or the injection of norepinephrine) relaxes the gallbladder, but only if the gallbladder has been previously stimulated with CCK or vagally. Smooth muscle of gallbladder contains both excitatory and inhibitory adrenergic receptors.

FACTORS IN GALLSTONE FORMATION

Gallstones are extremely common. Over 20 million Americans have them, and half a million patients undergo cholecystectomies every year. Gallstone formation indicates a failure of one or more components of the biliary system. Major factors in gallstone formation include alterations in composition of bile, reduced contractility of the gallbladder, infection, and possibly genetics. There are three major types of gallstones: cholesterol stones, which represent most (> 80%) of the gallstones in this country; black pigment stones; and brown pigment stones, which are also called mixed pigment stones. Factors involved in gallstone formation are outlined in Table 9-3.

Notes

Gallstones occur in more than 20 million Americans; more than 80% of them are cholesterol stones.

Table 9-3. Factors in Gallstone Formation

TYPE	FACTORS
Cholesterol stones	Increased cholesterol concentration in bile
	Estrogens
	Obesity
	Age
	Genetics
	Oral contraceptives
	High polyunsaturated fat diet
	Marked or rapid weight loss
	Decreased bile acid synthesis
	Age
	Genetics
	Reduced 7α-hydroxylase activity
	Ileal disease or bypass
	Primary biliary cirrhosis
	Cholestyramine treatment
	Decreased contractility of gallbladder
	Progestins
	Increased cholesterol in bile
Black pigment stones	Increase in levels of unconjugated bilirubin
	Congenital abnormalities
	Hemolysis
	Liver diseases
	Fasting
Brown pigment stones	Infection of biliary tree resulting from surgical or endoscopic procedure or stasis

Cholesterol stones form as a result of destabilization of the composition of bile. As noted earlier, normal bile is carefully composed to permit maximum solubilization of its lipophilic and water-insoluble components. When this balance is disrupted, such as when cholesterol content increases, a supersaturation of components may occur. The micelles and vesicles in bile can begin to crystallize on the mucosal layer of the gallbladder and, particularly, attach to the glycoprotein mucin. This process forms the nidus for crystal growth and gallstone formation and is enhanced under conditions in which gallbladder contractility is reduced. Women are more susceptible to gallstone formation than men, particularly if they are overweight, in early middle age, and still have menstrual cycles. Estrogen can increase cholesterol content of the bile by enhancing low-density lipoprotein cholesterol uptake at the receptor level, and progesterone can decrease the contractility of the gallbladder. Formation of gallstones in both sexes increases with age and body weight. Rapid weight loss may also lead to the formation of gallstones; therefore, treatment for morbid obesity must be accompanied by prevention and/or monitoring of gallstone formation.

Black pigment stones are formed when unconjugated bilirubin polymerizes in a reaction catalyzed by free radicals. A number of processes and diseases influence the level of unconjugated bilirubin. Congenital syndromes that result in low or absent activity of UDPGT or enhanced hemolysis of erythrocytes, such as in glucose 6-phosphate deficiency or hemolytic anemia, may increase the risk of black pigment stones. Black pigment stones are found less frequently in this country but are more common in populations with inborn enzymopathies or hemoglobinopathies (in India, Sardinia, and other areas). Crohn's disease and administration of total parenteral nutrition are also associated with the development of black pigment stones.

Brown pigment stones are caused by infection, such as contamination of the biliary tree with bacteria from the duodenum after surgical or endoscopic procedures or in patients with biliary stasis. In Asia, the most common cause is parasitic infection with *Clonorchis*.

CASE STUDY: *RESOLUTION*

Mr. W. is worried about the results of the laboratory tests, especially after his friends told him stories about being denied life insurance coverage because of elevated liver enzymes. He consented to undergo a liver biopsy, which showed moderate macrovesicular steatosis, but no fibrosis or inflammation was apparent.

Mr. W. was counseled to lose weight gradually and was instructed to restrict total calories and saturated fats. He was encouraged to participate in regular exercise to help with weight reduction and reduce stress.

REVIEW QUESTIONS

Directions: For each of the following questions, choose the one best answer.

 The rate-limiting enzyme in bile acid synthesis is

A 3-Hydroxy-3-methylgutaryl coenzymeA (HMG CoA) reductase
B Glucokinase
C 7α-Hydroxylase
D Malic enzyme

2 Bile pigments are composed mainly of

A bilirubin.
B taurocholic acid.
C glucuronidated steroid hormones.
D very concentrated mixed inorganic ions.

3 Which of the following factors is implicated in development of steatosis (fatty liver)?

A High-fat diet
B Obesity
C Progesterone replacement therapy
D Vitamin A therapy

4 Gallbladder contractility is inhibited by

A cholecystokinin (CCK)-8.
B Progesterone.
C an increase in the ionic content of the bile.
D the sphincter of Oddi.

5 Under which of the following circumstances is bile delivered to the duodenum during the interdigestive period?

A Only in pathologic conditions, such as cholestasis
B Only if the sphincter of Oddi is defective
C In conjunction with the migrating motor complex (MMC) of the GI tract
D When the gallbladder becomes maximally distended during storage of bile

 Delivery of bile into the duodenum during digestion results from

A simultaneous relaxation of the gallbladder and contraction of the sphincter of Oddi.

B the action of cholecystokinin (CCK) on smooth muscle of the biliary tract.

C fluid present in the duodenum.

D presence of trypsin in the duodenum.

7 The mode of action of cholestyramine as a cholesterol-lowering agent is

A inhibition of hepatic HMG CoA reductase.

B binding of bile pigments within the intestinal lumen.

C prevention of bile salt uptake by the enterohepatic circulation.

D to decrease intestinal transit time by increasing motility.

References

Behar J: Physiology of the biliary tract. In *Bockus Gastroenterology*, 5th ed. Edited by Haubrich WS, Schaffner F, Berk JE. Philadelphia, PA: W. B. Saunders, 1995, pp 2554–2572.

Johnson LR: *Gastrointestinal Physiology.* St. Louis, MO: Elsevier Science, Mosby, 2001.

Malet Pf, Rosenberg DJ: Cholelithiasis: gallstone pathogenesis, natural history, biliary pain, and nonsurgical therapy. In *Bockus Gastroenterology*, 5th ed. Edited by Haubrich WS, Schaffner F, Berk JE. Philadelphia, PA: W. B. Saunders, 1995, pp 2674–2729.

Rose RC: Absorptive functions of the gallbladder. In *Physiology of the Gastrointestinal Tract*, 2nd ed. Edited by Johnson LR. New York: Plenum Press, 1987, pp 1455–1468.

Ryan JP: Motility of the gallbladder and biliary tree. In *Physiology of the Gastrointestinal Tract*, 2nd ed. Edited by Johnson LR. New York: Plenum Press, 1987, pp 695-721.

Schiff L, Schiff ER: *Diseases of the Liver,* 9th ed. Philadelphia, PA: J. B. Lippincott, 2003.

Weinman SA, Kemmer N. In *Textbook of Gastroenterology*, 4th ed. Edited by Yamada T. Philadelphia, PA: Lippincott, Williams, & Wilkins, 2003.

10

Normal and Disordered Swallowing

▓ CHAPTER OUTLINE ▓

▓ LEARNING OBJECTIVES ▓

At the completion of this chapter, the reader should be able to:

- Identify normal esophageal function associated with deglutition.
- Describe the different phases of swallowing and the neuromuscular activity associated with each of the phases.
- List the clinical symptoms and objective test results and describe the pathophysiology associated with esophageal dysfunction.
- Identify the advantages and disadvantages of the diagnostic tests used in the evaluation of dysphagia.

Anatomy and Physiology of the Swallowing Mechanism

ANATOMY OF THE SWALLOWING MECHANISM

Upper Esophageal Sphincter (UES)

The UES is a tonically contracted group of skeletal muscles separating the pharynx from the esophagus (Figure 10-1). The major component of the sphincter is the cricopharyngeus muscle. Portions of the inferior constrictor muscle and the muscles of the proximal esophagus also contribute to this 2–3-cm UES. The posterior border of the cricoid also contributes a passive component to the sphincter. During the non-swallowing state, entrance of air into the GI tract from respiration is minimized by resting sphincter pressure. Equally important is its function to prevent material from refluxing from the esophagus into the pharynx. The UES relaxes with swallowing to allow the bolus to enter the esophagus. It also relaxes during belching and emesis to allow retrograde movement of material from the esophagus to the pharynx.

Esophageal Body

The esophageal body is a muscular tube extending 20–25 cm in length from its origin just caudal to the cricopharyngeus muscle to its termination at the gastric cardia (see Figure 10-1). The primary function of the esophageal body is passage of ingested material from the pharynx to the stomach. The longitudinal muscle layer and the circular muscle layer constitute the outermost and innermost layers spanning the length of the esophageal body, respectively. At the top of the esophageal body, both muscle layers consist of skeletal muscle fibers. Approximately 5 cm distal to the UES, nonstriated smooth muscle fibers begin to intermingle with the striated muscle. Generally, there are fibers of both skeletal and smooth muscle for about 10 cm distal to the cricopharyngeus muscle. The proportion of muscle that is smooth muscle increases proportionately with distance from the UES. Thus, in humans, the caudal half of the esophageal body including the lower esophageal sphincter (LES) is composed entirely of smooth muscle fibers from

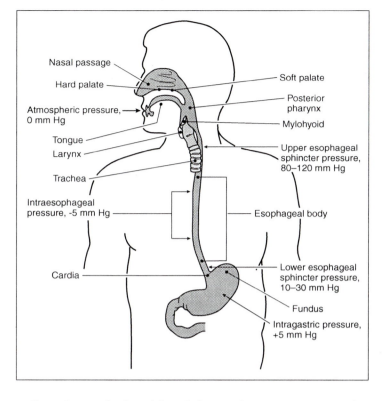

Fig. 10-1. Relationship of the Major Structures and Sphincters Constituting the Swallowing Mechanism

The normal pressure relationships of the upper esophageal sphincter, esophageal body, lower esophageal sphincter, and stomach are also shown. The pressures shown were derived by using atmospheric pressure at zero as a reference.

Notes

The **Z-line** is the squamocolumnar junction as seen on endoscopy.

both longitudinal and circular layers. The esophagus shortens by 10% on swallowing through longitudinal muscle contraction. Contraction of the circular muscle causes a squeezing motion required for peristalsis and sphincter control. Studies indicate that the esophagus is not merely a hollow conduit for food passage but, rather, has several active functions for acid control and mucosal protection. The esophageal body may secrete bicarbonate, possesses a cellular mechanism to transport hydrogen ions actively out of the epithelial cells, and secretes mucin and epidermal growth factor (EGF) in response to acid and pepsin.

LES

Gross and histologic examinations of the sphincter have failed to identify a specific sphincteric structure. Endoscopically, the squamous epithelium lining the esophagus appears pale and glossy and is distinguishable from the reddish, velvety columnar lining of the stomach. The junction between the squamous and columnar epithelium forms a circumferential line, often called the Z-line. The mucosal squamocolumnar junction, in the absence of disease, may correspond to the anatomic gastroesophageal junction. The position of this junction is variable and therefore may not be the optimal locator of the LES.

Notes

Basal LES tone is increased by ACh and drugs that act as ACh agonists.

Although the LES is difficult to define by gross observation, several physiologic characteristics distinguish it from adjacent, nonsphincteric muscles. Serially cut and stretched muscle strips from the esophageal body, LES, and stomach reveal that tension generated by similar increments in length produced substantially greater force in sphincteric than in nonsphincteric muscle. Because drugs that antagonize neural function do not affect this process, this increased force is likely myogenic. Furthermore, this increased force can be abolished using agents that inhibit muscle contraction. The myogenic tone of the sphincter is supported by aerobic mechanisms, in contrast to adjacent muscles of the esophageal body, which contract efficiently under anaerobic conditions. Mitochondria are larger and more centrally located in the muscle cells constituting the sphincter compared with those in the esophageal body.

Neural Innervation

LES. The sphincter muscle also possesses an increased sensitivity to many excitatory agents compared to that of the adjacent tissues, suggesting a greater influence on sphincter tone by nerves and hormones. Norepinephrine, for example, has a different effect on the sphincter than the adjacent muscles. It produces LES contraction and esophageal body relaxation. Basal sphincter tone is increased by agents that mimic acetylcholine (ACh) and by the GI hormone gastrin. Sphincteric tone is decreased by agents such as isoproterenol and prostaglandin E_1. Vasoactive intestinal peptide (VIP) and nitric oxide (NO) function as inhibitory neurotransmitters that relax the LES. Numerous pharmacologic agents and food products influence LES pressure (Table 10-1).

The vagus nerve carries preganglionic fibers, whose cell bodies lie in the dorsal root ganglion; these preganglionic fibers release ACh. Two types of postganglionic effector neurons are supplied by these preganglionic fibers. One of the effector neurons releases ACh and excites the

Table 10-1. Effect of Exogenous and Endogenous Agents on the LES

REDUCE LES TONE	INCREASE LES TONE
Chocolate	Protein meal
Peppermint	Acetylcholine
Caffeine	Phenylephrine
Alcohol	Serotonin
Fatty meals	Gastrin
Progesterone	Pancreatic polypeptide
Isoproterenol	Substance P
Secretin	Motilin
Vasoactive intestinal polypeptide	Neuropeptide Y
Nitric oxide	
Neurotensin	
Prostaglandin E_1	
Cholecystokinin	

smooth muscle fibers, whereas the other postganglionic neuron inhibits smooth muscle by releasing noncholinergic, nonadrenergic inhibitory neurotransmitters. Histochemical techniques have demonstrated the presence of nitric oxide synthase (NOS) in neurons supplying the circular muscle of the esophagus and the LES in the opossum. In vitro studies have shown that LES relaxation can be induced when muscle strips are bathed in a solution containing an NO donor. Similarly, these studies have also shown that NOS inhibitors markedly inhibit LES relaxation. Thus, the animal literature indicates that LES relaxation depends on NO as a final mediator. Relaxation results in human LES when muscle strips were treated with sodium nitroprusside, an NO donor. Cholecystokinin (CCK), a polypeptide hormone that is liberated by the upper intestinal mucosa on contact with gastric contents, stimulates both the smooth muscle cells and the inhibitory neurons in the wall of the esophagus. The weak, direct stimulatory effect of CCK on esophageal smooth muscle is opposed by the CCK-induced release of inhibitory neurotransmitters. The inhibitory effect predominates, and the net result of these disparate actions is a fall in LES pressure. NO and, to a lesser degree, VIP are the primary inhibitory neurotransmitters functioning in this mechanism.

Central Mechanism.   Deglutition, or swallowing, may be initiated voluntarily or reflexively. Once initiated, it proceeds as a coordinated involuntary reflex. Coordination occurs in the central nervous system (CNS) within the reticular formation of the brainstem. This area within the medulla portion of the brainstem has been identified as the "swallowing center." Normal swallowing requires complex interactions, involving structures of the oral cavity, pharynx, larynx, and esophagus. Cranial nerves V (trigeminal), IX (glossopharyngeal), and X (vagus) carry afferent impulses from the sensory receptors surrounding the oropharynx to their corresponding nuclei located in the brainstem. Efferent impulses from the nucleus ambiguus housed within the swallowing center are carried to the pharyngeal muscles via the motor portions of cranial nerves V (trigeminal), VII (facial), IX (glossopharyngeal), X (vagus), and XII (hypoglossal). The motor impulses arising from the nucleus ambiguus and traveling along these cranial nerves appear to be sequential, so the pharyngeal musculature is activated in a proximal-to-distal manner. The swallowing center also interacts with other areas of the brainstem and cortex involved with respiration and speech.

PROCESS OF SWALLOWING

The process of swallowing is typically divided into four consecutive phases: preparatory, oral, pharyngeal, and esophageal.

Preparatory Phase

In the preparatory phase, the bolus is processed through mastication into a cohesive bolus suitable for transport through the digestive tract. Inherent in this phase is a breakdown of the food to an appropriate

Notes

The trigeminal, facial, and hypoglossal cranial nerves operate during the oral phase of swallowing.

size, shape, and consistency to mix properly with saliva. Although movement of the jaw is an essential component of this phase, even more critical are the complex movements of the tongue. This activity functions to collect, control, and direct the bolus to the dorsum of the tongue for initiation of the oral phase of swallowing.

Oral Phase

In the oral phase of swallowing, a peristaltic wave is generated by sequential squeezing of the tongue, which propels the bolus from the oral cavity into the pharynx. More specifically, there is apposition of the jaws, the lips are together and relaxed, and the tip of the tongue contacts the hard palate. This configuration serves to thrust the food bolus against the palate until it reaches the oropharynx. The contraction of the mylohyoid muscle lifts the back of the tongue, thrusting the bolus into the posterior pharynx. Elevation of the soft palate and posterior portion of the tongue prevents nasal and oral regurgitation, respectively. Brief interruption of respiration, closure of the laryngeal inlet and vocal cords, and elevation and anterior displacement of the larynx prevent entrance of the bolus into the trachea, thereby preventing pulmonary aspiration. The oral phase of swallowing is under voluntary control and is dependent on cranial nerves V (trigeminal), VII (facial), and XII (hypoglossal). Because activity of the tongue is essential in this phase, the hypoglossal nerve and its supranuclear controlling pathways play a major role in the oral phase of swallowing.

Pharyngeal Phase

Unlike the oral phase, the pharyngeal phase of swallowing is controlled reflexively, involving protection of the airway and further propulsion of the bolus. The airway protective muscle functions include velopharyngeal closure to prevent the bolus from refluxing into the nose and laryngeal closure to prevent material from penetrating the larynx. The propulsion of food relies on pharyngeal peristalsis. During the pharyngeal phase of swallowing, approximation of the soft palate to the posterior nasopharyngeal wall accompanied by contraction of the superior constrictor muscles results in narrowing of the upper pharynx. Concurrently, the larynx is elevated and displaced forward, which causes relaxation of the cricopharyngeus muscle, or UES. Closure of the vocal cords, which follows UES relaxation, coupled with apposition of the base of the tongue to the posterior wall, increases the intrapharyngeal pressure, thus assisting in the propulsion of the bolus into the esophagus. Pharyngeal emptying is further accomplished by the contraction of the pharyngeal constrictors, which creates a peristaltic wave down the esophagus. The pharyngeal phase is completed by downward displacement of the larynx, contraction of the UES, and the resumption of respiration.

Esophageal Phase

The esophageal phase of swallowing is characterized by active peristalsis or sequential contraction of the esophagus and relaxation of the LES. Peristalsis is the aboral movement of a ring of muscular contraction (cranial to caudal). Distention of the esophagus by the bolus also acts as a stimulus for peristalsis. The bolus is propelled through the esophagus by a contraction above and relaxation below the bolus. This relaxation is referred to as descending inhibition. Primary peristalsis occurs when peristaltic activity is induced by a swallow, whereas secondary peristalsis is the initiation of a propagated contraction wave in the absence of a swallow. In this form of peristalsis, the movements are induced by stimulation of the sensory receptors in the esophageal body. Distention by a bolus, such as retained esophageal content that was not completely cleared by a primary swallow or refluxed gastric contents, provides adequate stimulation for the initiation of secondary peristalsis. It occurs only in the esophagus at or above the level corresponding to the location of the stimulus; it closely resembles peristalsis induced by a swallow, and it is also mediated by the swallowing center. Initiation of secondary peristaltic contractions is involuntary and normally is not sensed. The primary esophageal peristaltic wave is a continuation of the peristaltic wave that originated in the pharynx shortly after the initiation of a swallow. This wave passes from the pharynx to the striated muscle portion of the esophagus through the smooth muscle portion of the distal esophagus.

PHYSIOLOGY OF THE SWALLOWING SEQUENCE

The events associated with swallowing in the striated region occur very rapidly in a precisely timed manner. The beginning of the involuntary elements of the swallow, the apposition of the soft palate to the pharyngeal wall, is a contraction that lasts over 0.9 second and generates a pressure greater than 180 mm Hg. It is the beginning of a moving contraction front, pharyngeal peristalsis, that transverses the oropharynx and hypopharynx at about 15 cm/s to reach the UES in about 0.7 second. The timing of the bolus depends primarily on its volume and consistency. The tonically contracted musculature of the UES relaxes during the pharyngeal peristaltic sequence. The relaxation begins soon after the onset of swallowing and lasts 0.5–1.0 second, after which the muscles contract with a tone that may exceed twice the force of the resting contraction for another second before returning to baseline.

A caudally progressing front of contraction of the circular muscle layer begins at the top of the esophageal body, seemingly as a continuation of the UES that follows its relaxation. This contraction is preceded by a brief fall in intraesophageal pressure that begins about 0.2 second after the initiation of swallowing and is attributed to the entry of the swallowed bolus. The peristaltic contraction occurs and proceeds throughout the length of the esophageal body, with the velocity varying at different levels from 3 cm/s in the upper esophageal body, to 5 cm/s in the midesophageal body, to 2.5 cm/s just proximal to the LES. The contraction requires 5–6 seconds to traverse the

esophageal body. The force of the peristaltic contraction also varies among levels and is expressed as generated intraluminal pressure. The forces also vary with the age of the patient, bolus, volume, temperature, and intra-abdominal pressure. Generally, amplitudes of 53.4 ± 9.0 mm Hg can be obtained in the upper part of the esophageal body, 35.0 ± 6.4 mm Hg in the midesophageal body, and about 69.5 ± 12.1 mm Hg in the distal esophagus.

The LES is a specialized segment of smooth muscle in the distal esophagus that relaxes with swallowing, permitting entrance of the bolus into the gastric cavity and preventing gastroesophageal reflux in its resting state (see Figure 10-1). LES relaxation occurs at the time of deglutition or when the esophagus becomes distended. The relaxation lasts 5–7 seconds and is followed by a transient contraction, which may be twice the force of the resting tone. After this hypercontraction, which lasts about 2 seconds, the muscle tone returns to basal level. This brief hypercontraction seems to be a continuation or extension of the peristaltic contraction that sweeps the esophageal body.

Normal swallowing also involves the fundic portion of the stomach, which relaxes almost simultaneously with the onset of LES relaxation. Intragastric pressure falls just prior to the arrival of the swallowed bolus because of reactive relaxation of the smooth muscle cells of the stomach. After passage of the bolus, the pressure in the stomach returns to basal levels. This process, which has been named "receptive relaxation," is mediated by a reflex pathway involving afferent and efferent neurons. The neurotransmitter that mediates this process is unknown. Because relaxation happens with each swallow, large volumes can be accommodated dated with minimal rise in intragastric pressure.

ESOPHAGEAL MANOMETRY

Esophageal motility studies examine the static and dynamic functions of the pharyngeal and esophageal mechanisms responsible for swallowing. Pharyngeal manometry can be performed in conjunction with esophageal motility studies. Normally, the response of the oropharynx to swallowing has two components: (1) Compression of the catheter against the pharyngeal wall by the tongue results in a high, sharp-peaked amplitude pressure wave. (2) This is followed by a low-amplitude, long-duration wave, which reflects the initiation of pharyngeal peristalsis. A rapid, high-amplitude pressure upstroke ending in a single, sharp peak, followed by a rapid return to baseline, is produced by the contraction of the middle and inferior pharyngeal constrictor muscles to provide the midpharyngeal response to swallowing. Pharyngeal manometry is more difficult to study, however, and is poorly standardized.

Several factors are responsible for the variability in recordings of UES pressure. Rapid pressure changes that characterize pharyngeal motor function exceed the capacity of most systems to record. Normal reference values for pharyngeal pressure vary with catheter placement. Recorded pressure measurements from the UES fluctuate with both axial and radial shifts in catheter position, as well as with fluctuations in respiration and changes in intrathoracic pressure. Because of this wide variability in pressure measurements, the UES is generally assessed qualitatively as opposed to quantitatively. In general, mean amplitude and duration of peak pressures recorded from the oropharynx range from 100 to 150 mm Hg and 0.1 to 1.0 second, respectively. Those recorded from the hypopharynx range from 150 to 200 mm Hg and 0.3 to 0.5 second for amplitude and duration, respectively. Figure 10-2 illustrates a normal UES response to a swallow.

In a normal swallow, the contraction front moves sequentially from proximal to distal to create peristalsis. The amplitude of the esophageal peristaltic contraction wave ranges from about 60–120 mm Hg. A peristaltic contraction of at least 30 mm Hg is required to prevent retrograde movement of the bolus. Because the esophagus lies in the thoracic cavity, it is under negative pressure, that is, the intraesophageal pressure at rest is negative relative to atmospheric pressure referenced at zero. Normal intraesophageal pressure in the basal state has a pressure about 5 mm Hg below atmospheric pressure. Furthermore,

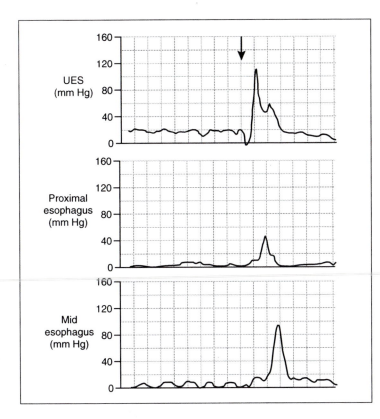

Fig. 10-2. Normal Upper Esophageal Sphincter (UES) Response to a Swallow

Relaxation of the UES from basal levels in response to a bolus (arrow) produces a U-shaped curve. This is a result of the decrease in pressure to esophageal baseline followed by a rise in pressure higher than original pressure and a return to basal UES pressure.

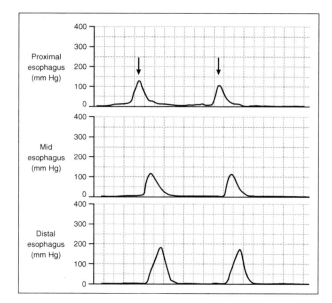

Fig. 10-3. Normal Esophageal Peristalsis

Esophageal motility recording with three pressure sensors placed in the esophageal body. Each arrow indicates a normal peristaltic sequence in response to a wet swallow.

intra-abdominal and, therefore, intragastric pressure is 3–6 mm Hg above atmospheric. Figure 10-3 illustrates normal esophageal peristalsis in response to a swallowed bolus.

Basal LES pressure is determined manometrically as a step up in pressure from gastric baseline (Figure 10-4). Normal values for LES pressure range from 10 to 30 mm Hg. After swallowing or with distention of the esophagus, sphincteric pressure falls to gastric baseline and remains at this level for about 5–7 seconds and is followed by a transient contraction, which may be twice the force of the resting tone. After this bound hypercontraction, the muscle tone returns to the basal pressure (see Figure 10-4).

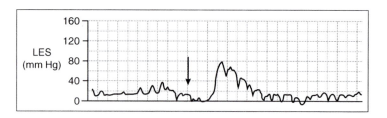

Fig. 10-4. Illustration of a Motility Recording from One Pressure Sensor Placed in the LES

The resting pressure is shown as 10–20 mm Hg above gastric baseline. In response to a wet swallow, the LES relaxes to baseline indicated by the arrow. Following the relaxation, there is a hypercontraction where the LES pressure exceeds basal level. Finally, LES pressure returns to its resting tone.

Dysphagia

The oropharyngeal swallowing mechanism is followed by primary and secondary peristaltic contractions of the esophageal body. This usually transports solid and liquid boluses from the mouth to the stomach within 10 seconds. When these orderly contractions fail to develop or progress, an ingested bolus may not clear the esophagus, resulting in intraluminal accumulation, distention, and discomfort. These symptoms associated with difficulty swallowing are known collectively as *dysphagia*. Dysphagia may result from functional motility disorders or mechanical obstructing lesions. Some individuals, especially patients with scleroderma, advanced diabetes, and pseudo-obstruction, demonstrate weak peristaltic activity that may be inadequate to clear the esophagus. Patients may also have primary or secondary motility disorders that disturb the orderly contractions of the pharynx or esophageal body. Finally, mechanical narrowing or inflammation may interrupt the passage of a bolus despite adequate peristaltic contractions. Patients frequently complain that food is sticking or is caught in the chest and will not go down. Associated symptoms include: chest pain, coughing, regurgitation, and heartburn. Because multiple mechanisms are responsible for inducing dysphagia, the clinical spectrum and presenting symptoms vary. For example, dysphagia resulting from a primary motility disorder may be intermittent, whereas dysphagia from an obstructing lesion is usually progressive, initially for solids and in the later stages for liquids. The severity of dysphagia frequently varies with the consistency of the ingested bolus, including solids, semisolids, thick and thin liquids, and secretions. Dysphagia is classifiable into two distinct types based on the anatomic site of disease: oropharyngeal, (or transfer dysphagia) and esophageal dysphagia. Table 10-2 lists typical etiologies of oropharyngeal and esophageal dysphagia.

CLASSIFICATION OF DYSPHAGIAS

Transfer Dysphagia

The term *oropharyngeal* (or *transfer dysphagia*) describes an inability to swallow because of a disease process affecting the oral or pharyngeal structures and the associated innervating pathways. Functional causes of transfer dysphagia result from abnormalities that affect the finely tuned neuromuscular mechanism of the pharynx and the UES. The patient may experience difficulty initiating a swallow or, once it is initiated, be unable to propel the bolus from the hypopharyngeal area through the UES into the esophageal body. Because this phase of swallowing is coordinated with respiratory activity, pulmonary aspiration is a frequent complication. Nasal regurgitation frequently accompanies swallowing if muscle weakness is the primary cause of dysphagia and if the weakness involves the muscles of the soft palate or superior constrictors of the pharynx. Poor pharyngeal propulsion or peristalsis may result in delayed or impeded movement of the

Two classifications of dysphagia are **oropharyngeal** (or **transfer dysphagia**) and **esophageal dysphagia**.

Table 10-2. Etiologies of Dysphagia

OROPHARYNGEAL	ESOPHAGEAL
Neurologic disorders	Motility disorders
Cerebral vascular accident	Achalasia
Head trauma	Diffuse esophageal spasm
Parkinson's disease	Nonspecific motility disorders
Amyotrophic lateral sclerosis	Mucosal lesions
Cranial nerve lesions	Reflux esophagitis
Poliomyelitis	Infectious esophagitis
Bell's palsy	Pill-induced esophagitis
Myoneural junction	Barrett's esophagus
Myasthenia gravis	Mass effect
Skeletal muscle disorders	Tumors
Dermatomyositis	Peptic stricture
Inflammatory myopathies	Diverticulum
Muscular dystrophies	Systemic illness
Mass effect	Scleroderma
Tumors	Amyloidosis
Zenker's diverticulum	Diabetes mellitus
Cervical webs	
Cervical osteophytes	
Systemic illness	
Sjögren's disease	

bolus, thus giving the patient a sensation that residual material remains in the pharynx after a swallow. Oropharyngeal dysphagia can also be caused by obstructing lesions, such as benign or malignant tumors, cervical rings or webs, or extrinsic compression by cervical osteophytes that narrow the lumen and impede bolus transit through the oropharynx. Oropharyngeal dysphagia can be divided into those abnormalities affecting the oral phases of swallowing and those affecting the pharyngeal stage.

Abnormalities Affecting the Oral Phase of Swallowing. Oral dysphagia may be divided into (1) disorders in the preparation and sizing of the bolus and (2) disorders in the transport of the bolus from the mouth to the pharynx. A normal oral phase requires adequate dentition, adequate salivary flow, intact neuromuscular control (particularly the corticobulbar connections), and the absence of painful oropharyngeal lesions. It is important to realize that over 400 commonly prescribed and over-the-counter medications decrease salivary flow and may contribute to oral dysphagia. The most common disease causing dysphagia as a result of decreased salivary flow is Sjögren's syndrome, an immunologic disease characterized by progressive destruction of the exocrine glands, resulting in mucosal and conjunctival dryness. The symptoms are subtle, and the diagnosis will be missed unless it is specifically considered.

A variety of inflammatory processes producing painful lesions of the mouth and pharynx may cause dysphagia. Most of these are brief and self-limiting, including canker sores and herpetic lesions. In immunocompromised hosts, such as patients who have received chemotherapy or radiation therapy or who have AIDS, the process may be so severe and prolonged as to seriously interfere with nutrition.

Neurologic disorders may cause defects in both the preparatory and propulsive phases of oral dysphagia. Neurogenic dysphagia involving the oral preparation phase may present with complaints of oral spills at the lips, commonly described as drooling or messy eating. There may be a history of difficulty with chewing, and patients often complain of an inability to initiate swallowing. There may be a sense of abnormal salivary volume, which may be excessive, as in tardive dyskinesia, versus minimal, as seen in Sjögren's syndrome or from drug use. Weakness of the muscles of the face and lips results in poorly mixed food, and chewing time may be increased, resulting in food restrictions or modifications. Nutritional intake may decline, with resultant weight loss.

Dysphagia occurring in the oral phase of swallowing produces symptoms associated with an inability to transfer food from the mouth to the pharynx. Patients may resort to compensatory techniques, such as moving food with the assistance of fingers or feeding utensils. They may employ "trick movements," such as voluntary flexing and neck extension to assist in the mechanical transfer of food.

Abnormalities Affecting the Pharyngeal Stage of Swallowing.
Pharyngeal dysphagia is frequently a result of (1) a failure of the driving force or propulsion, (2) obstruction to flow, or (3) a combination of these two causes. Failure of propulsive forces resulting in oropharyngeal dysphagia is generally due to defects in the brainstem, cranial nerves, myoneural junction, or muscles. Pharyngeal dysphagia resulting from an obstruction to flow is almost always due to a mass lesion or incomplete UES relaxation. Poor compliance of the UES can cause incomplete relaxation during swallowing, leading to a rise in hypopharyngeal pressure. As a result, a pharyngoesophageal or Zenker's diverticulum may develop. The clinical presentation of patients with an obstructing lesion is similar to that of those with a Zenker's diverticulum. Patients may present with dysphagia for both solids and liquids, regurgitation of undigested food, cough, and halitosis. Diagnosis is obtained by barium swallow with lateral views of the pharyngoesophageal junction.

Pharyngeal dysphagia is most frequently caused by CNS disease, such as cerebral vascular accident, Parkinson's disease, or amyotrophic lateral sclerosis. Swallowing disturbances may result from disease affecting the peripheral nerves, neuromuscular junction, and the muscle. These disturbances in swallowing may be diffuse or restricted to a focal function that depends on involvement of a particular nerve, such as in Bell's palsy. Some neurologic causes of pharyngeal dysphagia can be treated, such as myasthenia gravis and dermatomyositis.

Decompensation of the pharyngeal phase of swallowing results in leakage of material into the larynx and upper respiratory passages.

Notes

Pharyngeal dysphagia can result from a failure of the propulsive or driving force or an obstruction to the bolus.

There may be an initial involvement of the voice, which becomes distorted and "wet sounding," and patients may subsequently develop a habit of repeatedly clearing the throat. Food may escape through the nose; most alarming, retention of food in the pharynx may cause subsequent aspiration, resulting in coughing spells, choking episodes, and repeated bouts of pneumonia.

The clinical examination of a patient with suspected oropharyngeal dysphagia relies on the identification of abnormalities at both the upper motor neuron and lower motor neuron levels. The upper motor neuron components of the swallowing function include the cortex, subcortical structures, cerebellum, and brainstem. A careful neurologic evaluation is thus carried out to identify abnormalities referable to these regions. The lower motor neuron component includes structures innervated by the trigeminal, facial, glossopharyngeal, vagal spinal accessory, and hypoglossal nerves. Thus dysphagia may be associated with facial sensory loss, facial weakness, and disturbance of palatal and glossal function.

Finally, disturbances of swallowing may occur in the presence of cognitive dysfunction in which there is no obvious clinical disturbance of the swallowing mechanism. In situations where cognitive functions are impaired, apraxia, inattention, and lack of chewing and swallowing are possible. For example, a patient may sit for a meal unaware of his or her surroundings or that he or she has ingested food and make no attempt to continue with its passage.

Esophageal Dysphagia

Once a bolus of food successfully passes through the pharynx and enters the esophageal phase of swallowing, various motility disorders or mechanical obstructing lesions can cause esophageal dysphagia. Certain symptoms can help identify the cause of dysphagia as mechanical or the result of a neuromuscular defect. Of importance in the diagnosis of dysphagia is the consistency of what is ingested (liquid or solid), the nature of the symptoms (intermittent or progressive), and the presence of associated symptoms of heartburn, chest pain, or nocturnal coughing. Patients with motility disorders usually complain of slowly progressive dysphagia for liquids and solids from the onset. Conversely, patients with mechanical obstruction usually have dysphagia initially for solids only, and with worsening of disease symptoms become evident with liquids as well. Symptom onset is usually sudden in the case of mechanical obstruction.

For both motility disorders and obstructing lesions, patients commonly report the sensation that food appears to be "hanging up" in the mid or distal portion of the sternum. The site at which the patient localizes symptoms is frequently unreliable and is therefore of limited diagnostic value. Although symptoms localized to the epigastric or retrosternal area (just above the sternal notch) correspond fairly well to the site of obstruction, dysphagia localized by the patient to the neck is often referred from below.

ETIOLOGIES OF DYSPHAGIAS

Mechanical Lesions

The primary causes of progressive solid food dysphagia are peptic esophageal strictures and carcinoma. Because of the differences in treatment and prognosis, differentiating these etiologies is critical to the evaluation process. Peptic strictures are a complication of long-standing gastroesophageal reflux disease (GERD) that has often gone untreated. Therefore, patients with peptic strictures have a long history of heartburn and frequent use of antacids or over-the-counter histamine (H_2)-receptor antagonists. Radiographically, these strictures are smooth, of variable length, and usually located in the distal third of the esophagus. Patients with carcinoma of the esophagus (specifically squamous cell) differ from those with peptic strictures with respect to several historical characteristics. Generally, patients with cancer are older and give a history of rapidly progressive dysphagia. They usually do not have the long history of heartburn, although an association with reflux may occur. This is most often seen in the patient with Barrett's esophagus, where the esophageal mucosa undergoes metaplastic changes as a result of chronic gastroesophageal reflux (GER). Adenocarcinoma may later develop in the metaplastic esophageal mucosa. Patients with adenocarcinoma or squamous cell carcinoma of the esophagus frequently present with anorexia and significant weight loss. Although the history can help differentiate cancer from benign esophageal strictures, barium radiography followed by upper GI endoscopy are the main methods for diagnosis. Although a barium study may be very suggestive of the diagnosis, histologic confirmation of the cancer type can only be provided with a tissue sample and biopsy specimens, which can be readily obtained during endoscopy.

Patients reporting only intermittent dysphagia for solids may have an esophageal ring or web. A mucosal ring at the esophagogastric junction is frequently referred to as a Schatzki ring. The etiology of this ring has not been clearly defined. Historically, it was believed to be a congenital variant; a relationship to GER has been suggested. The incidence of these rings is estimated at 14% of the population; however, only those with a luminal narrowing of 13 mm or smaller in diameter are symptomatic. Characteristically, the dysphagia is episodic and not progressive. It is usually noted during a meal of meat or bread that is being consumed rapidly. The diagnosis is easily made with barium radiography. Muscular or contractile esophageal rings occur less frequently than Schatzki rings and are usually asymptomatic. However, in the rare cases where they are symptomatic, the symptoms are indistinguishable from those of a Schatzki ring. Esophageal webs are thin, transverse membranes of squamous epithelium, usually occurring in the upper and midesophagus. To avoid confusion of esophageal webs with rings, webs can be thought of as incomplete rings. Esophageal webs have been reported to occur in 7% of patients presenting with dysphagia.

Motility disorders that cause dysphagia include achalasia, diffuse esophageal spasm, and scleroderma.

Aperistalsis and absent or incomplete relaxation of the LES are required for the diagnosis of achalasia.

Functional Motility Disorders

Typical causes of motility disorders include achalasia, Chagas' disease, diffuse esophageal spasm, nonspecific motility disorders, and those secondary to other diseases, such as connective tissue disorders, most notably scleroderma.

Achalasia.   Achalasia is uncommon, with an annual incidence in the United States and Europe estimated at 1.1 per 100,000 population. It initially presents in individuals between 20 and 60 years of age. As in our case study, children may present with dysphagia. Men and women are affected equally. Classically, patients present with long-standing, slowly progressive dysphagia for both solids and liquids; however, dysphagia is more frequently associated with solids. Regurgitation is common and unprovoked, occurring during or shortly after a meal. Weight loss is common. Chest pain similar in nature to cardiac angina is frequently reported. Heartburn, defined as the reflux of gastric contents, is very rare. Patients do, however, complain of bitter or sour regurgitant material. This is a result of retained food in the esophagus, which may ferment, thus simulating GER. Because this regurgitation is primarily nocturnal, when gravity is not a factor, pulmonary aspiration frequently results.

Radiographic imaging has a clear role in the identification and diagnosis of achalasia. Unlike most causes of dysphagia, achalasia may be suggested by abnormalities on an upright chest x-ray. An air–fluid level within a dilated esophagus may be seen on a standard chest x-ray. The normally present gastric air bubble is frequently absent on posterior–anterior and lateral chest views in patients with achalasia. Barium esophagography is useful in the identification of achalasia. Early in the disease course, fluoroscopy may demonstrate abnormal peristalsis, such as frequent tertiary simultaneous contractions in the esophageal body. Most often there is complete absence of peristalsis in the esophageal body. The esophagus is usually dilated and often contains retained food, liquids, and secretions. The distal segment of the esophagus frequently tapers to a narrowing, giving the appearance of a "bird's beak," as shown in Figure 10-5. In those patients in whom the disease has been long-standing and untreated, as in the case study presented, esophageal dilation may become severe and attain a configuration similar to the sigmoid colon (Figure 10-6).

Esophageal manometry is a safe, relatively inexpensive test that provides the definitive diagnostic procedure in achalasia. Two abnormalities in the manometric study are required to make the diagnosis: first, an absence of peristalsis in the esophageal body and, second, incomplete or abnormal LES relaxation. Patients with achalasia frequently also have LES pressures greater than normal; however, this is not a necessary criteria for diagnosis. Patients often are found to have elevated intraesophageal pressures relative to gastric baseline. This is a result of retained material in the distal esophagus.

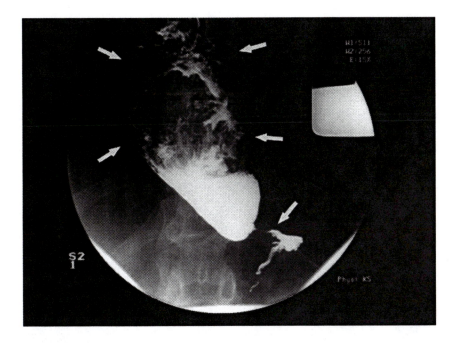

Fig. 10-5.

This barium esophagogram allows easy delineation of the dilated esophagus as shown by the thin arrows. The distal segment narrows at the LES, giving the appearance of a bird's beak as indicated by the thick arrow.

Although the etiology of achalasia is unknown, it is characterized by the degeneration of neural elements in the wall of the esophagus, particularly at the LES. A viral cause has been suspected; however, electron microscopy has failed to reveal viral particles in the vagus nerve or in the intramural plexuses. Genetic influences do not appear to have a significant role. Concurrence of the disease in first-degree relatives has been reported occasionally; however, there has been only a rare incidence of its occurrence in monozygotic twins.

Although abnormalities in both muscle and nerve components are detectable, the neural lesion is thought to be of primary importance. The pathogenesis is primarily due to a reduction in the number of ganglion cells in the myenteric plexus and secondarily to damage to the vagus nerve, most notably myelin degeneration. The degree of ganglion cell loss appears to be related to the duration of the disease. Ganglion cells are nearly absent in patients reporting symptoms for a minimum of 10 years. Although light microscopic examinations of the vagal branches to the esophagus appear normal, electron microscopy has demonstrated degeneration of myelin sheaths and disruption of axonal membranes. These changes are similar to those typically seen with experimental nerve transections and are referred to as *Wallerian degeneration*.

Physiologic studies have confirmed the presence of denervation of the smooth muscle segment of the esophagus in patients with achalasia. Muscle strips from the esophageal body contract in response to

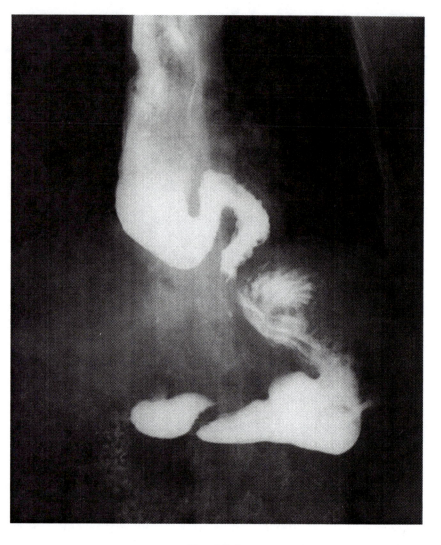

Fig. 10-6.

The barium esophagogram shown here was obtained from the patient in the case study. Note the severely dilated and tortuous esophagus, providing curves much like those seen in the sigmoid colon; hence the name "sigmoid esophagus."

direct stimulation with ACh but do not respond to direct stimulation with nicotine, suggesting a failure of neural stimulation. Likewise, muscle strips from the LES do not relax in response to ganglionic stimulation in patients with achalasia but do relax in normal controls. Neurotransmission has been found to be abnormal in the LES of patients with achalasia. Normally, CCK stimulation in the LES region produces an inhibitory response, resulting in relaxation or decreased LES pressure. In patients with achalasia, CCK produces an increase in LES pressure. This may represent a loss of inhibitory neurons in the LES region that normally produce the predominant response to CCK stimulation. Recently, evidence of the inhibitory neurotransmitter NO was located in the LES of animals and humans. NOS was not present, however, in the LES of patients with achalasia. Furthermore, NOS from donors elicited LES relaxation when applied to muscle strips obtained from patients with achalasia. Similar findings were reported in animal research. These studies indicate that NO is an inhibitory neurotransmitter that is absent in patients with achalasia, and it likely plays a critical role in the pathophysiology of this disease.

Denervated LES smooth muscle, primarily the result of a loss of the inhibitory innervation, produces the observed manometric and clinical findings. This chronic denervating process is irreversible, so that the only available treatments are palliative. Pharmacologic therapy with both nitrates and calcium channel blockers has been used to decrease LES pressure and relieve dysphagia. Although they are commonly used, the efficacy of these agents in the long-term treatment of achalasia is unclear. Furthermore, they often cause side effects of hypotension and tachycardia; therefore both are often poorly tolerated in otherwise healthy patients.

Endoscopic pneumatic dilations and surgical myotomies remain the primary therapies for achalasia. Prior to performing either of these procedures, an endoscopy is done to exclude other disease entities and diagnose possible complications. Pneumatic dilation involves the passing of a balloon, under fluoroscopic guidance, down the esophagus through the LES to the gastric cardia, allowing the balloon to straddle the LES. Inflation of the balloon to a pressure of 8–10 pounds per square inch (psi) and maintaining that pressure for a range of 15–60 seconds reduces basal LES pressure by the tearing of the muscle fibers. Although success rates are greater than 85% when the operator is experienced, complications, including esophageal perforation, average approximately 4%–8%, and symptomatic GER has been reported at a rate of about 2%–11%. Pneumatic dilations are significantly less expensive and associated with less morbidity and mortality than surgical therapy; however, 10%–15% of patients require a surgical procedure for persistent or recurrent symptoms. The most frequently performed surgical procedure is the Heller myotomy, which is a modification of the original procedure first performed in the early 1900s. Traditionally, this procedure uses a transthoracic or transabdominal approach, with 70%–90% of patients reporting good to excellent results. The most frequently reported complications are GER and its associated complications of esophagitis and peptic stricture formation. Because of the high incidence of postoperative GER, many surgeons also perform an antireflux procedure, such as a Belsey Mark IV procedure or a partial or loose fundoplication, at the time of the Heller myotomy. Infrequent but serious complications of this surgery include esophageal perforation, fistula formation, and infection, including a pleural empyema. The overall mortality of this procedure has been estimated at approximately 0.3%. In the past few years the Heller procedure has been further modified to use laparoscopic techniques rather than the standard laparotomy or thoracotomy.

Recent advances in the therapeutic management of achalasia include injections of botulinum toxin (botox) into the LES. *Clostridium botulinum*, an anaerobic organism, produces a toxin that exerts its

action by rapidly and strongly binding to presynaptic cholinergic nerve terminals. The toxin is then internalized, which ultimately inhibits the exocytosis of ACh release. Paralysis of affected cells and a nearly complete decline of miniature end-plate potentials occur within a few hours after the injection of botox. As a result, treated muscles become functionally denervated and atrophy. These effects gradually reverse as extrajunctional ACh receptors develop. In fact, within 2 days after muscle exposure to the toxin, the axon terminals begin to sprout, and the proliferating branches then form new synaptic contacts on the adjacent muscle fibers. Although best known for its effect on skeletal muscle, botox has been shown to also interfere with cholinergic signaling in the myenteric nervous system, where it affects smooth muscle motility. Several recent placebo-controlled trials have shown that intrasphincteric injections of botox into the LES of patients with achalasia resulted in symptomatic improvement, reduced LES pressure, and reduced esophageal retention of barium, compared with those receiving the placebo injections. The results of several trials have consistently shown that use of botox is a safe procedure and is successful 60%–75% of the time. The treatment, however, has only been shown to last 6–12 months, requiring repeat injections for continued symptomatic improvement. Following the success of the therapy in these trials, several investigations were performed to compare pneumatic dilation therapy to botox injections for the treatment of achalasia. Because of the limited duration of improvement, this therapy is generally reserved for the elderly or patients with comorbid medical illnesses who would otherwise not be considered operative candidates. Young or otherwise healthy patients should be treated with endoscopic pneumatic dilation and, if it is unsuccessful, be considered for a surgical myotomy.

Chagas' Disease. Chagas' disease, commonly known as American trypanosomiasis, is a zoonosis caused by the protozoan parasite *Trypanosoma cruzi* and is a major cause of morbidity and mortality throughout South and Central America because of its effect on the GI and cardiac systems. Patients may become infected via an insect bite or through seropositive blood products. Regardless of the route of transmission, if a patient experiences the acute form of the disease, characterized by high fever and marked edema, spontaneous resolution of the acute illness usually occurs. These patients may subsequently enter the indeterminate phase of *T. cruzi* infection, characterized by lifelong, low-grade parasitemia and an absence of symptoms. Most patients who harbor *T. cruzi* remain in the indeterminate phase for life. An estimated 10%–30% of persons in the indeterminate phase eventually develop symptoms related to the infection, but this generally does not occur until years or even decades after the infection is acquired. This latent form of the infection is manifested as chronic Chagas' disease, characterized by cardiac disease and enteromegaly. Megaesophagus, clinically indistinguishable from achalasia, and megacolon, presenting with infrequent bowel movements and chronic constipation, are the most common GI manifestations of the disease. The pathophysiologic mechanisms operating during this extended latent period and resulting in this form of digestive disease are not known. Infection with *T. cruzi* may cause lesions that result in a reduction in the number of autonomic nervous system neurons, leading to parasympathetic denervation. Megaesophagus resulting from *T. cruzi* infection may be treated in the same way as described for achalasia; however, in refractory cases esophagectomy may be performed.

Diffuse Esophageal Spasm.   Diffuse esophageal spasm (DES) is a well-described disorder of esophageal motility associated clinically with dysphagia and chest pain. The onset of the disorder may occur at any age, with the mean age of presentation occurring at about 40 years. A greater prevalence is seen in women. Anginalike chest pain is the most frequently reported symptom, occurring in up to 80%–90% of patients with manometrically confirmed DES. However, evidence suggests that DES may only account for 5%–15% of the esophageal motility disorders seen in patients with symptoms of noncardiac chest pain. The pain is generally retrosternal, lasting from minutes to hours, during which time swallowing is not usually impaired. The pain may radiate to the back and shoulders and be relieved with nitroglycerin, thus mimicking cardiac angina. The pain may be related to swallowing, but it may also occur independently of eating. Dysphagia is present in 30%–60% of patients with DES, but DES is the disease process in only 13% of patients presenting with dysphagia. Clinically, dysphagia is intermittent, with severity varying from mild to severe. Food impaction and weight loss occur very rarely.

The etiology of DES is not known, and there is a dearth of literature regarding the pathophysiology. Diffuse muscular thickening in the distal esophagus has been found in some patients with severe disease. Loss of ganglion cells in the intramural plexuses has not been demonstrated. Changes in vagal fibers have been found inconsistently by electron microscopy. Some of these changes resemble Wallerian degeneration, as reported in achalasia. The relationship of this inconsistent finding to the rare progression to achalasia in severe DES is unclear.

Manometric findings are limited to the smooth muscle segment of the esophagus. Nonperistaltic or simultaneous contractions following many or most swallows is the most consistent criterion in the definition of diffuse esophageal spasm. Less consistent but also observed are abnormalities of the contraction wave, such as increased amplitude or duration and intermittent episodes of repetitive contractions associated with increased baseline esophageal pressure. Abnormal esophageal motility is present when 15% or more of swallows are followed by nonperistaltic sequences. The diagnosis of diffuse esophageal spasm, however, is generally reserved for patients demonstrating nonperistaltic sequences in at least 30% of wet swallows. Regardless of disease severity, in all cases the unpropagated contractions are intermixed with normal peristalsis. An elevation in resting LES pressure

Table 10-3. Manometric Characteristics of Esophageal Motility Disorders

ACHALASIA

Esophageal aperistalsis
Absent or incomplete LES relaxation
Hypertensive (or high) normal LES pressure
Elevated intraesophageal pressures

DIFFUSE ESOPHAGEAL SPASM

Increased simultaneous or nonperistaltic contractions (> 30% of wet swallows)
Intermittent normal peristalsis
Duration of contractions increased (> 6 s)
High-amplitude contractions (±180 mm Hg)
Increased LES pressure or incomplete relaxation
Chest pain concurrent with abnormal contractions

NONSPECIFIC MOTILITY DISORDERS

Nontransmitted contractions (> 20% of wet swallows)
Hypertensive LES (basal LES > 45 mm Hg)
Increased duration of contractions
Retrograde contractions
High- or low-amplitude contractions
Absent peristalsis with normal LES pressure and relaxation

may be an associated finding. Table 10-3 summarizes the motility abnormalities most commonly seen in DES.

Barium radiographic studies of the esophagus are most often normal in DES. When abnormal, nonperistaltic contractions may indent the barium-filled smooth muscle portion of the esophagus. This distorted radiographic appearance has been described as a "corkscrew esophagus" or a "rosary bead esophagus." The presence of nonpropulsive circular muscle contractions (tertiary contractions) may be seen during the fluoroscopic examination. Nonperistaltic waves within the esophagus may result in barium being retained within a transient outpouching of the esophagus, giving the radiographic appearance of a diverticulum. Because this is not a result of an anatomic abnormality but of distorted motility, these changes are referred to as a pseudo- or transient diverticulum.

Nonspecific Esophageal Motility Disorders. A variety of other abnormalities may be found during esophageal motility testing in patients with dysphagia who have no evidence of other systemic diseases to explain the motility abnormalities. The manometric findings may show a variety of findings that are not found in normal individuals during wet swallows. These may include more than 20% of nontransmitted contractions, prolonged duration of contractions (> 6 seconds), triple-peaked contractions, retrograde contractions, reduced or exaggerated amplitude of contractions, hypertensive LES pressure, or absent peristalsis with normal LES relaxation. The term *nonspecific motility disorder* is most frequently used to categorize these findings. This diagnosis constitutes approximately 25%–50% of the abnormal motility studies performed in the diagnosis of dysphagia and noncardiac chest pain.

Diverticulum. As previously discussed, diverticula may also develop in the mid- or distal esophagus as a result of esophageal dysmotility. Esophageal diverticula are outpouchings of one or more layers of the esophageal wall. These diverticula occur primarily in three locations within the esophagus: (1) immediately above the UES (Zenker's diverticulum), (2) near the midpoint of the esophagus (traction diverticulum), and (3) immediately above the LES (epiphrenic diverticulum). Midesophageal diverticula are most often asymptomatic; however, complaints of dysphagia and rarely obstruction from a food impaction are reported. It is difficult to determine if dysphagia symptoms are caused by the presence of an epiphrenic diverticulum or from the associated motility disorder. Characteristic of these diverticula, however, is nocturnal regurgitation of large amounts of fluid that have presumably been stored within the diverticulum during the waking hours. Barium esophagography readily demonstrates the presence of these diverticula.

Progressive Systemic Sclerosis. Systemic diseases such as diabetes mellitus, amyloidosis, and most notably, progressive systemic sclerosis (PSS) can manifest esophageal dysmotility. In PSS, smooth muscle cells of the GI tract are progressively replaced with collagen infiltration and fibrosis. An estimated 50%–90% of patients with PSS have esophageal involvement. Esophageal motility studies reveal the characteristic findings of PSS to include reduced LES pressure, reduced amplitude of peristalsis in the distal two-thirds of the esophagus, or esophageal aperistalsis. Peristalsis is usually maintained in the striated or proximal portion of the esophagus, and UES pressure and relaxation are generally unimpaired. The esophageal dysmotility found in these patients—specifically, very low LES pressures combined with poor or absent esophageal peristalsis—may result in clinically significant GER. Thus, progressive dysphagia for solids and liquids may be a major complaint, but heartburn is most often the most prevalent symptom.

DIAGNOSIS OF DYSPHAGIA

History and Physical Examination

Taking a careful, thorough patient history is the first step in the diagnosis of dysphagia. As diagnostic tests become more available, complex, and expensive, the importance of the patient history cannot be overemphasized. Specific clues to the diagnosis become apparent from the patient's history. First, it is important to note if the patient has any coexisting medical illnesses. For example, dysphagia is part of the CREST syndrome (a variant of progressive systemic sclerosis with coexisting calcinosis, Raynaud's phenomenon, esophageal dysmotility, sclerodactyly, and telangiectasias), and other connective tissues diseases. If a patient had a recent cerebral vascular accident, the etiology of the dysphagia is very likely neurologic, and symptoms of transfer or oropharyngeal dysphagia should be elicited. It is critical to assess the nature of the food boluses with which the patient experiences difficulty. Patients with only solid food dysphagia are more likely to have esophageal dysphagia from an obstructing lesion. On the other hand, more difficulty with liquids is likely to indicate transfer dysphagia. Functional esophageal dysphagia is typically intermittent and is similar for both solids and liquids.

Evaluation of the frequency of the dysphagia should differentiate between those disorders that present intermittently and those that are constant in nature. The progression of the illness also provides clues as to the etiology of the presenting symptoms. A comprehensive assessment of the patient's prescribed and over-the-counter medications provides information critical to the diagnostic process. A cost-effective evaluation of a patient presenting with dysphagia begins with taking a complete medical, drug, and swallowing history. A comprehensive physical examination should, as always, be an integral part of the evaluation process. It should include a thorough evaluation of the oral cavity, head and neck, supraclavicular structures, and the abdomen. It should also include a thorough neurologic examination, particularly of the cranial nerves. In patients with suspected neurogenic dysphagia, the clinical neurologic examination should distinguish abnormalities at the upper motor neuron level from those resulting from lower motor neuron disease or myopathies.

Esophagography

Because normal swallowing requires the coordination of neuromuscular events in seconds, specialized approaches are often needed. A systematic approach to the diagnosis of disordered swallowing is essential. Malignant neoplasms, ulceration, and infection should first be excluded with flexible endoscopy. Endoscopy is of limited value in the examination of the coordination of the pharynx and hypopharynx; therefore, the evaluation of dysphagia usually begins with radiographic imaging of the pharyngeal and esophageal mechanisms. This mode of imaging is essential for the diagnosis of transfer dysphagia. Fluoroscopic observation is valuable for the investigation of motor activity of the pharynx. Videofluorography permits the evaluation of rapid motor sequences by slow-motion picture analysis. This is important in the oropharyngeal phase of swallowing because of the speed with which the bolus travels through this region. Major structural abnormalities, including webs, rings, and diverticula, that may affect swallowing in the pharyngeal phase can be seen with barium esophagography, especially if special attention is given to the cervical region. Barium esophagograms, however, provide little information regarding the presence, extent, and volume of reflux material and correlate poorly with more sophisticated measures of GERD. Esophageal transit time, that is, the amount of time for a bolus to navigate the esophagus and enter the stomach, can be calculated with fluoroscopic imaging. The importance of this measure is unclear, and it is not widely used in clinical practice. A modified barium swallow examination, when performed under the direction of a speech pathologist, is extremely useful in the diagnosis and management of transfer dysphagia. In this examination, the speech pathologist feeds the patient barium-labeled food and liquids of different consistencies. Using this technique, a speech pathologist can determine the consistency of bolus preparation that the patient can safely swallow. Laryngeal penetration and tracheal aspiration can also be closely monitored. Rings and webs not seen by a plain barium swallow can often be detected through the use of barium-impregnated solid food or capsules.

Fiber Optic Endoscopic Examination

Fiber optic endoscopic examination of swallowing safety (FEESS) is a new procedure used by otolaryngologists in the assessment of the pharyngeal stage of swallowing in patients with dysphagia. The pharyngeal area is intubated with a very narrow diameter (3.7 mm) flexible fiber optic nasopharyngolaryngoscope in those patients for whom the traditional videofluoroscopic evaluation may be difficult or impossible. This procedure can often be done at the bedside with minimal discomfort to the patient. This technique is used to detect aspiration and determine the safety of oral feeding in patients with probable oropharyngeal dysphagia. A clear and direct view of the hypopharynx and larynx can be obtained and studied without interfering with the function of the other structures.

Esophageal Manometry

Esophageal manometry is highly sensitive and specific for the detection of esophageal motility abnormalities. A polyvinyl catheter with multiple pressure sensors is passed transnasally, and the patient is instructed to perform a series of wet and dry swallows. Several measurements can be obtained from different sites within the LES and esophagus. LES pressure is measured at baseline and then in response to a swallow. Complete LES relaxation with a swallow is demonstrated by a decrease in pressure to gastric baseline for a duration of approximately 10 seconds. The catheter is then pulled into the esophagus by 1-cm intervals (station pull-through method) or rapidly (rapid pull-through method) until all ports have transversed the LES and entered the esophagus. Location of the catheter within the esophagus is indicated by a negative baseline pressure, reflecting intrathoracic pressure, and positive pressure waves should be present on swallowing. Peristaltic contractions are analyzed with respect to the amplitude, duration, and morphology of the wave form. UES pressure and relaxation can be measured by further withdrawal of the catheter until the pressure ports are located in the high-pressure zone of the proximal esophagus or the UES. A normal UES response to a swallow is a U-shaped drop to esophageal baseline, which is followed by a rise in pressure higher than the original pressure, followed by a return to UES pressure (see Figure 10-2). This examination is minimally invasive, causing only transient mild discomfort to the patient; complications are rare, and it is widely used in clinical practice, with well-established reference values.

Gastroesophageal Reflux Disease

The term *gastroesophageal reflux disease* (GERD) has been used to describe the full spectrum of disorders caused by GER. Although the prevalence of this disorder is difficult to establish, a study of normal individuals revealed that 7% of those questioned had typical symptoms of acid reflux, including heartburn, on a daily basis, and 36% had the symptoms at least once a month. A random study of 2000 subjects demonstrated a prevalence of 58.1% of white patients with symptoms of heartburn or acid regurgitation. The prevalence of weekly or more frequent episodes of heartburn or acid regurgitation was 19.4%.

PATHOPHYSIOLOGY OF GERD

GER is defined as the retrograde movement of gastric contents across the LES into the esophagus. Acid, pepsin, and bile are the toxic components of the refluxed material contributing to GER. There are several physiologic mechanisms that act to prevent and protect the esophagus from the damaging effects of GER. LES competence is the most important barrier to reflux. The LES is a localized region of tonically contracted smooth muscle at the gastroesophageal junction, which is best described as a 2–4-cm zone of increased pressure in the distal esophagus. The amplitude of this zone is altered by gut hormones, which receive information from excitatory and inhibitory neurons of the vagus nerve. The sphincter is affected by food, alcohol, smoking, drugs, and hormones (see Table 10-1). For example, progesterone has a major relaxation effect on this sphincter, as seen in pregnancy. Any dysfunction of this sphincter that causes the LES to be open or have reduced pressure may lead to GER. Mechanisms include (1) inappropriate or transient LES relaxation (TLESR); (2) increased abdominal pressure or stress-induced reflux; or (3) incompetent or reduced LES pressures or spontaneous free reflux. TLESR is now believed to be the main mechanism for GER in most patients with this condition. Esophageal clearance mechanisms may be an additional important factor in the control of GER. When gastric contents reflux into the esophagus, esophageal peristalsis clears the majority of refluxed material, whereas the swallowed alkaline saliva neutralizes residual acid. Gravity also affects esophageal clearance, returning refluxed materials to the stomach in the absence of peristalsis when the patient is in an upright position. The constant emptying of gastric contents ensures that gastric stasis and subsequent increases in gastric pressure, with resulting GER, do not occur. Table 10-4 lists the different mechanisms responsible for producing GER.

Table 10-4. Mechanisms of GER

Transient LES relaxations[a]
Reduced or incompetent LES pressures
Increased intra-abdominal pressure
Large hiatal hernia
Impaired esophageal peristalsis
Supine position
Reduced saliva production
Delayed gastric emptying

[a] Primary mechanism.

Normally, LES pressure is measured in mm Hg as the increase in the pressure gradient above intragastric pressure. The normal reference values vary from 15 to 35 mm Hg. A minimum level of 6–10 mm Hg is assumed to be necessary to prevent GER. At the time of swallowing, the LES relaxes, and LES pressures drops to gastric baseline, thereby permitting passage of the bolus. LES pressures frequently fall to levels that are incompetent for all or part of the day because of physiologic temporary relaxation and cyclic variations in pressure. These TLESRs represent a decrease in LES that is not associated with swallowing or primary or secondary peristalsis. Stress reflux results when intra-abdominal pressure exceeds LES pressure during coughing, Valsalva maneuver, straining, or wearing tight abdominal garments. Reflux episodes associated with increased intra-abdominal pressure are usually noted when LES pressures are relatively low and intra-abdominal pressure overcomes the LES pressure. Spontaneous free reflux occurs readily during periods of very low LES pressures. This form of reflux is most common in those patients with a hypotensive sphincter, usually with LES pressures of less than 10 mm Hg. TLESRs are the most important cause of GER, both in healthy individuals and in patients with esophagitis. TLESRs provide a measure for reflux in patients with normal sphincter pressures.

Severity of esophagitis is related not only to acid reflux but the ability to clear refluxed acid from the esophagus. Acid clearance is determined by esophageal motility, gravity, and swallowed saliva. Normally, esophageal peristalsis acts to protect the esophagus from refluxed gastric contents. The severity of the abnormalities in esophageal peristalsis is proportionate to the severity of esophagitis. Because esophageal peristaltic activity is the major mechanism of acid clearance, impairment of this important function results in a cyclical pattern of worsening esophagitis and decreased acid clearance. The duration of acid exposure to the esophagus can be measured by intraesophageal pH monitoring. The duration of acid exposure correlates better with the severity of esophagitis than the frequency of reflux events. Duration of acid exposure reflects the ability of the esophagus to clear acid. During the awake or upright period, pH tracings show that when patients are standing or sitting and are able to recognize

heartburn and swallow, the reflux episodes are quickly cleared and are short in duration. However, during sleep in the recumbent position, esophageal clearance mechanisms are impaired, and intraesophageal acid is cleared slowly. As previously discussed, saliva production may be impaired by medication or disease. During sleep the amount of saliva produced and the frequency of swallows are reduced, thus diminishing the availability of saliva to neutralize refluxed gastric contents.

Finally, hiatal hernias are common and are noted in 42% of patients with symptoms of reflux but in 60%–80% of patients with endoscopic esophagitis or peptic strictures. Recent studies indicate that patients with large hiatal hernias complicated by relatively low LES pressures are susceptible to reflux episodes following sudden increases in intra-abdominal pressure. These reflux episodes probably occur because the diaphragmatic crus does not contract completely following intra-abdominal pressure events, thereby permitting transmitted intragastric pressure to overcome the LES easily. Once GER occurs, esophageal peristalsis serves to clear the esophageal contents into the hiatal hernia, which then acts as a reservoir of gastric contents awaiting further intra-abdominal pressure events, TLESRs, or free reflux events to repeat the reflux cycle.

CLINICAL PRESENTATIONS OF GERD

GERD presents in several different ways. Patients may have mild disease that barely interferes with their lives, and thus they do not report any symptoms. Typical reflux symptoms occur commonly in healthy individuals and in 80%–85% of patients with esophagitis. Typical symptoms include heartburn and acid regurgitation. Both odynophagia (painful swallowing) and dysphagia are important but less frequently reported symptoms. Odynophagia is more commonly associated with opportunistic infections in the esophagus. Upper GI bleeding in the form of blood-tinged vomitus or iron-deficiency anemia are unusual presentations of GERD. The presence of these less common symptoms suggests that complications of reflux have developed. The term *atypical reflux* is used to describe acid reflux–induced symptoms in areas other than the esophagus, including the oropharynx and respiratory tract, and anginalike chest pain. Common atypical symptoms include hoarseness, globus hystericus, chronic throat clearing, cough, and asthma. The mechanisms believed to be responsible for these atypical reflux symptoms are only partially understood. The mucosal lining of these other structures are much more sensitive to damage than those of the esophagus. Frank aspiration of gastric acid into the trachea or larynx probably plays a small role in the pathophysiology of these atypical symptoms. More important may be microaspiration, in which minute amounts of gastric acid are aspirated into the trachea or larynx, stimulating the chemoreceptors located in these areas to respond by causing a broncho- or laryngospasm. Equally likely is the possibility of broncho- or laryngospasm resulting from the stimulation of esophageal chemoreceptors by refluxed gastric acid.

Classic and atypical symptoms are equally annoying to the patient, may result in serious complications, and are exacerbated in similar ways. Reflux symptoms are reported to be worse postprandially, when the patient is bending over or lying down, and may be improved by standing.

GERD not only results in symptoms, but the complications that develop from persistent GERD are more serious. The most common complications of GERD are ulceration, bleeding, and stricture. The severity of esophagitis graded during an endoscopic evaluation ranges from 1 to 4. Erythema in the distal esophagus is reported as grade 1 esophagitis. More severe grades are based on the presence of erosions, ulcerations, extent of inflammation, and the presence of peptic strictures or Barrett's esophagus.

Barrett's metaplasia is a compensatory change in the esophageal mucosa from the normal stratified squamous epithelium to specialized intestinal epithelium. It occurs in 10%–14% of patients with chronic symptoms of GER. Many patients with Barrett's, the most severe complication of GERD, have only mild heartburn, exhibit atypical symptoms, or may be asymptomatic for reflux. Barrett's metaplasia has the potential to progress from metaplasia to dysplasia and on to adenocarcinoma. The risk of esophageal cancer in patients with Barrett's is 30- to 40-fold higher than in the general population. Adenocarcinoma of the esophagus is almost exclusively from Barrett's esophagus. Its incidence is rising to such a degree that it has been described as being in epidemic proportions, especially in white men.

DIAGNOSIS OF GERD

Prolonged esophageal pH monitoring is the most reliable test for diagnosing GERD. This test requires passing a thin tube via the nares and into the esophagus. There are special sensors that can measure the pH, and some catheters have several sensors. Typically the pH sensors are placed above the LES and below the UES. The patient goes home with the tube in place and maintains a diary of symptoms and records meals, medications, and times when recumbent. The data are then analyzed to determine how often and how long the pH was lower than 4 and to determine if symptoms correlated with a drop in the pH. This test is especially useful in patients with atypical presentations. The sensitivity of the test in diagnosing GERD is around 90%. In addition, ambulatory monitoring devices permit evaluation of the temporal relationship between reflux episodes and atypical symptoms. Although this test is the most reliable procedure, it is relatively expensive, not available at all institutions, and may be uncomfortable for some patients. The addition of a pharyngeal probe to the single distal esophageal pH studies has improved the diagnostic accuracy of atypical reflux symptoms. Placement of the distal pH probe in both the standard and dual pH monitoring systems is 5 cm above the LES. Placement of the proximal probe has been less standardized, but generally they are placed 2–3 cm below the UES. Figure 10-7 is an example of a dual pH tracing.

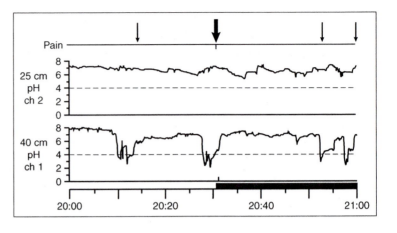

Fig. 10-7.

One hour during this 24-hour ambulatory pH recording from the distal and proximal esophagus shows several episodes of distal reflux (thin arrows). No episodes of proximal reflux were obtained during this 1-hour recording. The normal intraesophageal pH of 6.5–7.5 is maintained by swallowed saliva and esophageal secretions. In the second reflux episode shown in this tracing (heavy arrow), acid reflux into the distal esophagus was associated with heartburn, indicated here as pain. The dark bar indicates the time during which the patient was supine.

Acid perfusion tests, including the Bernstein test and acid reflux tests, are used less frequently today. The Bernstein test is a specific yet insensitive test for diagnosing substernal chest pain and dysphagia caused by GER. In these tests, acid or saline solutions are infused through a nasogastric tube in an attempt to elicit symptoms.

Radionuclide scanning is a very specific test for demonstrating GER or pulmonary aspiration; however, it is not sensitive, and it is expensive. Clearance of a technetium 99m radiolabeled meal from the esophagus can be documented by scintigraphy. The patient undergoes immediate scanning to document GER of labeled material. This may be followed by scanning the next morning to document pulmonary aspiration. In a recent study comparing scintigraphy to other modes of diagnosis, a sensitivity of only 36% was seen; however, the specificity was greater than 88%.

Upper endoscopy is the most specific test for identifying esophageal complications of GER, esophageal ulcers from other causes, infectious disorders, and neoplasms. Esophagitis may be seen in up to 40% of reflux patients, and Barrett's metaplasia will be found in 10%–15% of patients. Esophagoscopy has limited usefulness in demonstrating a relationship between GERD and atypical symptoms. The severity of esophagitis determined by endoscopy, however, is an important predictor of the response to medical therapy.

Table 10-5 summarizes the procedures used to diagnose GERD.

Table 10-5. Diagnostic Procedures Frequently Used for GERD

TEST	INDICATION
Videofluoroscopy with barium esophagography	Oropharyngeal or transfer dysphagia Structural lesions
Fiber optic endoscopic examination of swallowing safety (FEESS)	Pharyngeal dysphagia
Endoscopy	Esophageal mucosal lesions Structural lesions
Esophageal manometry	Esophageal motility disorders
Intraesophageal pH monitoring	Gastroesophageal reflux (GER)
Acid perfusion tests	GER-related symptoms
Radionuclide scanning	GER and pulmonary aspiration

TREATMENT OF GERD

Treatment of GERD involves three primary phases. Phase 1 consists primarily of behavioral modification with specific lifestyle and dietary changes and occasional antacid use. Phase 2 involves the addition of antisecretory therapy in the form of H_2-receptor antagonists, proton pump inhibitors (PPIs), or prokinetic agents. Advances in medical management, specifically in acid suppression with PPI therapy, have reduced the need for surgical management. Within medical therapies there has been great debate on whether to apply a step up (beginning with lifestyle modification) or step down (beginning with the PPIs) approach to therapy. Finally, phase 3 therapy involves antireflux surgery. Nissen fundoplication and the Belsey Mark IV repair are two commonly used surgical procedures for the treatment of idiopathic GERD. Both procedures involve the reduction of a hiatal hernia coupled with the construction of a wrap around the gastroesophageal junction. The Belsey repair creates a partial wrap, whereas the Nissen fundoplication creates a complete wrap. The success of this therapeutic approach is dependent on the degree to which the surgical wrap causes occlusion of the gastroesophageal junction. Laparoscopic procedures are now the standard for surgical therapy. Newer endoscopic therapies have also been developed. One such therapy applies an endoscopically placed suture. Another procedure (Stretta system) uses radiofrequency to promote thermal lesions in the LES where as the lesions heal, the tissue contracts which has resulted in decreased reflux episodes.

Non-GERD-Related Esophageal Mucosal Disease

Although esophageal mucosal injury is most often secondary to GERD, injury can also result from infectious agents and pill ingestion. The clinical presentation may be identical to GERD, including chest pain,

heartburn, and dysphagia. More frequently, however, odynophagia is the patient's primary complaint. Herpes simplex, cytomegalovirus, and *Candida* may invade or colonize the esophageal mucosa and cause inflammation of the mucosa. Clinically significant esophagitis is most commonly seen in immunocompromised patients.

Although not a common cause of esophagitis, muscosal injury as a result of ingested pills should be considered in the differential diagnosis of dysphagia and odynophagia. Potassium chloride, tetracycline, quinidine, and NSAIDs are most frequently implicated. Delayed esophageal transit resulting from esophageal dysmotility increases the amount of mucosal contact with the pill, thus increasing the likelihood of injury.

Summary

Normal swallowing requires the precise interaction of a number of structures and, when functioning properly, proceeds through an orderly sequence. A disruption at any point in the process can cause dysphagia. Disorders of structure resulting from masses, inflammation, or functional derangement as seen in motility abnormalities result in dysphagia. The clinical presentation, however, varies with the etiology of the disordered swallowing. The diagnostic assessment should be based on the presenting clinical symptoms. Likewise, treatment is varied, based on the nature and severity of the patient's dysphagia.

CASE STUDY: *RESOLUTION*

Pneumatic dilation was attempted twice unsuccessfully for this patient. Because of the severity of her disease and the massive dilation and tortuous nature of her esophagus, it was felt that any further endoscopic therapy would be futile. In the absence of esophageal peristalsis, a food bolus would be unable to transverse the curves and upward segments in this severely diseased esophagus. Consequently, a distal esophagectomy with a gastroesophageal anastomosis was performed. The patient did well during the postoperative period and was able to eat within a few of weeks of the surgery. She gained a significant amount of weight and did very well.

---

*R*EVIEW *Q*UESTIONS

Directions: For each of the following questions, choose the one best answer.

1 Which of the following substances increases lower esophageal sphincter (LES) pressure?

A Progesterone
B Nitric oxide (NO)

C Acetylcholine

D Vasoactive intestinal polypeptide (VIP)

2 The mechanism responsible for gastroesophageal reflux (GER) in most patients is

A transient lower esophageal sphincter (LES) relaxations.

B poor esophageal peristalsis.

C delayed gastric emptying.

D persistently weak LES pressure.

3 The diagnostic test considered the gold standard for measuring gastroesophageal reflux (GER) is

A endoscopy.

B 24-hour ambulatory pH monitoring.

C esophageal manometry.

D barium esophagography.

4 Which of the following is true about achalasia?

A The LES is hypotensive.

B It is most common in children.

C Apersistalsis is seen on manometry.

D The esophagus is usually strictured.

5 From among the following, choose the atypical manifestation of reflux:

A Cardiac chest pain.

B Shortness of breath.

C Postnasal drip

D Hoarseness

References

Annese V, Basciani M, Perri F, et al: Controlled trial of botulinum toxin injection versus placebo and pneumatic dilation in achalasia. *Gastroenterology* 111:1418–1424, 1996.

Cook I, Kahrilas P: AGA technical review on management of oropharyngeal dysphagia. *Gastroenterology* 1999;116: 455–478.

Dent J, Doddson J, Friedman RH, et al: Mechanisms of GER in recumbent asymptomatic human subjects. *J Clin Invest* 65:256–267, 1980.

Dodds WJ, Dent J, Hogan WJ, et al: Mechanisms of gastroesophageal reflux in patients with reflux esophagitis. *N Engl J Med* 81:376–394, 1982.

Dua KS, Ren J, Bardan E, et al: Coordination of deglutitive glottal function and pharyngeal bolus transit during normal eating. *Gastroenterology* 112:73–83, 1997.

Hsu JJ, O'Connor MK, Kang YW, et al: Nonspecific motor disorder of the esophagus: a real disorder or a manometric curiosity? *Gastroenterology* 104:1281–1284, 1993.

Jaradeh S: Neurophysiology of swallowing in the aged. *Dysphagia* 9:218–220, 1994.

Katz PO: Ambulatory esophageal and hypopharyngeal pH monitoring in patients with hoarsenses. *Am J Gastroenterol* 85:38–40, 1990.

Massey BI, Dodds WJ, Hogan WJ, et al: Abnormal esophageal motility: an analysis of concurrent radiographic and manometric findings. *Gastroenterology* 101:344–354, 1991.

Mearin F, Mourelle M, Guarner F, et al: Patients with achalasia lack nitric oxide synthase in the gastro-esophageal junction. *Eur J Clin Invest* 23:724–728, 1993.

Reynolds JC, Parkman HP: Achalasia. *Gastroenterol Clin North Am* 18:223–255, 1989.

Waring P: Surgical and endoscopic treatment of gastroesophageal reflux disease. *Gastroenterol Clin North Am* 31: S89–S109, 2002.

11

Peptic Ulcer Disease

▓ CHAPTER OUTLINE ▓

▓ LEARNING OBJECTIVES ▓

At the completion of this chapter, the reader should be able to:

- Explain the functional anatomy of the stomach.
- Describe the paracrine, endocrine, and neurocrine regulation of acid production.
- Classify the phases of gastric acid secretion.
- Correlate gastric physiology as it relates to peptic ulcer disease (PUD).
- Describe the aggressive and protective factors involved in the pathophysiology of PUD.
- Discuss the role of *Helicobacter pylori* and NSAIDs in PUD.
- Classify the medical treatments for PUD.
- Analyze the mechanism of action of the drugs used in treating PUD.
- Identify the surgical treatments for PUD.

PUD results from an imbalance of aggressive and protective factors within the lumen of the stomach and small intestine.

CASE STUDY: *INTRODUCTION*

S.A. was a 32-year-old second-year medical student at the Dyspepsia School of Medicine. She was in excellent health until the beginning of her anatomy course. At that time, she began to complain of intermittent abdominal distress, which was relieved by food. She described the symptoms as "horrible hunger pains," nonradiating, and unrelated to position or change in bowel habits. She took over-the-counter antacids, which offered short-term relief. She denied any vomiting, weight loss, fevers, dysphagia, melena, or bright-red blood per rectum.

Her medical history was quite benign. There was no history of GI problems. She had recently seen her gynecologist for menorrhagia and dysmenorrhea and was placed on birth control pills. Her only other medicines were NSAIDs for the dysmenorrhea. There was no surgical history, and she had never been hospitalized. She had no family history of GI problems or cancer except that her mother was always complaining of similar symptoms.

On examination, she was a healthy woman in no apparent distress. Her sclera were clear, and she had no oral ulcerations. Her lung and cardiac examinations were unremarkable. Her abdomen was soft and nontender, with good bowel sounds and no masses. On rectal examination, she had brown stool that was guaiac-negative. Her laboratory data revealed a normal hemoglobin.

Introduction

Peptic ulcer disease (PUD) is one of the most common GI diseases in the world today. It has been estimated that 15% of men and women in this country will be diagnosed with PUD at some time in their lives. According to a National Institutes of Health (NIH) report, the direct costs of ulcer disease have been estimated to be more than $2 billion annually, with indirect costs reaching at least $500 million. Although it is commonly thought that PUD is simply a disease related to abdominal pain, in fact, ulcers cause bleeding, GI obstruction, perforation, and death.

In the past, PUD was believed to be simply an "acid-related disease." It is now understood that PUD results from an imbalance of aggressive and protective factors within the lumen of the stomach and small intestine. However, to understand ulcers, one must still understand acid, and to understand acid, one must understand the anatomy, histology, and physiology of the stomach.

The stomach is more than just a reservoir that passes on digested food to the intestine; rather, it is an elegant organ with both exocrine and endocrine functions that initiates the breakdown of protein, facilitates the absorption of minerals and other food by-products, and prevents bacterial overgrowth in the intestine. Unfortunately, these

mechanisms that are important to health may also be involved in the pathogenesis of PUD.

The Stomach

ANATOMY

The stomach is generally described as consisting of three parts (Figure 11-1): (1) the fundus, which includes the portion of the stomach proximal to the gastroesophageal junction; (2) the corpus, which covers the fundus to the incisura; and (3) the antrum, which includes the incisura to the pylorus.

FUNCTION

Exocrine

The fundus and cardia contain cells that secrete hydrochloric acid (HCl), pepsin, and intrinsic factor. The fundus and cardia are lined by a simple columnar epithelium of surface mucous cells. The lower two-thirds of the gastric pits contain the parietal cells (source of HCl and intrinsic factor) and the chief cells (source of pepsinogen).

Endocrine

The antrum contains cells that secrete gastrin, somatostatin, and gastrin-releasing peptide. Pyloric glands are made up of mostly mucous

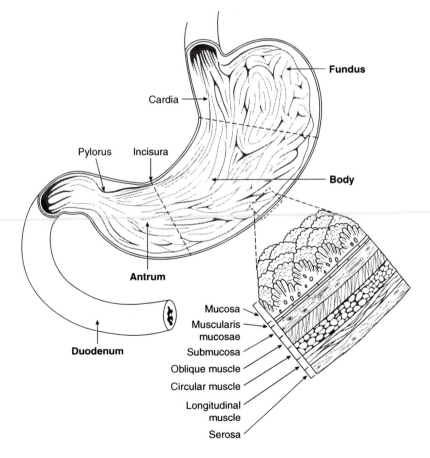

Cardia

Fundus

Pylorus Incisura

Body

Antrum

Duodenum

Mucosa
Muscularis mucosae
Submucosa
Oblique muscle
Circular muscle
Longitudinal muscle
Serosa

Fig. 11-1. Functional Anatomy of the Stomach

cells, G cells (gastrin-secreting cells), and D cells (somatostatin-secreting cells). Immunocytochemical stains have also identified nerve fibers containing gastrin-releasing peptide, serotonin, and histamine.

INNERVATION

Parasympathetic (Vagus Nerve)

The cell bodies of the vagus nerve, located in the medulla, are found on the floor of the fourth ventricle. These fibers contain 80% afferent and 20% efferent fibers.

Sympathetic (Thoracic Splanchnic Nerves)

The Lateral horn cells, located in the thoracic segments T-6 to T-10, give rise to axons that are carried by the thoracic splanchnic nerves to the celiac plexus.

Enteric (Meissner's and Auerbach's Plexuses)

Unique to the GI system are the enteric plexuses that are found both in the submucosal (Meissner's) and myenteric (Auerbach's) layer in the walls of the intestines. Their importance in gastric function is postulated to be less than that of their function in other areas of the intestine.

Transmitters identified in the gastric mucosa include the conventional nonpeptide transmitters, such as acetylcholine, serotonin, and γ-aminobutyric acid (GABA), as well as peptide transmitters, such as bombesin, vasoactive intestinal polypeptide (VIP), opioids (enkephalins), and tachykinins (substance P).

REGULATION OF ACID AT THE CELLULAR LEVEL

The parietal cell (the source of gastric HCl) is stimulated by three mechanisms: (1) neurocrine stimulation via the vagus nerve by *acetylcholine* (ACh), (2) endocrine stimulation via the bloodstream by *gastrin*, and (3) paracrine stimulation via the local circulation by *histamine.*

Although all three receptors can be found on the parietal cell (Figure 11-2A), the fact that H_2 blockers also block ACh- and gastrin-stimulated acid secretion suggests that ACh and gastrin can also stimulate acid secretion via histamine release (Figure 11-2B).

Control of acid secretion becomes even more complicated because gastrin release is also regulated. The G cell (the source of gastrin) is controlled by (1) neurocrine stimulation via the vagus nerve (ACh), (2) endocrine stimulation via the bloodstream (theory) (gastrin-releasing peptide [GRP]), and (3) paracrine inhibition via the local circulation (somatostatin).

Finally, the D cell is controlled by at least one known mechanism, neurocrine inhibition via the vagus nerve through ACh. It is theorized that GRP is responsible for endocrine stimulation via the bloodstream.

The control of HCl secretion by the parietal cell, which is also illustrated in Figure 11-3, can be summarized as follows: under

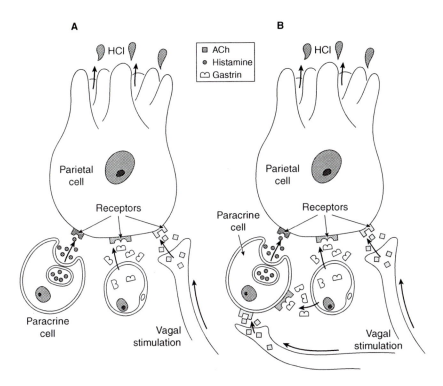

**Fig. 11-2. Regulation of Hydrochloric Acid
at the Cellular Level**

(A) Neurocrine, paracrine, and endocrine action directly on the parietal cell.
(B) Neurocrine and endocrine action on the paracrine cell and the parietal
cell. ACh = acetylcholine.

neurocrine control, ACh (1) directly stimulates production from the
parietal cell, (2) stimulates histamine secretion from the paracrine
cell, (3) stimulates gastrin from the G cell, and (4) inhibits somatostatin release from the D cell, resulting in stimulation of HCl secretion; under *paracrine control,* (1) histamine directly stimulates HCl
production from the parietal cell, and (2) somatostatin inhibits gastrin
release from the G cell; and under *endocrine control,* gastrin stimulates
(1) HCl secretion from the parietal cell and (2) histamine secretion
from the paracrine cell; and theoretically GRP (1) stimulates gastrin
secretion from the G cell and (2) inhibits HCl by stimulating somatostatin from the D cell.

Many of the cells also have a feedback mechanism related to the
concentration of intraluminal hydrogen ion (H^+): (1) in the D cell, H^+
stimulates somatostatin release, thus inhibiting HCl release from the
parietal cell; (2) in the G cell, H^+ inhibits gastrin release, thus blocking gastrin stimulation of parietal cell HCl production.

Finally, other peptides have been implicated in HCl production,
including cholecystokinin (CCK), secretin, gastrin inhibitory polypeptide (GIP), enteroglucagon, neurotensin, and peptide YY (PYY).

Gastrin binds to gastrin receptors, histamine to H_2 receptors, and
ACh to muscarinic M_1 receptors on the parietal cell surface. Once

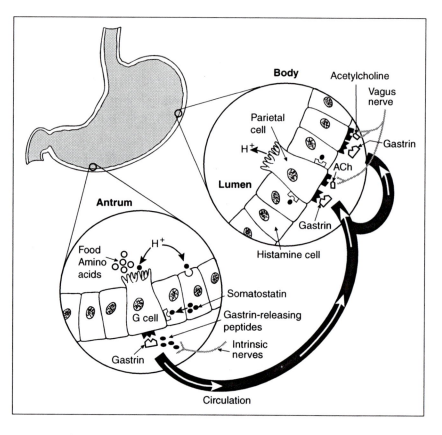

Fig. 11-3. Control of Hydrochloric Acid Secretion by the Parietal Cell

binding has taken place, secondary messenger systems are stimulated; intracellular calcium (Ca^{2+}) is mobilized when gastrin or ACh binds to its receptor and intracellular cyclic AMP (cAMP) elevates when histamine binds to its receptors. The end result is the activation of the H^+-K^+-ATPase, which produces acid secretion via the proton pump (Figure 11-4).

PHYSIOLOGY OF GASTRIC ACID SECRETION

Fasting (Basal)

It appears that tonic vagal stimulation is the principal means of regulation of interprandial acid secretion (vagotomy reduces this period of acid secretion). Circadian in nature, the rate of acid secretion is highest in the evening, with levels lower in the morning. Gastrin and histamine may also have minor roles (H_2 blockers reduce fasting acid secretion).

Prandial (Stimulated)

There appear to be three distinct phases of prandial acid secretin, with both stimulation and inhibition of gastric acid as end points.

Stimulation. Stimulation may be cephalic, gastric, or intestinal. In the *cephalic phase*, the thought, sight, smell, or taste of food can stimulate acid secretion. Physiologic changes (such as hypoglycemia) can

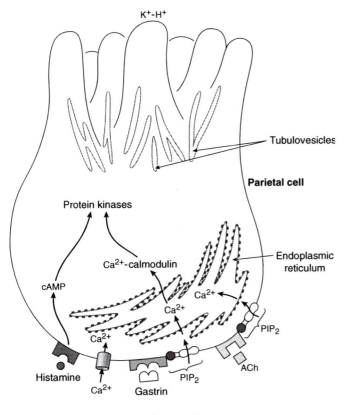

Fig. 11-4.

H$_2$ blockers that inhibit paracrine action of the parietal cell also reduce neurocrine and endocrine action of the parietal cell via the paracrine cell as noted. ACh = acetylcholine; cAMP = cyclic adenosine monophosphate; PIP$_2$ = phosphatidylinositol 4,5-bisphosphate.

also stimulate acid production and stimulation. The mechanisms are (1) vagal stimulation of HCl production by parietal cells, and (2) vagal stimulation of gastrin release from G cells. In the *gastric phase*, the entrance of food into the gastric cavity causes increased acid secretion. The mechanisms are as follows. (1) Distention of the gastric cavity activates stretch receptors in the gastric tissue, which in turn causes vagal stimulation of gastrin release. (2) Chemicals such as caffeine, alcohol, calcium, and products of protein digestion are though to stimulate HCl production via vagal stimulation of gastrin release and, possibly, release of other peptides such as CCK, secretin, GIP, and PYY. In the *intestinal phase*, the entrance of food into the duodenum activates HCl production. The mechanisms involved are as follows. (1) Distention activates acid production, although the precise mechanism is unknown; it is not inactivated by vagotomy. (2) Chemicals, such as products of protein digestion (peptides, amino acids), are thought to stimulate HCl production via gastrin or other humoral agents.

Inhibition.   Inhibition is also classified as cephalic, gastric, or intestinal. In the *cephalic phase*, the proposed mechanism is via bombesin.

Animals with bombesin injected into the brain were found to have inhibited gastric acid secretion. In the *gastric phase*, antral acidification (pH < 2) blocks the gastrin stimulation of HCl secretion. The *intestinal phase* is the predominant inhibitory phase, in which (1) acid, possibly via secretin or another unidentified hormone, decreases acid secretion in the stomach; and (2) fatty acids, possibly via enterogastrin, inhibit acid secretion.

Much of the data generated to describe and define the phases of gastric acid secretion, as well as the clinical applications of gastric acid secretion, require the knowledge of how gastric acid is measured. Aspiration of gastric juice using a small nasogastric tube is the most commonly used method of measuring gastric acid secretion in humans. The following measurements can be determined:

1. Basal acid output (BAO) estimates resting acid secretion. By means of the nasogastric tube, the gastric contents are collected for four consecutive 15-minute periods, and H^+ content is measured. BAO is expressed as H^+ mEq/hr and the normal range is 0–11 mEq H^+/hr.

2. Maximal acid output (MAO) or peak acid output (PAO) estimates maximal acid secretion in response to an exogenous secretagogue for HCl. Pentagastrin is used, either intramuscularly or intravenously, in doses that cause supraphysiologic stimulation of HCl from the parietal cell. Normal range is 10–63 mEq H^+/hr. The measurements are used to estimate the total number of parietal cells (parietal cell mass).

Although these measurements have been helpful in understanding PUD and diagnosing diseases of increased acid secretion, such as Zollinger-Ellison syndrome, these measurements actually underestimate gastric acid secretion. It is important to note that during these measurements acid is lost into the duodenum, H^+ diffuses back into gastric mucosa, and gastric HCO_3^- neutralizes acid.

Pathophysiology of PUD

DEFINITIONS

Superficial breakdowns of the GI lining not involving the submucosa are called *erosions*. These generally heal without scars. On the other hand, breakdown of the GI lining involving the muscularis and deeper layers are *ulcers*. Complications include pain, bleeding, perforation, obstruction, and death. Ulcers can be found anywhere in the GI tract, but PUD is used to describe one or more ulcers involving the stomach or duodenum, in the absence of a gastric or small intestine malignancy.

MECHANISM OF DISEASE

The Davenport model was the original description of the pathogenesis of ulcers: "no acid, no ulcer." This theory has been expanded to state that ulcers arise when there is an imbalance between aggressive factors and defensive factors. In general, the latter hypothesis applies equally to both type 1 (fundic and cardia ulcers) and type 2 (duodenal and prepyloric ulcers). However, some differences do exist; for example, type 2 ulcers are associated with an enhanced secretion of acid, whereas, in type 1 ulcers less acid may be secreted than normal. Two clinical examples where hyperacidity alone leads to PUD are Zollinger-Ellison syndrome and Cushing's ulcer.

- **Zollinger-Ellison Syndrome.** In this syndrome, there is a gastrin-secreting tumor that causes ulcers of the non–beta cell endocrine pancreas, which leads to hypersecretion of acid and multiple GI ulcers.
- **Cushing's Ulcer.** This is a hyperacidic state resulting from increased vagal tone. Patients in intensive care with CNS trauma or surgery are at great risk for these ulcers.

Mucosal Aggressive Factors

Pepsin. This proteolytic enzyme produced by H^+ activation of pepsinogen, which is secreted by the chief cells, has been suggested to cause proteolytic damage and mucosal injury in the duodenum of families that produce excessive pepsinogen I. Its role in the genesis of ulcers in the rest of the population is not well understood.

Bile. Lithocholic acid has been found to cause mucosal damage in patients who are known to have bile refluxing into the gastric cavity. This often occurs in patients with gastric motility disorders or abnormal gastric anatomy secondary to surgery. However, inhibition of acid secretion in these patients can result in healing of ulcers, suggesting that HCl, not bile, may be the true aggressive factor.

Alcohol, Tobacco, and Caffeine. Alcohol, tobacco, and caffeine have all been shown to be risk factors for PUD; however, their actual role in the generation of ulcers is unclear. Caffeine acts synergistically with histamine to stimulate gastric acid secretion. Nicotine may decrease HCO_3^- secretion (a gastric protective mechanism) in tobacco users; the rate of healing of ulcers is decreased in smokers. Alcohol can increase gastric acid production. Despite this research, it is still unknown if these chemicals can lead to ulcers without the presence of other aggressive factors.

H. pylori. There has been a clear causal association established between *Helicobacter pylori* infection and mucosal damage of the upper GI tract, primarily the gastric antrum and duodenum. *H. pylori* is an S-shaped, gram-negative rod flagellate and has been found in the antrum of more than 95% of patients with duodenal ulcers and at least 75% of patients with gastric ulcers. Unfortunately, 20% of healthy volunteers and 50% of patients with nonulcer dyspepsia are also infected; thus, most infected patients have no ulcers. One of the most important arguments in favor of a causal role of *H. pylori* in the

Infection with *H. pylori* has been shown to result in mucosal damage to the upper GI tract.

NSAIDs irritate the mucosa and inhibit prostaglandin production.

pathogenesis of PUD is the lower relapse rate of patients with duodenal ulcers in whom *H. pylori* was eradicated. Clearly, this is one of the predominant aggressive factors for peptic ulceration in the stomach and proximal small bowel. It has been suggested that *H. pylori* promotes peptic ulceration by disrupting the mucous barrier. *H. pylori* eradication is now one of the hallmarks of treating PUD.

NSAIDs. Ulceration is increased in patients taking NSAIDs, approximately 2%–4% patients/yr. Several factors appear to increase this risk, including family history of PUD, cigarette smoking, alcohol, and *H. pylori* infection. NSAIDs play a major role in ulcer formation. Many have a topical irritative effect on the GI mucosa, but more likely the problem is their ability to inhibit prostaglandin production. Cotherapy with prostaglandin analogs can prevent NSAID-induced complications. Studies have also found decreased mucous secretion and decreased HCO_3^- secretion in patients treated with NSAIDs. Because GI adverse events may result from treatment with NSAIDs, the use of cyclo-oxygenase-2 (COX-2)-specific inhibitors has increased. Patients experience approximately half the associated GI risks compared with nonselective NSAIDs. An alternative approach would be taking the NSAID in conjunction with a proton pump inhibitor (PPI), which will similarly reduce the GI risk. PPIs are more costly than the use of a generic NSAID alone, and COX-2 therapy is also more expensive than generic NSAIDs. The choice of therapy is also challenged with recent concerns about potential cardiovascular toxicity associated with COX-2-specific inhibitors.

Aggressive factors, albeit quite important, are only one set of factors involved in the pathogenesis of PUD; mucosal resistance factors, mucosal blood flow, and prostaglandins are just as important in the pathophysiology of ulcers.

Mucosal Resistance Factors

Mucus. There are two types of mucous cells: surface mucous cells and gastric pit mucous cells. Mucous cells are found throughout the upper GI tract, from the cardia to the duodenum. These cells secrete mucus, which is a glycoprotein, and are possibly regulated by cholinergic agonists. In general, the gastric epithelium is protected by the mucous gel that covers its entire epithelium. This barrier consists of an unstirred layer of mucus, HCO_3^-, phospholipids, and water. It is 0.2–0.6 mm in diameter, with a pH gradient extending from the lumen (pH 2) to the epithelial surface (pH 7). The actual role of mucus as a protective factor is controversial. The consequences of breaching this layer appear minimal. Substances such as aspirin that can disrupt the mucous layer can also cause damage to the underlining epithelium, so that the actual role of disrupting the mucous layer is unclear. Perhaps more important is the ability of mucus to restoring already damaged mucosa. It has been suggested that the mucous layer helps form a mucoid cap over a denuded area, protecting the underlying acid-sensitive basal lamina.

Bicarbonate. HCO_3^- is secreted throughout the stomach and duodenum surface mucous cells, Brunner's glands, and the pancreas. HCO_3^- secretion is controlled by a variety of mechanisms. (1) Under *endocrine* control, enteroglucagon, pancreatic polypeptide (PP), CCK, and VIP have all been shown to stimulate the secretion of HCO_3^-. (2) Under *neurocrine* control, HCO_3^- is stimulated via the vagus nerve by sham feeding and functional distention. (3) Under *paracrine* control, endogenous mucosal prostaglandins and luminal acid also stimulate the secretion of HCO_3^-. As discussed, mucosal HCO_3^- not only contributes to the mucous layer but also neutralizes acid in the lumen ($HCO_3^- \rightarrow H_2CO_3 \rightarrow H_2O + CO_2$). Despite all these mechanisms, the magnitude of the importance of HCO_3^- is difficult to ascertain. There are data to suggest that in patients with decreased HCO_3^- secretion (such as smokers with decreased duodenal and pancreatic HCO_3^- secretion), peptic ulcers are higher in incidence and take longer to heal.

Gastric ulcers in burn patients are examples of ulcers occurring due to decreased mucosal cytoprotection. Burn patients have an increased risk of ulcer disease. Acid output is normal, and the incidence of ulcerations is proportional to the surface area of the burn. Thus, it is presumed that the problem lies with inadequate defenses, not hyperacidity.

Mucosal Blood Flow. The high metabolic rate of the gastric and duodenal epithelium requires rapid blood flow to maintain oxygenation. The rate-limiting step for HCO_3^- transportation during H^+ production by the parietal cell is mucosal blood supply. The importance of mucosal blood flow thus becomes evident, but its exact role is not completely understood. In shock and other low-flow conditions, mesentery blood flow is shunted to the systemic circulation to maintain perfusion. This shunting is important in clinical situations in which stress-related mucosal disease is common, such as in patients in intensive care units. Animal studies in which arterial supply to the stomach was interrupted for as little as 30 seconds found a decreased pH in the mucoid cap, allowing an erosion to extend even deeper into the submucosa.

Prostaglandins. It appears that prostaglandin E (PGE) analogs can inhibit gastric acid secretion. They act on the parietal cell by inhibiting H^+ production via adenylate cyclase inhibition. In mucus-secreting cells, binding of PGE can also stimulate HCO_3^- secretion via adenylate cyclase stimulation. Finally, animal studies suggest that PGE also inhibits histamine release and enhances mucosal blood flow. Theoretically, these actions would all be protective mechanisms in the pathogenesis of PUD.

Genetics. There is a threefold increased risk of developing a duodenal ulcer in the first-degree relatives of duodenal ulcer patients. Males are represented more often than females in a ratio of 2:1. As discussed, families with increased levels of pepsinogen have an increased risk of duodenal ulcers. Blood group O patients are represented more often among duodenal ulcer patients than other blood groups. Finally,

Cessation of smoking is imperative in PUD treatment.

duodenal ulcer patients are more likely to be nonsecretors of ABH antigens in their saliva. The genetic data for gastric ulcers are similar: Sibling risk is increased threefold.

Treatment of PUD

Therapies for PUD can be classified as nonpharmacologic or pharmacologic. Included among the nonpharmacologic therapies are cessation of smoking because of its role as an aggressive factor in PUD and reducing and eliminating aspirin and NSAID usage because of the important role they play in the pathogenesis of PUD. The importance of drinking milk and the restriction of spicy foods in the treatment of PUD has been touted for years, but these therapies have never been shown to heal ulcers. Surgery remains an important therapy for some cases of PUD, though the increase in pharmacologic options has diminished its role as an elective treatment.

SURGICAL THERAPIES

As more efficacious pharmacotherapeutic agents become available for the treatment of PUD, the need for elective surgical treatment lessens; however, the incidence of emergent surgery has not changed over the past 15 years. Many different surgical approaches have been used for the treatment of PUD (Figure 11-5). These include gastroenterostomy, subtotal gastrectomy, and elective vagotomies.

Gastroenterostomy

This operation was performed to divert gastric acid from the duodenum to allow ulcer healing. This operation became obsolete 50 years ago; it is not used today.

Subtotal Gastrectomy

The rationale for this procedure is to reduce acid secretion by removing the entire antrum of the stomach, allowing the reduction of variable amounts of the parietal cell mass. Initially, 75% of the stomach was removed with significant side effects. Now 60%–65% is removed and results in much less morbidity. Depending on the state of the duodenum, a gastroduodenal anastomosis may be chosen (Billroth I) or a gastrojejunal anastomosis (Billroth II) (see Figure 11-5A and B).

Truncal Vagotomy

The intent of this surgery is to reduce basal acid secretion by 85% and MAO response to gastrin and histamine by 50% (see Figure 11-5C). Pepsin secretion by chief cells is also reduced. Unfortunately, vagotomy also destroys the afferent and efferent motor fibers to the stomach. The vagus is important in the regulation of gastric motor function, so vagotomy impairs gastric relaxation and pyloric sphincter relaxation. Thus, an accompanying drainage procedure is needed. Five are available, but the most common is pyloroplasty, in which a longitudinal incision is made across the pylorus. Other physiologic consequences of truncal vagotomy include (1) a decrease in the pancreatic basal enzyme

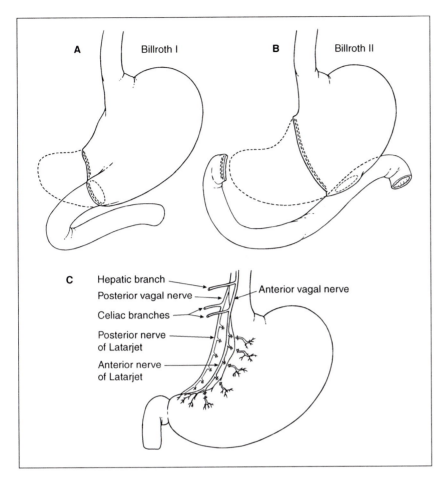

Fig. 11-5. Surgical Approaches to PUD

(A) Billroth I, in which the duodenum is anastomosed to the resected stomach;
(B) Billroth II, in which the resected stomach is anastomosed to the jejunum;
and (C) truncal vagotomy.

secretion and the loss of cephalic and gastric phases of pancreatic secretion, (2) the loss of the gastrocholecystic reflex and the possibility
of defective gallbladder contraction, and (3) postvagotomy diarrhea.
The cause of postvagotomy diarrhea is unknown, but rapid gastric
emptying, rapid small intestine transit, increased delivery of bile acids
and carbohydrates to the colon, and bacterial overgrowth of the upper
GI tract have all been implicated.

Selective Gastric Vagotomy

The extragastric vagal branches are spared to decrease the nongastric
physiologic consequences of a truncal vagotomy.

Highly Selective or Proximal Gastric Vagotomy

Only the parietal cell mass is vagally denervated. The antrum retains
its vagal input and motility is not affected; thus, no drainage procedure is required. Other advantages include (1) less risk of infection
because there is no entry into the GI tract by the surgeon, (2) few
long-term side effects, and (3) no suture lines. The major disadvantage

Notes

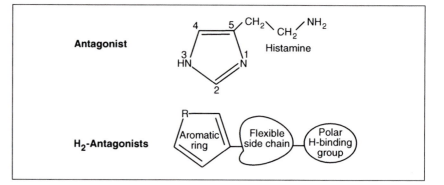

Fig. 11-6. H₂-Receptor Antagonists

is the requirement of highly specialized surgical skills; there is a high incidence of ulcer recurrence if the surgery is not done correctly.

PHARMACOLOGIC THERAPIES

Drugs used to treat PUD can be grouped by their mechanism of action: (1) decreasing the H^+ level in the stomach, (2) increasing gastric and small bowel protective mechanisms, and (3) eradicating *H. pylori*.

Therapies to Decrease Gastric Activity

H₂-Receptor Antagonists. H₂-receptor antagonists (see Figure 11-6) include cimetidine, ranitidine, famotidine, and nizatidine. These medicines block the effects of histamine by binding to H_2 receptors on gastric parietal cells. They inhibit the basal, nocturnal, and food-stimulated acid secretion by 90%. They have also been shown to decrease pepsin secretion. Clinically, H_2 blockers are well known to promote healing of peptic ulcers and decrease ulcer recurrence.

Rapidly absorbed, with peak half-lives between 2 and 2.5 hours, most H₂-receptor antagonists are eliminated in urine, although hepatic biotransformation does play an important role in some, and a portion can be found in plasma protein blood. The various H₂-receptor antagonists have many more similarities than differences and rapidly became the most common agents used in the treatment of PUD because of their ease of usage (two or four times per day) and the relative absence of side effects. H₂-receptor antagonists are now readily available over-the-counter in the United States and are widely advertised and used by consumers.

Side effects include drug interactions because these drugs use the cytochrome P-450 system. Cimetidine has been shown to cause gynecomastia, sexual dysfunction, and mental confusion in the elderly. Although the new H_2 blockers have fewer of these effects, they can still occur.

PPIs. PPIs (see Figure 11-7) include omeprazole, lansoprazole, esomeprazole, pantoprazole, and rabeprazole. They are the most powerful inhibitors of gastric acid secretion available. They have been shown to heal ulcers faster than other agents, and administration is one to two

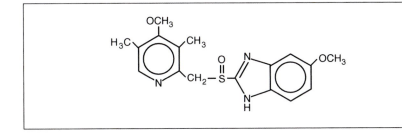

Fig. 11-7. H⁺-K⁺-ATPase Inhibitors

H_2 antagonists share similar structures with histamine, as noted. Differences in the flexible side chains and polar H-binding groups separate the different H_2 blockers now available.

times daily. They work by inhibiting H^+-K^+-ATPase (the proton pump), and thus inhibit histamine-, gastrin-, and ACh-stimulated acid secretion. This inhibition is irreversible, and cellular acid production can only occur when a new proton pump is formed.

PPIs are rapidly absorbed but must be protected from stomach acidity to do so. The half-life is 1 hour, but drug actions last 1–3 days. These drugs are completely eliminated by biotransformation.

Side effects have been observed in animals, where prolonged use of PPIs at high levels with resultant high levels of circulating gastrin have been shown to cause carcinoid tumors and parietal cell hyperplasia. This phenomenon has yet to be seen with doses used in humans. When first approved, these medications had a black box warning indicating they were recommended for a limited time only because the FDA was concerned about the increase in serum gastrin. This original warning was removed when additional safety data became available. Now one of the PPIs has been approved for the over-the-counter use.

Antacids. Rather than inhibiting secretion of acid, antacids decrease H^+ levels in the stomach by neutralizing the already secreted acid. They offer rapid symptomatic relief but require multiple dosing schedules (five to six times per day) for PUD treatment, which makes their usage difficult. There are over 30 antacids available on the market, but they can be grouped as products containing magnesium, aluminum, or calcium.

The *magnesium hydroxide* group is a potent one, with the major side effect of diarrhea. Some of the original dose is absorbed and rapidly excreted by the kidney, which can be toxic to patients with chronic renal failure.

The *aluminum hydroxide* group is less potent than the magnesium-containing antacids; these tend to cause constipation as a side effect. Patients can become phosphate-depleted when using these agents every 4 hours.

The *calcium carbonate* group offers excellent acid-neutralizing power. However, these drugs can prevent absorption of other drugs (e.g., tetracyclines), cause rebound acid hyposensitivity, and milk-alkali syndrome. They do offer a source of calcium to peri- and post-menopausal women.

Antimuscarinic Agents. Antimuscarinic agents (such as propantheline bromide) decrease basal and food-stimulated gastric acid secretion by 50% and 30%, respectively, much less than other acid inhibitors. They have limited clinical usage because of their side effects, such as dry mouth, tachycardia, urinary retention, and blurred vision.

Therapies to Increase Gastric and Small Bowel Protective Mechanisms

Sucralfate. In the stomach, this drug polymerizes into a sticky gel and can bind to an ulcer crater. It also directly binds and inactivates pepsin. In clinical trials, sucralfate promoted ulcer healing as effectively as cimetidine. Unlike acid-reducing agents, this drug is not absorbed systemically. The most frequent side effect is constipation. Its clinical usage is inhibited by its dosing schedule (four times per day).

Colloidal Bismuth Compounds. These agents coat ulcer craters with a thick layer. This appears to increase mucous production and inhibit pepsin. These drugs also have bacteriostatic activity against *H. pylori*. As with sucralfate, the dosing schedule is difficult (four times per day), but there are few side effects. These agents have been as effective as cimetidine in the treatment of PUD.

Prostaglandin Agonists. As described earlier, prostaglandins protect the gastric and small bowel mucosa by stimulating mucous secretion, increasing mucosal blood flow, and inhibiting gastric acid secretion. Misoprostol, a prostaglandin agonist, has been found to promote ulcer healing and decrease ulcer recurrence in patients using NSAIDs. Its usage has been limited by its major side effect, diarrhea. There is more recent clinical information that suggests a decreased dosage schedule (twice a day rather than four times) is just as effective and has fewer side effects.

Therapies to Eradicate H. pylori

The role of *H. pylori* in PUD has been clearly established, and its eradication is important in reducing its recurrence and may also heal active PUD. Numerous antibiotics and antibiotic combinations have been used. There are multiple FDA-approved treatment regimens for *H. pylori* with two to four medications taken over 10–14 days. Eradication is not 100% for any single regimen, and testing may be recommended to document eradication of *H. pylori* with breath testing, stool testing (noninvasive), or endoscopic biopsy.

CASE STUDY: *RESOLUTION*

S.A. was treated with an H_2 blocker twice a day. She immediately had relief, but her symptoms returned after 2 weeks, at which point she complained of maroon stools and presented to the emergency room. An endoscopy showed multiple erosions in her antrum with a 7-mm ulcer in the duodenal bulb that was actively bleeding. The bleeding was treated with injection therapy of epinephrine, and then electrocautery was applied with good coagulation noted. She was observed in the hospital and did well. A biopsy of the antrum done at the time of endoscopy showed that the patient was infected with *H. pylori*. She was treated with omeprazole and clarithromycin for 2 weeks, followed by omeprazole for another 2 weeks. She noted almost complete relief of symptoms over the next 10 days and had no further complaints of abdominal pain, bleeding, or other GI symptoms.

REVIEW QUESTIONS

Directions: For each of the following questions, choose the one best answer.

1 Which of the following mechanisms is involved in the stimulation of acid during the prandial phase of gastric acid secretion?

   A Bile reflux into the stomach stimulates acid secretion.
   B Entrance of bicarbonate (HCO_3^-) into the gastric cavity increases acid secretion.
   C Entrance of food into the colon activates hydrochloric acid (HCl) production.
   D Thought, sight, smell, or taste of food can stimulate acid secretion.

2 The pathogenesis of PUD is now felt to be an imbalance between aggressive and defensive factors in the mucosal lining of the stomach and small intestine. Which of the following mucosal aggressive factors is *most* important in the production of gastric ulcers?

   A Pepsin
   B Bile
   C *Helicobacter pylori*
   D Alcohol
   E Tobacco

3 A variety of pharmacologic therapies are now available for the treatment of PUD. The most powerful inhibitor of gastric acid secretion is

   A H_2-receptor antagonists
   B Sucralfate
   C K^+-H^+-ATPase inhibitors
   D Antacids

4 Despite the success of pharmacologic therapies to treat PUD, surgery is still required at times for patients with active ulcers. Truncal vagotomy is a commonly used surgical treatment. A possible side effect of a truncal vagotomy is

A an increase in pancreatic basal enzyme secretion.
B loss of the gastrocolonic reflex.
C postvagotomy diarrhea.
D somatostatin-producing tumors.

5 Which of the following statements best defines PUD?

A Superficial breakdown of the GI lining that does not involve the submucosa
B Breakdown of the GI lining that involves the muscularis and deeper layers in the setting of gastric cancer
C One or more ulcers involving the stomach and duodenum in the absence of a gastric or small intestine malignancy
D Stress-induced breakdown in the lining of the small intestine

References

Del Valle J, Chey WD, Schieman JM: Acid peptic disorders. In *Textbook of Gastroenterology*. Edited by Yamada T et al. Philadelphia, PA: Lippincott Williams & Wilkins, 2003, pp 1321–1376.

Hunt, RH. *Helicobacter pylori*: from theory to practice. Proceedings of a symposium. *Am J Med* 100(5A), 1996 (supplement).

Mezey E, Paklovitx M: Localization of targets for anti-ulcer drugs in cells of the immune system. *Science*, 258:1662–1665, 1992.

Molinoff PB: *Peptic Ulcer Disease: Mechanisms and Management*. Rutherford, NJ: Health Place, 1990.

Muller MJ, Defize J: Control of pepsinogen synthesis and secretion. *Gastroenterol Clin N Am* 19(1):27–40, 1990.

NIH Consensus Development Conference. *Helicobacter pylori* in peptic ulcer disease. *J Am Med Assoc*, 272:65–69, 1994.

12

Small Bowel Disorders

■ CHAPTER OUTLINE ■

■ LEARNING OBJECTIVES ■

At the completion of this chapter, the reader should be able to:
- Identify the major causes of malabsorption and their pathogenesis.
- Identify disorders of small bowel motility.
- Analyze how intestinal ischemia of the small bowel occurs.
- Enumerate small intestine neoplasms and risk factors for their development.
- Distinguish various small bowel disorders.

CASE STUDY: *INTRODUCTION*

At presentation, the patient, a 26-year-old man, complained of a 1-year history of weight loss (approximately 30 lbs), increasing frequency of bowel movements (five to seven times a day), and fatigue. He stated that the bowel movements were greasy and difficult to flush. He denied any abdominal pain but complained of abdominal bloating. The patient denied any loss of appetite, nausea, or vomiting. Over the week prior to admission, he noted increased swelling in both feet and in the left leg and pain and tenderness in the left calf. The patient denied taking any medication on a regular basis. He has not traveled outside of the country.

His medical and surgical history were insignificant. He was not sexually active at the time of his admission but was heterosexual and had tested negative for HIV about 6 months prior to admission. He was employed as a political consultant. He never smoked and very rarely drank alcohol. He denied any illicit drug use.

The patient was of Jewish descent, but the last several generations of his family lived in Ireland. There was no known family history of any GI disorders.

On physical examination, the patient appeared pale and chronically ill but in no acute distress. He was afebrile, and his pulse and blood pressure were normal. He was nonorthostatic. No skin lesions were noted. Examination of the head, eyes, ears, nose, and throat was notable for pale conjunctiva. Cardiovascular and respiratory examinations were normal. Abdominal examination revealed a bloated, slightly doughy abdomen. Bowel sounds were normoactive. There was no hepatosplenomegaly. His left extremity was swollen to the thigh with 2+ pitting edema of the skin. The right foot also had a 2+ pitting edema. Neurologic examination was normal.

Laboratory results were as follows: There was a normal white blood cell (WBC) count. Hemoglobin and hematocrit were depressed at 11.5 g/dl and 35%, respectively. Platelets were normal. The mean corpuscular volume (MCV) was 79 fl. Electrolyte blood urea nitrogen (BUN) and creatinine were normal. Liver function tests were normal. Albumin was 2.8 g/dl (low). Prothrombin time (PT) and activated partial thromboplastin time (APTT) were normal. A coagulogulation profile, antithrombin III, protein C, and protein S were normal. Stool cultures, ova and parasites, and *Clostridium difficile* were negative. Qualitative stool fat was positive for macrovesicular drops. Ferritin was 10 ng/ml (low). A small bowel endoscopy was notable for flat mucosa and subtotal villous atrophy.

Malabsorption Syndromes

Although carbohydrate and protein as well as fat can be malabsorbed, when speaking of clinical syndromes in the small intestine, one thinks most commonly of fat malabsorption. Fat malabsorption can be divided into three broad categories: (1) maldigestion of intraluminal contents, (2) malabsorption postmucosally as a result of lymphatic obstruction, and (3) malabsorption by the mucosa.

Intraluminal maldigestion may occur in several disorders. It occurs secondary to pancreatic exocrine insufficiency (which may occur in chronic pancreatitis), cystic fibrosis, or with somatostatinomas. Malabsorption may also occur with bacterial overgrowth secondary to stasis syndromes that cause brush-border damage or poor micelle formation, to name just a few of the mechanisms responsible. Finally, chronic liver disease and bile duct obstruction result in steatorrhea as a result of both bile salt and pancreatic insufficiency.

Postmucosal malabsorption due to lymphatic obstruction occurs in intestinal lymphangiectasia and can be either congenital or acquired (posttraumatic, lymphoma, carcinoma, Whipple's disease). These diseases cause a significant protein-losing enteropathy as well as significant steatorrhea.

This chapter focuses on mucosal malabsorption. Celiac disease, tropical sprue, Whipple's disease, abetalipoproteinemia, and immune system diseases are reviewed.

Before proceeding to a discussion of systemic disorders, readers should be aware that drugs such as cholestyramine, neomycin, para-aminosalicylic acid, and colchicine can cause steatorrhea, usually by causing enterocyte damage. A careful history can exclude pharmacologic causes. Infectious diseases are discussed elsewhere in this book, but when considering steatorrhea, it is important to exclude *Isospora* and *Giardia* as well as *Strongyloides* species as causative agents. These organisms cause steatorrhea by causing brush-border damage. Stool examination and small bowel biopsy generally exclude these treatable diseases.

CELIAC DISEASE

Celiac disease, also known as celiac sprue, nontropical sprue, or gluten-sensitive enteropathy, is generally considered the prototypical disease of mucosal malabsorption. It is a disease activated by the ingestion of wheat gluten (gliadin) and similar proteins called prolamins in rye, oats, and barley. These proteins cause damage to the mucosa of the small intestine, resulting in malabsorption. Newer data suggest strong genetic and immunologic components.

Celiac disease can be seen as a spectrum of disease, ranging from the clinically silent to active disease to the latent form seen with dermatitis herpetiformis. The prevalence in the United States is 1 in 3000 to 1 in 10,000. It used to be known as the Irish disease because the prevalence in western Ireland was 1 in 300, but the prevalence

Three Categories of Fat Malabsorption
1. Intraluminal maldigestion
2. Postmucosal malabsorption as a result of lymphatic obstruction
3. Mucosal malabsorption

Celiac Disease
Celiac disease is the prototypical disease of mucosal malabsorption. It is activated by wheat gluten and prolamins in rye, oats, and barley.

has been falling since 1975. It is relatively common in Northern Europe but less common in Central America, South America, the Middle East, and the Indian continent. It is very rare in Southeast Asia and Africa.

Pathogenesis

The disease usually presents after weaning, when grains are introduced into the diet, and sometimes goes into remission in adolescence. In adults, it often presents in the third decade and occasionally later. The pathogenesis of celiac disease is thought to be multifactorial, consisting of environmental, genetic, and immunologic factors.

Environmental Factors

One environmental factor is grain. Taxonomically, wheat, rye, oats, and barley activate the disease with their protein moieties of gliadin and prolamins (secalins, avenins, hordeins). There are 40 different types of gliadin, classified by electrophoretic function (α, β, γ, ω). The major disease-activating component is the α-gliadin.

A second environmental factor may be the role of human adenovirus in the pathogenesis of this disease. Both the α-gliadin protein and the E1b protein of human adenovirus serotype 12 have a region of amino acid similarity. This homology sequence may be an antigenic determinant for certain populations of patients with celiac disease. Some patients have been reported to have a significantly higher prevalence of serotype 12 adenovirus than controls.

Genetic Factors

Genetics also plays a role in the pathogenesis of celiac disease. In family and twin studies, this condition occurs in 5%–15% of first-degree relatives, and there is 70%–75% concordance for monozygotic twins.

Other genetic evidence for celiac disease is found in human leukocyte antigen (HLA) and non-HLA markers. Celiac disease is associated with HLA class IID region genes in the major histocompatibility complex (MHC) on chromosome 6. Within the HLA-D region, two DQ subregion alleles (*DQA1*0501* and *DQB1*0201*) code for a specific DQ2 molecule that is present in 95% of celiac disease patients from different geographic areas. These two alleles are inherited in a *cis* pattern on HLA-DR17 haplotypes versus a *trans* pattern on heterozygote DR11/DR7 or DR12/DR7 haplotypes. Other HLA haplotypes inherit these two alleles in a *cis* or *trans* pattern in a small number of individuals. The presence of the specific DQ molecule is necessary for susceptibility to disease, but it is not sufficient evidence for expression of the disease. Only 0.1% of people carrying the molecule develop clinically apparent disease. It also may be the gene dosage of *DQB1*0201* that increases susceptibility to celiac disease.

If the DQ2 molecule is not present, then the HLA-DR4 haplotype with alleles *DQA1*0301* and *DQB1*0302* encodes a DQ8 molecule. This evidence indicates that it is likely that more than one MHC-encoded gene contributes to the disease pathogenesis.

The HLA locus is not the only area that influences development of the disease. The fact that 25% of identical twins and 60% of siblings thought to be HLA identical do not develop disease points to other host background genes or environmental factors that influence the expression of the disease.

A second area of genetic susceptibility for celiac disease is thought to be the genes that encode the immunoglobulin G (IgG) heavy chain (Gm markers). Evidence for this exists in the fact that the G2m(n) allotype marker on IgG_2 has been associated with the persistence of antigliadin antibody in patients who are on a gluten-free diet. Other candidate genes modulating immune response are also thought to play a role in susceptibility to celiac disease.

Immunologic Factors

Humoral and cell-mediated immunity may also play a role in pathogenesis. Evidence for humoral factors is suggested by the fact that IgG and IgA antibodies to gliadin exist in patients with active celiac disease, in patients with partially treated disease, and in patients with asymptomatic disease. The IgG antibody can persist for long periods of time in clinically asymptomatic patients and in patients on a gluten-free diet. However, it can also be seen in other intestinal disorders. IgA titers are higher in untreated than treated celiac disease patients. It is not usually seen in healthy controls but can be seen in IgA mesangial glomerulonephritis.

Secretions of the small intestine also contain increased humoral factors. Most patients with this condition and 15%–20% of patients with other disorders have increased IgA and IgM antibodies. This increase is associated with increased numbers of IgG, IgA, and IgM cells in the lamina propria and thereby is thought to play a role in maintaining the inflammatory response in the mucosa of the patient with celiac disease. Approximately 2% of patients with celiac disease are IgA deficient. These patients produce increased amounts of IgM cells instead of IgA in the lamina propria. This fact must be taken into consideration in the serologic testing for diagnosis because a low titer of antibody may simply reflect IgA deficiency.

In addition to being found in increased amounts in celiac disease, antigliadin antibodies may play a role in pathogenesis by forming immune complexes. The formation of immune complexes may activate tissue effector mechanisms by stimulating the complement cascade and even by causing antibody-dependent, cell-mediated cytotoxic reactions. Often people with celiac disease have antibodies to other proteins, such as milk, soy, and egg, resulting in either increased permeability of the mucosa or an abnormality in immunoregulation of host responses to dietary antigens.

In terms of cell-mediated immunity, increased numbers of intraepithelial lymphocytes (IELs) have been noted in the small intestine mucosa. There is an increase in the proportion of IELs bearing the γ/δ T cell receptor to those bearing the α/β T cell receptor. However, it is the T cells bearing the α/β T cell receptor that are most activated by gliadin challenge; therefore, they are the cells most likely to release the cytokines that cause epithelial cell damage. The role of the γ/δ T cell receptor in the pathogenesis of celiac disease is not known. However, we do know the CD4 to CD8 ratio is similar in patients with celiac disease versus controls. The CD8 cells (suppressor cells) may also have decreased suppressor function.

Because of the villous atrophy in celiac disease, the class II DR molecules cannot be expressed in villous epithelial cells as they are in normal small intestine cells, and therefore are expressed in the epithelial cells in the crypt region. When exposed to gliadin challenge or active disease, increased levels of HLA-DQ molecules occur on mucosal mononuclear cells in the lamina propria. The role of this molecule in pathogenesis is not understood, but it is thought to present gliadin peptides to mucosal lymphocytes.

Diagnosis

Diagnosis is made by endoscopic biopsy. Grossly, on upper endoscopy, a decrease in mucosal folds is seen with scalloping of the edge of the folds. The duodenum is more affected than the jejunum, which in turn is more affected than the ileum. Histology depends on the severity of disease. In mild disease, there is an increase in IELs. As the disease increases in severity, this progresses to a loss of villous architecture with a loss of the brush border. As the villi are blunted or lost, there is an elongation of the crypts. In the lamina propria, there is an increase in inflammatory cells. Under electron microscopy, there is a decrease in the number of microvilli. The remaining villi are shorter than normal.

When celiac disease is treated and the patient is put on a gluten-free diet, there is a reversal of this process. Probably because of decreased exposure to the offending proteins, the mucosa improves faster distally than proximally. These changes occur over weeks to months, and residual abnormalities persist in 50% of patients for months to years.

As pointed out, oriented small bowel biopsy is the gold standard for the diagnosis of celiac disease. The biopsy, which is performed near the ligament of Treitz, should be done at the time of diagnosis and again 3–6 months later to demonstrate an improvement on a gluten-free diet. Certain laboratory tests can suggest malabsorption and contribute to the diagnosis. These include a decreased serum carotene, decreased albumin, increased prothrombin time, a complete blood count (CBC) demonstrating either a decreased MCV suggestive of iron deficiency, an increased MCV suggestive of folate, or, rarely, vitamin B_{12} deficiency. An upper GI series can be very suggestive of celiac disease when it shows a coarsened mucosal pattern, prolonged transit time, and dilation of the small bowel.

Recently, noninvasive laboratory tests have come into more general use to help make the diagnosis of this condition. They include: (1) antigliadin antibody, (2) transglutaminase antibody, and (3) antiendomysial antibody. Antigliadin antibody may be present in other GI disorders and consists of IgG and IgA antibodies. IgA has a greater specificity than IgG (95.5% versus 86%). With celiac disease, IgA antibody titers increase with increased gluten in the diet, and they decrease as the patient follows a gluten-free diet and the disease improves. The antireticulin antibody, which previously was used, has a poor sensitivity of 40%–50% but higher sensitivity. It is no longer commonly ordered because it has been superceded by testing for antiendomysial antibody and the transglutaminase (tTG) antibody. The demonstration that the antigen for EMA was tTG promoted the development of an enzyme-linked immunosorbent assay (ELISA) for both IgA and IgG tTG to screen for celiac sprue. The IgA assay has a sensitivity of 95% and specificity of 94% in untreated celiac patients. Antiendomysial antibody has very high sensitivity and specificity. There are increased levels of IgA endomysial antibodies in patients with clinically active disease who have villous atrophy. Titers decrease to normal as the mucosa improves.

The combined determination of all antibodies has a greater level of sensitivity and specificity than does each alone. Approximately 2% of celiac disease patients have IgA deficiency. For these patients, IgA antibodies may not be helpful, but IgG antibodies to gliadin may still be useful.

When the diagnosis is in doubt, absorption tests using a disaccharide to monosaccharide ratio, such as the lactulose to mannitol ratio, may be helpful. Finally, HLA typing may be helpful when the biopsy, antibody, or absorption tests are not. More than 95% of celiac disease patients have an HLA-DQ2 molecule encoded by class II alleles *DQA1*0501* and *DQB1*0201*.

Clinical Presentation

As already noted, celiac disease can occur in children or adults and can vary in severity from clinically silent to mild to severe. The classic presentation is that of a patient with steatorrhea, weight loss, and watery diarrhea. There is increased bloating or flatulence.

Following the pathogenesis of the disease, malabsorption of nutritional factors, such as iron, fat-soluble vitamins, and other nutrients, can result in extraintestinal manifestations. For instance, anemia can be secondary to folate or iron deficiency. Hemorrhagic manifestation such as ecchymosis, hematuria, epistaxis, and GI bleeding can occur with malabsorption of vitamin K. Osteogenic bone disease can occur because of malabsorption of calcium and vitamin D. Neurologic symptoms such as parathesias and sensory abnormalities, as well as proximal muscle weakness and ataxia, have been described. Depression, irritability, and mood changes have also been reported. Malnutrition can cause menstrual changes in women and impotence and infertility in men.

Physical findings also vary with the severity of the disease and include pallor, emaciation, ecchymoses, and a tympanitic, doughy,

Diagnosis of Celiac Disease by Noninvasive Laboratory Tests
1. Antigliadin antibody
2. tTG antibody
3. Antiendomysial antibody

Complications of celiac disease include ulcerative jejunoileitis, refractory disease, collagenous sprue, and small bowel malignancy.

protuberant abdomen. Peripheral edema and ascites, as well as neurologic defects, have been described. Vitamin A deficiency can cause keratosis follicularis, and vitamin B deficiency can cause cheilosis and glossitis.

Various disease disorders have been associated with celiac disease. Among these are insulin-dependent diabetes mellitus, Sjögren's syndrome, hyposplenism, nonspecific arthritis, mixed cryoglobulinemia with vasculitis, neurologic disorders, ulcerative jejunoileitis, primary biliary cirrhosis, and primary sclerosing cholangitis. Of patients carrying the diagnosis for 20–40 years, 10%–15% develop cancers of the GI tract. Fifty percent of these are small bowel lymphomas of T cell origin, and the other 50% are solid tumors (usually adenocarcinoma) of the esophagus, mouth, pharynx, or small intestine. Studies suggest that adherence to a gluten-free diet decreases the incidence of malignancy.

A gluten-free diet excluding wheat, rye, oats, and barley is the basis of therapy. All labels must be read carefully, and processed foods should be eliminated from the diet, because wheat is often used as an extender but may not be labeled as such. Only corn, rice, millet, buckwheat, and sorghum grains are allowed. Initially, the diet may need to be lactose-free as well because of the loss of brush-border enzymes. Supplementation with iron, folate, vitamin K, calcium, vitamin D, and zinc may also be necessary. Refractory celiac disease or ulcerative jejunoileitis may require treatment with steroids, azathioprine, cyclophosphamide, or cyclosporine. Response to therapy is generally over weeks to months.

Complications of Celiac Disease

Even patients who are compliant with a gluten-free diet often develop further complications. Ulcerative jejunoileitis may occur. Multiple ulcers may be seen, not only in the jejunum but also in the ileum. These ulcers can also perforate or bleed. Ulcers, it has been hypothesized, occur as a result of an autoimmune reaction to intestinal epithelial cells and as the result of the chronic inflammation of celiac disease.

The recurrence of symptoms after many years of compliance should also raise the suspicion of refractory disease or collagenous sprue. Patients with refractory disease may respond to treatment with corticosteroid or immunosuppressants, such as azathioprine, cyclosporine, or cyclophosphamide.

As the name suggests, collagenous sprue is characterized by the development of a thick band of collagenlike material beneath the epithelial cells. Whether or not this should be considered a separate entity has been questioned, but it appears that up to 36% of individuals with classic celiac disease and even tropical sprue have this characteristic subepithelial deposition of collagen.

Unfortunately, the recurrence of symptoms raises the most serious consideration of all—malignancy. Of patients with celiac disease,

10%–15% develop cancers. Both adenocarcinoma and lymphoma have been reported to occur in patients many years (usually 20–40) after diagnosis. Most of the lymphomas are of a T cell origin. Lymphoma makes up 50% of the malignancies in celiac disease. The remaining 50% are comprised of nonlymphoma solid tumors, such as carcinoma of the mouth, pharynx, esophagus, and small intestine.

DERMATITIS HERPETIFORMIS (DH)

DH is a skin disorder characterized by papulovesicular lesions. Generally, these are pruritic, burning lesions that can occur symmetrically on the elbows, knees, buttocks, sacrum, face, scalp, neck, and trunk.

Only 5% of patients with celiac disease have this skin lesion. However, more than 80% of patients with this skin disorder may have no intestinal symptoms, although isolated nutrient deficiencies have been seen. When biopsies of the small intestine are done in these patients, they show changes that resemble celiac disease but are patchy and vary in severity. As with celiac disease, there is an increased incidence of lymphoma.

Biopsies of the uninvolved skin of patients with DH show two different patterns of IgA deposits at the dermal–epidermal junction. The most common immunofluorescence pattern is a granular or speckled pattern, but a linear pattern is seen as well. The deposits consist of IgA and of complement components (C_3 and C_5). It is not understood whether these components are directed against specific skin and connective tissue proteins or against dietary proteins that cross-react with skin proteins. Another factor must induce the rash because the pattern is found in both involved and uninvolved skin.

Only the patients with a granular pattern have partial or total villous atrophy of the small intestine. This disorder is commonly associated with HLA-DQ2, which in most patients is encoded in *cis* pattern on the HLA-DR17 haplotype. A large number of DH patients also have evidence of previous exposure to adenovirus (Ad12). The precise nature of the relationship of DH to celiac disease is not understood. Treatment of the disorder is with dapsone, which treats the skin but not the small intestine. A gluten-free diet also helps both the skin and small intestine and gradually allows for tapering or stopping the dapsone.

TROPICAL SPRUE

This disease is histologically similar to celiac disease. It affects the entire small intestine but progresses in severity until it causes nutritional deficiencies. The disease may not become clinically apparent until months or years after moving to a temperate climate. However, it usually affects residents of tropical areas or people who have lived in these areas for as little as several weeks, but more typically for longer than 1 year. Implicated geographic areas are India, Southeast Asia, Puerto Rico, the Dominican Republic, Haiti, the Philippines, and the Middle East. Patients have also been seen from parts of Africa and Central America.

Tropical sprue seems to be caused by persistent contamination of the small bowel by coliform bacteria. The toxins they produce seem to cause structural abnormalities, and antibiotic treatment makes patients better.

The etiology of this process is thought to be secondary to persistent contamination of the small bowel by coliform bacteria. The supporting evidence for this is threefold. First, although a single organism has not been isolated as the causative one, studies of patients with the disease reveal overgrowth of *Klebsiella, Enterobacter cloacae,* or *Escherichia coli* in the jejunum. Second, these coliforms are not invasive, but the toxins they produce seem to result in structural abnormalities. Finally, when the bacteria are killed by treatment with antibiotics, many patients get better.

The factors responsible for persistence of the bacterial colonizations are not known. When observed by light or electron microscopy, it does not appear that the organisms are more adherent to the intestinal wall, but other evidence does suggest this may be a factor. There appears to be no defect in the immunologic protective system. However, it may be that a diet high in long-chain fatty acids, such as linoleic acid, may alter the intestinal flora, favoring coliform colonization.

Although persistent coliform colonization seems to be a factor in northern India, Asia, and the West Indies, it does not seem to be common in patients from southern India or South Africa. A viral etiology has been hypothesized in these areas.

Also, bacterial colonization cannot fully explain the role of folate deficiency that is commonly seen in this disorder. Normally, patients who have folate deficiency have abnormal small bowel structure or function. However, giving folate to patients with tropical sprue has resulted in histologic and clinical improvement. The hypothesis offered is that the coliform bacteria produce alcohol as a metabolic by-product and that the alcohol along with folate deficiency must cause the structural changes.

Clinically, patients present with watery diarrhea, abdominal cramps, and increased flatulence. Histologically, in the first few weeks, jejunal structure is normal or only slightly abnormal. After that, intestinal defects become more prominent, with the formation of brush-border abnormalities resulting in disaccharidase deficiencies, such as lactase deficiency. Some patients become intolerant of alcohol.

Jejunal malabsorption occurs 2–4 months later, resulting in the depletion of body folate, anorexia, and weight loss. Six months later, megaloblastic anemia with weakness and glossitis can develop. Approximately 10% of patients present with no GI symptoms and with anemia only. One needs to distinguish tropical sprue from tropical enteropathy, but this disease generally improves when the patient moves to a temperate climate. Tropical enteropathy seems to result from transient episodes of intestinal infection by varied pathogens.

The laboratory tests that physicians find helpful are generally those that reflect malabsorption, such as tests for iron, folate, vitamin B_{12}, PT, cholesterol, albumin, and others. Early in the course of this disease these results may be normal. As the disease progresses, one sees folate and vitamin B_{12} deficiency. Folate deficiency occurs because of impaired hydrolysis of the dietary polyglutamate form of the vitamin by the brush border and malabsorption of the monoglutamate form by the enterocyte. Vitamin B_{12} malabsorption is not corrected by intrinsic factor because impaired ileal transport is the usual cause. Vitamin B_{12} may also be low because it is taken up by bacteria in the intestine.

Hypocalcemia is seen because of impaired absorption and deficiency of vitamin D. Albumin is usually low because of its loss from the gut. Carotene and vitamin A can also be low. Increased PT is unusual. Steatorrhea occurs in 50%–90% of patients.

X-rays of the small intestine show the nonspecific finding of thickening and coarsening of the folds. Early on, small bowel biopsy will be positive only in the jejunum and later on in the entire small bowel. There will be lengthening of the crypts and broadening and shortening of the villi. The lamina propria is often infiltrated with chronic inflammatory cells. Less than 10% will have completely flat villi. A thickened basement membrane looks like collagen on hematoxylin and eosin staining.

Early on, the differential diagnosis must distinguish between *Giardia* and γ-enterocolitis; later, it must distinguish between sprue and tropical enteropathy.

The treatment of this disease is generally with folic acid, tetracycline, or both. In the early stage of the disease, 5 mg daily of vitamin B_{12} and folic acid may be sufficient. Even if treated in the early stage of the disease, it may take up to 2 years for the intestinal structure to return to normal. Generally, therapy consists of 5 mg folic acid daily, with 1000 mcg vitamin B_{12} injected weekly for several weeks, and 250 mg tetracycline four times a day for 3–6 months, depending on the severity of the disease.

WHIPPLE'S DISEASE

Like celiac disease and tropical sprue, Whipple's disease can present with diarrhea and malabsorption but is also more of a systemic disease. It can present with fever of unknown origin and a sarcoid-like illness. Arthralgias, CNS symptoms, pericarditis, or endocarditis may present years before the diarrhea.

Whipple's disease is seen primarily in Caucasians in America or Europe, with a 5:1 ratio of men to women. It has not been seen in Southeast Asia. The average age at diagnosis is 50 years.

Primarily, Whipple's is a bacterial disease. Polymerase chain reaction (PCR) techniques led to the identification of the bacterium *Tropheryma whipplei*, which stains positive with silver, periodic acid–Schiff (PAS), Gram, and Giemsa methods. The two most remarkable histologic features are, first, that the lamina propria is filled with macrophages containing bacilli in varying stages of digestion, and second, that free extracellular bacilli are present below the epithelial basal cell lamina. The hallmark signs are considered to be the PAS-positive macrophages on light microscopy and the electron microscopic appearance of the bacillus. The bacillus has been identified

The causative organism in **Whipple's disease** is *T. whipplei*. The hallmark is the PAS-positive macrophage with rod-shaped inclusions.

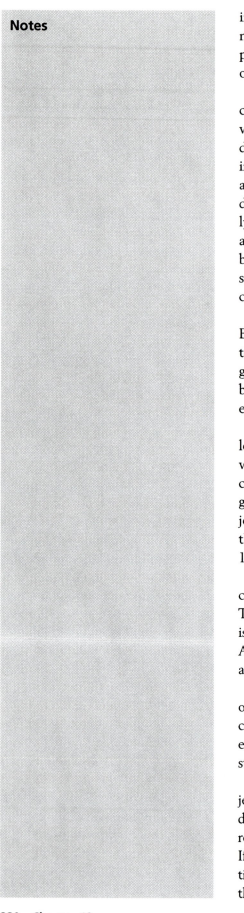

in virtually every tissue (e.g., liver, lymph nodes, heart, CNS, eye, kidney, and synovial tissue) as well as in the intestine. The organism appears to have a low virulence in humans because large numbers of the organism may be present before tissue damage is seen.

Why certain individuals become susceptible to the bacteria is not clear, but susceptibility has some unusual features. First, individuals with the disease seem immunodeficient. This may be secondary to decreased nutritional stores, obstructed lymphatic drainage from the intestine, or the transient anergy of infection. Even the patient who appears clinically healthy may have some subtle defect of immunodeficiency. Evidence of this is shown by the existence of a persistent lymphocytopenia (normal ratio of T cell helper to suppressor cells) and a decreased cutaneous response to antigens. T cells also seem to be less responsive to nonspecific mitogens. Monocyte defects may be secondary to decreased γ-interferon (γ-IFN) production and decreased IgG_2 serum levels.

Of patients with Whipple's disease, 26% were found to be HLA-B27-positive. The usual gene frequency in the population has been tested at 0.3%–7%. Nine percent of patients have been found to have granulomatous changes on biopsies from the liver, lymph nodes, brain, and intestines, as well as from the lung. This results in the disease being confused with sarcoidosis.

Clinically, the disease presents with fever (40%–50%), weight loss, diarrhea, arthralgias, and abdominal pain. The diarrhea can be watery or steatorrhea. Less often, the disease presents with cardiovascular or neurologic symptoms. Occult GI bleeding is common, but gross bleeding is occasionally seen. Migratory arthralgias of large joints can present as early as 9 years before more specific signs of the disease. Weight loss, diarrhea, and fever may precede diagnosis by 1–4 years.

On physical examination, weight loss and hypotension are most common. Peripheral lymphadenopathy is present in 50% of patients. Twenty-five percent have a palpable abdominal mass. Low-grade fever is present in 40%–50%, and 25% of patients have cardiac murmurs. About 33% have increased skin pigmentations, which may be associated with hyperkeratosis and purpura.

On laboratory examination, 90% of patients have anemia, most often of chronic disease but sometimes consistent with iron deficiency. Neutrophilia is present in 33%, and lymphocytopenia is expected. Hypoalbuminemia and increased PT are common, and steatorrhea has been reported to be as frequent as 93%.

X-rays of the small bowel reveal coarsening of the duodenal and jejunal folds. Increased retroperitoneal lymph nodes can cause the duodenal loop to be widened or the stomach to be displaced. Magnetic resonance imaging (MRI) of the head is needed to detect CNS lesions. If an abnormal D-xylose test (or a test for fat) suggests malabsorption, then the diagnostic test of choice is small bowel biopsy. Grossly thickened mucosal folds coated with yellow granular material with

1–2-mm yellow-white plaques are seen. The plaques can have a diffuse or patchy distribution. Under the microscope, one sees PAS-positive macrophages, which are often filled with rod-shaped inclusions. Various other diseases such as *Mycobacterium avium-intracellulare* (MAI), histoplasmosis, and macroglobulinemia can have prominent macrophages. However, in MAI, the macrophages are round and stain positive for acid-fast bacilli. In histoplasmosis, again the macrophages are round and contain encapsulated organisms. In macroglobulinemia, the macrophages are homogeneous without inclusion.

A number of patients present only with CNS disease and no GI symptoms. The most classic triad is dementia, ophthalmoplegia, and myoclonus. Occulomasticatory myorhythmia is rare, but it is unique to Whipple's disease. It consists of a rhythmic convergence of the eyes with chewing. In 50% of patients, joint symptoms precede intestinal symptoms and can do so by as much as 10–30 years. Sixty-five percent of patients have arthralgias or arthritis affecting ankles, knees, shoulders, elbows, or fingers. Often arthritis attacks have an acute onset and last hours to days. The occurrence of axial arthritis is not uncommon. From 20% to 30% of patients have radiologic sacroiliitis.

Pericarditis or endocarditis (50% with marantic valve lesions) is rarely of clinical significance and is usually discovered at autopsy. Pulmonary disease can mimic sarcoidosis, and the disease can present with nonproductive cough, dyspnea on exertion, and pleuritic chest pain.

In diagnosing Whipple's disease, the differential diagnosis may be very broad because of its many presentations. Depending on the symptoms, abdominal lymphoma, sarcoidosis, and collagen vascular disorders may all need to be considered.

Even with treatments, the long-term outlook is guarded. CNS relapse with dementia and death is not uncommon. Treatment often consists of double-strength trimethoprim-sulfamethoxazole twice a day for 1 year or intravenous penicillin for 10–14 days, followed by penicillin VK 250 mg four times a day for 1 year. Supplemental vitamins are given as necessary. If a relapse of symptoms occurs, the small intestine may be rebiopsied, or if appropriate, lymph node biopsy may be done via a surgical procedure or a CT-guided procedure. If CNS symptoms appear, examination of the cerebrospinal fluid (CSF) by lumbar puncture may be done. A recent study suggests that it may be helpful to examine the CSF with PCR both during treatment and with relapse. The study gives further support to the notion that even without neurologic symptoms many patients have CNS involvement. If there is known CNS involvement or failure to respond to treatment, then 250 mg chloramphenicol four times a day for 1 year, with or without the addition of intravenous ceftriaxone, may be instituted.

OTHER MALABSORPTIVE CONDITIONS

Other conditions that may cause malabsorption and that histologically resemble celiac disease are eosinophilic gastroenteritis, common variable immunodeficiency syndromes, and small intestine bacterial overgrowth. In addition, lymphoma can cause similar changes (discussed later in the chapter).

Eosinophilic Gastroenteritis

Eosinophilic gastroenteritis is characterized by diffuse eosinophilic infiltration of the GI tract, most commonly of the stomach, duodenum, and jejunum. Involvement of other organs, such as the esophagus, colon, bladder, and liver, has also been reported.

In children, the pathogenesis may be related to food allergy, particularly milk. In these cases, eczema and rhinitis may be present. Withdrawal of dairy products from the diet usually helps. In adults, the pathogenesis is less clear, and eggs, grains, beef, and chicken have been implicated. Also postulated as a mechanism of disease is a genetic predisposition to form IgE antibodies to specific food antigens. Older children also may have a different mechanism of disease because they show elevated IgE levels, systemic allergic reactions, and positive skin and radioallergosorbent tests, not seen in infants. Also, not all adults show elevated IgE levels. Therefore, different mechanisms may be operative within different subgroups.

Histopathology shows edema and eosinophilic infiltration. The pathophysiology of the disease can also explain the severity of symptoms. If there is merely mucosal involvement, malabsorption (particularly of protein), hypersecretion, and bleeding and ulceration may appear. With increasing penetration, deformity and nodularity occur, and alterations in the muscle layers lead to motility disturbances, commonly manifested by spasm or obstruction. Serosal involvement can result in ascites or adherence to adjacent bowel. The liver and spleen can increase in size secondary to infiltration.

Symptoms include diarrhea, abdominal pain, weight loss, bleeding, fever, and edema of the abdomen and legs. Itching, rhinorrhea, or wheezing may also occur. Charcot-Leyden crystals can be seen in the stool, and peripheral eosinophils of greater than 20% can be seen on a blood smear. Radiologic examination of the small bowel may vary. Thickened edematous folds may be seen, as well as bowel dilation, nodular defects with deformity, obstruction, or ulceration.

Treatment generally consists of withdrawal of proposed food antigens. Often, this is not sufficient, and corticosteroids are necessary. It is especially important, therefore, to rule out parasitic disease as a cause for the changes, especially *Strongyloides*.

Bacterial Overgrowth

Histologically, bacterial overgrowth may resemble celiac disease. The conditions that predispose to this are those that promote small bowel stasis (Table 12-1). The pathogenesis of this disorder is secondary to either mucosal injury or bacterial metabolism of intraluminal

Table 12-1. Conditions That Predispose to Bacterial Overgrowth

Advanced age

Immunodeficiency
    Primary or acquired
    Malnutrition

Stasis of the small intestine
    Small bowel motility disorders
    Anatomic
        Strictures
        Diverticulosis of the small intestine
        Surgery (e.g., Bilroth II, end-to-side enteric surgery, jejunoileal
           bypass)

Abnormal anatomic connection
    Fistulas secondary to cancer or Crohn's disease
    Ileocecal valve resection

Hypochlorhydria

substances. Bacterial overgrowth may also be seen in conditions of abnormal motility or stasis. It may be seen in connective tissue disease, such as scleroderma, or in diabetes mellitus. When diverticulosis of the small intestine is present, bacteria may overgrow in these outpouchings and produce symptoms and problems related to bacterial overgrowth.

Abetalipoproteinemia

When diarrhea of small bowel origin is either watery or steatorrhea, thought should be given to disorders of carbohydrate absorption, such as lactase deficiency, disorders of protein and amino acid transport, and disorders of fat malabosorption, such as abetalipoproteinemia, as well as miscellaneous defects. Although a full discussion of these disorders is beyond the scope of this text, abetalipoproteinemia deserves some attention.

Abetalipoproteinemia is an autosomal recessive disorder in which patients present at birth with acanthocytosis and fat malabsorption. The disorder is the result of a defect in the gene that produces microsomal triglyceride transfer protein. The defect results in the absence of plasma apolipoprotein β–containing lipoproteins, as well as in low concentrations of plasma cholesterol and triglycerides.

Clinical variants of this disorder exist, but acanthocytosis is absent and fasting triglycerides are normal. An autosomal dominant disorder called familial hypobetalipoproteinemia has been identified. The defect is different, and symptoms are often milder. Treatment of these malabsorption disorders consists of a fat-restricted diet and large doses of vitamins E, A, and K.

Most Common Malignant Tumors of the Small Bowel
1. Adenocarcinoma
2. Carcinoid
3. Lymphoma
4. Sarcoma

CASE STUDY: *CONTINUED*

A diagnosis of celiac disease was made on the basis of increased plasma cells, elongation of crypts, and villous atrophy. In addition, elevated IgG and IgA levels of antigliadin were noted. A tTG antibody was also positive. The patient was placed on a gluten-free diet. The diarrhea ceased, and he gained weight.

The patient remained well until age 41, when he presented again with a recurrence of weight loss, steatorrhea, and abdominal pain that was periumbilical and colicky and that often occurred 1–2 hours after eating. Antigliadin antibodies suggested that the patient was compliant with his diet. Biopsy of the small intestine showed patchy villous atrophy. No collagenlike material was noted under the intestinal epithelial cells. A small bowel series was performed and showed a 5-cm strictured area in the midjejunum with nearby ulceration, as well as diffuse thickening of the folds. An abdominal x-ray taken prior to the small bowel series failed to show any free air.

Small Bowel Malignancies

Small bowel tumors make up less than 1% of all GI malignancies. Malignant tumors make up 50%–65% of small bowel tumors and are usually fatal. The remainder are benign. Table 12-2 summarizes and classifies both benign and malignant small bowel tumors.

In descending order, the most common malignant tumors are adenocarcinoma, carcinoid, lymphoma, and sarcoma. The annual incidence varies from one to four cases per million, and tumors are more prominent in males as well as in patients over age 60. Carcinoma and carcinoid are more common in those patients of African descent, and lymphoma is twice as prevalent in Caucasians.

The relative rarity of small bowel tumors has caused much debate, and several reasons have been put forth to explain this phenomenon. First, the small intestine has very low bacterial counts, and anaerobic bacteria, thought to be a risk factor in colon cancer, are usually absent. The bacterial count in the jejunum is less than 10^4/g and less than 10^8/g in the ileum. The presence of detoxifying enzymes in the small intestine, such as benzopyrene hydroxylase, which can neutralize carcinogens, is also thought to play a role in the decreased incidence. In addition, the rapid transit time in the small intestine and the mostly liquid nature of the contents may explain a lower incidence of small bowel tumors. This means that digestive material, which includes toxic metabolites, is not in prolonged contact with epithelial cells as it is in the colon.

Furthermore, the phenomenon of apoptosis, the physiologic process of programmed cell death, is thought to be another mechanism by which the body protects itself. In the colon, expression of the

Table 12-2. Small Bowel Tumors and Neoplasms

BENIGN TUMORS

Adenomas
Leiomyomas
Lipomas
Hamartomas
Fibromas
Angiomas
Neurogenic tumors

MALIGNANT NEOPLASMS

Adenocarcinoma
Lymphoma
    Primary lymphoma: Western type or Mediterranean type
      (immunoproliferative small intestinal disease)
    Secondary lymphoma
Leiomyosarcoma
Carcinoid
Kaposi's sarcoma
Metastatic cancer: melanoma, breast, lung

BC12 gene prevents apoptosis and therefore allows aberrant cell survival. This rarely happens in the small intestine. A variety of clinical conditions is associated with an increased risk of small bowel tumors (Table 12-3).

Most benign tumors usually do not become symptomatic before the patient reaches age 50, and when they do, they usually present with fluctuating pain caused by intermittent small bowel obstruction. Malignant tumors usually became symptomatic during the sixth and seventh decades. Abdominal pain is also the most common initial symptom of malignant tumors. One-third of the patients develop partial or complete small bowel obstruction. About 50% present with weight loss or hemorrhage, usually occult. The distribution of the four major types of tumors, and their relative frequencies with 5-year survival, are summarized in Table 12-4.

ADENOCARCINOMAS

As noted, adenocarcinoma is the most common small bowel tumor. Several conditions are associated with adenocarcinoma, most notably celiac disease, Crohn's disease, and familial adenomalours polyposis (FAP). Approximately 30% of small bowel adenomas have malignant foci. About 40% of individuals with FAP who have had total colectomy have polyps in the upper GI tract. More than 90% of these are

Table 12-3. Clinical Disorders Associated with Small Bowel Tumors

TUMOR TYPE	DISEASE	USUAL SITE
Adenoma	Familial adenomatous polyposis	Duodenum
Adenocarcinoma	Celiac disease	Duodenum or jejunum
	Crohn's disease	Ileum
	Familial adenomatous polyposis	Duodenum
	Ileal conduit or ileocytoplasty	Adjacent to anastomosis
	Ileostomy after colectomy	Ileum
Kaposi's sarcoma	AIDS	Ileum
Leiomyoma	Ileostomy after colectomy	Ileum
Non-Hodgkin's lymphoma	Nodular lymphoid hyperplasia	Ileum
	AIDS	Ileum
Non-Hodgkin's B-cell lymphoma	Immunoproliferative disease	Jejunum
Non-Hodgkin's T-cell lymphoma	Celiac disease	Jejunum

duodenal, often at the ampulla of Vater. Like colonic polyps, there is thought to be an adenoma-to-carcinoma sequence. Diagnosis is often made by small bowel follow through or by enteroclysis (small bowel enema). Crohn's disease causing adenocarcinoma most often involves the terminal ileum. Endoscopy is most helpful when tumors are in the duodenum or ileum. Arteriography often shows a mass with encasement of tumor vessels. Surgery is indicated only when there are no extranodal metastases. Five-year survival is 10%–20% even after curative resection.

CARCINOIDS

Carcinoids are the second most common small intestine tumor. Seventy percent of carcinoids are found in the appendix, with the next most common site being the ileum. Approximately 70% are asymptomatic.

Table 12-4. Distribution of Malignant Tumors in the Small Bowel with Relative Frequency and 5-Year Survival (Based on Combined Studies)

TUMOR TYPE	DUODENUM	JEJUNUM	ILEUM	RELATIVE FREQUENCY	FIVE-YEAR SURVIVAL
Primary adenocarcinoma	40%	38%	22%	33%–50%	Resec. 10%–20% Unresec. <1%
Carcinoid	18%	4%	78%	17%–39%	50%
Primary lymphoma	6%	36%	58%	12%–24%	Resec. 40%–50% Unresec. <25%
Leiomyosarcoma	3%	53%	20%–50%	11%–20%	20%–50%

Source: Modified from Lance in Yamada 1995, p. 1699.

Overt metastases occur in one-third of symptomatic small bowel cases. Only 10% of patients with symptomatic small bowel carcinoids develop the classic carcinoid syndrome of flushing, diarrhea, and abdominal pain.

A significant proportion of these tumors present as small bowel obstruction. This is thought to be the result of an intense fibroblastic or desmoplastic response in the vicinity of the carcinoid tumor, which is attributed to a local elevation of serotonin. Mesenteric shortening and thickening results, which on small bowel series is seen as kinking or narrowing of the small intestine. On CT or arteriogram, a stellate pattern is seen in involved arteries.

Other methods of diagnosis include a 24-hour urine collection of 5-HIAA greater than 10 mg. Patients must be instructed to eliminate tomatoes, bananas, plums, and eggplants from the diet for 24 hours before and during urine collection. An octreotide scan may light up the areas of the carcinoid 10–30 minutes after injection. (Octreotide is a synthetic somatostatin analog.) Increased plasma or platelet serotonin levels may also be helpful in diagnosis. All carcinoids secrete serotonin, but it is known that the immunohistochemical and hormonal profiles of various carcinoids differ according to the tissues of embryologic origin. Tumors of foregut origin, lung, pancreas, stomach, and duodenum secrete other hormones.

If a carcinoid tumor is found without obvious metastatic disease, as with adenocarcinoma, the treatment is resection with 10-cm margins. Debulking is often recommended if there is metastatic disease. Other modalities of treatment with metastatic disease include hepatic artery embolization and chemotherapy with 5-fluorouracil (5-FU) and streptozocin. To control symptoms of the carcinoid syndrome, somatostatin (50–250 mg two to three times a day) is often used. The 5-year survival is 54%.

LYMPHOMAS

Lymphomas can be divided into several categories. Immunoproliferative small-intestinal disease (IPSID) is seen primarily in developing areas (Middle East, Africa, Southeast Asia, South Central America) and is associated with poor hygiene and increased incidence of enteric and parasitic infections. The major etiologic factor is thought to be microbial colonization of the small intestine.

With IPSID, there is a proliferation of IgA-secreting B cells, and alpha heavy chains are detectable in 20%–70% of patients, usually in the early stages. In the early stages, intestinal infiltration of mature plasma cells is seen. Later, these cells become dystrophic, and late in the disease there is frank lymphomatous proliferation.

IPSID usually presents in the patient's second or third decade with weight loss, abdominal pain, or diarrhea, which can range from watery to steatorrhea. The interval between symptoms and diagnosis can range from 1 month to 12 years. In the early stages, it appears that this disease can be reversed by treatment with tetracycline, which causes remission of the dystrophic changes. Later it becomes a diffuse lymphoma that is difficult to treat or cure but, like primary lymphoma, is treated with radiation therapy and chemotherapy. It has a 5-year survival of about 20%.

Various conditions are associated with an increased risk of primary lymphoma. HIV-1 increases the risk of developing non-Hodgkin's lymphoma. Nodular lymphoid hyperplasia, especially if diffuse, can be a prelymphomatous condition with or without an associated immunodeficiency syndrome. Celiac disease predisposes toward lymphoma of T cell origin. The etiology of malignancy in celiac disease has been suggested to be related to a variety of causes, from oncogenic viruses to increased mitotic activity to abnormalities in the mucosal immune system with in increased turnover of lymphoid cells in the mucosa.

Primary lymphomas are defined by an absence of palpable lymphadenopathy, normal total and differential leukocyte counts, the absence of mediastinal lymphadenopathy on chest x-ray, and grossly demonstrable disease confined to an affected segment or segments of the GI tract. Seventy percent of primary lymphomas are gastric. The remaining 30% are divided between the small and large intestines.

Most primary small bowel lymphomas are of the non-Hodgkin's type. Hodgkin's lymphoma is very rare. The stages of non-Hodgkin's lymphomas, using the Ann Arbor system, are shown in Table 12-5.

With the exception of those related to celiac disease, most primary small bowel lymphomas are of the B cell type. Researchers have noted a connection between malignant lymphomas of the salivary gland, lung, thyroid, and GI tract and have used the phrase mucosa-associated lymphoid tissue (MALT) to describe the histogenesis of these lymphomas. Having common clinical and histologic features, they all express a heterogeneous array of leukocyte differentiation antigens. They also share a characteristic feature called the centrocytelike cell. These centrocytelike cells are named for their resemblance to the small, cleaved cells of the follicle center cell lymphomas of peripheral lymph nodes.

It has been argued that primary small bowel lymphomas are reactive lesions like IPSID. The argument is based on the fact that, in

Table 12-5. Staging of Non-Hodgkin's Lymphoma

STAGE	
IE	Localized segment without nodal involvement
IIE	Localized segment with regional nodes
IIIE	Bowel and lymph nodes on both sides of the diaphragm (spleen may be involved [stage IIIES])
IV	Diffuse involvement of more than one extralymphatic organ or tissue with or without nodal involvement

these lymphomas, there are well-defined follicles, a long clinical course, and late dissemination to other parts of the body. Centrocyte-like cells have been thought to be key to the development of malignancy. They have been thought to be analogous to follicle center cells, and GI lymphomas have been thought to be follicular tumors.

Newer research suggests that the normal counterparts of the centrocytelike cells probably are derived from B cells that are external to the mantle zone of Peyer's patches in the dome epithelium. This evidence is derived from leukocyte antigen studies. Phenotype studies suggest that these cells may be identical to cells from the splenic marginal zone. Although they are known to circulate, these cells do not recirculate, and this could explain the indolence of primary small bowel lymphoma. Further evidence for the centrocytelike cell not being of follicular origin comes from molecular hybridization studies of the circular DNAs from the *BCL2* gene. A characteristic rearrangement of the gene that occurs in 75% of nodal follicular lymphomas was absent from primary small bowel lymphomas.

Small bowel lymphomas usually appear before patients reach age 10 or after they reach age 50. They most commonly present with abdominal pain, weight loss, and obstruction. One-third of patients have a palpable mass. Diagnosis is often made with a small bowel series. Most primary small bowel lymphomas have a restricted segment of disease in contrast to the more extensive disease seen in IPSID. If biopsy can be done, it is diagnostic in 85% of cases.

Generally, segmental resection of the small intestine and regional lymph nodes is recommended. Some specialists recommend liver biopsy, periaortic node sampling, and splenectomy for staging. Resection is potentially curative if the disease is stage IE or IIE.

If curative resection is not possible, palliative resection before chemotherapy is recommended, but chemotherapy alone has also been done. Palliative radiation therapy for extensive unresectable disease has been performed, usually with concomitant chemotherapy. The role of adjuvant radiation or chemotherapy in treating limited disease is not well defined.

The reported 5-year survival after surgical resection in stage IE or IIE is 24%–47%. The 5-year survival for unresectable disease is less than 25%. The prognosis is worse if the patient has celiac disease. Of patients with celiac disease who develop lymphoma, 55% die within 6 months of diagnosis, and only 10% survive 5 years.

LEIOMYOMATOUS TUMORS

The fourth most common small bowel tumor is leiomyoma (benign) or leiomyosarcoma (malignant). These tumors are derived from smooth muscle cells in the muscle layer of the bowel or from blood vessel walls that may project into the lumen or the serosa.

Leiomyosarcomas are staged from stage I through IV. Stage I is confined to the bowel wall, and stages I and II are difficult to distinguish from leiomyomas. The relative number of mitoses is used to distinguish the stages. In stage III and IV lesions, the resemblance to smooth muscle is lost. Stage IV lesions have local spread and distant metastases.

Both benign and malignant lesions can present with abdominal pain or obstruction, bleeding, and weight loss. Unless there is obvious metastasis, surgical resection is often needed to distinguish benign from malignant lesions. Leiomyosarcomas rarely present in individuals under age 50. Stage I lesions usually have a 75% 5-year survival, as opposed to 7% for stage IV lesions. Size is also a determining factor in survival; lesions smaller than 5 cm have a 71% 5-year survival versus 27% for lesions larger than 5 cm. Both palliative radiation therapy and chemotherapy are used to treat advanced stages of the disease. An aggressive surgical approach is urged for isolated pulmonary or hepatic metastases because of the low potential for lymphatic spread. The overall 5-year survival for this lesion is 20%–50%.

Small Bowel Ischemia

In discussing small bowel ischemia, it is important to remember that the digestive tract is nourished by three arterial trunks that branch from the abdominal aorta: the superior mesenteric artery, the inferior mesenteric artery, and the celiac axis. The celiac axis has three major branches: the splenic, left gastric, and hepatic arteries. The branches of the hepatic artery primarily feed the duodenum. These branches of the hepatic artery in turn form collaterals with smaller intestinal branches of the superior mesenteric artery. The collaterals feed the duodenum, as well as the jejunum and ileum. In addition to smaller intestinal branches, the superior mesenteric artery has three major branches: the middle colic, right colic, and ileocolic arteries. Only the ileocolic artery directly feeds the ileum of the small intestine.

The causes of mesenteric ischemia can be either occlusive or nonocclusive. The causes of occlusive ischemia can be further classified as arterial, venous, or a result of strangulation. Strangulation causes 20%–40% of occlusive mesenteric ischemia. It is the most common cause and usually occurs as a result of an adhesive band. The adhesive band causes lymphatic obstruction followed by venous obstruction. In addition, dilation of the bowel may cause strangulation by causing a volvulus, resulting in pinching off the vascular supply to the involved loop. Strangulation can result in a doubling of the 5%–10% mortality rate associated with small bowel obstruction.

Venous occlusion is a rare occurrence, and it usually occurs as a result of an acute thrombotic event. It can be idiopathic or secondary to a number of clinical disorders, such as protein C or S deficiency or antithrombin III deficiency. In addition to trauma, other hypercoagulable states or intraperitoneal irritation can be a cause. Severity can vary from unrecognizable to catastrophic.

Oral contraceptives have been reported to cause intestinal infarction, perhaps via mesenteric arterial occlusion or venous thrombus. Estrogens can produce both arterial and venous occlusion, whereas progesterone causes arterial occlusion. Proposed mechanisms of causation include endothelial proliferation, reduced venous blood flow in the mesenteric circulation, and hypercoagulability. Certain risk factors increase the risk of hormones having these effects. These include cigarette smoking, hypercoagulable states, hypertension, and collagen vascular disorders.

Arterial occlusion can be either acute or chronic. Acute ischemia can involve the whole small intestine and other parts of the GI tract (e.g., gastric, acalculous cholecystitis, ischemic colitis), or it can be segmental. Segmental occlusions are usually embolic, whereas global involvement can have thrombotic or embolic causes. Chronic occlusion is usually secondary to atherosclerotic disease, such as intestinal angina.

Arterial emboli usually originate from the heart and account for around 75% of cases. Atrial fibrillation is a common risk factor, as is a recent myocardial infarction with a mural thrombus. Patients with a history of stroke or peripheral vascular disease are also at risk. Clinical manifestations depend on adequacy of flow.

Arterial thrombus accounts for 10%–15% of all cases of acute mesenteric ischemia. It is often difficult to differentiate thrombus from embolus. A thrombus usually occurs at a site of previous damage or abnormality, such as a preexisting atherosclerotic lesion or an anatomic variation. Clinical manifestations depend on the adequacy of collateral flow. Typically, patients with this disorder have some sort of low-flow state, such as congestive heart failure (CHF), recent myocardial infarction, or preexisting atherosclerotic lesions at the origin of the superior mesenteric artery. Hypercoagulable states such as polycythemia vera, cancers, or trauma have been associated with mesenteric arterial thrombosis.

Nonocclusive causes account for 10%–20% of mesenteric ischemia. A distinct clinical and pathologic entity called nonocclusive mesenteric ischemia (NOMI) can result from a selective splanchnic vasoconstriction as a result of hypovolemia or cardiogenic shock. Humoral mediators, such as angiotensin II and vasopressin, directly mediate this response. Certain drugs are known to cause vasoconstriction or hypotension either in the splanchnic or systemic circulation. In addition, myocardial infarction, CHF, chronic dialysis, hypervolemia, and shock all predispose to NOMI.

Examples of drugs that cause ischemic damage are cocaine, ergotamines, or cardiac drugs. Cocaine and crack cocaine stimulate increased synthesis of dopamine and norepinephrine. There are also stimulatory effects on the CNS because of the inhibition of synaptic reuptake of dopamine, serotonin, and norepinephrine. The drugs may initially cause increased sympathetic stimulation, resulting in tachycardia and peripheral vasoconstriction, which in turn cause hypertension and nonocclusive intestinal ischemia. Rebound vasodilation can further compromise intestinal blood flow. Used in the prevention of migraine headaches, ergotamine in various forms (methylsergide,

methylergonovine, dihydroergotamine) can be a rare cause of nonocclusive splanchnic vasoconstriction.

Cardiac drugs are yet another nonocclusive cause of ischemia, either by arterial vasoconstriction or hypotension. This occurs more commonly when CHF already has compromised the splanchnic circulation. Diuretics and antihypotensive agents can induce ischemia by causing hypovolemia and hypotension. Drugs such as norepinephrine, dopamine, or vasopressin can reduce splanchnic blood flow by vasoconstriction. In patients with CHF, another drug that causes reduced splanchnic blood flow is digitalis, probably by causing low-flow states.

A rare form of nonocclusive ischemia is necrotizing enterocolitis (NEC). One form of NEC is acute jejunitis, also called dormbrand, pig-bel enteritis necroticans, and Pasini's regional jejunitis, to give just a few of its other names. It most often occurs in children in communities where there is protein deprivation in the diet, as well as poor hygiene, especially in food preparation. In New Guinea, this syndrome was discovered to be associated with the β-toxin of *Clostridium perfringens*. Further studies established the toxin as the cause; immunization against the β-toxin can prevent this disease.

Although neonatal NEC is very rare and its cause is unknown, it may be important because similar pathophysiologic mechanisms may be factors in adult necrotizing enteropathies. The initial insult is splanchnic vasoconstriction secondary to severe physiologic stress. This seems to start a two-step pathophysiologic process. It appears that vasoconstriction causes ischemia and thereby the initial mucosal injury. Subsequently, there is progression to transmural infarction related to such factors as enteral feeding formulas, bacterial overgrowth, and immune incompetence. Immaturity of the immune system allows a normally irreversible lesion to progress by bacterial invasion to an irreversible transmural infarction. Histologically, there is ischemic necrosis with the mucosa being preferentially affected. The pathogenic factors that appear to be important in neonatal enterocolitis are prematurity, intestinal ischemia, infectious agents, and enteral nutrition. The initiation of enteral nutrition is not absolute, and not all cases occur in low birth weight or premature infants. Bacterial colonization seems to be clinically and experimentally a significant factor.

Bacterial endotoxins stimulate the inflammatory cytokines that cause injury to the mucosa and may be mechanisms by which bacteria contribute to the development of NEC. Enteral feeding may be the factor through which bacteria are introduced to the GI tract. Intestinal ischemia and hypoxemia are thought to result from intestinal distention resulting from overfeeding. In addition, hypertonic fluids may cause direct mucosal injury, further predisposing the neonatal intestine to ischemic injury.

A very rare cause of splanchnic ischemia, celiac artery compression syndrome, usually occurs in younger patients and has a threefold predominance in women. In this disorder, chronic abdominal pain is caused by stenosis of the celiac artery. The stenosis is caused by fibrosis of the median arcuate ligament of the diaphragm compressing the vessel. Irritation of the visceral autonomic nerves has also been proposed as a cause. Cutting the ligaments relieves the pain but does not necessarily improve the blood flow. Perivascular sympathectomy or ganglionectomy is not recommended. Optimal treatment requires division of the crural fibers, excision of periceliac neural tissue, and celiac artery dilation or reconstruction.

In most adults a triad of acute abdominal colic, GI emptying (vomiting, defecation, or both), and cardiovascular disease should raise one's index of suspicion for mesenteric ischemia. The classic symptom associated with acute mesenteric ischemia is abdominal pain, which is out of proportion to abdominal tenderness on physical examination. Early on, signs of peritoneal inflammation are usually absent. Bloody diarrhea (signifying necrosis and sloughing of intestinal mucosa) does not usually appear for several hours. The absence of blood in the stool does not rule out intestinal ischemia.

Most laboratory tests, such as those for leukocytosis, increased amylase, increased creatinine phosphokinase, phosphate, and metabolic acidosis, are not helpful because they may not become abnormal until mesenteric ischemia becomes irreversible. Various radiologic modalities have been used for diagnosis. An abdominal flat plate may show thumbprinting, a sign of mucosal edema. Barium studies may be useful in ischemic colitis, and CT or MRI may be of benefit in mesenteric venous thrombosis, showing a clot or thickened bowel wall. Duplex ultrasound evaluation may be helpful in the assessment of both acute and chronic arterial mesenteric ischemia. However, diagnostic angiography may be crucial in confirming mesenteric ischemia, and it should be employed immediately when available.

Initially, if mesenteric ischemia is suspected and if sepsis is felt to be imminent, fluid resuscitation and antibiotics should be initiated. In drug-induced ischemia, certain drugs, such as calcium channel blockers and nitroprusside, may be helpful. If there is evidence of severe ischemic injury, laparotomy or laparoscopy may be indicated to see if there is gangrenous bowel or bowel that looks clinically compromised. Under these circumstances surgical resection is imperative. Some surgeons advocate a second-look laparotomy 24–48 hours later to assess the remaining bowel.

Disorders of Small Bowel Motility (Chronic Intestinal Pseudo-Obstruction)

The intrinsic and extrinsic nervous system control small bowel motility. GI hormones play a lesser role. For the most part, disorders of motility in the small intestine are caused by defects in the intrinsic and extrinsic nervous system, as well as by smooth muscle defects.

Small bowel motility disorders can be divided into those having primary and secondary causes. Primary causes that have been described

The triad of acute abdominal colic, GI emptying (vomiting, defecation, or both), and cardiovascular disease suggests **mesenteric ischemia.**

Small bowel motility disorders have primary or secondary causes. Primary causes include visceral myopathies or neuropathies; secondary causes are related to various underlying etiologies.

Table 12-6. Secondary Causes of Small Bowel Dysmotility

DRUGS

Phenothiazines
Narcotics
Clonidine
Tricyclic antidepressants
Antiparkinson's drugs
Ganglionic blockers

ENDOCRINE DISORDERS

Diabetes mellitus
Hypothyroidism or
  hyperthyroidism
Hypoparathyroidism

NEUROLOGIC DISORDERS

Chagas' disease
Parkinson's disease
Carcinomatosis-causing
  visceral neuropathy
Spinal cord injury
Neurofibromatosis

DISEASES AFFECTING SMOOTH MUSCLE CELLS

Collagen vascular disorders (e.g., systemic
  lupus erythematosus, scleroderma,
  progressive systemic sclerosis)
Muscular dystrophies
Amyloidosis

MISCELLANEOUS CAUSES

Celiac disease
Radiation enteritis
Diverticulosis of the small intestine
Postviral infection
Eating disorders
Jejunoileal bypass
Diffuse lymphoid infiltration of the small
  intestine

Source: Modified from Anuras and Hodges in
Yamada 1995, p. 1579.

are either visceral myopathies or visceral neuropathies. Both familial and sporadic types have been described. Secondary causes are those that are related to various conditions. Etiologies generally are related to the underlying disease. Table 12-6 lists the various causes.

Visceral myopathies are classified as childhood, familial, or sporadic. Childhood myopathies differ from familial myopathies in their clinical manifestations and modes of inheritance. Both types are caused by degeneration and fibrosis of GI smooth muscle. In some familial types and in all the childhood types degeneration and fibrosis occur in urinary smooth muscle as well.

The characteristic pathologic change is that of fibrosis and degeneration of smooth muscle cells. The change may involve the whole muscularis propria or be limited to the external layer. The degeneration gives the longitudinal or circular muscles a vacuolated appearance and makes them pale. Trichrome stain best highlights these changes.

Clinically, the visceral myopathies that present in childhood are the childhood type, whereas those that present in the teens or in middle age are the familial or sporadic types. Symptoms of these disorders include nausea, vomiting, obstruction, and abdominal pain. Additional symptoms may be present if the disease involves other organ systems.

Of the visceral neuropathies that are either familial or sporadic, one familial type, the myenteric plexus, shows a degeneration of argyrophilic neurons and a decrease in the number of nerve fibers.

The other familial type as well as the sporadic type show a reduction in the number of neurons; those neurons that remain are histologically very abnormal.

Sporadic neuropathies are generally more common than sporadic myopathies. The etiology of these neuropathies is thought to be secondary to drugs, chemicals, or viral infections. Clinically, the disorder can be asymptomatic or may cause nausea, vomiting, abdominal pain, constipation, or diarrhea.

Diagnostic studies to distinguish causes of intestinal motility include blood tests, radiologic studies, biopsies, and small intestinal manometry. In addition to routine blood tests such as a CBC and biochemical profile, an antinuclear antibody test, thyroid function test, and a blood test for Chagas' disease may be helpful. Radiologic tests include a plain abdominal film in patients with abdominal distention and appropriate contrast studies of the GI and genitourinary tract. Contrast studies usually show dilation of the affected organ. Other studies that may prove helpful are striated muscle biopsy to rule out muscular dystrophy or cultures of small bowel aspirates to rule out bacterial overgrowth. Full thickness biopsy shows the characteristic change in the smooth muscle or myenteric plexus on silver stain.

Finally, when available, small bowel manometry may show characteristic changes that help distinguish myopathic from neuropathic disease. A cyclic pattern of motility called the migrating motor complex (MMC) occurs during fasting. This is a three-phase cycle lasting 80–100 minutes, continuing until the subject is fed. The fed state is a pattern of frequent intermittent contractions lasting 4–7 hours.

In patients with visceral myopathic disorders, a decrease in both frequency and amplitude of contractions is seen in the affected segments. The increase is generally seen in both fed and fasting states. The same pattern may also be seen in patients with dermatomyositis, amyloidosis, late scleroderma, and muscular dystrophies.

Visceral neuropathic disorders produce dyscoordination and a lack of organization in the motor activity. Other secondary causes of small bowel dysmotility, such as neurologic diseases, diabetes mellitus, early scleroderma, and amyloidosis, may also produce similar manometric abnormalities.

For primary disorders of motility, treatment is primarily symptomatic and supportive. The goal is to relieve the symptoms of nausea, vomiting, bloating, and abdominal pain that are related to eating or to relieve obstipation. Promotility agents have not been found to be helpful. Surgery consisting of partial duodenal resection or side-to-side duodenojejunostomy of a megaduodenum may be helpful in treating the autosomally inherited familial type of visceral myopathy. This type of surgery may also be helpful in patients with secondary dysmotility, such as scleroderma or systemic lupus erythematosus. Where applicable, secondary causes of dysmotility may be ameliorated by treating the underlying disorder. Examples of this are celiac disease, hypothyroidism, or particular medications.

CASE STUDY: *RESOLUTION*

In this young man with celiac disease, an arteriogram showed no arterial occlusions. A laparotomy was performed, and the small bowel was resected. Pathology showed lymphoma with positive regional and para-aortic nodes. Evidence of lymphoma was also found in the spleen. The patient was treated with chemotherapy and radiation therapy. He survived for an additional 2 years but eventually succumbed to the lymphoma, an unfortunate but not uncommon complication of celiac disease.

REVIEW QUESTIONS

Directions: For each of the following questions, choose the one best answer.

1 A 35-year-old man presents for endoscopy with a 6-month history of steatorrhea, weight loss of 20 lbs, and abdominal bloating. At the onset of his illness, he was traveling in Central America. Although a biopsy demonstrates blunted villi with elongation of crypts consistent with celiac disease, his physician wishes to confirm the diagnosis. Which blood test would be most helpful in confirming the diagnosis of celiac disease?

A Antitreponemal antibody
B Angiotensin-converting enzyme (ACE)
C Antireticulin antibody
D Ferritin
E HLA typing

2 A 55-year-old man presents with a history of migratory arthritis. Over the past year, he has had watery diarrhea, a 25-lb weight loss, and abdominal pain. His physical examination is notable for occulomasticatory myorhythmia. An upper endoscopy is performed. Which biopsy result most closely fits this clinical history?

A Blunted villi with crypt elongation and increased inflammatory cells in the lamina propria
B Scattered blunted villi with crypt elongation, chronic inflammatory cells in the lamina propria, and a thickened basement membrane
C Scattered blunted villi with crypt elongation and PAS-positive macrophages with rod-shaped inclusion bodies
D Blunted villi with crypt elongation and a predominance of eosinophilic inflammatory cells in the lamina propria

3 A 26-year-old woman has just completed a 2-year stint as a Peace Corps volunteer. She gave a 6-month history of anorexia and weight loss. Recently, she noted diarrhea and abdominal cramps. A CBC is consistent with a megaloblastic anemia. The best treatment for this patient would be

A multivitamin therapy and a lactose-free diet.
B multivitamin therapy and a gluten-free diet.
C tetracycline therapy for 1 year.
D tetracycline and folic acid for 6 months and vitamin B_{12} injections for several weeks.

4 A 60-year-old man presents with a 3-month history of watery diarrhea, abdominal pain, and a 30-lb weight loss. A small bowel series is performed that shows a nodular stricturing in the distal ileum. A malignancy is suspected. Which of the following conditions would most likely be associated with this clinical picture?

A Small intestine bacterial overgrowth
B Crohn's disease
C Celiac disease
D Whipple's disease
E Necrotizing enterocolitis

5 A 40-year-old man presents with abdominal pain, nausea, and vomiting for 12 hours. In the several months prior to this episode, he has been experiencing flushing, diarrhea, and abdominal pain. A small bowel series shows kinking and narrowing in a 4-cm segment of the ileum. A CT scan demonstrates several filling defects in the liver and a stellate pattern in the involved arteries to the ileum. Which of the following is the most likely diagnosis?

A Adenocarcinoma
B Non-Hodgkin's lymphoma
C Ischemia
D Leiomyosarcoma
E Carcinoid

6 A 70-year-old woman with a history of CHF and atrial fibrillation presents to the emergency room with a history of severe periumbilical pain, nausea, and vomiting for several hours. She takes furosemide and digoxin. Over the past month, she has noted postprandial discomfort 1–2 hours after eating that has resolved spontaneously. Her abdominal examination is remarkable only for some mild periumbilical tenderness. Which of the following would be the diagnostic test of choice for this patient?

A Abdominal x-ray
B Arteriogram of the superior mesenteric artery
C CT scan of the abdomen
D Amylase, electrolyte profile, and CBC
E Abdominal sonogram with Doppler

7 A 30-year-old woman presents to the gastroenterologist's office with a 12-year history of increasing nausea and abdominal bloating. She has a bowel movement every 7–10 days and difficulty passing urine. A diagnostic workup is done, and it is notable for a small bowel biopsy showing intact nerve fibers and degeneration in the longitudinal and circular muscle fibers, with a pale vacuolated appearance on trichrome stain. Small bowel manometry shows a decrease in the frequency and amplitude of contractions in both fed and fasting states. This patient most likely has which of the following diseases?

A Diabetes mellitus

B Dermatomyositis

C Familial visceral myopathy

D Familial visceral neuropathy

E Late scleroderma

References

Anuras S, Hodges D: Dysmotility of the small intestine. In *Textbook of Gastroenterology*, 2nd ed. Edited by Yamada, T. Philadelphia, PA: J. P. Lippincott, 1995.

Bresalier RS, Ben-Menachem T: Tumors and neoplasms of the small intestine. In *Textbook of Gastroenterology*, 4th ed. Edited by Yamada T. Philadelphia, PA: Lippincott, Williams & Wilkins, 2003.

Camilleri M: Dysmotility of the small intestine. In *Textbook of Gastroenterology*, 4th ed. Edited by Yamada T. Philadelphia, PA: Lippincott, Williams & Wilkins, 2003.

Case record of the Massachusetts General Hospital: A 79-year-old female with anorexia, weight loss, and diarrhea after treatment for celiac disease (weekly clinicopathological exercise: case 15-199). *N Engl J Med* 334(20):1316–1322, 1996.

Ciclitira PJ: AGA technical review on celiac sprue. American Gastroenterological Association. *Gastroenterology* 120(6):1526–1540, 2001.

Ciclitira PJ, Ellis HJ: Celiac disease. In *Textbook of Gastroenterology*, 4th ed. Edited by Yamada T. Philadelphia, PA: Lippincott, Williams & Wilkins, 2003.

Lance P: Tumors and other neoplastic diseases of the small bowel. In *Textbook of Gastroenterology*, 2nd ed. Edited by Yamada T. Philadelphia, PA: J. P. Lippincott, 1995.

Marth T: Whipple's disease. *Lancet* 361(9353):239–246, 2003.

Panés J, Piqué JM: Intestinal ischemia. In *Textbook of Gastroenterology*, 4th ed. Edited by Yamada T. Philadelphia, PA: Lippincott, Williams & Wilkins, 2003.

von Jerbay A, Ditton HJ, et al: Whipple's disease staging and monitoring by cytology and polymerase chain reaction analysis of cerebrospinal fluid. *Gastroenterology* 113:434–441, 1997.

13

Acute and Chronic Pancreatitis

▨ LEARNING OBJECTIVES ▨

At the completion of this chapter, the reader should be able to:
- Recognize the presentation of acute and chronic pancreatitis.
- Differentiate among different causes of acute and chronic pancreatitis.
- Evaluate unique complications that can develop with acute and chronic pancreatitis.
- Identify appropriate tests to confirm or rule out the diagnosis of acute or chronic pancreatitis.
- Outline treatment options for acute and chronic pancreatitis.

CASE STUDY 1: *INTRODUCTION*

A 67-year-old man came to the emergency department with the abrupt onset of severe, stabbing, midepigastric pain that radiated to the middle of his back with nausea and vomiting. He had a medical history of chronic obstructive pulmonary disease and coronary artery disease. He denied use of alcohol. His temperature was 38°C, blood pressure, 150/60 mm Hg; pulse, 80 beats/min; and unlabored respiratory rate, 22 breaths/min. He lay still and was mildly diaphoretic. Both pulmonary and cardiac examinations were normal. His abdomen was moderately obese and nondistended with minimal bowel sounds. There was moderate tenderness in the epigastric region but no rebound. A serum amylase of 2340 IU/L (normal: < 115 IU/L) raised the suspicion of acute pancreatitis.

He was admitted to the hospital with the diagnosis of mild acute pancreatitis and treated conservatively with nothing by mouth and intravenous analgesics until the pain improved. Because of the suspicion of pancreatitis, a CT scan was performed (Figure 13-1).

Acute Pancreatitis

Acute pancreatitis is inflammation of the pancreas clinically characterized by the sudden onset of abdominal pain in association with elevation in blood or urine pancreatic enzyme activity. In acute pancreatitis, there is "autodigestion" of pancreatic cells and infiltration of

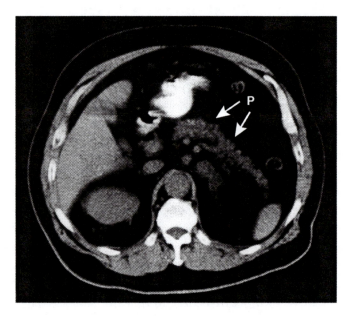

Fig. 13-1. CT Scan of the Abdomen

Early acute pancreatitis with normal-appearing pancreas (P).

inflammatory cells, with surrounding areas of fat necrosis and edema. This process may be extensive and includes peripancreatic and intra-pancreatic fat necrosis, hemorrhage, and parenchymal necrosis. These pathologic changes usually regress when the cause is removed, and the patient is asymptomatic following recovery. Acute pancreatitis is divided into *severe acute pancreatitis* and *mild acute pancreatitis*. This division is made on the basis of the following two factors: (1) the presence or absence of organ failure, and (2) the severity of local complications. The distinction between them is important because it alters treatment strategies.

PATHOLOGY

Although the causes of acute pancreatitis vary, the pathologic appearance and progression are similar for all cases. The examination of the pancreas during mild acute pancreatitis reveals spotty areas of pancreatic and peripancreatic fat necrosis, up to 1 cm in diameter. These areas resolve without sequelae in mild cases. In severe acute pancreatitis, however, larger areas of fat and pancreatic necrosis (> 1 cm) occur; these may liquefy and slowly resolve or may become "walled off" with granulation (scar) tissue, thereby forming a mature pseudocyst. In severe acute pancreatitis, there are larger areas of more intense inflammation involving the pancreas and adjacent structures, systemic complications, and various degrees of pancreatic gland necrosis.

Molecular Pathophysiology

In a healthy pancreas, digestive enzymes are produced as inactive enzymes (proenzymes). Proenzymes are secreted from the pancreas and activated in the small intestine. In acute pancreatitis, the proenzymes become activated within the acinar cells. Although the exact intracellular location and mechanism responsible for premature digestive enzyme activation are debatable, clearly activation of these enzymes promotes autodigestion of pancreatic cells and initiates the inflammatory reaction.

Once an episode of acute pancreatitis is triggered, a characteristic inflammatory reaction occurs. When acinar cells are damaged, they begin leaking activated digestive enzymes and other cellular elements into the interstitial space. This triggers an inflammatory response with the release of proinflammatory mediators including interleukins (IL-1, IL-2, IL-6, IL-8), tumor necrosis factor, and platelet-activating factor. If pancreatic injury is mild, the inflammatory response is self-limited and the process is contained. However, if pancreatic injury is more severe, a more intense inflammatory response ensues, which mediates a significant proportion of the local and systemic complications of acute pancreatitis.

ETIOLOGY

Determination of the etiology of acute pancreatitis may be very important for immediate treatment or for prevention of relapses. Gallstones

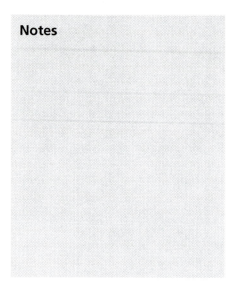

or alcohol abuse cause up to 80% of acute pancreatitis cases, although the etiologic factors vary among populations. About 10% of episodes are caused by metabolic derangements, trauma, infections, and drug reactions, although the latter category remains controversial. The final 5%–10% of cases remain idiopathic (Table 13-1).

CLINICAL ASSESSMENT

Determining the severity of acute pancreatitis is important for initiating appropriate therapy and anticipating complications. Eighty percent of these patients only suffer mild acute pancreatitis and will recover with supportive care. However, patients with severe acute pancreatitis require early institution of specific and intensive therapies to minimize morbidity and mortality. Thus, the initial goal of assessment is to determine if acute pancreatitis is mild or severe.

Table 13-1. Causes of Acute Pancreatitis

TYPE	ETIOLOGY	FEATURES
Toxic	Alcohol	Forms proteinaceous plugs in ducts and activates proteolytic enzymes, leading to pancreatic autodigestion
		Occurs after years of heavy alcohol use
		Recurrent attacks lead to chronic pancreatitis
Mechanical	Pancreatic cancer	May result in obstruction of ampulla of Vater with reflux of biliary and intestinal contents into pancreatic duct and localized duct obstruction
	Gallstone passage	Recurrent episodes of gallstone pancreatitis are virtually eliminated by cholecystectomy
Drugs	Anticonvulsants: valproic acid	Usually an idiosyncratic reaction
	Immunosuppressive agents: azathioprine, 6-mercaptopurine	Rechallenge of drug useful in cause and effect
	Antibiotics: sulfonamides, dideoxyinosine	
	Diuretics: thiazide, chlorthalidone	
	Others: steroids, L-asparaginase	
Trauma	Penetrating ulcer	Inflammation result of direct injury to acinar cells
	After surgery	
	Automobile accident	
	Endoscopic retrograde cholangiopancreatography	
Familial	Hereditary	Onset in childhood
		Caused by a mutation in cationic trypsinogen gene
		Increased risk of chronic pancreatitis
Metabolic	Hyperlipidemia	Hyperlipidemia-induced pancreatitis usually occurs with triglycerides > 1000
	Hypercalcemia	
Infection	Cytomegalovirus	Seen in many immunosuppressed patients (e.g., HIV)
	Epstein-Barr virus	
	Cryptosporidium	
	Microsporidium	

Evaluation of patients with suspected acute pancreatitis includes both establishing the diagnosis and ruling out other diseases. Typically, acute pancreatitis patients develop symptoms of steady epigastric pain that radiates to the back and vomiting that does not improve. On physical examination, the abdomen is tender; in half of the cases, guarding is present. Ileus, peritoneal signs, fever, hypotension, and tachycardia are seen in more severe cases. Ecchymosis around the umbilicus (Cullen's sign) and in the flanks (Turner's sign) are suggestive of hemorrhagic pancreatitis but are seldom seen except in severe cases. Almost all patients presenting with acute pancreatitis have elevated serum amylase levels. However, other disorders may present with elevated serum amylase or abdominal pain, including mesenteric ischemia or infarction, intestinal obstruction, acute cholecystitis, peptic ulcer disease with perforation, choledocholithiasis, and dissecting abdominal aortic aneurysm. Acute, severe, left upper quadrant pain and rigidity indicate more severe acute pancreatitis, although perforated peptic ulcer, subphrenic abscess, jejunal diverticulitis, spontaneous rupture of the spleen, ruptured aneurysm, or perinephric abscess may cause similar symptoms. Laboratory abnormalities of acute pancreatitis cases include elevated serum amylase and lipase levels. Amylase usually rises within 2–12 hours after the initiating insult and remains elevated for 3–5 days. Lipase level, although less sensitive, is more specific and remains elevated longer than amylase. Serum lipase levels may be useful in making a diagnosis when the patient presents as an episode of acute pancreatitis that is resolving and when the amylase has already normalized.

Establishing the correct diagnosis requires evaluating the patient's history, pattern of pain, and serum amylase and lipase levels. Imaging studies can provide supporting evidence. Both chest and abdominal x-rays are helpful in excluding other disorders (e.g., perforated viscus) and in identifying nonspecific but helpful signs of acute pancreatitis. These signs include a sentinel loop (dilated loop of small intestine in the vicinity of the pancreas), generalized ileus, obscure psoas shadow, or pancreatic calcifications. Ultrasound examination may be useful in identifying an edematous pancreas, peripancreatic fluid, pancreatic pseudocyst, or stones in the gallbladder or common bile duct. Ultrasound is often limited by overlying intestinal gas, however. Contrast-enhanced CT (CECT) may be the most useful imaging modality because it is unaffected by overlying intestinal gas. In addition, it is possible to grade the severity of pancreatitis and identify local complications on a CECT scan; however, a delay in its use for at least 24 hours should be considered unless another diagnosis is being ruled out. This delay is suggested because of concern that CECT may worsen acute pancreatitis. The CECT scan may appear nearly normal in mild pancreatitis or very early in the course of more severe pancreatitis, as is demonstrated by the clinical case.

CASE STUDY 1: CONTINUED

Initial laboratory values included hematocrit, 47.5 ml/dl; white blood cell (WBC) count, 12,300/mm³; blood urea nitrogen (BUN), 18 mg/dl; creatinine, 1.1 mg/dl; glucose, 250 mg/dl; calcium, 9.4 mg/dl; lactate dehydrogenase, 234 IU/L; aspartate transaminase (AST), 96 IU/L; alkaline phosphatase, 122 IU/L; total bilirubin, 1.5 mg/dl; albumin, 3.1 g/dl; amylase, 2340 IU/L; and lipase, 1000 IU/L. In the emergency room, the patient had a Glasgow score of 4.

Within 48 hours of admission, the patient developed the following Ranson's criteria: hematocrit decrease of 15%, BUN increase of 10 mg/dl, serum calcium of 7.8 mg/dl, arterial Po_2 of 52 mm Hg, base deficit of 2.9 mEq/L, and fluid sequestration of 10 L. Thus, his Ranson score was 6. Both the Ranson and Glasgow scores suggested severe pancreatitis.

Ranson and Glasgow Scores

Ranson made a significant contribution toward improving patient evaluations by proposing a series of 11 commonly available clinical signs and laboratory tests obtained during the first 48 hours of admission (see Table 13-2). Classifying patients according to the number of positive signs stratifies them into groups with well-defined probabilities of significant morbidity and mortality (e.g., rate of mortality is 25% with more than four signs; see Table 13-3). However, one major limitation is that 48 hours are required to complete this scoring system.

Table 13-2. Ranson's Criteria

ON ADMISSION	FIRST 48 HOURS
Age > 55 years	Hematocrit decreases > 10%
Leukocyte count > 16,000/mm³	BUN rises > 5 mg/dl
Blood glucose > 200 mg/dl	Serum calcium < 8 mg/dl
Serum LDH > 350 IU/L	Pao_2 < 60 mm Hg
SGOT/AST > 250 IU/dl	Base deficit > 4 mEq/L
	Estimated fluid sequestration > 6 L

Note: Criteria are used to assess the severity of chronic pancreatitis 48 hours after presentation. Score is calculated by adding all criteria together. AST = aspartate aminotransferase; BUN = blood urea nitrogen; LDH = lactate dehydrogenase; Po_2 = oxygen partial pressure; SGOT = serum glutamic-oxaloacetic transaminase (now called AST).

Table 13-3. Ranson's System

	0–2	3–4	5–6	7–8
Number of signs				
Percent mortality	0.9	16	40	100
Percent morbidity (> 7 days in ICU)	3.7	40	93	100

Note: Risk of morbidity and mortality depends on patient's score at 48 hours.

Table 13-4. Glasgow Criteria

Age > 55 years
WBC > 15,000/μl
Glucose > 180 mg/dl
BUN > 45 mg/dl
Po$_2$ < 60 mm Hg
Albumin < 3.2 g/dl
Calcium < 8 mg/dl
LDH > 600 IU/L

Note: Number of criteria correlates with severity of acute pancreatitis. Presence of more than three criteria signifies significant pancreatitis.

The *Glasgow score* (see Table 13-4), like the Ranson score, was developed specifically for assessment of acute pancreatitis. Each of the criteria is given 1 point, and the score is calculated by adding for the total number of criteria present. Many physicians now favor the Glasgow score because the calculations are completed at the time of admission. With either system, a score of 3 or more places the patient in a category of high risk for serious complications or death.

The Ranson and the modified Glasgow criteria were developed specifically for pancreatitis; there are additional scoring systems such as the APACHE II (Acute Physiology and Chronic Health Evaluation) and SAPS (Simplified Acute Physiology) scores. Scoring systems are 70%–80% accurate in predicting mild versus acute pancreatitis; because they are not perfect, each patient's clinical course must be assessed carefully.

Radiologic Evaluation

Abdominal x-ray films are obtained to rule out perforated viscus. Sentinel loop or colon cutoff sign may also be seen with acute pancreatitis. CECT or ultrasound will show diffuse enlargement of the pancreas in 70%–90% of acute pancreatitis cases and can usefully rule out other diagnoses with similar presentations (e.g., perforated ulcer, bowel obstruction, bowel infarction) as well as reveal possible complications (e.g., pseudocyst). A CECT should therefore be performed when the case is either (1) clinically severe acute pancreatitis without improvement in 72 hours, (2) showing signs of complications (such as fever and increasing WBC count), or (3) in need of evaluation for local complications or pancreatic necrosis. Magnetic resonance cholangiopancreatography may play a role as a noninvasive test to assess the biliary tree, detecting or excluding choledocholithiasis.

CASE STUDY 1: *CONTINUED*

Diagnosis of acute pancreatitis was made, and the patient was admitted to the hospital. He was treated with intravenous fluids and meperidine for pain. Blood cultures were obtained, and he was started on broad-spectrum antibiotics. Early on the day of admission, CT of the abdomen revealed a normal liver, gallbladder, and common bile duct; a normal-appearing pancreas; and no gallstones (see Figure 13-1).

TREATMENT

Mild Acute Pancreatitis

Usually, mild edematous pancreatitis resolves within several days; therefore, the treatment is supportive (Table 13-5). Treatment includes avoidance of oral intake to prevent stimulation of the exocrine pancreas, intravenous fluids to prevent dehydration and maximize vascular perfusion, and meperidine for pain control. Meperidine is used because it is thought to cause less contraction of the sphincter of Oddi than does morphine. If early feeding causes pain or an increase in amylase or if the episode of pancreatitis is severe enough to last more than 2–3 days, nutritional support is indicated. Enteral feeding is the preferred method and can be administered successfully through an enteral feeding tube placed beyond the ligament of Treitz. The use of total parenteral nutrition (TPN) is also acceptable. Finally, frequent clinical reassessment is advisable, because unexpected complications can be life-threatening.

Severe Acute Pancreatitis

Because the pathophysiology of severe acute pancreatitis is complex, treatment strategies are multifaceted and dynamic. Early life-threatening complications include *cardiovascular collapse* and *respiratory failure*, whereas later complications include *sepsis* and *multiorgan system failure*. Therefore, patients with physiologic signs of severe acute pancreatitis should be closely monitored in an intensive care unit (ICU) or step-down unit.

There are several important interventions to consider. The first involves optimizing hemodynamics. Monitoring central venous pressure and providing adequate volume replacement are appropriate. Because of associated systemic inflammatory response, with resultant leakage of fluid into lungs and the risk of developing adult respiratory distress

Table 13-5. Treatment for Acute Pancreatitis

TREATMENT	INDICATION
Meperidine	Pain
Intravenous fluids	Volume depletion
Nothing by mouth	"Pancreatic rest"
Nasogastric suction	Ileus, nausea, and vomiting

syndrome, monitoring the patient's respiratory status is important so that supportive measures, such as oxygen and ventilatory support, can be initiated if the arterial oxygen partial pressure (PaO_2) decreases. Next, nutritional support should be considered. The body has limited energy stores, and patients with severe acute pancreatitis cannot eat, which leads to rapid depletion of energy stores, especially in this hypermetabolic state. Depletion of energy stores contributes to multiorgan systemic failure. Therefore, nutritional support (enteral or parenteral) should be initiated within 48–72 hours. One of the most severe late complications is infection, especially infected pancreatic necrosis. Infected pancreatic necrosis rarely responds to antibiotics; thus, if significant necrosis is visualized on CECT, prevention of infected necrosis is attempted with broad-spectrum antibiotics such as imipenem or cefuroxime. In gallstone pancreatitis, impacted stones cause common bile duct (CBD) obstruction and the complications of cholangitis, sepsis, and worsening pancreatitis. Endoscopic retrograde cholangiopancreatography (ERCP) offers a way of extracting CBD stones as well as severing pancreatic duct and CBD sphincter fibers, resulting in resolution of the obstruction. Therefore, in severe gallstone pancreatitis, ERCP can reduce the risk of cholangitis and sepsis and reduce the risk of associated mortality. ERCP is also indicated as a diagnostic procedure if a patient has had two or more episodes of idiopathic pancreatitis, but this is usually delayed until after the acute phase.

CASE STUDY 1: *CONTINUED*

The severity of the pancreatitis was obvious by the third hospital day, with worsening pain, increasing serum amylase, and progressive fluid sequestration. On that day, CECT demonstrated an enlarged, hypodense pancreatic head, body, and tail with peripancreatic fat inflammation and peripancreatic fluid collection. This confirmed the diagnosis of acute pancreatitis without significant pancreatic necrosis. ERCP demonstrated pancreatic duct disruption with communication between the ducts and an extrapancreatic fluid collection. There was no evidence of gallstones. Because there was persistent leukocytosis and low-grade fever, CT-guided aspirations from the peripancreatic fluid collections were performed for Gram staining and culture (Figure 13-2).

COMPLICATIONS

Local complications arise from severe inflammation that disrupts the anatomy or function of the pancreas or local structures. Historically, many different terms and classifications of complications were proposed, but attempts at classification suffered from confusing and

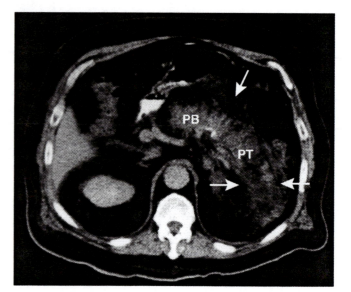

Fig. 13-2. CT Scan of the Abdomen

Acute pancreatitis showing enlarged edematous pancreas body (PB) and pancreatic tail (PT) and peripancreatic fat inflammation (arrows).

conflicting definitions. In 1992, 40 international experts met and agreed on terms and a classification system for acute pancreatitis.

There are also some local complications that involve organs adjacent to the pancreas. These complications include pancreatic ascites, pleural effusion, bile duct obstruction, and colonic obstructions or strictures. Systemic complications are also possible (Table 13-6).

Table 13-6. Systemic Complications of Acute Pancreatitis

CARDIOVASCULAR

Hypotension and shock
ECG changes
Pericardial effusion and tamponade

PULMONARY

Hypoxia
Atelectasis, pneumonia
Pleural effusion
Adult respiratory distress syndrome
Respiratory failure

METABOLIC

Hypocalcemia
Hyperglycemia
Hypertriglyceridemia
Metabolic acidosis

RENAL

Oliguria
Azotemia
Acute tubular necrosis
Renal artery or vein thrombosis

HEMATOLOGIC/COAGULATION

Vascular thrombosis
Disseminated intravascular
 coagulation
GI bleeding

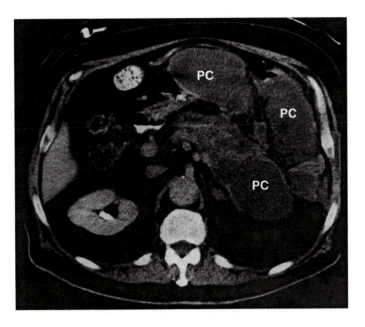

Fig. 13-3. CT Scan of the Abdomen

Multiple pseudocysts (PC) filling a significant portion of the abdominal cavity.

Acute Fluid Collection

These acute fluid collections occur early in the course of acute pancreatitis, are located in or near the pancreas, and always lack a wall of granulation or fibrous tissue. The fluid is usually rich in pancreatic enzymes. More than half of these cases resolve spontaneously; in the others, however, acute fluid collections may become pseudocysts.

Pseudocyst

Collection of fluid within or around the pancreas (pseudocyst) results from disruption of the ductal system and is usually (but not always) rich in pancreatic digestive enzymes (Figure 13-3). These collections evolve from acute fluid collections by development of a nonepithelial wall or capsule as the result of an inflammatory reaction in the periphery. Pseudocysts are distinguished from true cysts by lack of an epithelial lining. However, they also differ from simple peripancreatic fluid collections or effusions in that they have a well-defined fibrous wall. About half resolve spontaneously, whereas the rest may remain asymptomatic or may enlarge and cause such complications as pain, infection, hemorrhage, and bile duct or bowel obstruction. Treatment is indicated if complications occur, which involves draining the pseudocyst through endoscopic drainage (Figure 13-4), radiologic intervention, or surgery.

Pancreatic Necrosis

Pancreatic necrosis is a diffuse or focused area of nonviable pancreatic parenchyma, which is typically associated with peripancreatic fat

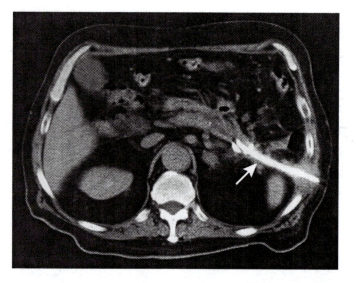

Fig. 13-4. CT Scan of the Abdomen

Drainage of pseudocysts by CT-guided percutaneous catheter (arrow).

necrosis. Identification of areas of pancreatic necrosis are usually made with rapid-bolus CECT scans. Pancreatic necrosis can either be sterile or infected.

Pancreatic Abscess

A pancreatic abscess is a circumscribed intra-abdominal collection of pus, usually in the proximity of the pancreas, containing little or no pancreatic necrosis. It should be distinguished from infected necrosis, which has twice the mortality rate of pancreatic abscess. The treatment is drainage, as the infected area has undergone liquefaction.

Infected Necrosis

Necrotic tissue, usually in pancreatic or peripancreatic fat, becomes infected. Because necrotic tissue is incompletely liquefied, it cannot be drained and requires surgical debridement.

SUMMARY: ACUTE PANCREATITIS

A typical patient with acute pancreatitis presents with acute mid-epigastric abdominal pain radiating to the back, associated with nausea and vomiting. The diagnosis of pancreatitis is confirmed by laboratory tests, radiographs, and excluding other diseases with a similar presentation. An evaluation for the etiology of pancreatitis is important, because this impacts on treatment and counseling of the patient. Assessing the severity of pancreatitis by the Glasgow scale or Ranson's criteria assists the anticipation of complications. Treatment involves close monitoring and supportive measures. ERCP is indicated for therapeutic purposes only, during the active phase of pancreatitis.

CASE STUDY 1: *RESOLUTION*

The patient was treated with intravenous fluids, oxygen, and TPN. The initial CT-guided fluid aspiration produced sterile fluid, and prophylactic broad-spectrum antibiotics were continued. A long, complicated hospital stay ensued, and the patient developed several common late complications. Multiple large pseudocysts developed. Because of their size, persistence, and compression of the stomach, they were drained by placement of percutaneous drainage catheters under CT guidance. In addition, a cystcolonic fistula developed. The fistula closed after conservative treatment with long-term TPN and octreotide. The patient eventually made a complete recovery. A cholecystectomy was eventually performed to prevent a recurrence.

CASE STUDY 2: *INTRODUCTION*

A 35-year-old man presented to the outpatient clinic because of chronic abdominal pain that had acutely worsened. His medical history was significant for repeated episodes of severe epigastric abdominal pain radiating to the back. These episodes were associated with nausea, vomiting, and elevated serum amylase and lipase levels. He frequently required admission to the hospital during severe episodes. On admission, he was treated with intravenous fluids and pain medication while receiving nothing by mouth. These episodes began occurring every few weeks. He was unable to work because of his illness, which was treated at home with bed rest and fasting or with hospitalization. Over the previous 6 months, the pain had become constant and notably worsened with food. The inability to eat without pain and frequent illness led to a 30-lb weight loss to his present weight of 135 lbs. He noted increased stool frequency and bulk but denied passing blood or oil.

Physical examination revealed a cachectic-appearing man who appeared to be in pain. Vital signs included normal blood pressure, pulse, respiratory rate, and temperature. The lung fields were clear to auscultation, and cardiac examination was normal. Abdominal examination revealed normal bowel sounds, a normal liver edge, absence of organomegaly, and moderate epigastric tenderness without rebound pain or guarding.

Laboratory tests values included the following: hemoglobin, 11 g/dl (normal: 13–18 g/dl); WBC count, 12,000/mm^3 (normal: 4000–11,000/mm^3); AST, 60 IU/L (normal: 1–36 IU/L); alanine aminotransferase (ALT), 30 IU/L (normal: 1–45 IU/L); alkaline phosphatase, 260 IU/L (normal: 45–115 IU/L); amylase, 250 IU/L (normal: 25–125 IU/L); and lipase 300 IU/L (normal: 10–140 IU/L).

Chronic Pancreatitis

Chronic pancreatitis is a necrotic-inflammatory condition of the pancreas resulting in the permanent loss of pancreatic exocrine function. Clinically, chronic pancreatitis is characterized by recurrent or persistent abdominal pain, although it presents without pain in 15%–20% of patients. In more advanced cases, patients suffer loss of pancreatic exocrine function, leading to maldigestion of nutrients, and loss of endocrine functions, leading to diabetes mellitus. Morphologically, chronic pancreatitis results in areas of fibrosis, with loss of exocrine parenchyma in focal, segmental, or diffuse patterns and is usually associated with ductal changes.

PATHOLOGY

Early Chronic Pancreatitis

Examination of the pancreas in early chronic pancreatitis reveals areas of induration, with other areas appearing nearly normal. Duct irregularities with occasional stones are present, as are areas with pseudocysts, recent necrosis, and scarring. Microscopically, varying degrees of fibrosis, necrosis, and atrophy of the acinar cells develop within distinct lobules (Figure 13-5). Infiltration of inflammatory cells, including lymphocytes, plasma cells, and macrophages, occurs within affected lobules. The islets of Langerhans often escape early destruction, so diabetes mellitus rarely develops during the early stages of chronic pancreatitis (see Figure 13-5).

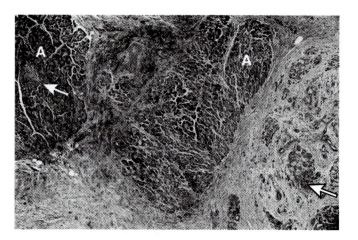

Fig. 13-5. Low-Power Photomicrograph of Surgical Specimen from a Patient with Chronic Pancreatitis

Note the progressively worsening severity of acinar damage proceeding from left to right. The acinus on the left appears normal. The acinus in the middle is surrounded by fibrosis. The acinus on the right is severely damaged, with few surviving acinar cells and scattered dilated ducts. Note that the islets of Langerhans (arrows) are relatively spared. A = acinus; F = fibrosis.

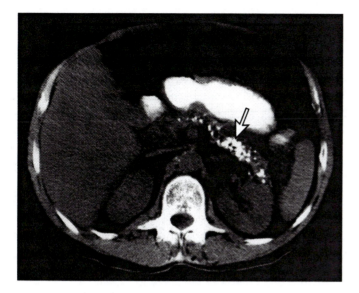

Fig. 13-6. CT Scan from a Patient with Chronic Pancreatitis

Non-contrast-enhanced CT scan of the abdomen at the level of the pancreas. Note the many stones and the dilated pancreatic duct extending through the body and tail of the pancreas (arrow).

Advanced Chronic Pancreatitis

In advanced chronic pancreatitis, the gland appears shrunken and deformed and becomes firm. The ducts are dilated and distorted to varying degrees. In some cases, marked alterations appear in the main pancreatic duct (large-duct disease), whereas in other cases the main pancreatic duct is relatively spared (small-duct disease) (Table 13-7). Other features include fibrosis, pancreatic duct stones, protein plugs, and thick-walled pseudocysts, which are present in about one-quarter to one-half of all cases (Figure 13-6). Extrapancreatic pathologic manifestations include CBD stenosis, duodenal stenosis, and thrombosis of the splenic vein or other vessels. Microscopically, the fibrosis becomes widespread, with distortion of pancreatic ducts, blood vessels, and nerves. The islets of Langerhans become sparse, and nerve trunks become prominent and, in many cases, surrounded by inflammatory cells.

Table 13-7. Small-Duct Disease Compared with Large-Duct Disease

DISEASE	PREDOMINANT SYMPTOMS	ETIOLOGY	TESTING
Small-duct disease	Pain and mild to moderate pancreatic exocrine dysfunction	Idiopathic	Functional (secretin stimulation)
Large-duct disease	Pain with endocrine and exocrine function impairment	Alcohol	Structural endoscopic ultrasound/ endoscopic retrograde cholangiopancreatography

ETIOLOGY

In the United States and other developed countries, heavy alcohol use is responsible for most cases of chronic pancreatitis. However, in some developing countries, tropical chronic pancreatitis leads the list of causes. Although the factors associated with chronic pancreatitis are often identified, the pathophysiologic mechanisms connecting these factors with pancreatic injury remain under investigation.

Alcohol-Induced Chronic Pancreatitis

Alcohol-induced chronic pancreatitis develops after years of heavy alcohol use. Alcohol ingestion may cause injury by one or more mechanisms. It is believed that acinar cell injury results from the direct cytopathic effect of alcohol and its metabolites, leading to recurrent episodes of acute pancreatitis. Inflammation and scarring damages the ductal system, leading to strictures, protein precipitation, stone formation, ductal obstruction, and areas of high ductal pressure. These changes perpetuate a cycle of pancreatitis, inflammation, and further scarring. Another possible mechanism may be a change in the protein concentration in the pancreatic juice, with associated changes in pancreatic stone protein, resulting in precipitation of proteins and calcium with ductal obstruction, which then evolves into chronic pancreatitis.

Tropical Chronic Pancreatitis

Tropical chronic pancreatitis presents in children and young adults from sub-Saharan Africa and India. Some experts hypothesize that this form of chronic pancreatitis results from malnutrition combined with an unknown toxin; however, this hypothesis is unproven, and the cause remains obscure. Macroscopically and microscopically, tropical pancreatitis is indistinguishable from chronic pancreatitis from other causes.

Hereditary Chronic Pancreatitis

Hereditary chronic pancreatitis is an autosomal dominant trait that primarily affects families of European ancestry, although cases on other continents have been reported. Heredity chronic pancreatitis is caused by a mutation in the cationic trypsinogen gene. Normally, trypsin remains in the inactive trypsinogen form until it reaches the duodenum, where it is activated by enterokinase. Premature activation of trypsin in the pancreas may lead to pancreatic autodigestion and pancreatitis. However, within the pancreas, up to 10% of the potential trypsin can be inactivated by pancreatic secretory trypsin inhibitor. When more trypsin is prematurely activated than can be inhibited by pancreatic secretory trypsin inhibitor, the trypsin digests itself, starting at a trypsin-sensitive site in the chain connecting the two globular domains of the trypsin molecule. In hereditary pancreatitis, the cut site is mutated so that the mutant trypsin is resistant to self-digestion. Loss of this site leads to continued activation of other enzymes by mutant trypsin, autodigestion, and acute pancreatitis. Eventually, the recurrent episodes of acute pancreatitis and scarring lead to chronic pancreatitis.

Senile Chronic Pancreatitis

Senile chronic pancreatitis describes the common observation of pancreatic exocrine failure in elderly patients. Senile chronic pancreatitis is most likely due to obstructions of small ductal tributaries by nonneoplastic duct epithelial changes and intraductal stone formation.

Cystic Fibrosis

Cystic fibrosis is an inherited form of chronic pancreatitis and the most common cause of chronic pancreatitis in children in the United States. Cystic fibrosis is caused by a variety of mutations in the chloride channel in pancreatic duct cells, termed the cystic fibrosis transmembrane regulator (CFTR). The loss of CFTR function impedes ductal bicarbonate (HCO_3^-) and fluid secretion, resulting in the formation of protein plugs in the pancreatic ducts. The disruption of the normal Cl^- transport system eventually results in pancreatic fibrosis and exocrine insufficiency.

Pancreas Divisum

Pancreas divisum is a result of failure of the embryonic dorsal and ventral pancreas to fuse, resulting in pancreatic body and tail draining through the minor papilla. This minor papilla results in a relative ductal stenosis, which may lead to high duct pressure, episodes of acute pancreatitis, and eventually chronic pancreatitis. Pancreas divisum is a common variant of normal pancreatic ductal anatomy, which is present in as many as 10% of patients.

Idiopathic Chronic Pancreatitis

Between 10% and 20% of cases of chronic pancreatitis are idiopathic and may be painless. However, this group includes all cases of chronic pancreatitis in which no cause has been identified; therefore, it is heterogeneous. A subset of these patients are women who present in midlife with nonspecific abdominal pain. They have nearly normal duct morphology on ERCP (small-duct disease) but have evidence of pancreatic insufficiency on pancreatic function tests. Others develop a pattern of chronic pancreatitis that is identical to alcoholic or hereditary pancreatitis without the use of alcohol or a typical family history.

Other

Hyperlipidemia and hypercalcemia, like other causes of acute pancreatitis, occasionally progress to chronic pancreatitis. Furthermore, recent evidence suggests that any cause of acute pancreatitis in the head of the pancreas may initiate a process leading to chronic pancreatitis, as described with alcoholic chronic pancreatitis.

CLINICAL ASSESSMENT

Chronic pancreatitis should be considered in patients with chronic abdominal pain and associated risk factors or in patients with symptoms of pancreatic insufficiency. In contrast to acute pancreatitis, serum pancreatic enzyme levels may be normal in chronic pancreatitis until late in the disease, when levels may fall well below the normal range.

Clinical Features

There are four classic clinical hallmarks of chronic pancreatitis: (1) pain, (2) weight loss, (3) pancreatic calcifications, and (4) diabetes. The severity and chronicity of pain and other signs and symptoms may become debilitating and result in frequent hospitalizations, loss of employment, narcotic dependence, and depression.

Pain

Pain is the presenting symptom in 80%–90% of patients with chronic pancreatitis. The nature of the pain may vary from a dull, constant, epigastric pain radiating to the back and upper abdomen to a sharp, piercing, or burning pain exacerbated by food. Weight loss occurs usually due to fear (sitophobia) of this painful reaction to food. There are at least five theories regarding the causes of pain in chronic pancreatitis. It must be recognized, however, that in any given patient, pain may arise from multiple causes.

1. Increased intraductal pressure is clearly associated with pain. The increased pressure arises from obstruction of the pancreatic ducts by strictures or intraductal stones. This theory is supported by the observation that once an obstruction is relieved by surgical or endoscopic drainage, there is amelioration of pain.
2. Increased pancreatic pressure may cause pain in some patients. This pressure develops when viable pancreatic tissue is encased in fibrosis with blockage of normal drainage. When pancreas secretion is stimulated, the parenchymal pressure rapidly rises and pain develops, as seen in compartment syndrome.
3. The stimulated pancreas is one of the most metabolically active organs in the body, and it requires a rich blood supply. In chronic pancreatitis, arterioles and other blood vessels become distorted and stenotic as they pass through fibrotic areas or are compressed in areas of elevated pancreatic parenchymal pressure. A reduction in blood flow may lead to ischemia and pain

through mechanisms similar to those of the chest pain of ischemic heart disease.

4. Acute and chronic inflammation of the pancreas with release of cytokines also causes pain.
5. Pain arises from chronic perineural inflammation, which results in accumulation of eosinophils, with associated disintegration of perineural sheaths and edema of nerve bundles. Perineural inflammation has been identified in the resected pancreas of patients with chronic pancreatitis and severe, constant, unrelenting pain. It is hypothesized that perineural inflammation destroys the normal barrier between nerves and pancreatic tissue, with resultant exposure of nerve cells to inflammatory cytokines, which continually drive the pain sensation.

The exacerbation of pain in Case Study 2 was caused in part by mild acute pancreatitis superimposed on chronic pancreatitis. The physician must remain aware of other causes of pain in addition to chronic pancreatitis. These include pancreatic cancer, stenosis of the common bile duct, and other extrapancreatic complications of pancreatitis. Pain in chronic pancreatitis is not associated with elevated serum pancreatic enzymes (amylase and lipase).

Pancreatic Calcification

In chronic pancreatitis, protein precipitation occurs in pancreatic ducts. This results in plug formation within the ducts and is frequently followed by calcification that occurs by surface accretion. Acinar cell necrosis and atrophy develop, and more protein precipitation occurs in pancreatic ducts, which is followed by further calcification. Pancreatic calcification is apparent on abdominal radiography in up to 30% of patients with chronic pancreatitis.

Maldigestion and Weight Loss

Maldigestion occurs when the pancreas fails to produce sufficient digestive enzymes to hydrolyze dietary nutrients. Usual signs are large, bulky stools or diarrhea. Amylase deficiency results in carbohydrate maldigestion and is associated with increased luminal gas and diarrhea as bacteria metabolize the carbohydrates in a manner similar to lactose intolerance. Steatorrhea (increased fecal fat) occurs in the later stages of disease, after lipase secretion has dropped to less than 10% of normal (~30,000 IU/meal). Passage of droplets of oil is therefore a sign of advanced chronic pancreatitis. Azotorrhea occurs with protein maldigestion but is rarely of clinical significance. Maldigestion of nutrients further contributes to weight loss.

Endocrine Insufficiency

Glucose intolerance is common in the early stages of chronic pancreatitis and progresses to diabetes in later stages of the disease as the islets of Langerhans are destroyed. Approximately 30% of patients eventually develop diabetes.

The patient's CT scan demonstrated pancreatic atrophy, ductal dilation, cystic changes, and pancreatic parenchymal calcification. In addition, a fasting serum glucose was 220 mg/dl in the absence of a history of diabetes (see Figure 13-6). The results of these tests confirmed the suspicion of chronic pancreatitis and diabetes and suggested that the condition was advanced. During his hospitalization, the patient's pain subsided, and he began eating. However, he required insulin therapy to control his diabetes.

DIAGNOSIS

In patients exhibiting the hallmark of chronic pancreatitis, confirmation of the diagnosis relies on identification of structural changes in the pancreas or on documenting diminished pancreatic function.

Structural Evidence

The goal of structural testing of the pancreas is to identify changes in pancreatic size, shape, duct morphology, calcifications, or pseudocysts that are associated with chronic pancreatitis. The major imaging techniques, given in descending order of sensitivity, include endoscopic ultrasound (EUS), ERCP, CT, transcutaneous abdominal ultrasound, and plain abdominal film (Table 13-8). EUS represents one of the latest advances in imaging technology and has the advantage of virtually always demonstrating diagnostic changes in the pancreas of patients with advanced chronic pancreatitis as well as identifying characteristic changes in most patients with minimal ductal change on ERCP (i.e., small-duct disease). However, EUS is still not universally available. ERCP provides the best test of duct structure and adds the advantage of potential therapeutic interventions. The CT scan provides both superior assessment of many of the complications of chronic pancreatitis, including pseudocysts that do not communicate with the main pancreatic duct, and imaging of various extrapancreatic

Table 13-8. Structural Tests for Chronic Pancreatitis

TEST	SENSITIVITY (%)	RISKS AND DRAWBACKS
Endoscopic ultrasound (EUS)	90	Available only in major medical centers
Endoscopic retrograde cholangiopancreatography (ERCP)	85	Invasive procedure with higher risk of complications than noninvasive tests
Computed tomography (CT)	80	—
Transabdominal ultrasound	70	—
Plain abdominal film	30–40	—

complications (see Figure 13-6). Magnetic resonance imaging (MRI) is another imaging option. Magnetic resonance cholantiopancreatography is a noninvasive modality to visualize the pancreatobiliary system and may be used to support a clinical diagnosis in early chronic pancreatitis. Transabdominal ultrasound is inexpensive and noninvasive, but a complete examination of the pancreas may be precluded in many patients by overlying bowel gas. In each of these imaging modalities, attention should be directed to the diameter of the pancreatic duct, because the size of the duct may dictate therapeutic options. Plain abdominal film is inexpensive but insensitive. However, identification of calcification in the pancreas (using bone technique) may be helpful in making a diagnosis.

Functional Evidence

The goal of the pancreatic function test is to determine whether the stimulated output of pancreatic HCO_3^- or pancreatic enzyme is normal or diminished. Pancreatic function tests include the "tubed" secretin stimulation test, the bentiromide test, carbon 14-olein absorption test, dual Schilling's test, fecal chymotrypsin or elastase, serum trypsin level, and fecal fat (Table 13-9). The secretin or cholecystokinin (CCK) stimulation test requires placing a sampling tube into the duodenum for recovery of pancreatic juice. (It is sometimes called the tubed secretin test to distinguish it from the secretin test used to diagnose Zollinger-Ellison syndrome). A properly performed secretin stimulation test is considered the most sensitive and specific test of chronic pancreatitis because it measures pancreatic function directly. However, because this test is complex, cumbersome, and unpleasant for the patient, it is not widely available, and other indirect pancreatic function tests have been developed. These other indirect tests of pancreatic function all suffer from the same limitations: good sensitivity in severe chronic pancreatitis but poor sensitivity in mild and moderate chronic pancreatitis.

Table 13-9. Functional Tests for Chronic Pancreatitis

TEST	SENSITIVITY (%)	MEASURES	RISKS AND DRAWBACKS
Secretin stimulation	85	Pancreatic HCO_3^- production after intravenous injection of secretin	Requires placement of a nasoduodenal tube False positives can be seen with maldigestion resulting from intestinal disease
Serum trypsin	Low in early stages of disease	Decreased serum trypsin level (present in late stages)	—
Bentiromide	75	Action of chymotrypsin (indirectly); decreased chymotrypsin manifested by decreased serum and urine p-aminobenzoic acid (PABA) level.	—

CASE STUDY 2: *CONTINUED*

Six months later, the patient returned to the clinic with a chief complaint of worsening, persistent, increased abdominal pain and sharp pain in his back causing shortness of breath. He appeared uncomfortable, was leaning forward and to the left, and had shallow breathing at a rate of 20 breaths/min. Physical examination revealed a supraumbilical abdominal mass and tenderness, decreased breath sounds in the left base with a pleuritic rub on inspiration and with dullness on percussion. Chest x-ray confirmed the presence of a left pleural effusion, and an abdominal CT scan identified a pseudocyst in the body of the pancreas. A thoracentesis was performed, and pleural effusion amylase was 1125 IU/L compared to a serum amylase of 70, which suggested a pancreatic-pleural fistula. An ERCP demonstrated a dominant proximal pancreatic duct stricture, continuity of duct with pseudocyst in the body of the pancreas, and a fistula between the tail of the pancreas and the left pleural space. An endoscopic stent was placed across the dominant stricture to decompress the pancreatic duct and pseudocyst, and the patient was started on TPN, given nothing by mouth, and treated with somatostatin to minimize pancreatic exocrine secretion. Over the next 6 weeks, the pleural effusion resolved, the pseudocyst shrank, and the pain decreased, although the patient required narcotics for control of abdominal pain.

The patient had a distal pancreatectomy with splenectomy for pain control. Postoperatively he had good pain relief and was off all narcotics. He developed steatorrhea, maldigestion, and foul-smelling stool, consistent with pancreatic insufficiency. He was treated with pancreatic enzyme supplements and the maldigestion symptoms resolved.

COMPLICATIONS

A number of common complications of chronic pancreatitis are encountered. A mechanical obstruction of the CBD or duodenum may occur. The obstruction may be caused by pancreatic pseudocyst, acute inflammation, or retroperitoneal fibrosis. Approximately 5%–10% of patients develop CBD obstruction and present with jaundice, right upper quadrant pain, or cholangitis. Duodenal obstruction is less common and presents with postprandial nausea and vomiting.

In chronic pancreatitis, as opposed to acute pancreatitis, pseudocysts rarely resolve spontaneously. Pseudocysts in chronic pancreatitis may remain asymptomatic or may enlarge and cause such complications as pain, infection, hemorrhage, and bile duct or bowel obstruction. Pseudocysts can be seen in up to 25% of patients.

Pancreatic ascites, a rare complication, occurs when pancreatic enzymes leak into the peritoneal space, elevating ascitic fluid amylase.

This may also be associated with pleural effusion. If pleural effusion is present, one must consider the presence of pancreatic-pleural fistula. This can be confirmed by measurement of pleural fluid amylase and lipase, which should be higher than serum levels.

The prevalence of pancreatic cancer increases in chronic pancreatitis. Frequently, this is a difficult diagnosis as pancreatic head enlargement and fibrosis are difficult to differentiate from adenocarcinoma radiographically, and biopsies have a low sensitivity.

TREATMENT

Goals of treatment in chronic pancreatitis are alleviation of pain and treatment of maldigestion and complications, such as pseudocyst and diabetes. Pain management in chronic pancreatitis patients remains one of the more challenging problems in medicine. This problem reflects the multiple etiologies of chronic pancreatitis pain, the difficulty in pinpointing the source of pain, and limited ability to control visceral pain. Therefore, pain management often requires a multidisciplinary approach. In contrast to pain, maldigestion responds well to pancreatic enzyme supplementation. Diabetes may require insulin treatment.

Management of Pain

Pain management is divided into three progressive phases.

Stage 1. Pain in patients with early chronic pancreatitis often responds to therapy directed at removing the underlying cause and controlling the symptoms. In the alcoholic patient, abstinence from alcohol may alleviate pain. Likewise, drugs that are known to cause acute pancreatitis should be stopped when possible. Addition of pancreatic enzymes with gastric acid suppression may alleviate pain in some patients. It is believed that the delivery of sufficient proteases to the duodenum results in the digestion of a luminal CCK-releasing peptide, causing a reduction in the release of CCK from mucosal endocrine cells and thereby reducing the hormonal stimulation to the pancreas. To date, only enzyme preparations that are fully active in the duodenum have been shown to reduce pain, with the best result seen in mild or early idiopathic pancreatitis. Oral analgesics may be required to control pain. Acetaminophen or NSAIDs should be the first line of therapy, but narcotics may be required to control pain in more severe cases. Care must be taken, because patients with a history of alcohol abuse frequently become dependent on narcotics.

Stage 2. If alcohol abstinence, enzyme supplements, and analgesics fail, more invasive attempts to control pain are initiated. To guide therapy, a CT or ERCP should be performed to identify treatable causes of pain and formulate a treatment plan. Delineation of pancreatic ductal anatomy helps distinguish between large- and small-duct disease.

Patients in whom the main pancreatic duct is dilated beyond 5 mm have several therapeutic options. Endoscopic therapy, including stone extraction and dilation or stenting of ductal stenosis, result in significant improvement of pain in about 75% of patients for up to 6 months. However, pain relief rate drops with time to about 50% after 3 years of treatment. Because stents frequently become clogged over time and can cause obstruction, periodic ERCP with pancreatic stent changes is indicated.

Surgical options for large-duct disease include lateral pancreatico-jejunostomy (Puestow procedure) and two types of duodenum-preserving resections of the pancreatic head (Beger and Frey procedures). The Puestow procedure alleviates pain in 70% of cases for at least 6 months after surgery. However, the success rate of the Puestow procedure for pain alleviation decreases to 50% at 5 years after surgery. If the duct disease is segmented, other surgical options may be useful. Subtotal pancreatic resection is an option in patients with dominant ductal stricture in the body or tail of the pancreas (as in Case Study 2); however, it worsens pancreatic insufficiency. When the disease is prominent in the head of the pancreas, resection of the head of the pancreas by modified Whipple or duodenum-sparing procedure may alleviate pain in up to 85% of patients. Resection increases the risks of diabetes and maldigestion.

Management of pain in patients with small-duct disease presents a more difficult problem. Celiac plexus and splanchnic nerve blocks have generally offered short-term amelioration of pain. EUS-guided celiac plexus block is currently being studied.

Frequently, pseudocysts require drainage for alleviation of intractable pain or bile duct or duodenal obstruction. Pseudocysts can be drained by surgical means, by ERCP placement of stents through the transpapillary route, by nasocystic drainage tubes, or by cystenterostomy. Often the drainage of a pseudocyst results in significant relief of pain. Recurrence of pseudocysts is seen in 10%–20% of surgical or ERCP drainage methods.

Stage 3. In patients with intractable pain, total pancreatic rest with nothing by mouth, TPN, or jejunal enteral feeding with octreotide occasionally results in significant pain improvement. Total pancreatectomy is the final option for patients who continue to have abdominal pain despite stage 2 interventions. However, total pancreatectomy results in brittle diabetes in 100% of patients, steatorrhea in 100% of patients, and a high mortality rate, and pain relief is achieved in only about 80% of these patients. Diabetic management is very difficult after total pancreatectomy; therefore pancreatic islet cell autotransplantation should be seriously considered.

Management of Maldigestion

Steatorrhea and carbohydrate and protein maldigestion are effectively treated with pancreatic enzyme replacement. Two important problems must be considered for effective pancreatic enzyme replacement. The first is that *pancreatic enzymes are destroyed in the low-pH environment of the stomach.* The second is that *pancreatic enzyme activity is required in the duodenum and jejunum:* 30,000 IU/meal of lipase for fat absorption (remembering that free fatty acids are absorbed in the proximal small intestine, whereas bile acids are absorbed in the *distal* small intestine) and "significant" protease activity to digest the CCK-releasing factors. Two approaches to these problems have been used. (1) If nonenteric-coated pancreatic enzymes are used, sufficient gastric acid suppression prevents pancreatic enzyme destruction and active enzymes are delivered to the proximal small intestine. (2) Acid suppression with histamine (H_2)-receptor antagonists is an effective choice in many patients, but therapeutic failures may occur in patients with high meal-stimulated acid secretion. Higher doses of a H_2-receptor antagonist or use of a proton pump inhibitor (PPI) may be necessary for pancreatic enzyme protection in these patients. The second approach is to protect the pancreatic enzymes in enteric-coated microspheres that release the enzymes at a safe pH. However, gastric emptying of large microspheres (>1 mm in diameter) is significantly delayed compared to that of the meal so that the utility of the enzyme supplement in the proximal small intestine is diminished. Furthermore, in patients with diminished HCO_3^- secretion (especially in cystic fibrosis), the pH of the proximal small intestine may be lower than normal. Therefore, the enteric coatings that release the pancreatic enzyme at a pH near 7 may not be released in the proximal small intestine until late. Thus, enteric-coated preparations with a smaller microsphere size and enzyme release at a pH near 5.5 may be preferable. Use of H_2-receptor antagonists or PPIs does not preclude the use of enteric-coated preparations. However, to date, only nonenteric-coated enzyme supplements have been of proven benefit for pain control.

SUMMARY: CHRONIC PANCREATITIS

A typical patient with chronic pancreatitis presents with recurrent or chronic midepigastric pain that radiates to the back and weight loss due to sitophobia and maldigestion. Pain is usually exacerbated by eating. The diagnosis is confirmed by structural or functional pancreatic testing as well as by excluding other diseases with a similar presentation. Treatment involves alleviation of pain and treatment of maldigestion and complications, such as pseudocyst and diabetes.

CASE STUDY 2: *RESOLUTION*

After 18 months, the patient returned to the office. Since his surgery, he regained the lost weight, reentered the workforce, and married. He continued to take his insulin and an enteric-coated pancreatic enzyme supplement with occasional over-the-counter analgesics for mild abdominal pain. The reason for his visit was to let you know just how well he had been doing and to say, "thank you!"

REVIEW QUESTIONS

Directions: For each of the following questions, choose the one best answer.

1 A 70-year-old man with chronic pancreatitis and small-duct disease presents to clinic with a chief complaint of epigastric pain radiating to the back for the last 3 months. The pain is exacerbated by eating. He is concerned about the pain and recent weight loss. What would be an appropriate next step?

A Oral narcotics for pain control
B Hospital admission for bowel rest and intravenous analgesics
C Nonenteric-coated pancreatic enzyme with acid suppression therapy
D The Puestow procedure

2 A 15-year-old boy with history of recurrent pneumonia is complaining of watery diarrhea, failure to gain weight, and chronic fatigue. He appears cachectic. Stool Sudan stain is positive for fat. The next step in the diagnosis of this patient is

A sweat chloride test.
B secretin stimulation test.
C endoscopic retrograde cholangiopancreatography (ERCP).
D abdominal CT scan.

3 A 33-year-old man with a history of chronic pancreatitis secondary to alcohol abuse whose pain had been well controlled with ibuprofen 600 mg three times a day is seen in a clinic because of jaundice, right upper quadrant pain, and fever. Laboratory tests show WBC count, 18,000/mm^3; alkaline phosphatase, 600 IU/L; total bilirubin, 9 mg/dl; AST, 60 IU/L; ALT, 50 IU/L. Abdominal ultrasound shows dilated CBD. The next best action for this patient would be to

A admit to ICU for antibiotics and close observation.
B perform emergent ERCP for treatment of ascending cholangitis.
C perform endoscopy to assess for ulcers induced by NSAIDs.
D perform abdominal CT scan to assess for cancer in head of the pancreas.

4 A 44-year-old woman presents with 6 hours of severe epigastric pain radiating to the back and associated nausea and vomiting. She denies use of alcohol. Vital signs are normal. On examination, she has severe upper abdominal tenderness without guarding. Normal bowel sounds are present. Laboratory assessment is significant for amylase of 1200 IU/L, lipase of 490 IU/L, AST of 124 IU/L, ALT of

160 IU/L, total bilirubin of 1.2 mg/dl, and alkaline phosphatase of 600 IU/L. The best course of action would be to

A admit the patient to the ICU and start TPN.

B admit patient to the ward, order nothing by mouth, administer intravenous fluids, and obtain abdominal ultrasound.

C perform emergent ERCP with stone extraction.

D perform emergent surgery for pseudocyst drainage.

5 A 34-year-old man presents with 3 days of epigastric pain radiating to the back. Pain increases postprandially and is associated with nausea and vomiting. Physical examination is significant for a young man in moderate distress. Abdominal examination reveals decreased bowel sounds with periumbilical tenderness and voluntary guarding but without rebound tenderness. Amylase level is checked because of suspicion for pancreatitis and is 80 IU/L. Serum is noted to be turbid and lipemic. Abdominal CT scan is significant for mild edema in the head of the pancreas. The next step should be to

A repeat serum amylase level in a diluted sample.

B proceed with emergent ERCP.

C repeat amylase test.

D perform endoscopy to assess for peptic ulcer disease.

6 A physician is asked to evaluate a 66-year-old man who was admitted to the hospital 1 week ago with a diagnosis of severe alcohol-induced pancreatitis. His pain has improved with supportive measures, nothing by mouth, intravenous fluids, and TPN. Over the last 2 days he became jaundiced. Temperature was 40°C last night. Blood pressure is 100/60 mm Hg, pulse is 110, with a respiratory rate of 24. Abdomen is tender in the epigastric and right upper quadrant region. Amylase has decreased from 1000 IU/L on admission to 180 IU/L. Total bilirubin is 8 mg/dl, alkaline phosphatase is 400 IU/L, and AST is 120 IU/L. What is the next best step?

A Perform emergent ERCP and administer antibiotics for treatment of cholangitis

B Obtain abdominal CT scan to assess for pseudocyst

C Start antibiotics for cholangitis

D Start antibiotics for infected pancreatic necrosis

7 A 30-year-old woman with a history of ulcerative colitis is seen in the clinic on routine follow-up. She complains of 1 week of diffuse abdominal pain and nausea with postprandial vomiting. She has been unable to hold any food down for 5 days. Medications are azulfidine 1 g three times a day, prednisone 10 mg/d, and azathioprine 100 mg/d. Vital signs are blood pressure of 90/60 mm HG, pulse of 100, respiratory rate of 20. Her abdomen is diffusely tender with voluntary guarding without rebound tenderness. Bowel sounds are

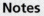

decreased. Serum amylase is 1500 IU/L. Appropriate management would be to

A obtain abdominal CT scan to evaluate for pancreatic necrosis.

B stop azathioprine, admit to hospital, start intravenous fluids, order nothing by mouth, and order an abdominal ultrasound to assess for gallstone pancreatitis.

C perform emergent ERCP with therapeutic intervention.

D check amylase isoenzymes.

8 A 35-year-old alcoholic man presented to the emergency room with severe epigastric pain that started exactly 35 minutes prior to presentation. He complained of nausea and vomiting. Vital signs: pulse, 120; blood pressure, 90/60 mm Hg; respiratory rate, 24; and temperature, 38.4°C. He was in severe distress and lay still in bed. His abdomen was silent, with diffuse tenderness, guarding, and rebound. Abdominal x-rays showed free air under the right diaphragm. Amylase was 200, WBC count was 14,000/mm^3. The next best action would be to

A admit to ICU and treat for severe pancreatitis.

B perform emergent surgery for perforated viscus.

C admit to the hospital and start antibiotics for diverticulitis.

D perform emergent ERCP for extraction of stone from ampulla.

References

Banks PA: Practice guidelines in acute pancreatitis. *Am J Gastroenterol* 92:377–386, 1997.

Bradley E: A clinically based classification system for acute pancreatitis. *Arch Surg* 128:536–590, 1993.

Cappel MS, Das KM: Rapid development of acute pancreatitis following reuse of 6-mercaptopurine. *J Clin Gastroenterol* 11:679–681, 1989.

DiMagno EP: Laboratory assessment of pancreatic impairment. In *Bockus Gastroenterology*, 5th ed. Edited by Haubrich WS, Schaffner F, Berk JE. Philadelphia, PA: W. B. Saunders, 1995, pp 2835–2850.

DiMagno EP, Go VLW, Summerskill WHJ: Relations between pancreatic enzyme outputs and malabsorption in severe pancreatic insufficiency. *N Engl J Med* 288:813–815, 1973.

Dominguez-Munoz JE, Carballo F, Garcia MJ, et al: Evaluation of the clinical usefulness of APACHE II and SAPS systems in the initial prognostic classification of acute pancreatitis: a multicenter study. *Pancreas* 8:682–686, 1993.

Fan S-T, Lai ECS, Mok FPT, et al: Early treatment of acute biliary pancreatitis by endoscopic papillotomy. *N Engl J Med* 328:228–232, 1993.

Fayad LM: MR cholangiopancreatography: evaluation of common pancreatic diseases. *Radiol Clin North Am* 41(1):97–114, 2003.

Freeny PC: Incremental dynamic bolus computed tomography of acute pancreatitis. *Int J Pancreatol* 13:147–158, 1993.

Frey, CF: Current management of chronic pancreatitis. *Adv Surg* 28: 337–370, 1995.

Gerzoff SG, Banks PA, Robins AH, et al: Early diagnosis of pancreatic infection by computed tomography-guided aspiration. *Gastroenterology* 93:1315, 1987.

Kloppel G, Maillet B: Pathology of acute and chronic pancreatitis. *Pancreas* 8:659–670, 1993.

Kloppel G, Maillet B: Pathology of acute and chronic pancreatitis. *Pancreas* 13:818–829, 1993.

Malfertheiner P, Dominguez-Munoz JE: Prognostic factors in acute pancreatitis. *Int J Pancreatol* 14:1–8, 1993.

McArthur KE: Drug-induced pancreatitis (review article). *Ailment Pharmacol Ther* 10:23–33, 1996.

Mulvihill SJ, Debas HT: Surgical treatment of pancreatitis and its complications. *Semin Gastrointest Dis* 2:194–202, 1991.

Sainio V, Kemppainen E, Puolakkainen P, et al: Early antibiotic treatment in acute pancreatitis. *Lancet* 346:663–667, 1995.

Singer ML, Gyr K, Sarles H: Revised classification of pancreatitis (Report of the Second International Symposium on Classification of Pancreatitis in Marseille, March 28–30, 1984). *Gastroenterology* 89:683–685, 1985.

Slaff J, Jacobson D, Tillman CR, et al: Protease-specific suppression of pancreatic secretion. *Gastroenterology* 87:44–52, 1984.

Soergel KH: Pancreatitis. In Goldman C: *Textbook of Medicine*, 21st Ed. Philadelphia, PA: W.B. Saunders, 2000, pp 752–759.

Toskes PP: Medical therapy of chronic pancreatitis. *Sem Gastrointest Dis* 2:188–193, 1991.

Whitcomb DC, Gorry MC, Preston RA, et al: Hereditary pancreatitis is caused by a mutation in the cationic trypsinogen gene. *Nat Gene* 13:141–145, 1996.

Whitcomb D, Martin SP: Complicated acute pancreatitis. *Gastroenterol Endoscopy News* 45(5):8–19, 1994.

14

Functional Bowel Disorders

■ LEARNING OBJECTIVES ■

At the completion of this chapter, the reader should be able to:

- Define functional bowel disease, name several forms of functional disease of the GI tract, and explain the difference between functional and organic disease.
- List the Rome II criteria for diagnosis of irritable bowel syndrome (IBS).
- Describe the motility and neurologic abnormalities seen in IBS.
- Describe nonulcer dyspepsia and discuss the motility disorders seen in this entity.
- Discuss appropriate evaluation and possible treatment methods for the functional bowel diseases.
- Describe Oglivie's syndrome.
- List the factors that maintain normal continence and describe how problems with any one factor can lead to incontinence.

CASE STUDY: *INTRODUCTION*

A 35-year-old woman was referred to a physician's office with a 20-year history of intermittent abdominal discomfort, diarrhea, and flatulence. She had seen several other generalists and specialists and after an upper GI series with small bowel follow-through, CT scan of the abdomen, two separate air-contrast barium enemas, esophagogastroduodenoscopy (EGD), and colonoscopy had simply been told "it's all in your head." She had not experienced weight loss with the diarrhea, had no rashes or arthralgias, and had never noted blood in her stools. On prompting, she did note that her symptoms worsened in times of stress and that in college during each examination period, she experienced diarrhea, which resolved after completion of finals.

The patient described the pain as diffuse, cramping pain over her lower abdomen. The pain resolved with bowel movements, and she had up to six bowel movements per day during one of her attacks. Occasionally, she was troubled by constipation, for which she took an over-the-counter laxative. She was never awakened from sleep by pain or the urge to defecate.

Recently, an aunt had died of colon cancer, and she was concerned that "something has been missed." She also noted that the symptoms were troublesome to her at her job as a realtor. When eating fast food in the car, she could not drive more than 15–30 minutes after lunch without urgent need of a restroom.

Her physical examination was unremarkable except for left lower quadrant discomfort on palpation. What studies and laboratory tests should be added to this "million dollar workup?" What suggestions would improve this patient's condition?

Introduction

The diagnosis of a functional bowel disorder carries with it negative connotations, primarily because of our own poor understanding of the pathophysiology and limited therapeutic options. Although the pathophysiology of this group of disorders remains nebulous, there are clearly abnormalities in motility of the small and large intestines, as well as in the sympathetic and parasympathetic nervous systems that have been identified in the most common and most studied of the functional diseases: irritable bowel syndrome (IBS). The hallmark of functional disorders of the gut is an abnormal awareness of what generally is unnoticed daily gut activity—one should be unaware of the reflexive activities of the GI tract except for feelings of satiety and the need to defecate. This phenomenon of heightened awareness is known as visceral hyperalgesia.

Functional GI disorders, those relating to motility to the nervous system, may involve any portion of the gut. Gastroesophageal reflux

Organic disease represents disease associated with histologic, structural, or biochemical findings. **Functional disease** (which previously implied psychosomatic etiology), now indicates the disorders of motility or central nervous system (CNS)-mediated abnormalities of function. Absence of GI symptoms interrupting sleep is a classic clinical indication of functional disease.

disease (GERD), now known to be primarily due to disordered motility functions of the esophagus, is examined in detail elsewhere (see Chapter 10). Other GI disorders labeled nonorganic in etiology include noncardiac chest pain (largely due to GERD), chronic pelvic pain syndrome, biliary dyskinesia, fecal incontinence, pelvic floor dysfunction, and sphincter of Oddi dysfunction. In this chapter, we address and discuss the known physiology of the most common and most poorly understood group of diseases: IBS, nonulcer dyspepsia, Ogilvie's syndrome, and fecal incontinence.

The first study to address diagnostic criteria for IBS was a working team report published in 1989 on behalf of the 1988 International Congress of Gastroenterology in Rome. Following this, the Rome criteria were developed. Documents published in the *Gastroenterology International Journal* from 1992 to 1995, as well as the Rome I book are referred to as Rome I. Committees working on these criteria were expanded, and a series of articles were published in 1999 in a supplement of *Gut*. These are considered the Rome II criteria. The committees are now working on Rome III, which is due for publication in 2006. Table 14-1 indicates the functional bowel disorders that were identified by the Rome II committee. The clinical

Table 14-1. Rome Functional Bowel Disorders Identified by the Rome II Committee

A. Esophageal disorders
  A1. Globus
  A2. Rumination syndrome
  A3. Functional chest pain of resumed esophageal origin
  A4. Functional heartburn
  A5. Functional dysphagia
  A6. Unspecified functional esophageal disorder
B. Gastroduodenal disorders
  B1. Functional dyspepsia
    B1a. Ulcerlike dyspepsia
    B1b. Dysmotilitylike dyspepsia
    B1c. Unspecified (nonspecific) dyspepsia
  B2. Aerophagia
  B3. Functional vomiting
C. Bowel disorders
  C1. Irritable bowel syndrome (IBS)
  C2. Functional abdominal bloating
  C3. Functional constipation
  C4. Functional diarrhea
  C5. Unspecified functional bowel disorder
D. Functional abdominal pain
  D1. Functional abdominal pain syndrome
  D2. Unspecified functional abdominal pain
E. Biliary disorders
  E1. Gallbladder dysfunction
  E2. Sphincter of Oddi dysfunction

F. Anorectal disorders
  F1. Functional fecal incontinence
  F2. Functional anorectal pain
    F2a. Levator ani syndrome
    F2b. Proctalgia fugax
  F3. Pelvic floor dyssynergia
G. Functional pediatric disorders
  G1. Vomiting
    G1a. Infant regurgitation
    G1b. Infant rumination syndrome
    G1c. Cyclic vomiting syndrome
  G2. Abdominal pain
    G2a. Functional dyspepsia
    G2b. IBS
    G2c. Functional abdominal pain
    G2d. Abdominal migraine
    G2e. Aerophagia
  G3. Functional diarrhea
  G4. Disorders of defecation
    G4a. Infant dyschezia
    G4b. Functional constipation
    G4c. Functional fecal retention
    G4d. Nonretentive fecal soiling

Table 14-2. Rome II Criteria for IBS

At least 12 weeks, which need not be consecutive, in the preceding 12 months of abdominal discomfort or pain that has two of three features:

1. Relieved with defecation
2. Onset associated with a change in frequency of stool
3. Onset associated with a change in form (appearance) of stool

The validity of the symptom criteria for IBS is supported by studies of IBS patients, the analysis of factors affecting non-IBS patients, and the long term follow up of IBS patients.

Migrating Motor Complex
During fasting, the small intestine on manometric study reveals a distally propulsive cycle (the MMC), which is disrupted by eating with more irregular contractions.

value of separating the functional GI symptoms into these discrete conditions is to focus diagnostic and therapeutic strategies.

IBS

IBS is a distinct syndrome with diagnostic criteria developed by Rome II (Table 14-2), but may have broad overlap with the other functional disorders. The criteria for the diagnosis of IBS as determined by Rome II may be found in Table 14-2. In addition, Table 14-3 offers a list of supportive symptoms that can be used to help classify patients into diarrhea- or constipation-predominant IBS.

Causes for abdominal pain in IBS have been investigated for over 20 years. It has been well documented that colonic distention with balloon inflation requires a lower volume to induce pain in patients meeting criteria for an IBS diagnosis. Studies of GI tract motility in IBS reveal that the migrating motor complex (MMC) periodicity in diarrhea-variant IBS patients is shorter than in control groups and that ileal propulsive waves and clusters of jejunal propulsive activity are also more common. Cramping discomfort with prolonged contractions was common after intraduodenal infusion of a fatty meal (which could account for IBS patients' intolerance of fatty or fast-food meals). In addition—and of unclear significance—is the lower rectal compliance with balloon distention in diarrhea-variant IBS, as well as repetitive motor activity induced by that balloon distention. Exaggerated small bowel motor response to pain, stress, and balloon distention of the ileum has been noted.

Table 14-3. Supportive Symptoms Consistent with the Diagnosis of IBS

1. Fewer than three bowel movements a week
2. More than three bowel movements a day
3. Hard or lumpy stools
4. Loose (mushy) or watery stools
5. Straining during a bowel movement
6. Urgency (having to rush to have a bowel movement)
7. Feeling of incomplete bowel movement
8. Passing mucus (white material) during a bowel movement
9. Abdominal fullness, bloating, or swelling

Diarrhea-predominant: 1 or more of 2, 4, or 6 and none of 1, 3, or 5
Constipation-predominant: 1 or more of 1, 3, or 5 and none of 2, 4, or 6

IBS patients have increased visceral pain sensation but do not exhibit hypersensitivity to noxious somatic stimuli.

Attempts to measure the distress or the motility disorders of IBS may lead to additional distress or alterations in motility.

Clinical studies of IBS are hampered by disease heterogeneity and the possibility that the testing itself may cause stress and discomfort that could alter test results.

However, disordered motility alone cannot account for the pain experienced by patients with IBS, because these motility abnormalities are also identified in normal, pain-free controls. The question of gut hypersensitivity to noxious stimuli (balloon distention) has been extensively evaluated, and it appears that selective hypersensitivity of the mechanoreceptors of both the large and small intestines are present in IBS, leading researchers to hypothesize a central dysfunction of viscerosomatic pain referral. Although normal control subjects can and do feel abdominal discomfort to balloon distention, patients with IBS experience discomfort much more diffusely over their abdomen. Patients with IBS, do not, however, appear to have increased sensitivity to noxious somatic stimuli.

Studies have identified abnormalities in vagal (cholinergic) function in the constipation-variant IBS population, as opposed to sympathetic adrenergic dysfunction in the diarrhea-variant group. This finding may have great implications in further studies and treatment of IBS, as it further reveals the inhomogeneity of the study population, which has not been addressed in earlier studies.

A confident diagnosis after careful history and physical examination and appropriately tailored work-up, patient education, and appropriate reassurance are all part of the therapeutic plan. A graded approach should be taken, considering the dominant symptoms, their severity, and psychosocial factors.

Clinical studies of IBS relating to both pathophysiology and treatment are challenged by several variables. Subsets of IBS (diarrhea-versus constipation-variant) are not homogeneous on motility studies, and the "diagnosis of exclusion" of IBS may be problematic. Motility studies of either the small or large bowel are unappealing to both patients and controls because catheter placement is uncomfortable. Control subjects who are asymptomatic often reveal manometric findings similar to those of their affected counterparts. In addition, the discomfort and psychologic stress influences the motility tracings of IBS (stress and discomfort being common in experimental trials). Because it is difficult to identify and monitor responses in the IBS population, it is also difficult to establish the utility of the limited therapeutic armamentarium. Thus the motility and neurologic evaluations of the patient with IBS remain only theoretical and in the research realm, with little clinical application.

Therapy may include the use increased dietary fiber, such as wheat bran or bulking agents for constipation, loperamide or diphenoxylate for diarrhea, and anticholinergic/antispasmodic agents or low-dose antidepressants for pain. Newer medications are now available and in development. The use of alosetron, a 5-HT3 antagonist, for diarrhea-predominant IBS was met with challenges due to adverse effects in some patients. After FDA approval and then removal from the market, it is now available when prescribed by qualified providers. Tegaserod, a 5-HT4 agonist, has been approved for use in

Table 14-4. Intervention in IBS

Patient Education
Dietary counseling/fiber/food diary
Drugs
    Antispasmodics
    Prokinetic agents
    Antidepressants
    Laxatives
    Antidiarrheal agents
    5 HT3 antagonist
    5 HT4 agonist
    Drugs studied in clinical trials
Psychologic treatments
Behavioral therapy

Diarrhea may be defined as an increase in stool weight to greater than 250 g/d. Patients may define diarrhea in terms of increased stool liquidity or increased frequency of bowel movements.

Stool studies may include examination for enteric pathogens, Gram stain, ova and parasite evaluation, and qualitative fecal fat.

women with constipation-predominant IBS. Psychological or behavioral treatments may also help some patients.

With the uncertain utility of the medicinal interventions, it is important to educate the patient about his or her disease, providing reassurance and prescribing dietary restrictions of fats and increased dietary fiber. Patients may assist in monitoring their symptoms in diary form to limit inciting events. In some patients, behavioral treatments greatly improve their ability to cope with a lifelong disease that is associated with chronic intermittent discomfort (Table 14-4).

Chronic Diarrhea (NON-IBS)

Some patients exhibit chronic diarrhea—that is, diarrhea that fails to resolve in 3 weeks, is of obscure etiology, and is not accompanied by the discomfort faced by the IBS patient. The attempt to determine the cause then is truly a diagnosis of exclusion, when a thorough history, physical examination, complete stool evaluation, and search for diseases such as malabsorption, thyrotoxicosis, IBS, and cancer are without yield. Additional tests that might be ordered include testing for giardiasis and other stool testing, small bowel biopsy, or D-xylose test to exclude small bowel malabsorption, and stool electrolytes and osmolality to exclude secretory or osmotic diarrhea. Hydrogen breath testing, using different substrates, can be useful in determining carbohydrate malabsorption or bacterial overgrowth. When thorough endoscopic evaluation and small bowel radiographic studies (always done last, because barium impedes examination of the stool for paracytic ova) also prove negative, therapeutic trials are employed to exclude missed diagnoses.

Therapeutic trials are based on clinical suspicions aroused by the medical history. Metronidazole might be employed in a patient in whom giardiasis or antibiotic-associated diarrhea is suspected. Pancreatic enzymes might be useful in a patient with suspected insufficiency, and cholestyramine resin (brand name Questran) and other bile salt–binding agents in patients with suspected bile salt diarrhea. Broad-spectrum antibiotic agents might eliminate suspected bacterial overgrowth syndrome. Antispasmodics and fiber therapy, the mainstays of IBS treatment, should not be neglected. A careful dietary history is crucial and the use of a diary may be beneficial.

Should therapeutic trials fail to establish this frustrating diagnosis, symptomatic improvement may be achieved by use of clonidine. Loperamide hydrochloride (brand name Imodium), diphenoxylate hydrochloride and atropine sulfate (brand name Lomotil), or octreotide (brand name Sandostatin) may also be employed long-term to check diarrhea of uncertain etiology (Table 14-5).

Nonulcer Dyspepsia

Nonulcer dyspepsia is a heterogeneous collection of upper abdominal functional symptoms, such as pain or discomfort, bloating, gas, nausea, and early satiety, without organic findings on upper GI barium study or endoscopy. These symptoms are episodic, persistent, and often related to eating. Research has revelaed that 50% of these patients have delay in gastric emptying. Antral hypomotility has been documented, and a syndrome of gastric hyperalgesia, with a lower perception threshold for gastric balloon distention, has been seen. A high rate of colonization of the gastric mucosa with *Helicobacter pylori* has been noted (up to 60%); however, treatment of bacterial infestation does not improve the patient's symptoms. Therapeutic options in the treatment of this disorder should be targeted to the suspected underlying pathophysiology.

GASTROPARESIS

Gastroparesis, delayed emptying from the stomach, is not uncommon, occurring in 30%–50% of patients with diabetes and 40% of patients with GERD. The phenomenon is felt to be due to a vagal autonomic neuropathy; there is found to be a loss of phase 3 interdigestive migratory motor complex (IMMC). Although gastroparesis is generally idiopathic if not diabetic in nature, evaluation for electrolyte abnormalities

Table 14-5. Antidiarrheal Agents

TRADE NAME	GENERIC NAME	MODE OF ACTION
Clonidine	Catapres	Alpha agonist
Imodium	Loperamide hydrochloride	Slows intestinal motility by direct effect on circular smooth muscle and affects water and electrolyte movement through the bowel wall
Lomotil	Diphenoxylate hydrochloride with atropine sulfate	Direct effect on circular smooth muscle with enhanced segmentation and prolonged transit time; subtherapeutic atropine added to discourage deliberate overdose
Sandostatin	Octrectide	Inhibits release of serotonin, gastrin, vasoactive intestinal polypeptide, secretin, motilin, and pancreatic polypeptide

Table 14-6. Intervention in Gastroparesis

Patient education
Low-residue diet
Prokinetic agents
　Metoclopramide
　Erythromycin
　Motilinlike agents
Alternative feeding route (severe gastroparesis)
　Nasoenteral feeding
　Feeding jejunostomy with or without venting gastrostomy

and hypothyroidism and evaluation for outflow obstruction by endoscopy are indicated. Definitive diagnosis of gastroparesis with no gastric outlet obstruction is made by abnormal scintiscan data (solid-phase nuclear medicine gastric emptying study). Treatment includes optimization of glycemic control, low-residue diet, and treatment with prokinetic agents, such as metoclopramide (brand name Reglan), or erythromycin. In severe cases of gastroparesis, nasoenteric feeding or, in rare patients, venting gastrostomy and feeding jejunostomy might be indicated for this frustrating disease (Table 14-6).

Ogilvie's Syndrome and Chronic Intestinal Pseudo-Obstruction

Ogilvie's syndrome, named for the surgeon who, in 1948, noted massive colon distention in two patients who were later found to have tumor invasion of the celiac plexus, has now come to represent all idiopathic colonic ileus. Generally associated with severe medical illness or postoperative state, the condition generally subsides spontaneously, allowing little time to explore the pathophysiology. Generally in such cases, the patient's electrolytes are reviewed, and an x-ray is obtained to assess cecal diameter. If this diameter approaches 14 cm, up until recently a colonoscopy for decompression with endoscopic placement of a tube was performed to avoid an imminent perforation. There have been several studies over the past few years using neostigmine, a parasympathomimetic drug, as an effective therapy to treat this condition.

Chronic intestinal pseudo-obstruction (CIP) is the clinical picture of recurrent episodes of obstruction resulting from the failure of intestinal peristalsis to overcome resistance to flow. Because the disorder is difficult to differentiate clinically from mechanical bowel obstruction, these patients may be subject to multiple surgeries without cause.

CIP has been associated with the finding of antibodies against cell nucleus antigen (anti-PCNA) in scleroderma patients, digital arches in fingerprints, mitral valve prolapse, joint laxity, and constipation since the age of 10. These associations might direct treatment away from surgical intervention.

Notes

Biofeedback may be effective treatment for patients with fecal incontinence.

Although patients might benefit from selective and directed surgery, trials of erythromycin and octreotide have been shown to be of benefit in the relief of nausea and abdominal pain in some patients. The etiology of CIP is still being explored.

Fecal Incontinence

Fecal incontinence may be idiopathic but is commonly due to trauma in females (episiotomy, multiple pregnancies, or large-birth-weight babies) or to diabetic impairment of the nervous system. Normal continence depends on structural integrity and function of nerves and muscles, normal rectal compliance, normal sensation, and psychologic motivation. Any disruption of these normal mechanisms may result in the impaired ability to maintain continence. Evaluation consists of thorough history (with careful attention to the gynecologic history in female patients) and physical examination, followed by manometric evaluation to assess internal and external anal sphincter tone and rectal sensation. Transcutaneous electromyography may be used to measure external sphincter function, and anal endosonography may show muscle structure. Pudendal nerve conduction studies are used to assess the integrity of nerve function or the presence of a pudendal neuropathy that might predict poor surgical prognosis.

Biofeedback training may be an important intervention in appropriate candidates, with good outcome seen to range from 50%–92%. Why biofeedback training works is unclear, but it is believed to lead to improvement in both motor and sensory functions of the anorectum. Diet and bulking of stools may be helpful. Surgery is sometimes indicated, especially in cases of rectal prolapse. Newer interventions with perianal injection of fat, collagen, or synthetic gel and implantation of an artificial sphincter are in study.

CASE STUDY: *RESOLUTION*

The patient's films from previous radiographic and endoscopic evaluations were ordered for review, and some additional studies were ordered. The patient was started on a high-fiber, low-fat diet and instructed that a faster gastrocolonic reflex could be expected with ingestion of a fatty, fast-food meal. On the patient's return, she was again reassured that review of her good-quality radiographs had revealed no missed lesions. On diagnosis of a modest degree of lactose intolerance, dietary counseling was given. The patient began a food-and-incident diary, which further assisted in the management of her symptoms.

With the addition of an antispasm drug for intermittent use, the patient learned to live with her IBS.

REVIEW QUESTIONS

Directions: For each of the following questions, choose the one best answer.

1 Fecal incontinence may be idiopathic in etiology but may also be seen in association with

   A hypertension.
   B diabetes.
   C peptic ulcer disease.
   D hypothyroidism.

2 A 32-year-old woman comes to the physician's office with complaints of early satiety. The physician is concerned about gastric emptying delay. Which of the following tests would be most helpful in this situation?

   A Barium swallow
   B Upper GI endoscopy
   C Scintigraphy
   D Drug challenge with an anticholinergic agent

3 Which of the following factors may be part of the Rome II criteria for IBS?

   A A negative endoscopy
   B A negative breath test for lactose intolerance
   C Abdominal pain associated with a change in stool frequency
   D Abdominal pain associated with a change in stool color

4 Which of the following statements *best* describes functional and organic diseases of the GI tract?

   A Functional diseases are always readily diagnosed and treated.
   B Organic disease is often cryptic and hard to diagnose.
   C Organic disease is real; functional disease is not.
   D Functional disease is psychosomatic.
   E Functional disease lacks biochemical and histologic markers.

5 Which of the following is a physiologic finding of IBS as compared to normal controls?

   A Higher rectosigmoid distention threshold for pain
   B Longer migrating motor complex (MMC) periodicity
   C Higher rectal compliance to balloon distention
   D Ileal propulsive waves

6 Which of the statements concerning CIP is correct?

A It requires surgical intervention.
B It is easily differentiated from mechanical obstruction.
C It is clearly related to a bacterial infection.
D It may be associated with antibodies against cell nucleus antigen (anti-PCNA) in scleroderma.

References

Camilleri M, Prather CM: The irritable bowel syndrome: mechanisms and a practical approach to management. *Ann Intern Med* 116:1001–1008, 1992.

Christenson J: Pathophysiology of the irritable bowel syndrome. *Lancet* 340:1444–1447, 1992.

David D, Mertz H, Fefer L, et al: Sleep and duodenal motor activity in patients with severe non-ulcer dyspepsia. *Gut* 35:916–925, 1994.

Drossman DA: The functional gastrointestinal disorders and the Rome II process. *Gut* 145(Suppl 2):II1–II5, 1999.

Drossman DA, Camilleri M, Mayer EA, et al: AGA technical review on irritable bowel syndrome. *Gastroenterology* 123:2108–2131, 2002.

Drossman DA, Thompson WG: The irritable bowel syndrome: review and a graduated multicomponent treatment approach. *Ann Intern Med* 116:1009–1016, 1992.

Fine KD, Schiller LR: AGA technical review on the evaluation and management of chronic diarrhea. *Gastroenterology* 116:1464–1486, 1999.

Horowitz M, Fraser RJL: Gastroparesis: diagnosis and management. *Scand J Gastroenterol Suppl* 213:7–16, 1995.

Lind CD: Motility disorders in the irritable bowel syndrome. *Gastroenterol Clin North Am* 20:279–295, 1991.

McIntyre PB, Pemberton JH: Pathophysiology of colonic motility disorders. *Surg Clin North Am* 73:1225–1243, 1993.

Olden KW: Irritable bowel syndrome: an overview of diagnosis and pharmacologic treatment. *Cleve Clin J Med* 70:S3–S7, 2003.

Spiller RC: Postinfectious irritable bowel syndrome. *Gastroenterology* 124:1662–1671, 2003.

Stanghellini V, Ghidini C, Maccarini MR, et al: Fasting and postprandial gastrointestinal motility in ulcer and non-ulcer dyspepsia. *Gut* 33:184–190, 1992.

Thompson WG, Longstreth GF, Drossman DA, et al: Functional bowel disorders and functional abdominal pain. *Gut* 45(Suppl 2):II43–II47, 1999.

Turegano-Fuentes F, Munoz-Jimenez F, Del Valle-Hernandez E, et al: Early resolution of Ogilvie's syndrome with intravenous neostigmine: a simple, effective treatment. *Dis Colon Rectum* 40(11):1353–1357, 1997.

Verne GN, Sninsky CA: Chronic intestinal pseudo-obstruction. *Dig Dis Sci* 13:163–181, 1995.

15

The Mucosal Immune System

■ LEARNING OBJECTIVES ■

At the completion of this chapter, the reader should be able to:
- Distinguish immunologic from nonimmunologic mucosal defenses.
- Describe the basic components of the immune system and how they participate in mucosal immunity.
- Classify mucosal lymphoid tissue.
- Detail the effects of inflammation on the GI tract and inflammation results in GI disease.
- Describe the concept of oral tolerance.
- Explain the basis for food allergies.

The GALT possesses lymphoid cells (B and T lymphocytes) and myeloid cells (macrophages, neutrophils, eosinophils, and mast cells) and represents one of the largest immunologic compartments of the body.

A **nonspecific response** is an immediate reaction to all foreign material. A **specific response** is a delayed reaction that is possible only after previous antigen exposure.

CASE STUDY: *INTRODUCTION*

The patient is a 50-year-old woman who was well until 1 year prior to her presentation at the clinic. She presented with complaints of persistent diarrhea, which she described as containing droplets of fat, foul smelling, and often floating. She was also bothered by frequent gas and bloating, and although she denied abdominal pain, she had experienced a 20-lb weight loss over the last year. The patient noted that her symptoms became worse when she ate bread or baked goods and that she was no longer able to tolerate milk.

Introduction

The function of the body's immune system is to differentiate its own material, or "self," from foreign material, or "nonself," and protect the body from harmful foreign material. This is accomplished in part by the process of foreign antigen recognition performed by the immune cells. Although the immune cells in the blood are protected from exposure to most foreign antigens by the thick epithelial layers of the skin, the mucosal immune system is directly exposed to thousands of foreign antigens that pass through the gut in the form of food and enteric flora. The challenge for the mucosal immune system is thus made even greater by the sheer number and diversity of foreign antigens to which it is exposed. It must not only recognize self, it must also recognize nonself-nonharmful antigens and develop a tolerance to these antigens. To deal with this massive antigen exposure, the gut possesses an abundance of both lymphoid and myeloid cells, which are collectively known as the gut-associated lymphoid tissue (GALT). The mucosal immune system of the GI tract is one of the largest immunologic compartments in the body.

Basis of Immunity

The immune system possesses two types of reactions to foreign material: The first is a nonspecific, immediate response that rapidly reacts to all foreign material, and the second is a specific acquired response that manifests a delayed reaction only to those antigens to which the system has been previously exposed.

NONSPECIFIC MUCOSAL DEFENSE SYSTEM

The nonspecific mucosal defense system of the GI tract is comprised of both immunologic and nonimmunologic barriers. The nonimmunologic barriers to foreign material include chemical factors, such as gastric acid, digestive enzymes, lysozymes, bile, and mucus. Mechanical barriers, such as gut peristalsis, tight junctions of the intestinal epithelial cells, and indigenous gut flora, also provide a nonimmunologic mucosal defense. Nonspecific immunologic reactions to foreign material are mediated by phagocytes, the complement system, and natural killer cells, which are preformed and provide an immediate response to antigen exposure. Cytokines also provide a nonspecific immunologic response, but it is a delayed response because they are formed by macrophages after antigen exposure.

SPECIFIC MUCOSAL IMMUNITY

Specific mucosal immunity is an acquired response, requiring previous exposure to the antigen. The initial response is delayed, yet specific for each antigen. After the initial response, a clonal expansion of the antigen-specific lymphocytes occurs, which then creates an immunologic memory of that antigen. Subsequent exposure to the same antigen activates this memory, resulting in a more rapid and amplified immunologic response. Mast cells are capable of creating an immediate, specific immune response because previous antigen exposure results in the formation of immunoglobulin E (IgE), which remains in the bloodstream and causes immediate degranulation of mast cells when activated.

Acquired immunity is composed of both humoral responses, which are carried out by antibodies, and cellular responses, which are carried out by lymphocytes. The humoral response is enacted by B lymphocytes, which produce antibodies that provide extracellular protection from foreign antigens. The cellular response is enacted by T lymphocytes and macrophages, which produce cytokines that signal other cells to engage in the immune response. Both B and T lymphocytes possess cell surface receptors that are specific for certain epitopes found on foreign antigens. During maturation of B and T cells, those cells with receptors that react to self are deleted, and those with receptors that react to foreign antigens are promoted, thereby producing a lymphocyte population that is self-tolerant. If an inappropriate recognition of and response to self were to occur, autoimmunity would result.

Components of the Immune System

T LYMPHOCYTES

T lymphocytes coordinate the immune defense via their regulatory action on other cell populations. They arise from pluripotent stem cells in the bone marrow and migrate to the thymus, where they mature and acquire a tolerance to self. These self-tolerant T cells then populate the primary lymphoid organs—the spleen, lymph nodes, and tonsils. They also populate the secondary lymphoid organs—the intestine, lung, and skin. For T cells to recognize an antigen fragment, the fragment must be presented on an antigen-presenting cell in conjunction with components of the major histocompatibility complex (MHC).

T cells are separated into functional subtypes based on their expression of molecules known as cluster of differentiation (CD) antigens. T cells can be broadly divided into two categories: those that express the CD4 molecule (T helper cells) and those that express the

T-cell activation requires:
1. The adherence of a T cell to the antigen-presenting cell.
2. An antigen-specific signal and antigen-independent signal from cell surface molecules.

CD8 molecule (T suppressor cells). CD4 cells help coordinate immune responses and recognize antigens in the context of class II MHC molecules. CD8 cells play a role in the suppression of the immune response and recognize antigens in the context of class I MHC molecules.

T cell activation requires two events: (1) adherence of the T cell to the antigen-presenting cell and (2) reception of two intracellular signals from cell-surface molecules, one of which is antigen-dependent and the other antigen-independent. If the second intracellular signal is not received, either tolerance to the antigen or cell death occurs. The requirement of receiving two signals is likely inherent in antigen-specific interactions and plays an important role in avoiding autoimmunity.

B LYMPHOCYTES

B lymphocytes originate from hematopoietic stem cells in the bone marrow and fetal liver. Pre–B cells lack surface immunoglobulins. They therefore develop independently from antigen exposure because they are unable to recognize antigen. Further maturation of these cells in the bone marrow leads to the development of B cells that have surface immunoglobulins M and D (IgM and IgD), are antigen-responsive, and express the same variable (V) region or idiotype. The binding of surface membrane IgM with antigen activates IgM cell surface transport and signal transduction.

B cell subsets may also be identified by the presence of various markers. For example, CD5 (a T cell marker) is expressed on 5%–10% of B cells. These CD5 B cells can mature outside of the bone marrow within the peritoneal cavity. In this immunoprotected environment, the cells are unlikely to be exposed to antigens and therefore are not stimulated to produce antibodies. Furthermore, these cells are prone to replication in autoimmune disease states, and this suggests that under certain circumstances they may be activated to produce autoantibodies.

Stimulation of mature B cells by antigens outside the bone marrow results in a clonal expansion of these cells. A secreted form of the membrane-bound IgM is produced, which possesses the same V region and antigen specificity as the membrane-bound IgM. Some of these clonally expanded cells differentiate into memory cells. Antigen-specific T cells release cytokines to signal these B cells, causing them to convert to IgG isotypes in the periphery and IgA isotypes in the GALT, where they then differentiate into plasma cells. The GALT-associated plasma cells then secrete very high levels of immunoglobulin A (IgA).

IMMUNOGLOBULINS

Each B cell expresses an immunoglobulin molecule on its surface, and each immunoglobulin molecule contains a hypervariable region that determines its antigenic specificity, or idiotype. When expressed on the B cell surface, these immunoglobulins function as receptors, similar to those present on T cells. When a surface immunoglobulin binds its specific antigen, it initiates a series of events within the B cell that

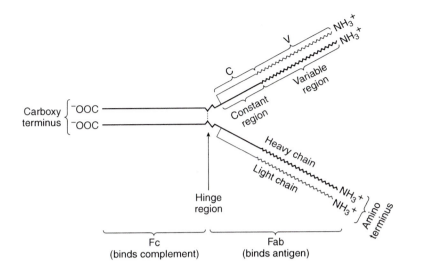

Fig. 15-1. Structure of Immunoglobulins

A simplified model for an IgG human antibody molecule, showing the four-chain basic structure. The thick black lines represent the heavy chains, and the thin black lines represent light chains. The wavy lines represent the variable region, which determines antigen specificity. Solid lines represent the constant region, which determines the subclass (IgG, IgA, IgE, IgD, IgM) of the antibody. *Source:* Modified from Goodman in Stites et al. 1987, p. 28.

causes clonal proliferation and plasma cell production. The plasma cells then secrete immunoglobulins that are specific for the initial antigen bound to the surface immunoglobulin.

The immunoglobulins that are secreted are known as *antibodies* (Figure 15-1). They are composed of two identical light chains, linked by disulfide bridges to two identical heavy chains. There are five immunoglobulin isotypes: IgG, IgM, IgA, IgE, and IgD. IgA contains two subtypes (IgA1, IgA2) and IgG contains four subtypes (IgG1–4). The Fc portion of the isotype is responsible for complement fixation, whereas antigen specificity is determined by the amino terminus of the heavy and light chains. The most polymorphic region of the amino terminus is the V region, which is further divided into three hypervariable regions known as complementary determining regions (CDR1–3). The structure of this region is complementary to that of the bound antigen and thus is very important for antigen binding. After recombination has taken place, the diversity of immunoglobulins is increased by somatic mutation of the gene sequence, which encodes the V region. This ability of the V region to mutate accounts for the "affinity maturation," which increases the ability of an immunoglobulin to bind a specific antigen the second time it is encountered.

CYTOKINES

Cytokines are protein hormones, which are secreted by both immune and nonimmune cell types. They play an important role in nonspecific

Secreted immunoglobulins are known as antibodies. They contain two identical light chains and two identical heavy chains.

Purpose of the Mucosal Immune System
1. It provides a barrier to harmful toxins, antigens, and infections.
2. It decreases the systemic immune response to benign antigens, such as food and normal gut flora.

immunity, regulation of lymphocyte function, regulation of leukocyte growth, and activation of inflammatory cells. Most cells produce several cytokines, and although significant redundancy exists within the system, a pattern may be found between the different cytokines and the cells that produce them. Helper T cells coordinate immune responses via the cytokines and the cells they produce. Helper T cells can be divided into two types: TH1 cells and TH2 cells. TH1 cells predominantly secrete interleukin-2 (IL-2) and interferon-γ (IFN-γ), which are important in early B and T cell development, as well as in cellular immunity. TH2 cells secrete IL-2, IL-4, IL-5, IL-6, and IL-10; all are cytokines that are important in humoral immunity. The effects of cytokines depend on the receptors present on the cells targeted by the cytokines. The presence of receptors is determined by the cell's level of maturation and previous cytokine exposure.

Mucosal Immune System

The mucosal immune system is responsible not only for providing a barrier to harmful intraluminal toxins, antigens, and infections but also for decreasing systemic immune responsiveness to common environmental antigens, such as food and normal gut flora. It is functionally divided into an afferent (information intake) and efferent (information output) limb (Figure 15-2). The afferent limb, composed

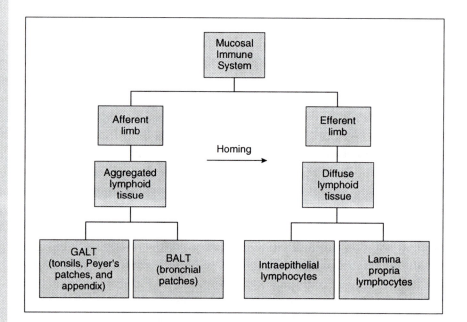

Fig. 15-2. Functional and Anatomic Organization of the Immune System

The mucosal immune system is organized into distinct functional limbs with corresponding anatomic parts. The afferent limb (located in the aggregate lymphoid tissue) gathers information on antigens, and the efferent limb (located in the diffuse lymphoid tissue) gives a response that is specific for certain antigens.

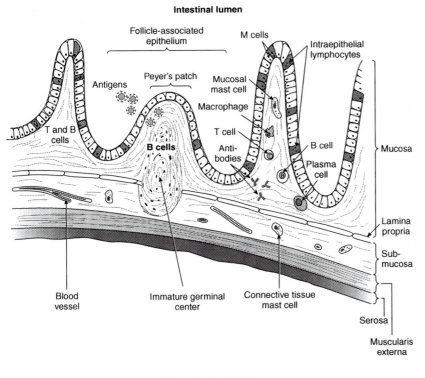

Intestinal lumen

Follicle-associated
epithelium

M cells

Antigens

Peyer's patch

Intraepithelial
lymphocytes

Mucosal
mast cell

Macrophage

T and B
cells

B cells

T cell

Anti-
bodies

B cell

Plasma
cell

Mucosa

Lamina
propria

Sub-
mucosa

Blood
vessel

Immature germinal
center

Connective tissue
mast cell

Serosa

Muscularis
externa

Fig. 15-3. GALT

The GALT consists of the cells of the mucosal immune system, which are
located between the intestinal lumen and the serosa of the intestine

of the aggregated lymphoid tissue, is responsible for sampling intraluminal antigens. The efferent limb is made up of the diffuse lymphoid
tissue, that is, mature lymphocytes, which have developed a memory
for specific intraluminal antigens and can migrate to various mucosal
sites where they provide immunity by reacting to these antigens.

AGGREGATE LYMPHOID TISSUE

The aggregate lymphoid tissue is the site where intraluminal antigens
first come into contact with the mucosal immune system. It is composed of lymphoid follicles known as Peyer's patches and the overlying follicle-associated epithelium (Figure 15-3). Peyer's patches are
present in the lamina propria of the small intestine and are more numerous in the ileum than the jejunum (Figure 15-4). They contain
an immature germinal center and regulatory T cells, as well as B cells
expressing IgM, IgG, IgA, and IgE. The ratio of T cells to B cells is
about 70:30. A T cell–dependent region is adjacent to the follicle.

The follicle-associated epithelium that overlies the Peyer's
patches contains microfold (M) cells. These M cells selectively
pinocytize and phagocytize intraluminal particles in the gut and
transport these antigens to the Peyer's patches. While en route, the
antigens come into contact with lymphocytes and macrophages,
where they are processed for antigen presentation to lymphocytes in
the Peyer's patches. Antigen presentation to naive lymphocytes in the

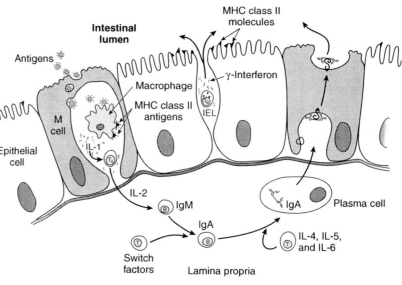

Fig. 15-4. Peyer's Patch

The Peyer's patch contains an immature germinal center, T cells, and B cells, which express IgM, IgG, IgA, and IgE. M cells transport intraluminal antigens to the Peyer's batch, where they are processed for presentation to lymphocytes, thereby initiating the process of lymphocyte differentiation.

Peyer's patches begins the process of differentiation of lymphocytes into mature effector cells. Infectious agents, such as HIV, reoviruses, cholera, and microbacteria, are known to be transported by M cells to the Peyer's patches. Larger molecules, such as horseradish peroxidase, ferritin, and various lectins, are also transported by M cells.

Absorptive intestinal epithelial cells can also function as antigen-presenting cells because they express MHC class II molecules. Although the epithelial cells of the small bowel consistently express MHC class II antigens, colonic epithelium may only express measurable levels of MHC class II molecules in the setting of inflammation. Although there is in vitro evidence that intestinal epithelial cells express class II MHC molecules and can present antigens, they preferentially engage and stimulate CD8+ cells and suppressor activity. This may contribute to the usual role of suppression of reactivity to antigens played by the small intestine.

After the M cells present selected antigens to the B cells in the Peyer's patches, the next step in the mucosal immune response occurs: Regulatory T cells within the Peyer's patches promote B lymphocytes to switch their immunoglobulin isotype from IgM to IgA. Activation by these "switch T cells," in addition to the antigen-presenting events, results in B cells that can be terminally induced to differentiate into IgA-secreting cells. About 85% of B cells are primarily focused on IgA synthesis, 5% on IgG synthesis, and 10% on IgM and IgE synthesis. T cells present in the aggregated lymphoid tissue are naive cells that develop into memory cells when antigen is presented to them.

DIFFUSE LYMPHOID TISSUE

The diffuse lymphoid tissue constitutes the efferent limb of the mucosal immune system. It is made up of a subcompartment of T lymphocytes called intraepithelial lymphocytes, which are B and T cells found diffusely throughout the lamina propria and plasma cells. Approximately 40% of the lymphocytes are B cells derived from precursors in the Peyer's patches. Resting B cells are activated by IL-4 and IL-5 to divide and grow. IL-6 is essential for the terminal differentiation of IgA plasma cells and stimulates secretion of large amounts of IgA.

Around 60% of the lymphocytes in the lamina propria are T cells, with CD4+ (helper) and CD8+ (killer) T cells present in a 2:1 ratio. Representing the majority of T cells present, the CD4+ and CD8+ T cells provide memory cells that help in IgA production when exposed to antigen, as well as cells that secrete cytolytic effectors aiding in lysis of virally infected target cells. Although cytotoxic effectors are present, the diffuse lymphoid tissue is generally a poor mediator of cell-mediated cytotoxicity.

IgE receptor-bearing mast cells are also present in the diffuse lymphoid tissue and become activated in immediate hypersensitivity reactions. Nerves that are closely positioned to mast cells can release neuropeptides, such as vasoactive intestinal peptide (VIP), substance P, and somatostatin, thereby triggering histamine release. Mast cell products are able to kill parasites directly, and they indirectly increase host response to these infections by inducing vascular permeability, thereby allowing more rapid antibody and complement-mediated reactions.

Activated B and T lymphocytes leave the intestinal tract and migrate into afferent lymphatics, which drain into the mesenteric lymph nodes. From there, they enter the efferent lymphatics of the mesenteric lymph nodes, pass into the thoracic duct, and then pass into the peripheral blood. Mature B and T lymphocytes then "home in" on various mucosal sites, including the breast, lung, eye, and bronchioles, as well as the GI mucosa. Homing occurs because there is a strong affinity between specific homing antigens on the lymphocytes and specific receptors on the surface of the endothelial cells at destination mucosal sites. These receptors are known as vascular addressins, and they are present on vessels known as high endothelial venules.

In chronic inflammatory states, the number of high endothelial venules is increased, especially in areas that are close to developing granulomas. Cytokines, such as IL-1, IFN-γ, and tumor necrosis factor (TNF), are also released in such states, and they increase lymphoblast adherence to endothelial cells by enhancing the expression of endothelial adhesion molecules. Once B lymphocytes reach these mucosal sites, they mature into IgA-secreting plasma cells and provide protective immunity by secreting antigen-specific antibodies. Thus, bacteria in a mother's GI tract induce an immune response that can be passively transferred through the secretory IgA in breast milk to a

Common Mucosal Immune System
This is a term used to describe the body's ability to develop immunity to an antigen encountered at one mucosal surface and then transfer this immunity to other mucosal surfaces.

IgA secretion is the major component of immunity for the intestinal tract. Over 70% of the immunoglobulin-producing cells in the body are found in the intestine.

nursing child, who will then gain immunity to these same organisms. The ability to develop a specific immune response to an antigen initially encountered at one mucosal surface (such as the GI tract) and then transfer this immunity to another mucosal surface (such as the respiratory tract), and vice versa, is known as the common mucosal immune system.

IMMUNOGLOBULIN SECRETION

Once IgA is secreted by mucosal immunocytes in the lamina propria, it is selectively transported across the mucosal epithelium to function in the external secretions. Immunoglobulin secretion is a major component of protective immunity for the intestinal tract, and the intestine contains over 70% of the immunoglobulin-producing cells in the body. Although the lamina propria B cells also produce IgG and IgM antibodies, the predominant antibody secreted is IgA.

Secretory IgA is the product of plasma cell–derived IgA and mucosal epithelial cells (Figure 15-5). Plasma cells produce IgA in either a monomeric or polymeric structure. IgA monomers are joined by a "J" chain. The J chain participates in the transport of polymeric IgA across intestinal epithelial cells, where it binds to the specific transport receptor, termed the secretory component (SC), of the epithelial cell. The IgA–SC complex is then endocytosed and transported in

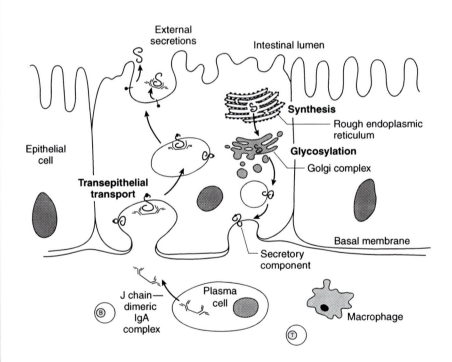

Fig. 15-5. Formation of Secretory IgA

SC is synthesized in the rough endoplasmic reticulum and ultimately fuses with the basal membrane to form a vesicle. The J chain–dimeric IgA complex then fuses with the SC vesicle, and the entire complex is transported across the epithelial cell, then secreted into the intestinal lumen.

endoplasmic vesicles to the apical, luminal membrane where the SC is partially cleaved, releasing the IgA with a portion of the bound secretory piece into the lumen. SC may prevent degradation of the secretory IgA molecule when it is secreted into an environment containing proteolytic enzymes, bacteria, and other substances that can cause degradation. The main action of secretory IgA is to provide protection against bacteria, viruses, and luminal antigens by inhibiting their adherence to epithelial cells and preventing effective colonization and proliferation.

INTRAEPITHELIAL LYMPHOCYTES

In addition to the lymphocytes found in the lamina propria, there is another specific population of lymphocytes that resides between the epithelial cells along the basolateral surfaces. They are predominantly (> 90%) T lymphocytes, and most (> 80%) express CD8 receptors characteristics of the suppressor-cytotoxic T cell subpopulation. They recognize only a small number of antigens and function biologically as cytotoxic effectors. These cells are regionally specific and are thought to play an important role in immunosurveillance against abnormal epithelial cells. They represent a first line of defense against adverse epithelial changes, and their numbers are markedly increased in such diseases as gluten-sensitive enteropathy, intestinal graft-versus-host disease (GVHD), AIDS, and protozoal infections such as Cryptosporidium and Isospora. Although immediate protection against deleterious events is provided by resident effector cells, this response may be boosted by specific cytotoxic T cell effectors, which are derived from precursors in the Peyer's patches and migrate to the epithelial cells.

Inflammation in the GI Tract

Inflammation in the GI tract is similar to that in other organ systems. In acute inflammation, there is an influx of granulocytes. These cells produce several inflammatory mediators, which directly damage surrounding tissue and release chemotactic peptides, which in turn recruit more inflammatory cells to the area. An influx of lymphocytes, mast cells, eosinophils, and macrophages is then seen as chronic inflammation begins. These cells are integral in protecting the intestine from potentially harmful bacteria, viruses, and other luminal agents. Although a normal inflammatory reaction to pathogens is essential for host survival, ongoing chronic inflammation can eventually be destructive to the intestine. In direct response to the acute effects of inflammation, the healing mechanisms that repair the damaged tissue are activated. This enhanced stimulation of collagen generation can lead to stricture formation and eventually intestinal obstruction. GI diseases that have a major component of chronic inflammation include reflux esophagitis, gastritis, pancreatitis, diverticulitis, celiac disease, ulcerative colitis, Crohn's disease, and multiple infectious processes.

Ongoing inflammation in the intestine can cause scarring with stricture formation and eventual obstruction.

Notes

Oral tolerance is defined as systemic hyporesponsiveness to orally ingested antigens.

Many causes of intestinal damage, such as ischemia, radiation, inflammatory bowel disease, and bacterial infections, produce a similar appearance in the bowel. The mucosa becomes inflamed and edematous, a hallmark of acute intestinal inflammation, suggesting that this is a final common pathway for the effects of many diseases. Some of the soluble mediators of inflammation, such as histamine and prostaglandin E_2 (PGE_2), are vasodilators and account for the hyperemia and erythema. Leukotriene B4, platelet-activating factor (PAF), bradykinin, and PGE_2 enhance vascular permeability, causing mucosal edema.

These cytokines and mediators of inflammation also induce the expression of adhesion molecules on the surfaces of circulating leukocytes and vascular endothelial cells in the gut. This facilitates the movement of leukocytes from the circulation into the inflamed intestine. The bonds between the leukocytes and the endothelial cells are formed by adhesion molecules called selectins. The bonds are relatively weak, and they act to slow down the leukocytes and cause them to roll along the endothelial surface. Later, stronger bonds form between the integrins on the leukocytes and the receptors expressed on the endothelial cells. These bonds immobilize the leukocytes and allow them to bind tightly to the endothelium. After adhering to the endothelial cells, the leukocytes migrate between the endothelial cells and enter the inflamed mucosa. The mix of cytokines then determines further proliferation and differentiation of inflammatory cells, activating processes ranging from phagocytosis of bacteria to wound healing.

Oral Tolerance

Although the majority of immunologic cells are directed against foreign antigens, a small subpopulation of autoreactive T cell and B cell clones is maintained within the body's immune system. This population is suppressed by a process of negative selection as the B cells mature in the bone marrow and the T cells mature in the thymus. It is thought that these autoreactive cells are necessary for the recognition of microbial peptides that mimic the peptides of normal self-antigens to which a person may be exposed. The constant need for the GI tract to mount an immune response against various bacteria, viruses, and other antigens raises the possibility that in forming antibodies to those foreign antigens that closely resemble self-antigens, an activation of these self-reactive T and B cells may occur. In a genetically predisposed host, this may lead to the development of autoimmune disease.

To prevent the continued activation of self-reactive T cells, the GI immune system must develop a tolerance to the many dietary antigens found in the GI tract. Systemic hyporesponsiveness to orally ingested antigens is known as oral tolerance, and it occurs when oral ingestion of an antigen leads to systemic antigen-specific unresponsiveness, specifically a lack of B cell or T cell responsiveness. This state of anergy holds only for that specific antigen and depends on the type of antigen, the amount, and the frequency of exposure to the antigen. Systemic immune tolerance may be accompanied by mucosal immune tolerance or a concurrent activation of mucosal immunity, as plasma cells locally secrete IgA. Oral tolerance allows the GI tract to be exposed to a variety of antigens, mount an appropriate response to infectious organisms, and simultaneously render the host unresponsive to subsequent challenge by these antigens. This prevents numerous bacterial and viral antigens, as well as food components, from initiating immunologic reactions that could result in uncontrollable food-induced allergic reactions.

Although the mechanisms that result in oral tolerance are not well understood, two theories have been developed: T cell suppression and clonal anergy. Low doses of antigen presentation to the intestine appears to induce CD8+ suppressor T cells and CD4+ helper T cells in the Peyer's patches and mesenteric lymph nodes. These cells migrate to a variety of tissues where they inhibit the production of antigen-specific effector cells. When antigen-specific TH1 cells are not activated, they undergo clonal anergy or apoptosis.

Oral tolerance has been used to treat several autoimmune diseases. In murine models, the ingestion of myelin basic protein, collagen type II, retinal autoantigen, porcine insulin, and class II MHC peptides can suppress allergic encephalitis, collagen-induced arthritis, allergic uveitis, and organ transplant rejection, respectively.

Food Allergy

In discussing food allergies, or hypersensitivity, it is important to distinguish this state from food intolerance. A true food allergy is a reaction that is mediated by the immune system. Food intolerance may closely resemble an acute allergic reaction, but it is not mediated by the immune system. True food allergies are actually relatively uncommon. Although community surveys indicate that 20%–40% of persons believe they have had an allergic reaction to a specific food, when tested objectively, these reactions cannot be reproduced. The true prevalence of food allergy in children is thought to be between 0.3% and 7.5%, and it declines with age.

Hypersensitivity to food represents a breakdown in oral tolerance. Although penetration of dietary antigens through the mucosal barrier under normal circumstances results at most in a merely local secretory IgA antibody response, a systemic response is seen with food allergy. IgE-mediated and delayed-type hypersensitivity responses are the immune responses most easily suppressed by orally ingesting proteins, and thus, these reactions mediate food allergy.

Most food allergies are caused by a fairly small number of foods: milk, eggs, nuts, fish, shellfish, soybeans, and wheat (gluten). Several of the specific allergens have been isolated for these foods. They are generally of low molecular weight (10–70 kDa) and have the appropriate size for bridging IgE on the surface of mast cells.

Food Hypersensitivity Reactions
1. Immediate hypersensitivity reactions (type I) are mediated by IgE.
2. Delayed hypersensitivity reactions (type II) are mediated by cellular activity or immune complexes.

CASE STUDY: *CONTINUED*

On physical examination, the patient appeared thin but otherwise well. Skin examination was notable for patchy areas of dryness and erythema. HEENT (head, ears, eyes, nose, throat) examination was unremarkable, as was the chest and cardiovascular examinations. The abdomen was soft and nontender with normoactive bowel sounds. No hepatosplenomegaly was present. There was no perianal disease, and rectal examination showed watery, heme-negative stool. Stool cultures were all negative; but 24-hour fecal fat was elevated at 12 g. Hemoglobin was low at 8.2 mg/dl with a decreased hematocrit of 25.6%. The white blood cell (WBC) count was 8.0 cells per microliter with a differential of 50% polys and no bands. Albumin was 3.0 mg/dl.

PATHOGENESIS

There are two major categories of food hypersensitivity reaction: immediate, also known as type I, which is an IgE-mediated reaction; and delayed, or type II, which is a late-phase IgE immune complex or cell-mediated reaction. Most food reactions are immediate, with the exception of gluten-sensitive enteropathy, which is a delayed hypersensitivity reaction.

Immediate Hypersensitivity Reactions

Mast cells play a key role in immediate hypersensitivity reactions (type I). They are abundant in the gut, and evidence suggests that mucosal mast cells are functionally distinct from mast cells in nonmucosal tissue. Unlike those in nonmucosal tissue, mucosal mast cells are unresponsive to certain antiallergenic medications. Food-specific IgE antibodies are present on the surface of these mast cells; when cross-linked by an allergen, they trigger degranulation of the mast cell. This central role of mast cell degranulation in the pathogenesis of food allergy is supported by the fact that plasma levels of histamine rise significantly in patients with cutaneous, GI, and respiratory symptoms elicited by a food challenge. An increase in IgE-bearing cells in the intestine of patients with cow's milk allergy has also been reported, providing further evidence for the role of mast cells in immediate hypersensitivity reactions.

Delayed Hypersensitivity Reactions

Gluten-sensitive enteropathy is an example of a delayed hypersensitivity reaction (type II) to a dietary antigen (see also Chapter 12). The active component in gluten is gliadin, which is found in wheat, barley, rye, and oats. In genetically predisposed individuals, exposure to the gliadin antigen results in an ongoing destructive mucosal immunologic reaction. Between 70% and 85% of patients with gluten-sensitive enteropathy bear human leukocyte antigens (HLA) HLA-B8 and HLA-DR3, and 90% of patients have HLA-DQw2.

In reacting to a gluten challenge, the lamina propria becomes infiltrated mainly with lymphocytes, the majority of which are B cells and IgA-containing plasma cells. The number of intraepithelial lymphocytes is also dramatically increased within hours of gluten ingestion, representing an early event in the reaction to gliadin. Although the event that initiates the immune response seen in gluten-sensitive enteropathy is unknown, recent studies have focused more on the intraepithelial lymphocyte. The concentration of intraepithelial lymphocytes is increased in a dose-dependent fashion, according to the degree of the gluten challenge. Specifically, an increase in lymphocytes bearing gamma or delta T cell receptors is seen, and these cells are known to possess a marked cytotoxic potential.

CASE STUDY: *CONTINUED*

An upper endoscopy was done with advancement to the second portion of the duodenum, where biopsies were obtained. The upper endoscopy was essentially normal with no evidence of ulceration or inflammation. Review of the biopsies revealed changes consistent with gluten-sensitive enteropathy. Serum IgG and IgA antibodies to gliadin were positive, as was the transglutaminase antibody. A colonoscopy was also done and found to be normal, with no evidence of mucosal disease or obstruction.

PATHOLOGY

Administration of food antigens directly to the gastric mucosa of allergic individuals results in erythema, edema, and even petechial hemorrhages, which can be seen on endoscopic evaluation. In gluten-sensitive enteropathy, mucosal changes are most marked in the duodenum and jejunum but can be seen throughout the entire small intestine, depending on the severity of disease. Villus atrophy and crypt hyperplasia result in a decrease in the villus–crypt ratio and are responsible for the flattened appearance of the mucosa. The epithelial cells lose their usual columnar morphology and become cuboidal in appearance. The mucosa becomes infiltrated with intraepithelial lymphocytes, plasma cells, and eosinophils, whereas the submucosa and muscularis are relatively spared (Figure 15-6).

CLINICAL MANIFESTATIONS

Symptoms of food allergy may occur within minutes of ingestion or may not become evident for several hours. Systemic anaphylaxis is the most serious manifestation and in rare cases can be fatal. Usually, the clinical manifestations are less severe. Skin, respiratory tract, and gut are the organs primarily affected, resulting in eczema, urticaria,

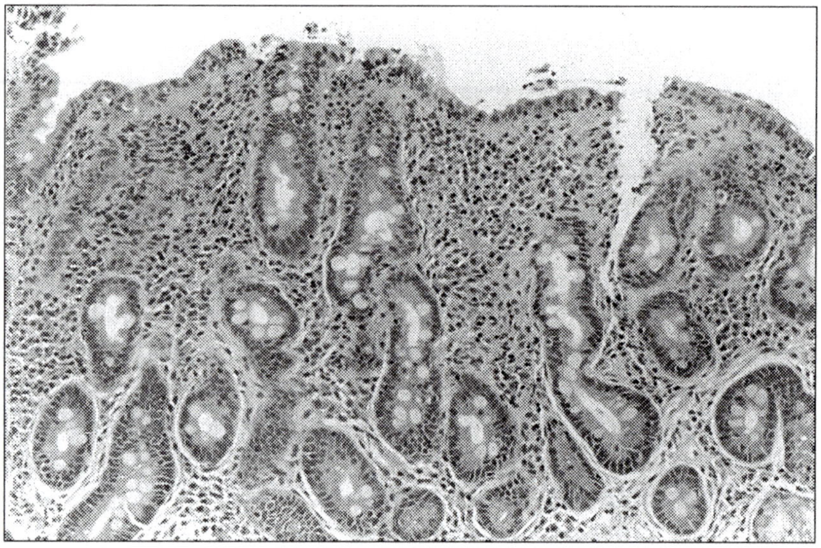

Fig. 15-6. The Pathology of Celiac Disease

The mucosal surface is flat, indicating total villus atrophy. The lamina propria contains a moderately intense chronic inflammatory infiltrate, which is more dense in the superficial half of the mucosa (H&E, 250×).

rhinitis, asthma, and diarrhea. In gluten-sensitive enteropathy, malabsorption can cause weight loss and diarrhea consisting of fatty stools.

EVALUATION

The degree to which the diagnosis of food allergy is pursued depends on the patient's age and ability to comply with testing, the nutritional importance of the suspected food, and the severity of the symptoms. For example, patients with only episodic symptoms triggered by uncommon foods can be instructed to avoid those foods, whereas patients with suspected allergy to several major food groups require a complete evaluation.

Confirmation that an adverse reaction to a specific food is immunologically mediated involves the demonstration of IgE antibodies that have specificity for the implicated food allergen. Food-specific mast cell–bound IgE antibodies can be detected easily using direct skin testing. The prick technique compares the reaction to the suspected food extract with the reaction to a control; production of a wheal that is more than 3 mm larger than the control is a positive test. A positive test confirms the presence of sensitizing antibodies, which can then be confirmed to represent a true food allergy by a positive food challenge. Skin testing should not be used if the clinical history suggests a possible anaphylactic reaction to the suspected food. Commercially available radioallergosorbent tests (RASTs) and enzyme-linked immunosorbent assays (ELISAs) are in vitro assays for the presence of serum IgE antibodies to several of the known food allergens and can be used when a severe reaction is expected. Cytotoxicity food allergy tests, which attempt to show the death of leukocytes in the serum of allergic patients when incubated with food extracts, are of no proven value and are not used in the evaluation of food allergy.

CASE STUDY: *CONTINUED*

After a review of the small bowel biopsies, the patient was started on a gluten-free and lactose-free diet. Her symptoms did not improve, and she was subsequently started on 10 mg prednisone per day.

After 4 weeks, the patient's symptoms improved dramatically, and she was weaned off the steroids. A second small bowel biopsy performed 2 months after beginning the gluten-free diet demonstrated resolution of the villus atrophy. After 6 months on the gluten-free diet, the patient regained her lost weight, and her anemia resolved.

TREATMENT

The only effective treatment for food allergy is avoidance of the culpable food. Instruction by an experienced dietitian can help prevent inadvertent ingestion of food allergens. Antihistamines and corticosteroids cannot be used to prevent adverse reactions; they are useful only secondarily to treat symptoms resulting from accidental ingestions. Although there is no evidence that hyposensitization is effective in treating an existing food allergy, there is some evidence that breastfeeding until an infant is 6 months old may have a protective effect against the development of a food allergy.

CASE STUDY: *RESOLUTION*

This was a case of a 50-year-old woman who presented with diarrhea and weight loss. She had no abdominal pain or history of fevers. Her description of her stools was consistent with malabsorption. At this point, evaluation on an outpatient basis was appropriate to investigate for colitis, infectious diarrhea, and celiac disease (also known as gluten-sensitive enteropathy, idiopathic steatorrhea, and nontropical sprue).

The physical examination was remarkable only for weight loss. A CBC revealed anemia, though her stool was negative for occult blood. Anemia in the absence of bleeding can indicate malabsorption and suggests a workup for celiac disease. The low albumin is also indicative of malabsorption and indicates a prolonged process. The stool cultures were all negative, ruling out an infectious etiology, but the 24-hour fecal fat was elevated, indicating fat malabsorption.

The upper endoscopy did not show any overt mucosal abnormalities, which is often the case in celiac disease. A small bowel biopsy is the procedure of choice for the diagnosis of celiac disease. The biopsies were consistent with celiac disease, showing the characteristic blunting or atrophy of villi, infiltration with intestinal lymphocytes, and crypt hyperplasia. Serum antibodies to gliadin and transglutaminase antibody were positive and thus confirmed the diagnosis of celiac disease.

After a diagnosis of celiac disease was made, the patient was started on a gluten-free diet, but her symptoms did not improve. A gluten-free diet is the treatment for celiac disease, and when strictly followed, it restores the intestinal mucosa to its normal morphology. Less than 10% of patients with classic celiac disease fail to respond to a gluten-free diet, but those who do not respond can show a dramatic clinical and histologic response to 10–40 mg prednisone. After 4 weeks on prednisone and a gluten-free diet, the patient's symptoms improved. Repeat biopsies confirmed improvement, and she was able to regain her lost weight. Failure to improve after 4–6 weeks of prednisone raises the possibility of lymphoma or some other extraintestinal block to the absorptive process, and this should be actively investigated.

*R*EVIEW *Q*UESTIONS

Directions: For each of the following questions, choose the one best answer.

1 Which of the following statements concerning microfold (M) cells is *true*?

A They are responsible for transporting antigens to the diffuse lymphoid tissue.

B They are macrophages located in the mucosa overlying the lymphoid follicles.

C They possess major histocompatibility complex (MHC) class II antigens and function as antigen-presenting molecules.

D They "selectively sample" intraluminal antigens.

2 Which of the following statements concerning intraepithelial lymphocytes is *true*?

A Most intraepithelial lymphocytes are T cells.

B They function as helper cells in mucosal immunity.

C Their population size generally remains stable in most mucosal inflammatory states.

D They are not specific to any one region.

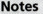

3 Secretory IgA has which of the following characteristics?

A It is protected from degradation in the lumen by the presence of secretory component (SC).
B It is transported across the epithelial cell in a monomeric form.
C It accomplishes immune protection by activating complement.
D It activates adherence of bacteria to epithelial cells.

4 Which of the following substances does *not* trigger histamine secretion by mast cells?

A Cholecystokinin
B Gastrin
C Insulin
D Vasoactive intestinal peptide (VIP)

5 A nonimmunologic mucosal barrier to infection is

A secretory immunoglobulin A (IgA).
B macrophages.
C interleukin-1 (IL-1).
D tight junctions of intestinal epithelial cells.

6 A 25-year-old woman presents for the evaluation of a suspected food allergy. She states that for the past year she has noticed that soon after the ingestion of eggs, she begins to experience skin eruptions (urticaria) and a runny nose (rhinitis). Her medical history is remarkable only for eczema. Physical examination and review of systems are normal. Which of the following tests would be most appropriate for the initial evaluation of this patient?

A Oral food challenge with eggs
B Skin testing with egg extract
C In vitro cytotoxicity food allergy testing
D RAST or ELISA

References

Blumberg RS, Stenson WF: The immune system and gastrointestinal inflammation. In *Textbook of Gastroenterology,* Edited by Yamada T. Philadelphia, PA: J. B. Lippincott, 2003, pp 117–150.

Ciclitira PJ: AGA technical review on celiac sprue. American Gastroenterological Association. *Gastroenterology* 120(6):1526–40, 2001.

Ernst PB, Underdown BJ, Bienenstock J: Immunity in mucosal tissues. In *Basic and Clinical Immunology.* Edited by Stites DP, Stobo JD, Wells JV. Norwalk, CT: Appleton & Lange, 1987, pp 159–166.

Feighery C: Intestinal immune system—a hidden symphony. In *Gastrointestinal Immunology and Gluten-sensitive Disease. Proceedings of the*

Sixth International Symposium on Coeliac Disease. Edited by Feighery C, O'Farrelly C. Dublin, Ireland: Oak Tree Press, 1994, pp 1–13.

Goodman JW: Immunoglobulins I: structure and function. In *Basic and Clinical Immunology.* Edited by Stites DP, Stobo JD, Wells JV. Norwalk, CT: Appleton & Lange, 1987.

MacDonald TT, Spencer J: Cell-mediated immune injury in the intestine. *Gastroenterol Clin N Am* 21:367–386, 1992.

Shanahan F: Gastrointestinal manifestations of immunologic disorders. In *Textbook of Gastroenterology.* Edited by Yamada T. Philadelphia, PA: J. B. Lippincott, 2003, pp 2705–2721.

Taylor KB, Thomas HC: Gastrointestinal and liver disease. In *Basic and Clinical Immunology.* Edited by Stites DP, Stobo JD, Wells JV. Norwalk, CT: Appleton & Lange, 1987, pp 457–480.

Wershil BK, Walker WA: The mucosal barrier, IgE-mediated gastrointestinal events, and eosinophilic gastroenteritis. *Gastroenterol Clin N Am* 21:387–404, 1992.

Notes

16

Inflammatory Bowel Disease

▓ CHAPTER OUTLINE ▓

▓ LEARNING OBJECTIVES ▓

At the completion of this chapter, the reader should be able to:
- Distinguish the clinical, pathological, and therapeutic interventions for Crohn's disease versus ulcerative colitis (UC).
- Describe the demographic and epidemiologic features of inflammatory bowel disease (IBD).
- Identity pathogenetic factors in the etiology of IBD.
- Detail the potential complications of IBD.
- Assess the extraintestinal manifestations of IBD.
- Compare and contrast medical versus surgical treatments for IBD.

CASE STUDY: *INTRODUCTION*

The patient, a 24-year-old female medical student, was well until 4 weeks prior to admission. At that time, she developed mild abdominal pain, lasting for 1 week. The episode of pain was followed by the onset of diarrhea, which progressed to a bowel movement every 15 minutes. She also noted blood in the stool. Over the 4-week period, her appetite decreased, and she lost 13 lbs. She also complained of intermittent fever.

Introduction

By definition, inflammatory bowel disease (IBD) includes any process that can result in inflammation of the GI mucosa. These are not limited to but may include infectious processes, toxic or radiation injury, or other conditions; however, when the term IBD is used, it very often refers to the two forms of idiopathic intestinal inflammation, namely, Crohn's disease and ulcerative colitis (UC). This chapter concentrates on delineating the similarities and differences between these two conditions.

DEFINITIONS

Crohn's disease and UC, although similar in many aspects, are two distinctive diseases clinically and histologically. The exact etiology of these two forms of idiopathic IBD is still unknown, and because they may be distinct in some of the initial pathogenic events, it is also likely that both diseases share common pathophysiologic mechanisms. There remain at least 10% of patients who have unclassified IBD because it is difficult to distinguish between UC and Crohn's.

Crohn's disease is also known as regional enteritis, Crohn's ileitis, and granulomatous colitis. Any part of the GI tract may be affected, from the mouth to the anus. In contrast, UC is a disorder confined to the colon. Although the disease is continuous starting from the rectum, it may involve just a short portion of the colon, the entire colon to the cecum, or any length in between. UC and Crohn's disease are usually characterized by periods of exacerbation and remission. The clinical manifestations depend on the extent and location of the disease as well as on any of the associated extraintestinal manifestations.

EPIDEMIOLOGY OF IBD

The incidence by age of both of these diseases is in a bimodal distribution with a peak occurrence from the late teenage years into the early thirties and a smaller yet significant peak in the sixth decade.

Women and men are affected similarly overall in IBD, but 20% more women are afflicted with Crohn's disease than men, whereas 20% more men than women suffer with UC. IBD affects the white population in greater proportion compared to the nonwhite population.

IBD can be found worldwide, but the highest incidence occurs in the Northern Hemisphere. Among Jewish populations, those of Eastern European descent (Ashkenazi Jews) have higher rates of both UC and Crohn's.

The incidence of UC has remained relatively stable while the incidence of Crohn's disease has risen over the past 30 years. Smokers have a twofold increased risk of developing Crohn's. In contrast, smokers have approximately half the risk of developing UC. There have been reports of UC presenting shortly after the cessation of smoking in some individuals. Oral contraceptives have also been implicated as a possible cause of Crohn's disease. As noted, incidence rates for Crohn's are higher for women. It is interesting that a family history for IBD is found in 8%–11% of those afflicted, implicating a genetic predisposition at least in part.

The impact of these diseases in terms of the morbidity and the clinical significance of IBD as a chronic disease have received increasing recognition.

Pathogenesis of IBD

The increased prevalence of IBD among first-degree relatives of patients and the increased incidence among certain ethnic populations favors a genetic contribution to the pathogenesis of IBD. Twin studies reveal that there is a high rate of concordance among monozygotic twins, particularly with Crohn's disease (and seen to a lesser degree in UC), when compared to dizygotic twins. The exact genetic contribution has not been identified. It may be that aberrant genes encode an immune regulatory product or factor that contributes to a structural alteration in the GI tract in patients with IBD.

The role of genetics in the pathogenesis of IBD is complex. There appears to be more than one single susceptibility locus, incomplete penetrance, and probable gene–gene and gene–environment interactions. Only modest associations have been documented in studies between IBD and genetic variants in the human leukocyte antigen (HLA) genes and a limited number of other genes that are involved in immune regulation and the inflammatory response. Crohn's disease–associated *NOD2* genetic variants have been identified that appear to alter the innate immune response to bacteria. A new discovery is that a version of the NFKB1 gene is an important risk factor for UC. This gene contains the DNA sequence for nuclear factor kappa B (NF-kappa B) protein, which is a regulator of the immune system and programmed cell death. Researchers also found that a version of another gene, MDR1, is strongly associated with Crohn's disease and possibly UC as well. The importance of these findings and the prospect of future discoveries, especially with completion of the Human Genome Project, holds great promise for better therapies and strategies for prevention.

UC patients are more likely to exhibit perinuclear antineutrophil cytoplasmic antibodies (p-ANCA) than either controls or patients

with Crohn's. The p-ANCA UC patient is more likely to be positive for HLA-DR2, whereas p-ANCA-negative UC patients often are HLA-DR4. Crohn's patients are most often p-ANCA-negative with HLA-DR1 and HLA-DQw5. There is also an association of IBD with HLA-B27 in patients with ankylosing spondylitis.

Infectious agents have been implicated in the development of IBD. It has been hypothesized that environmental toxins or infectious agents may cross the intestinal barrier and initiate a sequence of events in susceptible individuals. To date, there is no single agent that has been consistently associated with either form of IBD.

It has also been proposed that IBD may reflect an exaggerated physiologic inflammatory response. Several alterations in immune regulation have been indentified in IBD. IBD patients appear to have increased numbers of immunoglobulin G (IgG)-bearing cells. Increased IgG has been found in both peripheral blood and intestinal mucosa of patients. Deposition of complement components in the GI tract mucosa of IBD patients has been found. It has also been proposed that IBD is associated with a fundamental alteration in antigen-presenting activity. This is supported by the induction of the expression of major histocompatibility complex (MHC) class II antigens in intestinal epithelial cells.

CASE STUDY: *CONTINUED*

On admission to the hospital, the patient was orthostatic with a rapid pulse. Head, eyes, ear, nose, and throat (HEENT) were negative for lesions. Heart and lung examinations were normal. Abdominal examination showed a soft and flat abdomen with tenderness in the right lower quadrant. There was no perianal disease, and a rectal examination showed heme-positive mucus in the rectal vault.

Clinical Features of IBD

CROHN'S DISEASE

Crohn's disease and UC may present with similar or different clinical manifestations, depending on the extent and involvement of the disease (Table 16-1). Crohn's disease may involve any area of the digestive tract from the oral cavity to the anus. Pathologically, the inflammatory process is transmural. Macrophages aggregate and may lead to the development of noncaseating granulomas. These granulomas are pathognomonic for Crohn's, but most often they are not found on routine biopsies (Figure 16-1). Endoscopically, one may see deep linear ulcerations. One may also see inflammation in the setting of normal intervening mucosa. The clinical presentation is widely variable and depends on the site of tissue involvement as well as the extent of inflammation. Pain, diarrhea, obstructive symptoms, fever, weight loss, and (in children) failure to grow may all be the presenting symptoms.

Table 16-1. UC versus Crohn's Disease

	FAVORING UC	FAVORING CROHN'S
Clinical	Six or more bowel movements daily, usually bloody	Variable patterns of stools Pain Perianal disease
Endoscopic	Continuous disease Rectum involved Microscopic ulcers	Segmental disease No rectal disease Aphthous ulcers Macroscopic ulcers
X-ray	Continuous disease Ulcerations No small bowel disease	Patchy disease Strictures Involvement of terminal ileum Fistulas
Histology	Mucosal changes Ulcers	Transmural changes Granulomas

Notes

UC is a continuous disease always involving the rectum. Crohn's disease may involve any area of the digestive tract.

In Crohn's disease, there may be several mechanisms for the development of diarrhea. Diarrhea may result from mucosal destruction and malabsorption, malabsorption of bile salts, partial bowel obstruction, bacterial overgrowth, and rapid transit. It is therefore important to define the disease involvement and characteristics of the diarrheal illness in the patient with Crohn's disease.

UC

UC involves a mucosal inflammatory process that begins at the rectum and extends proximally in a continuous fashion. The disease is usually defined by the anatomic extent of inflammation: proctitis, proctosigmoiditis, left-sided colitis, and pancolitis (involvement of entire colon). The disease manifestations usually reflect the pathologic

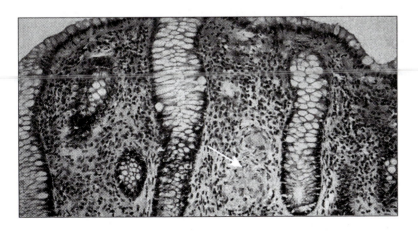

Fig. 16-1. Granuloma in Crohn's Disease

Granulomas (arrow) are present only in Crohn's disease and are not seen in UC. The absence of granulomas does not preclude Crohn's disease because they are found in less than 15% of biopsies in patients with Crohn's colitis. Courtesy of Dr. Sydney Frinkelstein.

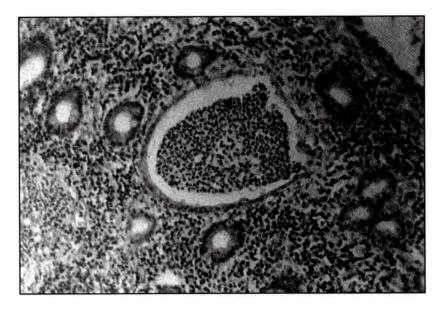

Fig. 16-2. Crypt Abscess in UC

Crypt abscesses, which may be seen in UC, are focal collections of polymor-phonuclear leukocytes within the lower part of the crypts. Courtesy of Dr. Sydney Finkelstein.

process of inflammation. On microscopic examination, microab-scesses may be found within the crypts, and depletion of mucin from the goblet cells may be evident (Figure 16-2). The lamina propria is densely populated with neutrophils, lymphocytes, and other con-stituents of acute and chronic inflammation. Superficial mucosal ul-ceration may develop. Endoscopically, one may see mucosal granular-ity, mucosal friability, and ulceration with mucopurulent exudate. There is no normal intervening mucosa. Patients often present with bloody diarrhea. Watery diarrhea may occur as a result of impaired ab-sorption of water and electrolytes caused by mucosal damage. Patients may experience tenesmus or painful urgency to defecate, usually re-lated to severe inflammation of the rectum.

Both Crohn's and UC are chronic and recurring illnesses. Long-term remissions may occur. The course for any individual may be variable.

CASE STUDY: *CONTINUED*

Stool studies for culture and sensitivity, *Escherichia coli* 0157:H7, ova and parasites, and *Clostridium difficile* were all negative. Hematocrit was 35.6% and hemoglobin was 12.6 mg/dl; white blood cell (WBC) count was 9500/μl with 27% polymorphonu-clear leukocytes (polys) and 53% bands. Albumin was 3.1 g/dl, and erythrocyte sedimentation rate (ESR) was 23 mm/hr. The patient had a flexible sigmoidoscopy to 10 cm, which showed discrete ulcerations with inflamed intervening mucosa.

Diagnosis of IBD

The diagnosis of IBD is based on clinical presentation and evaluation of the GI tract for evidence of inflammation in the absence of identifiable infectious agents. Initial evaluation should include stool cultures to rule out an infection and therefore a self-limited process. Laboratory evaluation may reveal leukocytosis, elevated ESR, and anemia. The differential diagnosis may include infectious colitis, diverticular disease, ischemic colitis, radiation colitis, lymphoma, appendicitis, GI neoplasm, and irritable bowel syndrome (IBS).

The diagnosis of Crohn's disease may be confirmed by endoscopy, radiologic studies, or both (Figure 16-3). If colonic disease is present, the mucosa may appear erythematous and friable with ulcerations, often in a linear pattern and surrounded by normal mucosa.

This appearance has been referred to as "cobblestone." In a patient with perineal involvement, a perianal examination may show fissures, fistulas, and perianal abscesses. In the patient with obstructive symptoms, a plain film may show dilated loops of small bowel consistent with obstruction. However, this finding can be found in any patient with a small bowel obstruction and therefore is not specific for Crohn's disease. Barium studies of the colon may show areas of ulceration or narrowing. Fistulas, which are abnormal connections between different parts of the intestine or between the intestine and another organ (such as a rectovaginal fistula), may also be evident. It is important to visualize the terminal ileum because this is the most common site of involvement. A small bowel series or enteroclysis,

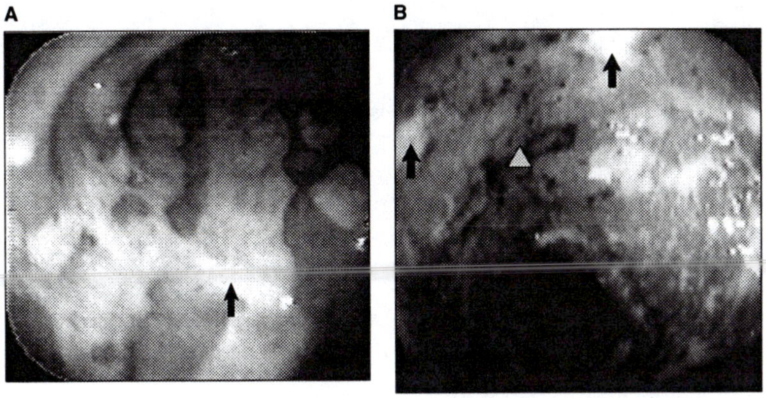

Fig. 16-3. Endoscopic Photographs of Crohn's and UC

(A) The photograph on the left shows linear ulcerations (arrow) that may be seen in Crohn's colitis. These would appear as white stripes in the middle of the colonic mucosa. In Crohn's disease, it is not unusual to see ulcerations, either linear or aphthous, in the setting of otherwise normal mucosa. (B) In contrast, the photograph on the right is an example of UC. There are diffuse ulcerations (arrows). The darkened area (triangle) is an area of hemorrhage. There is no normal mucosa in this region. Crohn's photograph courtesy of Dr. Richard Kim, Moon Township, Pennsylvania. UC photograph, courtesy of Dr. Paul Basuk.

Notes

Differential Diagnosis of IBD
Infectious colitis
Diverticular disease
Ischemic colitis
Radiation colitis
Lymphoma
Colon cancer
Appendicitis
IBS

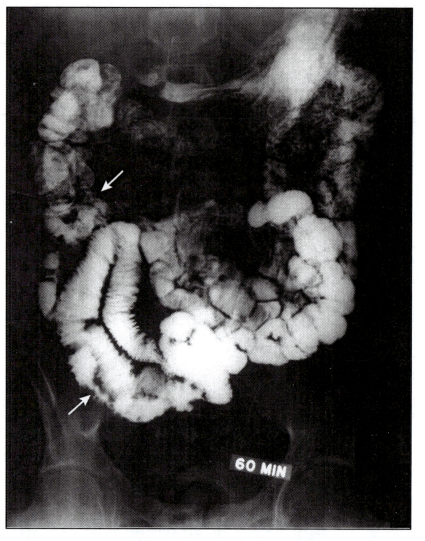

Fig. 16-4. Terminal Ileal Crohn's Disease

This small bowel study in a patient with Crohn's disease shows ileal disease (arrows) in the right lower quadrant with narrowing of the lumen, mural thickening, and cobblestone appearance of the mucosa. Courtesy of Dr. Susan Teeger.

which is a small bowel enema with barium given through a nasogastric tube, may show strictures, inflammation, or both anywhere in the small bowel. The "string sign" refers to a narrowed and scarred terminal ileum (Figure 16-4).

The diagnosis of UC may also be confirmed by endoscopy (see Figure 16-3) or barium studies. Biopsies should be obtained to confirm the diagnosis. Grossly, the mucosa of the involved area loses the normal pink, glistening appearance with its characteristic normal-appearing blood vessels. The affected mucosa appears granular and may be friable with ulcerations apparent. Pseudopolyps, which appear as small nodules, may also be present. A full colonoscopy may be useful to define the extent of the disease. It is also necessary that the patient, after 7–10 years duration of the disease, undergo a complete colonoscopy on a regular basis for surveillance biopsies for cancer. When severe pain is present, plain films of the abdomen are necessary to rule out perforation and evaluate for toxic megacolon, a severe complication of UC (see Complications of IBD). Barium studies of the colon may define the extent of disease. Barium studies are occasionally ordered to distinguish UC from Crohn's by evaluating the terminal ileum. Barium enema may show ulcerations, granular appearance with loss of haustral markings, and pseudopolyps.

CASE STUDY: *CONTINUED*

After review of the biopsies, the patient was treated with sulfasalazine and intravenous steroids. An upper GI and small bowel series were normal. The patient improved and was discharged on oral prednisone. Over the next 3 months, she was completely weaned off the steroids.

At age 27, the patient had a recurrence of abdominal pain, bloody diarrhea, and weight loss. She also complained of left knee and right elbow pain. It was also noted that she had developed a lesion on her right leg that was painful and necrotic, measuring 2 cm in diameter. Stool cultures were negative, and laboratory studies indicated an elevated ESR, an elevated WBC count, and anemia. A colonoscopy revealed pancolitis with ulcerations. The patient was given steroids but continued to have pain and bloody diarrhea.

The patient was admitted to the hospital 2 weeks later with a hemoglobin of 9.6 mg/dl, a hematocrit of 28.5%, a WBC count of 19,800/μl, with 76% polys and 6% bands. Albumin was 2.6 g/L (decreased). An abdominal x-ray showed dilated large bowel with thumbprinting and no free air. She was allowed nothing by mouth and was started on total parenteral nutrition (TPN) and intravenous steroids. Cyclosporine was considered. The patient developed a fever and was started on antibiotics.

Complications of IBD

TOXIC MEGACOLON

Toxic megacolon is a serious complication of IBD, occurring in 1%–2.5% of patients. This condition is associated with systemic manifestations of toxicity, including fever, tachycardia, leukocytosis, and a change in mental status. The diagnosis is made clinically. Dilation of the colon beyond 6 cm, most often evident as a dilated transverse colon, may be seen on a plain film of the abdomen (Figure 16-5). Initial treatment would include nothing by mouth, TPN, intravenous fluids, nasogastric suction, steroids, and broad-spectrum antibiotics. It is very important to avoid anticholinergic agents and opiate antidiarrheals, as they may predispose to or worsen toxic megacolon.

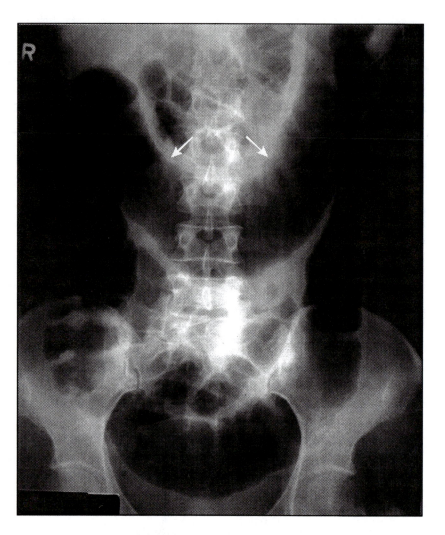

Fig. 16-5. Abdominal X-Ray in Toxic Megacolon

This plain x-ray of the abdomen in a patient with UC shows a dilated colon. There is loss of the normal haustral fold markings consistent with colitis. There is also evidence of edema of the bowel wall (arrow). Courtesy of Dr. Susan Teeger.

Colonoscopy should be avoided in cases of toxic megacolon because, even in UC, the inflammation becomes transmural and increases the risk of perforation. Surgical consultation is essential early in the diagnosis, and surgery is indicated if the patient does not respond to conservative medical management.

COLON CANCER

The prevalence of colorectal cancer (CRC) in patients with UC is estimated to be 3.7% overall, and 5.4% for those with pancolitis. The incidence rate is approximately 3 per 1000 person-years duration. The factors that the increase risk for developing CRC in UC include: (1) duration of colitis, (2) extent of colonic involvement, (3) family history of CRC, (4) primary sclerosing cholangitis, and (5) in some studies young age of IBD onset. The most important risk factor, as evidenced in many studies, is the duration of colitis. CRC rarely occurs before 7 years duration of IBD, the risk rises thereafter, with a cumulative risk for CRC in a patient with UC of 2% at 10 years, 8% at 20 years, and 18% at 30 years. Pancolitis is clearly a risk factor, but it appears that patients with left-sided disease may also be at increased risk. Surveillance colonoscopy, with its limitations, is beneficial for detecting earlier stage cancers and appears to promote mortality reduction. Patients with Crohn's colitis are also at greater risk for CRC than the general population. When long-standing, anatomically significant Crohn's colitis is evaluated, the risk of CRC is similar to that of UC. Although we are awaiting additional studies on CRC in Crohn's, it is recommended that a surveillance strategy similar to that for UC is initiated for patients with at least eight years of Crohn's colitis involving at least one-third of the colon.

GI BLEEDING

Massive GI bleeding is rare in IBD, but chronic GI blood loss is common and may lead to chronic anemia.

NUTRITIONAL DEFICIENCIES

Nutritional deficiencies are more frequent in Crohn's disease and may be from multifactorial etiologies. Inadequate dietary intake may be a cause in patients who are ill. Often malabsorption of folate and lipid-soluble vitamins may occur. Terminal ileal disease may result in vitamin B_{12} malabsorption and bile salt deficiency, which may contribute to diarrhea. Bacterial overgrowth may occur with stagnation as a result of fistulas or strictures.

PERFORATION

Perforations may occur in IBD but are rare and usually associated with toxic megacolon.

STRICTURES

Colonic strictures may occur in either UC or Crohn's. Malignancy needs to be ruled out. Small bowel strictures may occur in Crohn's disease and may result in small bowel obstruction. Inflammatory strictures may respond to anti-inflammatory treatment, whereas repetitive inflammation may result in fibrosis or scarring, which may require surgical intervention.

FISTULA FORMATION

Fistulas may complicate Crohn's disease and may be enteroenteric, enterovesical, enterocolonic, enterovaginal, or enterocutaneous. These fistulas may lead to malabsorption syndromes and bacterial overgrowth. Fistulas may become obstructed and result in abscesses.

Extraintestinal Manifestations of IBD

Extraintestinal manifestations occur often in patients with IBD (Table 16-2). They may precede, accompany, or follow the IBD

Table 16-2. Extraintestinal Manifestations of IBD

EXTRAINTESTINAL SITES	MANIFESTATIONS
Musculoskeletal	Peripheral arthritis, spondylitis, sacroiliitis, and hypertrophic osteoarthropathy
Ocular	Episcleritis, uveitis, cataracts, keratopathy, corneal ulcerations, central serous retinopathy, and iritis
Skin	Erythema nodosum, pyoderma gangrenosum, and oral lesions
Hepatobiliary	Pericholangitis, primary sclerosing cholangitis, cirrhosis, gallstones, and pancreatitis
Renal	Calculi, ureteral obstruction, and vesical fistulas
Vascular	Thromboembolic events
Cardiac	Pericarditis
Bronchopulmonary	Granulomatous lung disease, bronchiectasis, interstitial fibrosis, lymphocytic alveolitis, pneumonitis, vasculitis, apical fibrosis, and chronic suppurative bronchitis
Other	Growth retardation and amyloidosis

symptoms. The pathogenesis of these manifestations remains unclear, but immunologic phenomena are likely involved.

MUSCULOSKELETAL COMPLICATIONS

Arthritis complicates IBD in 4%–23% of patients. Four types of arthritis have been described. Peripheral or colitic arthritis is seen in 15%–20% of IBD patients. It is migratory and asymmetric, affecting the large joints of the lower extremities. Spondylitis is seen in 3%–6% of IBD patients. Asymptomatic sacroiliitis may be seen in 4%–8% of patients with IBD. Hypertrophic osteoarthropathy presents with clubbing, periostitis with pain and new bone formation, synovitis and burning of the palms and soles.

OCULAR COMPLICATIONS

In IBD patients, there are many different ocular manifestations, with a reported incidence of ocular complication of 4%–10% in both Crohn's and UC. The common complications include episcleritis, uveitis, cataracts, keratopathy, marginal corneal ulcerations, and central serous retinopathy. Iritis and uveitis are uncommon but more serious. Patients may present with acute onset of blurred vision and headache.

SKIN LESIONS

Erythema nodosum is associated with IBD, occurring more commonly in children with Crohn's disease, and is characterized by raised, red, tender nodules. It usually appears early in the course of the disease and is most often associated with a peripheral arthropathy. Pyoderma gangrenosum is an ulcerative skin lesion associated more often with UC, having a reported incidence of 1%–5%. The incidence associated with Crohn's is 1%–2%. Skin lesions are ulcerations with a necrotic center and violaceous skin surrounding the lesion, occurring often on the pretibial region, but they may be seen anywhere on the body. Oral lesions occur in IBD and may be seen in 6%–20% of Crohn's patients.

HEPATOBILIARY COMPLICATIONS

There are many different hepatobiliary disorders seen in patients with IBD. Fatty liver is a nonspecific lesion that has been reported in up to 80% of patients. It is usually macrovesicular, and the pathogenesis is unknown but is likely multifactorial.

Pericholangitis is an inflammatory lesion of the portal tract. This usually occurs in patients with extensive colonic disease.

Primary sclerosing cholangitis (PSC) is characterized by fibrosing inflammation resulting in bile duct obliteration, biliary cirrhosis, and ultimately hepatic failure. PSC occurs in 2.4%–7.5% of IBD patients, and 75% of the cases are associated with UC. This disease is more common in young males but may be seen in both men and women at any age.

Cirrhosis associated with IBD occurs in 1%–5% of patients. Other hepatobiliary diseases that may occur in association with IBD include pericholangitis, steatosis, chronic hepatitis, cryptogenic cirrhosis, cholangiocarcinoma, and gallstone formation. Gallstones occur in patients with Crohn's disease involving the terminal ileum and in patients after ileocolectomy. The incidence of choleithiasis in these patients ranges from 13% to 34% and correlates with the length of ileum involved, the history of ileal resection, and the duration of disease.

Bile duct carcinoma has been reported in as many as 1%–4% of patients with IBD. This occurs more commonly in association with UC but has been seen in patients with Crohn's. The risk of bile duct carcinoma is increased in patients with PSC. Of those patients with PSC, with or without UC, 8%–15% develop adenocarcinoma of the bile duct, with the highest incidence occurring in those patients with long-standing colonic disease and cirrhosis secondary to PSC.

Pancreatitis, although rarely seen in IBD, has been reported in two subpopulations of patients. One group includes those patients with duodenal Crohn's, in which reflux of duodenal contents into the pancreatic duct through an incompetent ampulla may occur. The other group includes those patients with UC, PSC, or pericholangitis, diseases known to be associated with pancreatitis.

RENAL COMPLICATIONS

Genitourinary complications have been reported in 4%–23% of patients with IBD. The most common of these include urinary tract calculi, ureteral obstruction, and fistulization to the urinary tract. These complications occur more commonly in Crohn's patients. Most renal stones are calcium oxalate, but uric acid stones do occur and are found more frequently in these patients than in the general population. Hyperoxaluria is a result of increased absorption of oxalate.

Right hydronephrosis has also been described in Crohn's disease and may result from the obstructing effect of inflammation surrounding the terminal ileum.

VASCULAR COMPLICATIONS

Thromboembolic complications in IBD have been reported in 1.3%–6.4% of patients. IBD has also been reported to be associated with vasculitis. The etiology of thrombosis in IBD is postulated to be from a hypercoagulable state.

CARDIAC COMPLICATIONS

Pleuropericarditis is an uncommon complication of IBD with an unknown etiology.

BRONCHOPULMONARY COMPLICATIONS

Granulomatous lung disease, bronchiectasis, interstitial fibrosis, lymphocytic alveolitis, and sulfasalazine pneumonitis are among the pulmonary diseases associated with Crohn's disease. Several respiratory diseases have been reported in association with UC, including vasculitis, apical fibrosis, chronic suppurative bronchitis, and bronchiectasis.

OTHER MANIFESTATIONS

Hematologic abnormalities have been seen in association with IBD. Growth retardation has been noted in children. Amyloidosis has been reported in Crohn's disease and may involve the kidneys, resulting in nephrotic syndrome and renal failure in some cases.

Treatment

MEDICAL THERAPY

Patients should be evaluated on initial presentation and with each subsequent exacerbation to rule out other etiologies of the symptoms or exacerbating factors, such as superimposed infection. Every effort should be made to stabilize the patient, replete fluid and electrolyte losses, and monitor hemodynamic parameters. It is important to note that sometimes initially and very often later in the course of the disease, issues relating to the emotional impact of the presence of a chronic disease must be addressed. Some patients may benefit from support groups and counseling.

Anti-inflammatory therapies have been used for a long time to treat both UC and Crohn's (Table 16-3). Corticosteroids were first used to treat IBD in the 1940s and since then have proven to be efficacious in the treatment of acute disease. Steroids are not effective in maintaining remission of either Crohn's or UC. Corticosteroids may be useful in patients with moderate to severe UC or Crohn's. Although there has been an impression that they may be useful in Crohn's colitis, they have been shown to be efficacious only in patients with small bowel involvement of Crohn's. Steroids do not appear to affect the rate of recurrence in patients with either UC or Crohn's in remission. Controlled or delayed ileal release formulations of budesonide have been successful in the treatment of mild to moderate Crohn's disease involving the ileum and right colon. Because of first-pass metabolism in the liver, budesonide, which is a significantly more potent glucocorticoid than prednisone, has 10%–15% systemic bioavailability and minimal steroid side effects.

Topical hydrocortisone has been useful in treating distal proctocolitis. However, preparations of increased potency have been associated with systemic effects due to general absorption of the drug. Prolonged use of steroids may lead to complications related to this medication.

Sulfasalazine is a dimer of 5-aminosalicylic acid (5-ASA), linked by an azo-bond to sulfapyridine. 5-ASA is released in the distal ileum and colon by bacterial azoreductases. 5-ASA is now known to be the therapeutic moiety of this drug. Sulfasalazine is an inhibitor of prostaglandin synthase and 5-lipoxygenase, thus leading to reduced production of prostaglandins and leukotrienes. Sulfasalazine blocks the chemotactic activity of formylated bacterial peptides, which may recruit polymorphonuclear netrophils to the bowel. It also acts as a scavenger of oxygen-free radicals.

Sulfasalazine reduces the frequency and severity of recurrent excerbations in UC but has not shown to be of prophylactic benefit once acute disease has been controlled in Crohn's disease. Up to 20% of patients may develop hypersensitivity to this drug. As noted, the

Table 16-3. Medications Used in the Treatment of IBD

MEDICATIONS	MECHANISM OF ACTION	COMPLICATIONS OF THERAPY
Corticosteroids	Anti-inflammatory modulation of phospholipase A_2, interleukin-1 (IL-1), tumor necrosis factor (TNF)-α, endothelial leukocyte adhesion molecule-1, intercellular adhesion molecule-1, and lysis of lymphocytes and eosinophils	Multiple potential complications
5-ASA agents (sulfasalazine and others)	5-ASA moiety, inhibitor of prostaglandin synthesis, and 5-lipoxygenase	Headaches, upper GI symptoms, and hypersensitivity
Azathioprine and 6-mercaptopurine	Affect natural killer cell activity and humoral responsiveness	Bone marrow depression, infections, pancreatitis, and allergic reactions
Methotrexate	Folic acid antagonist, interferes with cytokines involved in IBD pathogenesis	Liver enzyme elevation, leukopenia, nausea, vomiting, diarrhea, hypersensitivity, and pneumonitis
Cyclosporine	Inhibits transcription of IL-2, helper T-cell function, and interferon-γ	Hypertension, nephrotoxicity, tremors, gingival hyperplasia, hirsutism, rare hepatic dysfunction, and seizures
Infliximab	Chimeric monoclonal antibody to TNF: binding of free and membrane-bound TNF, potential of IgG_1 chimeric antibody to activate complement	Development of antichimeric and anti-DNA antibodies, lupus, acute and delayed infusion reactions

Note: 5-ASA = 5-aminosalicylic acid.

Notes

Surgical decisions for Crohn's disease must be made with the knowledge that there is a high likelihood of recurrence.

therapeutic activity of this drug results from its 5-ASA part. The sulfapyridine moiety is responsible for the hypersensitivity and intolerance to this drug. Newer agents with active 5-ASA but different compounds for drug delivery are available. Topical 5-ASA given as an enema is effective in control of distal proctocolitis.

Azathioprine and 6-mercaptopurine (6-MP) may be useful therapies. 6-MP has been effective in patients with refractory Crohn's. Azathioprine and 6-MP may (1) lead to improvement in refractory patients, (2) allow for reduction in steroid doses, (3) result in closure of fistulas, and (4) help maintain remission. Benefits from these medications do not result for months. Potential adverse effects include bone marrow depression, infections, pancreatitis, and allergic reactions. There has also been a concern regarding secondary malignancies in patients treated with these agents.

In low doses, methotrexate has been reported to be of benefit in patients with refractory UC and Crohn's. Cyclosporine may be of benefit in Crohn's and UC; however, toxicity may limit its utility. It has been used in efforts to postpone or defer colectomy in patients with severe colitis. Metronidazole has been shown to be effective in perineal fistulas. Infliximab is a chimeric monoclonal antibody to TNF. It is effective in the treatment of fistulous Crohn's disease.

The role of TPN as treatment for IBD has been controversial. TPN is especially useful in repleting nutrients, in the management of short bowel syndrome, and in restoring the growth spurt in adolescent patients with Crohn's. The role of an elemental diet in Crohn's disease has similarly sparked much controversy.

SURGICAL THERAPY

It should be remembered that proctocolectomy is curative for patients with UC, but surgical decisions for Crohn's disease should be made with the knowledge that there is a high likelihood of recurrence.

An ileoanal anastomosis following proctocolectomy in patients with UC is the preferred procedure for appropriate candidates requiring surgery for intractable UC or cancer prophylaxis. This surgery is inappropriate for Crohn's disease patients because of the high incidence of recurrences and perineal complications. A conventional proctocolectomy and ileostomy procedure is appropriate for patients with Crohn's disease requiring total colectomy, for elderly patients with UC, or for patients who for anatomic reasons are not candidates for the ileoanal anastomosis. Complications of the ileoanal anastomosis include frequency, incontinence, and pouchitis. The Kock continent ileostomy in general is no longer being performed because complications from this procedure have been reported in up to 30% of patients.

A conservative approach to surgery in Crohn's patients is prudent. Operations to preserve the length of bowel, strictureplasty, are considered if appropriate. This procedure may be useful in cases of multiple small bowel strictures, because it may help avoid the complications of multiple resections, including short bowel syndrome.

Summary

IBD is a chronic GI illness characterized by periods of remission and exacerbation. The clinical presentation depends on the involvement and extent of disease. Newer therapeutic options are available for treatment. Although complications and extraintestinal manifestations may occur, with appropriate follow-up most patients with IBD can experience a good quality of life and a normal life expectancy.

CASE STUDY: *RESOLUTION*

On the second day in the hospital, the patient continued to have pain and fever and became increasingly lethargic. She was taken to surgery for a subtotal colectomy and temporary ileostomy. Over the next 2 weeks, the patient completely recovered. Six months later, she underwent a proctectomy and ileoanal anastomosis and has done well since that time.

REVIEW QUESTIONS

Directions: For each of the following questions, choose the one best answer.

1 A 38-year-old man with a 7-year history of UC (involving the entire colon) has been having intermittent flares for the past 3 months. He is brought to the emergency room by his family because of increased lethargy, fever, bloody diarrhea, and abdominal pain. The physician on duty should

A administer anticholinergic agents to relieve spasm.
B administer opiate antidiarrheals in significant doses to relieve the diarrhea.
C feed the patient to see if it makes him feel better.
D get an abdominal x-ray and upright film.

2 Which of the following is an extraintestinal manifestation of IBD?

A Primary biliary cirrhosis   C Rheumatoid arthritis
B Primary sclerosing cholangitis   D Erythema infectiosum

Directions for questions 3–7: Select the most likely condition associated with the description.

A Ulcerative colitis   C Both diseases
B Crohn's disease   D Neither disease

3 Pathologically, the inflammatory process is usually transmural.

4 Fistulas are characteristic.

5 Surgery is the initial treatment of choice.

6 Granulomas may be seen.

7 Pathologically, the process is mucosal.

References

Balan V, LaRusso: Hepatobiliary disease in inflammatory bowel disease. *GI Clin N Am* 24:647–669, 1995.

Banerjee S: Inflammatory bowel disease. Medical therapy of specific clinical presentations. *Gastroenterol Clin North Am* 31(1):185–202, 2002.

Brant SR, Panhuysen CIM, Nicolae D, et al: MDR1 Ala893 Polymorphism is associated with inflammatory bowel disease. *Am J Hum Genet* 73:1282–1292, 2003.

Duerr RH: The genetics of inflammatory bowel disease. *Gastroenterol Clin* 31:63–76, 2002.

Eaden J, Abrams KR, Mayberry JF: The risk of colorectal cancer in ulcerative colitis: a meta-analysis. *Gut* 48:526–535, 2001.

Harrison J: Medical treatment of Crohn's disease. *Gastroenterol Clin North Am* 31(1):167–184, 2002.

Itzkowitz SH: Cancer prevention in patients with inflammatory bowel disease. *Gastroenterol Clin North Am* 31(4):1133–1144, 2002.

Jani N: Medical therapy for ulcerative colitis. *Gastroenterol Clin North Am* 31(1): 147–166, 2002.

Karban AS, Okazaki T, Panhuysen CIM, et al: Functional annotation of a novel *NFKB1* promoter polymorphism that increases risk for ulcerative colitis. *Hum Mol Genet* 13:35–45, 2004.

Lashner, BA: Epidemiology of inflammatory bowel disease. *GI Clin N Am* 24:467–474, 1995.

Podolsky DK: Inflammatory bowel disease. *N Engl J Med* 325:(part 1) 928–937, (part 2)1008–1016, 1991.

Su CG: Extraintestinal manifestations of inflammatory bowel disease. *Gastroenterol Clin North Am* 31(1):307–327, 2002.

17

Infectious Disorders of the GI Tract

■ LEARNING OBJECTIVES ■

At the completion of this chapter, the reader should be able to:
- Identify the clinical presentation, diagnosis, and therapy of bacterial, viral, and parasitic infections of the GI tract.
- Differentiate between infections in immunocompetent and immunosuppressed hosts.
- Identify the site of action in the GI tract for a particular organism or infection.
- Explore epidemiologic factors in the development of infections of the GI tract.
- Develop strategies to evaluate the patient with a GI tract infection.

A 36-year-old man with a history of AIDS and a CD4 count of 25 presented with nausea and vomiting for 2 weeks. The patient also reported that he had difficulty swallowing food. He noted that there was also a slight amount of pain with swallowing. His weight had decreased by 10 lbs in the previous month. He had fever but no night sweats. His major infectious complication from HIV was *Pneumocystis* pneumonia.

This patient had seen his primary care provider, who ordered a barium esophagogram, which revealed a large ulcer in the distal esophagus. He also reported the onset of abdominal pain and diarrhea in the previous 3–4 days. There was no visible blood in the stool. He was having five to six bowel movements a day. He denied recent travel or drinking well water. The patient recalled taking penicillin for a tooth infection 1 month before. The primary care provider had sent a stool sample to the laboratory.

Introduction

Infections of the GI tract are common disorders that may be associated with significant morbidity and mortality. People with deficient immune systems (e.g., with AIDS, with bone marrow or solid-organ transplants, receiving cancer chemotherapy) are especially susceptible to certain organisms not usually seen in immunocompetent patients. In this chapter, we discuss infectious diseases by organ and compare immunocompetent and immunocompromised individuals (Table 17-1).

Esophageal Infections

Infections of the esophagus can occur in immunocompetent patients but are more common in those who are immunocompromised. These infections are encountered more frequently as more patients are subject to immunosuppression from such aggressive therapies for malignant neoplasms as high-dose chemotherapy and bone marrow transplantation (BMT). In such situations, esophageal infections cause significant morbidity. Patients with AIDS are also at risk for developing esophageal infections, especially as their T cell counts fall below critical levels. Patients with mildly impaired immune function, as in diabetes, may also develop infectious diseases of the esophagus.

The most common clinical manifestations of infectious esophagitis include dysphagia (difficulty swallowing) and odynophagia (pain with swallowing) (see Chapter 10). Less common symptoms are weight loss, nausea, vomiting, chest pain, and fever. Some patients with esophageal infection may have no symptoms.

IMMUNOCOMPETENT HOSTS

Infections of the esophagus are unusual in immunocompetent patients. Persons who are on corticosteroids, are elderly, or are alcoholic

Table 17-1. Summary of Pathogens by Organ

ORGAN	IMMUNOCOMPETENT HOST	IMMUNOCOMPROMISED HOST
Esophagus	HSV	CMV
	Candida	HSV
		Candida
Stomach	*Helicobacter pylori*	CMV
	Treponema pallidum	*Mycobacterium avium* complex
Small intestine	Adenovirus	*Cryptosporidium*
	Rotavirus	Microsporida
	Norwalk virus	*Isospora belli*
	Vibrio cholerae	*M. avium* complex
	Giardia lamblia	
Large intestine	*Shigella*	CMV
	Salmonella	HSV
	Campylobacter	*M. avium* complex
	Clostridium difficile	
	Escherichia coli (EIEC, 0157:H7, ETEC)	
	Yersinia	
	Entamoeba histolytica	
	Schistosoma	

Note: Pathogens seen in immunocompetent persons are also seen in immunocompromised persons. CMV = cytomegalovirus; HSV = herpes simplex virus.

The main etiologic agents in esophageal infections are *Candida albicans*, HSV type 1, and CMV.

are susceptible to esophageal candidiasis. Patients with gastric surgery, prolonged acid suppression (treated with H_2 blockers or proton pump inhibitors), abnormal esophageal motility (e.g., achalasia) or structure, or on prolonged antibiotic therapy are also susceptible to *Candida* esophagitis. Esophageal infection with cytomegalovirus (CMV) in immunocompetent hosts is extremely uncommon. Herpes simplex virus (HSV), however, is seen with relative frequency. Clinical presentation does not differ from that of immunocompromised patients.

IMMUNOCOMPROMISED HOSTS

Candida *Esophagitis*

Candida albicans is a ubiquitous fungus that forms budding yeast and pseudohyphae. It is the most common human fungal pathogen. *C. albicans* is often found in the flora of the oral cavity and GI tract of immunocompetent hosts but usually does not cause esophageal disease in this group. Predisposing factors to esophageal fungal infection include impaired cellular immunity (e.g., T lymphocyte, granulocyte function), dysmotility, altered flora, and achlorhydria.

Clinical Presentation. Dysphagia and odynophagia are the initial symptoms in patients with *Candida* esophagitis. Occasionally, patients note only substernal chest pain. Oral *Candida* infection (thrush) is often an indicator of esophageal infection in patients with swallowing symptoms; however, its absence does not exclude esophageal *Candida*.

Diagnosis. The diagnosis of *Candida* esophagitis should be suspected in any immunocompromised patient with dysphagia or odynophagia. Radiologically, a barium esophagogram may be helpful in evaluating for *Candida* esophagitis. *Candida* esophagitis classically appears as plaquelike lesions with irregular filling. Less often, the esophagogram may appear normal or may have nonspecific findings, such as strictures, ulcers, polyps, or masslike lesions. However, endoscopy with brushings and biopsy is the most sensitive method for making a definitive diagnosis of *Candida* esophagitis. Endoscopic appearance may show raised, white exudates. Ulcers, inflammation, or stricture may be seen less commonly. Histologically, the presence of budding yeast cells, hyphae, and pseudohyphae are best seen by silver stain, periodic acid–Schiff (PAS) stain, or Gram stain and are diagnostic of *Candida* infection.

Therapy. Patients with esophageal candidiasis should receive fluconazole. Intravenous amphotericin B is available for patients who are unable to swallow or who do not respond to fluconazole. Patients with decreased granulocyte function, such as cancer patients after chemotherapy, are at risk for disseminated fungal disease and should be treated with intravenous amphotericin.

CMV

CMV is a ubiquitous herpesvirus that is seen in 80% of the world's adult population. In normal seropositive adults, CMV can be seen in its latent form in most body organs. Both the cellular and humoral immune systems are important in controlling CMV infections. Impaired cellular immunity for prolonged periods places seropositive patients at high risk for reactivation of latent infection. Primary CMV infection (in those without prior CMV infection) tends to be more severe in patients with depressed immune function.

Clinical Presentation. Unlike other esophageal infections, CMV in the esophagus may present with nonesophageal symptoms, such as nausea, vomiting, anorexia, diarrhea, weight loss, or fever. However, dysphagia or odynophagia are the most common presenting symptoms in patients with CMV esophagitis. Mixed infections with HSV or *Candida* can occur.

Diagnosis. Barium esophagogram may reveal small, superficial ulcers or a large, coalescent singular ulcer, but the radiologic findings are not specific. Endoscopy with biopsy is the best test to confirm a diagnosis. Endoscopically, lesions may begin as superficial erosions or coalesce into large, shallow ulcers. Biopsy specimens should be taken from the center of the ulcer crater because CMV often infects endothelial cells but not squamous epithelia found at the ulcer margins. Histologically, large cells with intranuclear inclusions are seen in the subepithelial layer. The most sensitive method for detecting CMV is viral culture of the biopsy sample.

Therapy. Ganciclovir and foscarnet are antiviral drugs that effectively treat CMV. They have significant side effects, which may limit their usefulness. Ganciclovir may suppress the bone marrow, whereas foscarnet may affect renal function and produce electrolyte disturbances. There is also a high recurrence rate after discontinuation of therapy.

HSV

HSV, like CMV, is a member of the herpesvirus family. There are two types of HSV: type 1, which causes nasolabial, oropharyngeal, and esophageal infection, and type 2, which causes genital and perianal herpes. HSV causes initial acute infection followed by latency. HSV may remain latent in the trigeminal root ganglion and the autonomic ganglion of the superior cervical and vagus nerves.

Clinical Presentation. Patients typically present with odynophagia, which may be severe, as well as with dysphagia. Patients may also experience constant retrosternal pain, nausea, vomiting, or hematemesis. It is uncommon for HSV to cause systemic disease, since it infects only squamous epithelia.

Diagnosis. Endoscopically, vesicles may rarely be seen early in the course of infection. More often, discrete 1–2-mm ulcers with raised borders may be seen. If the disease has progressed, larger coalescent ulcers may be seen (Figure 17-1). Biopsies or brushings must be done at the ulcer edge because that is where infected squamous epithelial cells are located. Histologically, HSV may produce multinucleated

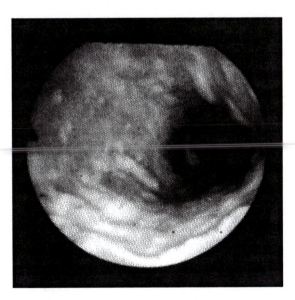

Fig. 17-1.

This endoscopic photograph shows ulcerations in the esophagus from HSV. Note raised borders. In this progressive case, a larger coalescent ulcer is seen. Courtesy of Dr. George MacDonald.

giant cells and intranuclear inclusions. Biopsy specimens should also be sent for viral culture, because this test is more sensitive than histologic examination. An esophagogram may suggest the diagnosis of HSV esophagitis when small superficial ulcers in the midesophagus are present, but the findings are nonspecific.

Therapy. Acyclovir is a nucleoside analog that is a mainstay of therapy for HSV esophagitis; it should be administered for 7–10 days.

Gastric Infections

HELICOBACTER PYLORI

In the past 15–20 years, Warren and Marshall discovered that chronic active gastritis and ulcer disease (duodenal and gastric) are due to a gram-negative, spiral bacterium known as *Helicobacter pylori*. It is a flagellated organism that resides below the mucous layer next to gastric epithelium. *H. pylori* is able to burrow through the mucous layer and attach to epithelia. It also produces urease, an enzyme that breaks down urea to ammonium (NH_4^-) and bicarbonate (HCO_3^-). NH_4^- provides an alkaline environment, which helps the bacterium protect itself from acid injury. HCO_3^- is secreted into the blood and is excreted as carbon dioxide, which can be detected (see Diagnosis). *H. pylori* has been associated with 80% of gastric ulcers and 95% of duodenal ulcers. Prior to this discovery, it was felt that excess acid was the main criterion required for ulcer formation. *H. pylori* infection has been epidemiologically linked to gastric cancer and lymphoma. Infection with this organism is the most common cause of gastritis in humans.

The prevalence of *H. pylori* is directly related to age, lower socioeconomic class, and living in a developing country. For example, more than 60% of children in developing countries are colonized by age 20, whereas those living in industrialized countries are rarely infected by this bacteria. In the Western world, 40%–60% of people are colonized by age 60. Those living in smaller, crowded spaces and those living with infected persons are more likely to acquire *H. pylori*, suggesting person-to-person transmission. There are also racial differences; for example, African Americans are noted to have a significantly higher prevalence of *H. pylori* than white Americans.

Clinical Presentation

The clinical presentation of *H. pylori* infection is quite variable. Most individuals are asymptomatic. A small percentage develop symptoms or complications of a gastric or duodenal ulcer, such as intractable pain, bleeding, or ulcers, and others do not. The organism may alter host defense mechanisms, such as mucosal HCO_3^- secretion, or it may stimulate postprandial gastrin secretion, rendering the patient susceptible to ulcer disease. Persons with acute *H. pylori* infection may present with symptomatic gastritis.

Diagnosis

H. pylori can be diagnosed by either invasive or noninvasive methods.

Antibodies to *H. pylori* immunoglobulin G (IgG) can be detected in the serum; however, its presence does not necessarily indicate an active infection. IgG antibody titers may decrease over time (6–12 months) in patients who have been successfully treated.

The urea breath test is a noninvasive test that detects radiolabeled carbon dioxide excreted in the breath of persons with *H. pylori* infection because orally administered urea is hydrolyzed to carbon dioxide and NH_4^- in the presence of urease. This test is commonly used to document success of therapy after treatment.

Endoscopy is required to obtain biopsy specimens. The rapid urease test involves placing a biopsy specimen from the stomach on a test medium that contains urea. The urea is hydrolyzed by urease, and the NH_4^- formed increases the pH, which is manifested by a color change in the medium. The sensitivity of the test is 70%–90%. Microscopic examination of the tissue obtained by biopsy is another method by which the diagnosis of *H. pylori* infection of the stomach can be made. The typical histologic appearance of *H. pylori* gastritis is characterized by inflammatory infiltrate with mononuclear cells, neutrophils, and occasionally eosinophils in the surface and foveolar epithelia. Routine hematoxylin and eosin staining may be adequate in identifying the organism epithelia, but special stains are often used to help detect the presence of *H. pylori* (Figure 17-2). The bacteria may be seen lining the surface epithelium. The sensitivity for histologic examination is 70%–90%. Culture for *H. pylori* is insensitive and unnecessary, as other less time-consuming and more sensitive methods for detection are available. Stool analysis for *H. pylori* is also available.

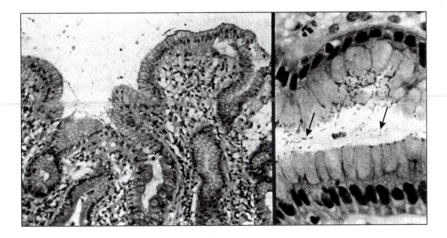

Fig. 17-2.

This photomicrograph shows gastritis with a mononuclear and neutrophilic inflammatory infiltrate (left). The higher power view (right) shows Helicobacter pylori organisms (arrows) on the surface epithelium of the gastric mucosa. Courtesy of Dr. Robert Genta.

Therapy

Elimination of the organism has been clearly shown to reduce the recurrence rate of ulcers dramatically.

Presently, antibiotics combined with either H_2 antagonists or proton pump inhibitors (PPIs) are the mainstays of therapy for *H. pylori*. See Chapter 10.

TREPONEMA PALLIDUM

Gastric syphilis is caused by infection with *Treponema pallidum*. Symptomatic gastritis occurs in less than 1% of patients with secondary or tertiary syphilis. This underestimates the true prevalence of syphilitic gastritis, as most patients are asymptomatic. The incidence of syphilis has increased since 1977 after a steady decline since 1943.

Clinical Presentation

Most patients with endoscopic evidence of syphilitic gastritis are asymptomatic. Symptomatic patients often have skin manifestations of secondary syphilis. Common GI symptoms are epigastric pain, nausea, and vomiting, as well as weight loss.

Diagnosis

Syphilitic gastritis should be suspected in any patient with syphilis and GI symptoms. The diagnosis can be made when three criteria are met: presence of gastric mucosal lesions, serologic evidence of active syphilitic infection, or *T. pallidum* in a mucosal biopsy specimen. On endoscopy, secondary syphilis of the stomach appears as erosive gastritis. Lesions of tertiary syphilis (gummas) in the stomach appear as masslike or infiltrating lesions and are almost indistinguishable from gastric carcinoma. Histologic evaluation requires that a pathologist be aware of the possibility of syphilis as the diagnosis because special stains are required.

Therapy

Penicillin is the treatment of choice for gastric syphilis. For penicillin-allergic patients, doxycycline is an adequate alternative.

Infections of the Small Intestine

IMMUNOCOMPETENT HOSTS

Viral Gastroenteritis

Viral gastroenteritis is the most common GI disease worldwide. It is a significant cause of morbidity and mortality in developing countries, especially among young children. In a 1-year period from 1977 to 1978, 5–10 million deaths from diarrhea occurred in Africa, Asia, and Latin America. In developed countries, viral gastroenteritis is an important cause of morbidity. In the Cleveland Family Study, it accounted for 16% of 25,000 illnesses over a 10-year period. Most cases of viral gastroenteritis are self-limited and require only oral rehydration.

Worldwide, rotavirus is the most common infectious cause of diarrhea in young children. Generally it is seen in children under 2 years of age. Rotavirus, like other pathogens transmitted by the fecal–oral route, spreads most easily in crowded areas with poor hygiene. Outbreaks have occurred on pediatric hospital wards and in day care centers. Adults may develop rotavirus diarrhea; however, the disease is most often mild or even asymptomatic.

Adenovirus is the second most common cause of viral diarrhea in children. Worldwide it is seen typically in children under 2 years of age. Transmission occurs by the fecal–oral route. Like rotavirus, adenovirus occurs commonly in day care centers.

Norwalk virus infection is a common cause of diarrhea in all age groups. The virus is transmitted by the fecal–oral route. It is highly infectious and has an attack rate of 50%. Infection with this virus is seen worldwide. Outbreaks are frequently attributed to contaminated water or food and can be seen in nursing homes, day care centers, and cruise ships.

Clinical Presentation. The most common presenting features of rotavirus infection are vomiting, diarrhea, and dehydration. Rarely, patients may develop necrotizing enterocolitis or hemorrhagic gastroenteritis. The condition is usually self-limited; however, a small percentage of patients, usually in developing countries, die from dehydration.

Adenovirus infection is characterized by watery diarrhea, occasionally accompanied by fever, vomiting, and dehydration. Diarrhea may occasionally last longer than 2 weeks in some patients. In immunocompromised patients, adenovirus may cause a severe enteritis, which can be fatal.

Norwalk virus infection is characterized by watery diarrhea accompanied by vomiting. Patients may also have abdominal pain and fever. The illness is usually mild and resolves in 1–2 days.

Diagnosis. Detection of the rotavirus in the stool establishes the diagnosis. Gel electrophoresis, enzyme immunoassay, latex agglutination, and polymerase chain reaction (PCR) are the techniques most often used to detect rotavirus. Adenovirus may be detected in the stool by enzyme-linked immunosorbent assay (ELISA), electron microscopy, or latex agglutination. Norwalk is detected by radioimmunoassay, ELISA, and electron microscopy. Most of these techniques are not used clinically.

Therapy. Treatment of viral gastroenteritis focuses on oral rehydration. In severe cases, intravenous hydration is necessary. Most often the condition is self-limited. Immunodeficient children with chronic rotavirus infection have been successfully treated with milk containing rotavirus antibodies. Antidiarrheal medications and bismuth salts may help reduce the volume of diarrhea. Measures such as hand washing should also be undertaken to limit transmission in high-risk settings, such as hospitals and day care centers.

Cholera

Vibrio cholerae can cause a severe diarrhea that may lead to rapid dehydration and death in less than a day. Infection primarily occurs in Africa and Asia; however, an increasing incidence has been noted in Central and South America. Transmission is by the fecal–oral route and via contaminated food and water. Cholera infection in North America occurs in tourists who acquire the bacteria while traveling to endemic areas. Epidemics in Latin America have been related to contaminated seafood.

The main virulence factor of *V. cholerae* is cholera toxin. The toxin binds to epithelial cells and stimulates the production of cAMP via adenylate cyclase. This in turn leads to the release of chloride (Cl^-) from the epithelial cells. Cl^- release is followed by sodium (Na^+) and water secretion, which leads to the large-volume diarrhea.

Recognized risk factors for acquiring cholera include low gastric acidity as a result of surgery, H_2 blockers, or atrophic gastritis. Children in endemic areas between the ages of 2 and 15 who have not been exposed to the bacterium are at risk. It appears that prior exposure may confer lifetime immunity.

Clinical Presentation. Most individuals with *V. cholerae* infection are asymptomatic or have mild infection that is indistinguishable from other causes of infectious diarrhea. However, some develop severe infection (cholera gravis) characterized by vomiting, voluminous diarrhea up to 1 L/hr, electrolyte imbalance, and dehydration leading to shock and death. Some may present with mild disease that can lead to massive diarrhea and death within hours. Fever and abdominal pain are not seen in cholera infection.

Diagnosis. The diagnosis of cholera infection can be made by examination of the stool by dark-field microscopy. Gram stain may reveal sheets of gram-negative organisms. Direct plating of stool specimen on selective culture media such as thiosulfate citrate–bile salts–sucrose is sufficient to isolate the organism. Rapid laboratory diagnosis can be made by agglutination of organisms in stool with cholera antisera and fluorescent antibody techniques.

Therapy. Therapy consists of rehydration and correction of electrolyte abnormalities as the mainstays of therapy. Antimicrobials may reduce stool volume and shorten the duration of disease. Tetracycline, doxycycline, fluoroquinolones, trimethoprim-sulfamethoxazole, and chloramphenicol are efficacious.

Giardia lamblia

Giardiasis is the most common waterborne pathogenic intestinal protozoan disease in the United States. It is seen worldwide and is most prevalent in areas with poor sanitation. In developed countries, campers and backpackers who drink untreated water can develop

Giardia infection. Transmission may also occur between homosexual males as a result of oral–anal sexual practices and in day care centers and institutions by fecal–oral spread.

When ingested, *G. lamblia* cysts enter the duodenum and transform into trophozoites. Bile salts and lipids promote the growth and multiplication of the organisms. They then colonize the upper small bowel and attach to (but do not invade) the epithelial lining. The pathogenesis of diarrhea in patients with giardiasis is not well understood. Hypotheses include decrease in diasaccharidase activity and impaired mucosal absorptive function. Bile salt deconjugation does not likely play a role in diarrhea and malabsorption. It is plausible that *G. lamblia* provides a mechanical barrier to absorption.

Clinical Presentation. The clinical spectrum of *Giardia* infection varies from asymptomatic colonization to severe chronic diarrhea. Most patients present with mild, watery diarrhea. The acute clinical syndrome may last for several months, and some patients can develop malabsorption and steatorrhea. Stools may be foul-smelling and greasy. Other symptoms include cramping epigastric pain, weight loss, anorexia, nausea, flatulence, and belching.

Diagnosis. The clinical manifestations are nonspecific. The diagnosis is established by detection of *G. lamblia* trophozoites or cysts in stool (Figure 17-3). Techniques allow for detection of particular *Giardia* antigens in the stool. Diagnosis may also be made by detection of organisms on duodenal fluid aspiration or biopsy. Serologic tests are usually not beneficial as patients in endemic areas may have antibodies without clinical infection.

Therapy. Metronidazole is the treatment for *Giardia* infection. Furazolidone is often used in children because it is available in suspension form.

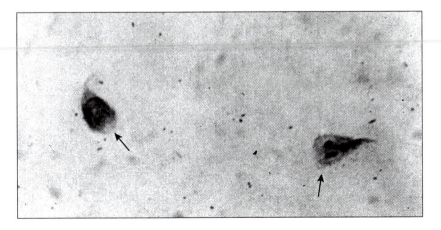

Fig. 17-3. *Giardia lamblia*

Trophozoite forms of *G. lamblia* are shown by the arrows.

IMMUNOCOMPROMISED HOSTS

Cryptosporidium

Cryptosporidia are protozoal parasites that are found worldwide. They can cause significant morbidity and mortality in immunocompromised hosts, particularly those with AIDS. Immunocompetent patients often have a mild, self-limited course. *Cryptosporidium* infection has been linked to a waterborne outbreak of diarrheal disease in Wisconsin in 1993, where over 400,000 cases were reported in a 2-month period. *Cryptosporidium* has also been linked to outbreaks in day care centers and crowded urban settings. Calves are a reservoir of *Cryptosporidium*, and up to 44% of dairy farmers in one study had serologic evidence of prior infection. Household cats and dogs, rodents, and sheep are other reservoirs of infection.

Clinical Presentation. The predominant symptom is watery diarrhea, often accompanied by cramps. Diarrheal volumes average 2–3 L/d, but volumes greater than 10 L/d have been reported. Prolonged infection may lead to malabsorption. Abdominal pain, nausea, vomiting, and weight loss may also be prominent findings. In AIDS patients, prolonged diarrhea may lead to severe dehydration, electrolyte imbalance, and even death.

Diagnosis. The diagnosis of *Cryptosporidium* infection is made by stool examination. A modified acid-fast stain colors the organisms red. Serologic tests are not useful in establishing the diagnosis in an acute infection.

Therapy. Supportive measures remain the mainstay of therapy for persons with chronic diarrhea. Fluid replacement and correction of electrolyte abnormalities are essential. Antimotility agents such as loperamide and diphenoxylate with atropine may be helpful in reducing diarrheal volumes. Octreotide, a somatostatin analog, may also reduce diarrheal volumes. Drug therapy against *Cryptosporidium* infection has generally been disappointing. Spiramycin appears to be effective in only a minority of infected patients. Paromomycin and other medications may show some promise.

Microsporida

Microsporida are obligate intracellular protozoa that commonly cause diarrhea in patients with AIDS, especially in those with CD4 counts of less than 100. The incidence of microsporida infection in this group varies from 6% to 50%. There is a single report of microsporida infection in an immunocompetent host. Microsporida infection occurs worldwide and is likely transmitted via contaminated food and water as well as the fecal–oral route. *Enterocytozoon bieneusi* and *Septata intestinalis* are the primary disease-producing microsporidian species.

Clinical Presentation. Diarrhea is the most common clinical manifestation of infection with microsporida. It is frequently accompanied by bloating, dehydration, and weight loss. Fever is not a common finding. Weight loss and wasting may be due to malabsorption. A minority of infected individuals may harbor microsporida without symptoms.

Diagnosis. Examination of a stool sample with a modified trichrome stain may quickly lead to the diagnosis of microsporida infection. Light microscopy of an endoscopic biopsy specimen may identify the organism in the enterocyte. There may also be villus atrophy and crypt hyperplasia. Electron microscopy is the gold standard for establishing the diagnosis; however, it is not widely available.

Therapy. Therapeutic options for microsporida infection are limited. Those infected with *S. intestinalis* have been reported to have excellent responses to albendazole. No effective treatment has been found for *E. bieneusi*, although albendazole may reduce the frequency or severity of diarrhea in some.

Isospora belli

Isospora belli, like *Cryptosporidium parvum*, is an intestinal protozoan parasite that can cause severe diarrhea in immunocompromised hosts. Infection with *I. belli* can occur worldwide; however, it is most common in tropical regions, such as Haiti, South America, Africa, and Southeast Asia. The organism is acquired by ingestion of fecally contaminated food or water. Direct person-to-person transmission has occurred, but it is uncommon.

Clinical Presentation. Isosporiasis resembles both *Cryptosporidium* and *G. lamblia* infection. Diarrhea is the predominant complaint, which may be accompanied by abdominal pain, nausea, vomiting, fever, and weight loss. Eosinophilia is also often present. Dehydration, electrolyte imbalance, and weight loss due to prolonged diarrhea may lead to death in patients with AIDS.

Diagnosis. Examination of stool samples for oocytes or modified acid-fast staining may provide the diagnosis. Multiple samples may be required (at least three) to establish the diagnosis. Acid-fast stains of mucosal biopsy specimens of the small intestine may identify the organism.

Therapy. *I. belli* responds readily to antibiotics. Trimethoprim-sulfamethoxazole is the drug of choice. Patients with AIDS require maintenance therapy to prevent recurrence.

Infections of the Large Intestine: Infectious Colitis

The most common symptoms of colitis are abdominal pain and diarrhea (which may be bloody). Nausea, vomiting, fever, chills, and cramps may also be seen in patients with colitis. Infectious-type colitis (or acute self-limited colitis) must be distinguished from inflammatory bowel disease (IBD; Crohn's or ulcerative colitis) because therapies and prognoses differ drastically. Acute self-limited colitis

Patients with colitis tend to have frequent, small-volume stools; in contrast, small bowel infections cause large-volume diarrhea.

generally presents and resolves in less than 4 weeks. IBD usually has a more insidious onset. Other clues suggesting infection include a history of recent travel, ingestion of certain foods, similar symptoms in close contacts, and recent use of antibiotics.

Bacteria and less frequently parasites cause infectious colitis. Many of the organisms causing infectious colitis in immunocompetent hosts also cause colitis in immunosuppressed patients, but infections may be more severe or protracted in the latter. Fungi and viruses generally cause colitis only in immunocompromised hosts (Figures 17-4 and 17-5).

IMMUNOCOMPETENT HOSTS

Shigella

Shigella infection occurs worldwide and is an important cause of diarrhea in developing nations. In developed countries, *Shigella* is uncommon; however, since the 1980s, the number of reported cases has increased. *Shigella* has the ability to survive the acidic environment of the stomach, and this likely contributes to the low number of organisms needed to cause infection. As few as 10 ingested organisms can cause disease. *Shigella* infection has a tendency to occur in epidemics. Infections are most common in young children (1–4 years of age), homosexual men, travelers, and individuals in institutions. Person-to-person spread is the most important mode of transmission. Foodborne outbreaks and contaminated water sources have also been identified.

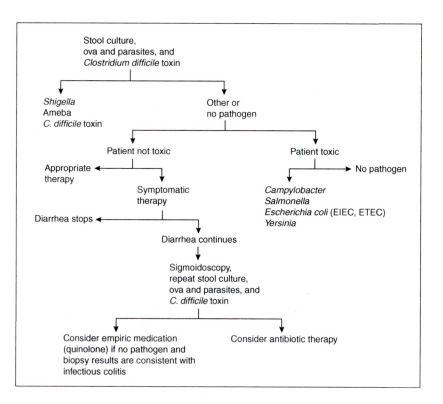

Fig. 17-4. Algorithm for Evaluation of Colitis (Immunocompetent Host)

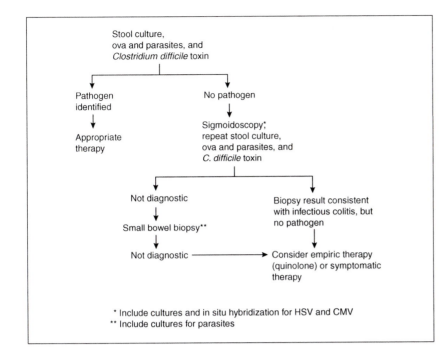

**Fig. 17-5. Algorithm for Evaluation of Colitis
(Immunocompromised Host)**

Human infection can result from one of four species: *S. dysenteriae*, *S. flexneri*, *S. boydii*, and *S. sonnei*. The virulence of *Shigella* is due to tissue invasion and toxin production. First, the bacteria invade superficial epithelial cells, causing cell death. Tissue invasion may be the reason for the intense inflammatory response and high fevers. Shiga toxin is released from *S. dysenteriae* and has several effects that could augment the symptoms caused by tissue invasion. It can inhibit protein synthesis in eukaryotic cells by cleaving the 60S ribosomal subunit. The toxin can kill colonic epithelial cells and cause fluid secretion from the ileum.

Clinical Presentation. The presentation of shigellosis varies according to species. *S. sonnei* usually causes a self-limited diarrhea. *S. dysenteriae* and *S. flexneri* produce a dysenteric illness. Patients often have fever, malaise, abdominal cramps, and a secretory diarrhea for 1–2 days followed by bloody diarrhea. Tenesmus and systemic toxicity may accompany the bloody diarrhea. In children, systemic toxicity can be seen as seizures, delirium, or obtundation. In severe cases, toxic megacolon and perforation can occur. Obstruction is rare, but when it is present, mortality is increased. Shigellosis may also be associated with hemolytic uremic syndrome. Untreated infection lasts about 1 week, although this can vary from 1 to 30 days. Most mortality from shigellosis is seen in children under 15 years of age and is primarily due to dehydration.

Diagnosis. Stool culture is the primary means of diagnosing *Shigella*. It is nonlactose-fermenting and can be grown on MacConkey agar as well as *Salmonella-Shigella* agar. Fecal leukocytes may be seen, but their absence does not exclude *Shigella* infection.

Therapy. Shigellosis is among the few bacterial diarrheas in which antibiotic therapy is of unequivocal benefit. Antibiotics reduce the duration of disease and reduce fecal excretion in convalescence. Fluoroquinolones are the preferred drugs to treat shigellosis; however, resistance has increased. Trimethoprim-sulfamethoxazole, ampicillin, and the tetracyclines are also effective. Children and pregnant women should not receive tetracycline because of the risk of tooth discoloration, and quinolones should be avoided because of potential osteotoxicity in this group. Supportive therapy (such as fluid replacement and reversal of malnutrition) is also important.

Campylobacter

Campylobacter species are a major cause of infectious diarrhea in the United States. The species that cause diarrhea are *C. fetus*, *C. intestinalis*, *C. veneralis*, and *C. jejuni*. *C. jejuni* is transmitted by the fecal–oral route or by contaminated milk, poultry, eggs, or water. *Campylobacter* infection has a peak incidence in preschool children and a second peak in young adults. It causes tissue injury in the jejunum, ileum, and colon by invasion of epithelial cells. Virulence mechanisms of these bacteria are not well defined.

Clinical Presentation. *Campylobacter* usually causes watery or bloody diarrhea accompanied by nausea, anorexia, or cramping. Headache, myalgia, or fever (up to 104°F) may precede the diarrhea. The incubation period is 2–4 days. Symptoms usually last 1–7 days.

Diagnosis. Stool cultures are necessary to make the diagnosis. Blood cultures should be obtained from patients at risk for bacteremia or with persistent fever at the time of positive stool cultures. On sigmoidoscopy, edema, erythema, ulcers, and friability may be visualized. On biopsy, colitis with neutrophilic infiltration of the epithelium may be seen. These findings are not specific to infection caused by *Campylobacter*.

Therapy. Treatment is recommended for patients with severe enterocolitis lasting more than 1 week. Erythromycin, tetracyclines, and quinolones are effective therapies. Antibiotics may hasten clearance from the stool. Patients with *Campylobacter* bacteremia should be treated with two parenteral antibiotics until susceptibilities are known. Gentamicin or a third-generation cephalosporin can be given along with erythromycin. It is recommended that patients have confirmed clearance of *Campylobacter* from the stool prior to returning to group settings.

Salmonella

Salmonella is an increasingly common cause of diarrhea in industrialized nations. There are over 2000 serotypes of *Salmonella*, which can be divided into three groups. Group 1 consists of *S. typhimurium, S. enteritidis, S. heidelberg,* and *S. newport;* group 2: *S. choleraesuis;* and group 3: *S. typhi. S. typhi* causes typhoid fever and infects only humans. *S. choleraesuis* and group 1 *Salmonella* can infect both humans and animals.

Transmission of *Salmonella* species is from contaminated water and food (especially poultry and eggs and sometimes beef, dairy products, and pork). Infection from infected food handlers is uncommon. Infection is seen most commonly in children under 5 years of age.

Colonization in the GI tract occurs after the ingestion of a large number of organisms. *Salmonella* can invade ileal M cells and then penetrate into Peyer's patches. *Salmonella* may be phagocytosed by monocytes and then, depending on the strain and host, disseminate to various sites.

Clinical Presentation. *Salmonella* most often presents with non-bloody diarrhea. Diarrheal volume may be quite large. Diarrhea may be preceded by nausea, vomiting, myalgias, headache, and abdominal pain. Some patients develop bloody diarrhea associated with fever, tenesmus, and small-volume diarrhea. Bacteremia occurs in a small percentage of cases; it is often self-limited and without extraintestinal seeding.

Extraintestinal seeding occurs most often in children under 3 months of age. Meningitis is the most severe complication of *Salmonella* infection. Other potential sites of infection include the biliary tree, liver, spleen, heart (endocarditis and pericarditis), and urinary tract. A reactive arthritis may occur in HLA-B27-positive persons; urethritis or conjunctivitis may accompany the reactive arthritis. Osteomyelitis, osteoarthritis, and arteritis are other complications of *Salmonella* infection.

Diagnosis. The diagnosis can be established by culturing the appropriate body substance. Stool cultures are the appropriate initial step in the evaluation. Blood cultures should be checked in immuno-compromised patients and those under 6 months of age. Once *Salmonella* is isolated, it is important to determine if the isolate is *S. typhi* because antibiotics are efficacious in its treatment.

Therapy. Antibiotic use in *Salmonella* infection is controversial because it may prolong the carrier state and has not been shown to reduce the duration and symptoms of infection. Those in whom the risk of extraintestinal disease is greater than being a carrier, such as those with cancer, AIDS, hemoglobinopathies, and children under 6 months of age, should be treated with antibiotics. *S. typhi* and *S. choleraesuis* should always be treated.

Trimethoprim-sulfamethoxazole and quinolones appear to be the most effective antibiotics. It has been recommended that children under 6 months of age receive amoxicillin if they are carriers because of the risk of developing meningitis. Patients with severe *S. typhi* infection may benefit from high-dose dexamethasone therapy.

Notes

A *Salmonella* carrier state may develop in some people. It may last up to 12 weeks in children under 5 years of age and up to several years in adults.

Notes

Outbreaks of *E. coli* 0157:H7 have been traced to unpasteurized milk and juices and undercooked ground beef.

Escherichia coli

There are five groups of *Escherichia coli* that can cause diarrhea. Three affect the small bowel: enteroadherent, enteropathogenic, and enterotoxigenic *E. coli*. Two others affect the colon: enteroinvasive and enterohemorrhagic *E. coli* 0157:H7.

Enteroinvasive *E. coli* (EIEC) produces signs and symptoms clinically indistinguishable from *Shigella*. The main pathogenetic mechanism of EIEC is its ability to invade epithelial cells. The clinical presentation is essentially the same as *Shigella*, with fever and small-volume bloody diarrhea with fecal leukocytes. The diagnosis should be considered in individuals who present with a syndrome of bloody diarrhea in whom a culture is negative. It is unknown if antibiotics alter the clinical course.

E. coli *0157:H7*

Outbreaks of this organism have made it a well-known cause of bloody diarrhea. It was first recognized in 1982. Infection occurs most frequently in children under 5 years of age. Cattle are a reservoir for this organism. *E. coli* 0157:H7 has been isolated in beef, poultry, and pork. The organism can be transmitted from person to person as well as in water. Most cases of *E. coli* 0157:H7 occur sporadically. The organism causes disease by releasing a toxin (verotoxin I or II) similar to Shiga toxin.

Clinical Presentation. Infection with *E. coli* 0157:H7 can cause several different clinical syndromes. Typically, patients have crampy abdominal pain and bloody diarrhea. Fever is not a prominent symptom. The clinical picture mimics ischemic colitis when seen in elderly patients. It simulates IBD or intussusception when seen in children. Infection with *E. coli* 0157:H7 has been associated with hemolytic uremic syndrome (HUS), a microangiopathic hemolytic anemia with low numbers of platelets and renal failure.

Diagnosis. *E. coli* 0157:H7 is not usually isolated on routine culture; therefore, a specific request must be made to look for this organism. It can be isolated on MacConkey sorbitol agar medium. *E. coli* 0157:H7 can be identified by immunofluorescence or rapid particle latex agglutination.

Colonoscopy and biopsy help in the diagnosis if cultures are negative. The mucosal findings of edema, erythema, and friability are nonspecific and can mimic ischemia. Histologically, there is preservation of normal architecture with acute inflammatory changes that distinguish it from IBD, where there is architectural distortion in the crypts.

Therapy. Although *E. coli* 0157:H7 is sensitive to most antibiotics, it is unclear if they alter the clinical course of the disease or prevent the development of HUS.

Clostridium difficile

Clostridium difficile is the most common cause of hospital-acquired diarrhea. It has been associated with outbreaks in nursing homes and rehabilitation centers. Acquisition of *C. difficile* is most commonly associated with antibiotic use; however, patients receiving chemotherapy for cancer and others not receiving antibiotics can develop infection. Any antibiotic can cause *C. difficile* diarrhea. Other predisposing factors include extended hospitalization, older age, and surgery.

The main virulence factors for *C. difficile* infection are an enterotoxin (toxin A) and a cytotoxin (toxin B). Toxin A causes injury by direct epithelial cell damage and recruitment of inflammatory cells and causes a hemorrhagic exudate. Toxin A can also induce intestinal fluid secretion. Toxin B works synergistically with toxin A and causes cytopathic effects on epithelial cells.

Clinical Presentation. The spectrum of disease with *C. difficile* infection varies from asymptomatic carriage to fulminant colitis with toxic megacolon and perforation. Patients may have watery diarrhea with few other symptoms. More severe cases are associated with dehydration, fever, abdominal pain, tenderness, leukocytosis, and bloody diarrhea. Patients may present with *C. difficile* infection up to 8 weeks after the end of a course of antibiotics.

Diagnosis. The diagnosis of *C. difficile* should be suspected in hospitalized patients and those receiving antibiotics who develop diarrhea. The diagnosis is made by detection of the cytotoxin in the stool. A rapid latex agglutination test is available but detects other clostridial antigens and is not specific for toxin. It can be used as a rapid screen. Enzyme immunoassays for toxin A and toxin B provide a rapid alternative to classic cytotoxicity assays.

Diagnostic pseudomembranes can easily be visualized on sigmoidoscopy. A minority of patients may have isolated right colon disease that would be missed on sigmoidoscopy.

Therapy. The initial treatment should be discontinuation of the offending antibiotic. The two most commonly used antibiotics for treating *C. difficile* infection are oral metronidazole (500 mg four times a day) and oral vancomycin (125 mg four times a day) for 10 days. If the patient cannot take the medicine orally because of ileus, vancomycin can be given by nasogastric tube or enemas, and intravenous metronidazole (500 mg every 6–8 hours) can be added. Asymptomatic carriers do not require therapy. Treating patients with *Saccharomyces boulardii* is of interest because it seems to inhibit the effects of toxins A and B on the human colonic mucosa.

Yersinia

Yersinia enterocolitica and *Y. pseudotuberculosis* can cause acute or chronic colitis in humans. Infection is often seen in Northern Europe, but it is uncommon in North America. *Yersinia* is most frequently found in contaminated milk, water, and pork. Clinically, infection may present as ileitis and mesenteric lymphadenitis (pseudoappendicitis syndrome) and may mimic appendicitis or Crohn's disease.

Yersinia has the ability to invade epithelia. It also has the ability to resist phagocytosis and lysis mediated by complement.

Clinical Presentation. Abdominal pain, fever, and diarrhea are the most common presenting symptoms of *Yersinia* infection. The pain may occur in the right lower quadrant, simulating acute appendicitis or Crohn's disease. Extraintestinal manifestations include pharyngitis, arthralgia, and erythema nodosum. Bacteremia may occur, especially in patients with chronic liver disease, diabetes, and malnutrition.

Diagnosis. The organism can be cultured from stool, but a special cold-enrichment technique is necessary. Blood and suppurative mesenteric nodes seen at laparotomy should be cultured. Colonoscopic features include aphthoid ulcers; ileoscopy reveals edema, ulcers, and round elevations of the mucosa. Serologic tests with elevated titers may be useful in the appropriate clinical setting.

Therapy. *Yersinia* species are susceptible to tetracyclines, trimethoprim-sulfamethoxazole, third-generation cephalosporins, fluoroquinolones, and chloramphenicol. Resistance is seen against first-generation cephalosporins, penicillin, and ampicillin and is mediated by β-lactamases. Persons with bacteremia should be treated with two antibiotics.

IMMUNOCOMPROMISED HOSTS

Mycobacterium avium *Complex (MAC)*

MAC is a common cause of diarrheal disease in AIDS patients. It is likely acquired through the ingestion of contaminated water. On entering the body, the bacteria are quickly phagocytosed by macrophages, which are unable to lyse the organism. The infected macrophages may infiltrate tissues, especially in the abdomen, stimulate cytokine release, and cause clinical disease.

Clinical Presentation. The clinical presentation is characterized by diarrhea, fever, and progressive wasting. Severe fatigue, abdominal pain, and organomegaly may also be present. Malnutrition likely results from some degree of malabsorption, anorexia, and metabolic derangements. Many patients may become bacteremic after GI infection. The disease is usually seen late in the course of AIDS when the CD4 count is extremely low (< 50).

Diagnosis. The diagnosis is usually established by blood culture or mucosal biopsy. Stool examination by culture or acid-fast stain may reveal MAC, but the clinical significance of this finding is unknown. Blood culture is sensitive and may detect infection prior to the onset of symptoms.

Therapy. MAC tends to be more resistant to antibiotics than *M. tuberculosis*. Most therapeutic regimens rely on combinations of antibiotics including macrolides, fluoroquinolones, rifabutin, rifampin, ethambutol, and aminoglycosides.

Infections of the Large Intestine: Parasites

Immunocompetent Hosts

Entamoeba histolytica

Entamoeba histolytica is a protozoan parasite that causes amebiasis. It is a commonly isolated pathogen in diarrheal disease and is the third leading parasitic cause of death. Most of the severe cases are found in developing countries in Africa, India, and Central and South America. Pregnant women, people on steroids, the elderly, and very young people tend to have more severe clinical manifestations. The organism is acquired by ingestion of fecally contaminated food or water or by oral–anal sexual contact. Primates and humans are the only known reservoirs of disease.

Infection is initiated by the ingestion of amebic cysts. The cysts reach the small bowel and release eight trophozoite forms, which colonize the colon. Trophozoites produce adhesive molecules that augment attachment to epithelial cells. They also produce proteases and collagenases that help mediate epithelial injury.

E. histolytica is the only pathogenic ameba. Other nonpathogenic strains include *E. coli*, *E. hartmanii*, *Endolimax nana*, and *Iodamoeba buetschlii*. Isolation of nonpathogenic strains in stool does not require treatment.

Clinical Presentation. *E. histolytica* can cause a variety of conditions, ranging from asymptomatic carriage to amebic peritonitis secondary to perforation. Acute proctocolitis is characterized by bloody diarrhea and abdominal pain and occasionally by fever and weight loss. Some people may develop chronic nondysenteric disease, which may simulate ulcerative colitis. Others with focal disease may develop a stricture and symptoms of obstruction. A small percentage of people with amebic colitis may develop a mass of granulation tissue in the cecum or ascending colon called an *ameboma*. Toxic megacolon is a rare but serious complication of amebic colitis and is characterized by fever, abdominal pain with peritonitis, tachycardia, and fever.

Diagnosis. Three separate stool specimens should be collected as part of the initial workup of suspected amebic colitis. A wet preparation of a fresh stool specimen (< 30 min old) should be performed as well as a formalin-ethyl acetate concentration step to identify cysts. Barium, bismuth, castor oil, and hypertonic and soapsud enemas can interfere with the ability to detect *E. histolytica* in the stool and should be avoided until a stool specimen has been collected.

Colonoscopy is an important tool in diagnosing amebic colitis. Sigmoidoscopy may miss isolated disease in the cecum and ascending colon. Ulcers with raised edges may be seen, and biopsy tissue should be taken from the edges. Radiologic findings are nonspecific. Toxic megacolon, however, is clearly seen on abdominal x-ray.

Therapy.   Therapy is based on the severity of the clinical manifestation. Patients with asymptomatic infection should probably not receive antibiotics to limit the spread of the organism. Patients with amebic dysentery should be treated with metronidazole (750 mg three times a day for 10 days) with or followed by iodoquinol (650 mg three times a day for 20 days). Patients with perforation or toxic megacolon should be started on intravenous metronidazole while awaiting surgical evaluation.

Schistosomiasis

Schistosomiasis, one of the world's most prevalent infectious diseases, has affected 200 million people. Most cases in humans are caused by *Schistosoma haematobium*, *S. japonicum*, and *S. mansoni*. *S. haematobium* is endemic to Africa and the Middle East. *S. japonicum* is seen exclusively in Asia, specifically along river basins in China. *S. mansoni* is prevalent in Africa and is the only cause of schistosomiasis seen in the Western Hemisphere—Brazil, West Indies, and Puerto Rico. In endemic areas, the prevalence of disease is highest between the ages of 15 and 20 years. Beyond age 30, the prevalence may fall. People from nonendemic areas acquire the infection while traveling to endemic areas, where they come into contact with freshwater sites.

The life cycle of most schistosomes is very similar. Eggs are passed from urine and stool into water, where they hatch. Larvae called miracidia then penetrate snails and multiply and develop into sporocysts. These emerge from snails as cercariae. The cercariae then penetrate human skin, enter veins, and implant into various tissues. The organisms lay eggs, some of which reach the intestinal lumen and are released in the stool, thus completing the life cycle.

Clinical Presentation.   Initial penetration through the skin does not usually cause symptoms; however, in some cases a mild pruritic dermatitis may occur. Approximately 4–10 weeks after initial exposure some patients may develop a serum sickness–like condition characterized by fever, chills, nausea, vomiting, abdominal pain, diarrhea, headache, and cough. Hepatomegaly and lymphadenopathy may also be seen. This condition (Katayama syndrome) may last up to several months.

Chronic schistosomiasis results from the inflammatory response to the eggs that are released into the intestine or that reach the liver and lungs via the portal and venous systems. The severity of disease depends on the worm burden and the immune response to the eggs. Infection in the intestinal tract may lead to diarrhea with blood or mucus in the stool, abdominal cramps, and fatigue from resulting iron-deficiency anemia. Late in the disease some patients may develop polyps or strictures in the colon. Chronic infection in the liver may lead to cirrhosis and complications of portal hypertension, including esophageal varices and ascites.

Diagnosis. The diagnosis is best established by isolation of the eggs. This may be done by stool examination, either by direct or Kato thick smears. Examination of biopsy material for eggs is also useful. Serologic tests are useful in patients with mild disease when eggs are not easily isolated.

Therapy. Praziquantel is the treatment of choice for all schistosomal species. Oxamniquine is an alternative for patients with *S. mansoni*. Stools should be checked for 3–6 months after therapy; if viable eggs are still being excreted, repeat treatment is indicated.

Infections of the Large Intestine: Viruses

IMMUNOCOMPROMISED HOSTS

CMV

CMV is an uncommon pathogen in immunocompetent patients; however, in immunocompromised hosts it can cause an enteritis or colitis. After an initial exposure, the virus can be reactivated at times of depressed T cell function. Infection most commonly occurs in persons with AIDS, those receiving chemotherapy for hematologic malignancy, or transplant patients.

Clinical Presentation. CMV infection most often occurs in the colon, although small-bowel disease can be seen. If the small bowel is involved, patients may have watery diarrhea and protein-losing enteropathy. Focal colitis may occur and presents as fever, diarrhea, bleeding, and weight loss. Rarely, CMV may produce ulcers in the colon that can perforate.

Diagnosis. Diagnosis of CMV infection is best made by mucosal biopsy. Histologic examination of biopsy specimens may reveal intranuclear inclusions, usually in the vascular endothelial cells in the bases of ulcers. Additional immunohistologic and in situ hybridization techniques as well as PCR may be helpful. Viral culture should also be performed on biopsy specimens.

Therapy. Ganciclovir is the treatment of choice for CMV infection. In ganciclovir-resistant cases, foscarnet is an adequate alternative. Relapse may occur after treatment is discontinued.

HSV

HSV is an uncommon cause of intestinal disease in both immunocompromised and immunocompetent patients. It was seen in gay men before the AIDS epidemic. Complications are most commonly seen in patients with HIV. HSV can cause severe proctitis with anorectal pain, tenesmus, malaise, fever, and rectal discharge that may be bloody. Diagnosis is made by recognition of typical intracellular inclusions or multinucleated giant cells on rectal biopsy. Acyclovir shortens the duration of disease and is the treatment of choice.

Notes

Most immunocompromised patients with CMV infection have serologic evidence of prior exposure to the virus.

CASE STUDY: *RESOLUTION*

The patient presented with several problems—nausea, vomiting, dysphagia, and diarrhea. In individuals with AIDS, these problems may be caused by one process or may have distinct etiologies.

Nausea and vomiting are nonspecific symptoms that have many possible causes. In a person with AIDS who also presents with dysphagia, an infectious process must be placed high on the list of differential diagnoses. The esophagogram demonstrated an ulcer, which could have been due to CMV or HSV. The ulcer might also be related to reflux of acid or be idiopathic. The most likely cause in this patient was CMV because of the associated symptoms of nausea, vomiting, and fever. The only way to prove it is with endoscopy and biopsy of the ulcer. The histologic finding for CMV is intranuclear inclusions in the subepithelial layer. Viral culture of the biopsy specimen is very sensitive in detecting CMV. The treatment of choice is ganciclovir. Foscarnet is an adequate alternative.

Diarrhea in patients with AIDS presents difficult diagnostic challenges for the clinician and causes significant morbidity in those affected. A careful history and physical examination may narrow the spectrum of potential diagnoses. It is important to ask about travel, antibiotic use, and drinking untreated water. The initial test should be evaluation of a stool sample for *C. difficile* toxin, ova and parasites, and culture. If this initial testing is negative, a sigmoidoscopy and upper endoscopy should be considered. In this patient, the key piece of information was the use of antibiotics.

This particular patient had diarrhea resulting from *C. difficile* confirmed by stool culture and toxin B in the stools. CMV also had to be considered because of the low CD4 count. Diagnosis of CMV colitis requires biopsy; a negative stool culture does not exclude this as the diagnosis.

*R*EVIEW *Q*UESTIONS

Directions: For each of the following questions, choose the one best answer.

1 Which of the following statements about *H. pylori* infection is *true*?

   A It is associated with 80% of gastric ulcers and 95% of duodenal ulcers in the absence of NSAIDs.
   B Positive serology indicates the presence of ulcers.
   C Residence in developing countries is not a risk factor for infection.
   D Elimination of the organism has no effect on the recurrence of ulcers.

2 Which of the following statements concerning giardiasis is *true*?

A Serology is the best test to ascertain the diagnosis of *Giardia*.
B Diarrhea is due to mechanical barrier of epithelial cells in the small bowel.
C Organisms may invade epithelial cells.
D The treatment of choice for *Giardia* infection is metronidazole.

3 Which of the following conditions is *rarely* seen in immunocompetent hosts?

A CMV esophagitis
B Schistosomiasis
C *E. coli* 0157:H7 colitis
D Cryptosporidia

4 *C. difficile* diarrhea is associated with which of the following risk factors?

A Radiation therapy
B Antibiotics
C *Shigella* infection
D Contaminated water

5 Antibiotic therapy is not indicated in the treatment of

A *G. lamblia* diarrhea.
B *C. difficile* diarrhea.
C *E. coli* 0157:H7 colitis.
D *Shigella*.

References

Baehr PH, McDonald GB: Esophageal infections: risk factors, presentation, diagnosis and treatment. *Gastroenterology* 106:509–532, 1994.

Butterman JR, Calderwood SB: *Vibrio cholerae 01*. In *Infections of the Gastrointestinal Tract*. Edited by Blaser MJ, Smith PD, Ravdin JI, et al. New York: Raven Press, 1995, p 653.

Cohen J: Infectious diarrhea in human immunodeficiency virus. *Gastroenterol Clin North Am* 30(3):637–664, 2001.

Cover TL, Aber RC: *Yersinia enterocolitica. N Engl J Med* 321:16–24, 1989.

Frierson JG: Colonic parasitic diseases. In *Gastrointestinal and Hepatic Infections*. Edited by Surawicz C, Owen RL. Philadelphia, PA: W. B. Saunders, 1995, pp 267–274.

Goodgame RW: Understanding intestinal spore-forming protozoa: cryptosporidia, microsporidia, isospora and cyclospora. *Ann Intern Med* 124:429–441, 1996.

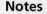
Graham DY, Malaty HM, Evans DG, et al: Epidemiology of *Helicobacter pylori* in an asymptomatic population in the United States: effect of age, race and socioeconomic status. *Gastroenterology* 100:1495–1501, 1991.

Gray JR, Rabeneck L: Atypical mycobacterial infection of the gastrointestinal tract in AIDS patients. *Am J Gastroenterol* 30:497–504, 1989.

Hook EW: *Salmonella* species. In *Principles and Practice of Infectious Disease*. Edited by Mandell GH, Douglas RG, Bennet JE. New York: Churchill Livingstone, 1990, pp 1700–1716.

Ilnyckyj A: Clinical evaluation and management of acute infectious diarrhea in adults. *Gastroenterol Clin North Am* 30(3):599–609, 2001.

Kelly CP, Lamont JT: *Clostridium difficile* colitis. *N Engl J Med* 330:256–262, 1994.

Midthun K, Kapikian AZ: Viral gastroenteritis. In *Gastrointestinal and Hepatic Infections*. Edited by Surawicz C, Owen RL. Philadelphia, PA: W. B. Saunders, 1995, pp 75–90.

NIH Consensus Development Conference: *Helicobacter pylori* in peptic ulcer disease. *J Am Med Assoc* 272:65–69, 1994.

18

Viral Hepatitis

▣ LEARNING OBJECTIVES ▣

At the completion of this chapter, the reader should be able to:
- Distinguish among the major types of viral hepatitis by their clinical course, serologic response to infection, epidemiology, prevention, and management.
- Identify the most likely etiology of the viral hepatitis in a clinical scenario by considering the epidemiologic aspects of transmission as well as understanding the immunologic markers of the different hepatitides.
- Recognize the importance of prevention of the various types of hepatitis viruses, given their limited responses to treatment.

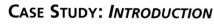

CASE STUDY: *INTRODUCTION*

M.S. was a 35-year-old Pakistani woman who had been living in California for the past 10 years. Her history was significant for intravenous drug use and alcohol abuse. She had a cholecystectomy 3 years previously during which she received two units of packed red blood cells (RBCs). At the time of presentation, she was taking no medicine. Her boyfriend with whom she had had unprotected intercourse, had "some kind of hepatitis." She works on a fishing boat and regularly eats raw fish and oysters from the Pacific Ocean. She had been sent to a gastroenterologist by her primary care physician after complaining of chronic fatigue and abdominal pain of several months' duration.

On examination, her vital signs were normal. She had mild scleral icterus, clear lungs, and a normal heart examination. Her abdominal examination revealed normoactive bowel sounds, a soft and nondistended abdomen, and mild tenderness in the right upper quadrant; the liver span was increased. No spleen was palpable. She had trace peripheral edema.

Laboratory reports from the referring physician revealed the following serum values: aspartate aminotransferase (AST, SGOT), 212 U/L (normal: 0–45 U/L); alanine aminotransferase (ALT, SGPT), 250 U/L (normal: 0–45 U/L); alkaline phosphatase, 168 U/L (normal: 30–110 U/L); lactate dehydrogenase (LDH), 135 U/L (normal: 80–225 U/L); total bilirubin, 3.5 mg/dl (normal: 0.2–1.3 mg/dl); direct bilirubin, 2.5 mg/dl (normal: 0.1– 0.4 mg/dl); and indirect bilirubin, 1.0 mg/dl (normal: 0.1– 0.8 mg/dl).

She revealed to the physician that she was now pregnant and was concerned about passing on "some infectious disease" to her infant.

Introduction

Viral hepatitis can be caused by a variety of infectious agents and afflicts over 500 million people worldwide. Viruses can cause a wide spectrum of systemic manifestations with different immunologic responses. The manifestations of viral hepatitis are varied, ranging from subclinical to chronic disease, often resulting in long-term sequelae.

The pathophysiology of hepatitis A, B, C, D, E, F, and G is reviewed to give a basic understanding of the effect of these viruses on the liver. The viruses vary in their immunologic responses as well as in seriousness of effect and prognosis. Table 18-1 summarizes the differences among these at once similar and diverse viruses.

Hepatitis A

Hepatitis A virus (HAV) is a single-stranded RNA *Enterovirus* of the family Picornaviridae. Transmitted by the fecal–oral route, HAV

Table 18-1. Comparison of Viral Hepatitides

VIRUS	TYPE	MODE OF TRANSMISSION	PROGRESSION TO CIRRHOSIS	NOTES
A	RNA	Fecal–oral	No	Common in milk and dairy products
B	DNA	Blood	Yes	Potentially carcinogenic
C	RNA	Blood	Yes	Most common reason for liver transplantation
D	RNA	Blood	Yes	Dependent on HBV coinfection
E	RNA	Fecal–oral	No	Most dangerous during pregnancy
G	RNA	Blood	?	Unknown relevance

Note: DNA = deoxyribonucleic acid; RNA = ribonucleic acid; HBV = hepatitis B virus.

Notes

The infectious stage of HAV has usually passed by the time the patient seeks medical attention.

causes only acute hepatitis and, with the exception of triggering auto-immune hepatitis, is not associated with chronic liver disease. Several major strains have been identified throughout the world, with only minor differences noted in their nucleotide and amino acid sequences. Of all the hepatitis viruses, only HAV has been cultured in vitro (Figure 18-1).

Humans are the primary host of HAV. It has been found in hepatocytes, blood, bile, and feces of infected individuals. However, the virus is rarely detected, given its transient viremia. The major risk of transmission occurs when the virus is shed in the feces. This generally occurs during the incubation period before symptoms are present, sometimes as early as 1–2 weeks after the host's exposure to the virus. By the time the infected individual seeks medical attention, he or she is usually no longer infective, and little if any fecal excretion is present.

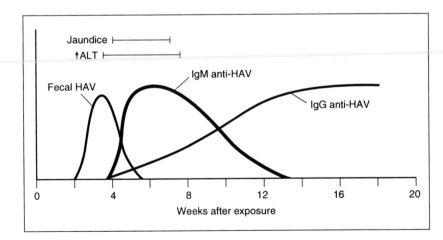

Fig. 18-1. Clinical Course of HAV Infection after Exposure

ALT = alanine aminotransferase; IgM anti-HAV = immunoglobulin M against HAV; IgG anti-HAV = immunoglobulin G against HAV.

Notes

Shellfish and fresh vegetables grown with night soil as a fertilizer are often implicated in HAV infection.

MARKERS

The best serologic marker for disease is detection of the humoral immune response (anti-HAV) by ELISA (enzyme-linked immunosorbent assay). The body's first response, immunoglobulin M (IgM) anti-HAV, is predominant for at least 3 months after onset. It can persist for as long as 12 months. It is a reliable marker of current or very recent HAV infection. Immunoglobulin G (IgG) anti-HAV increases during convalescence and persists indefinitely. A patient with acute hepatitis with IgG anti-HAV but without IgM anti-HAV can be ruled out for acute HAV infection.

DISTRIBUTION AND TRANSMISSION

HAV is a worldwide disease and is most common in areas of overcrowding and poor hygiene and sanitation. Contamination of food and water also play a role in transmission. HAV infection has occured in huge epidemics as well as in sporadic cases. In developing areas, HAV infection is almost universal in early childhood. Those at highest risk for HAV infection are residents of institutions, those in day care facilities, military personnel, and those with promiscuous sexual behavior. Several outbreaks have been associated with undercooked shellfish and fresh vegetables grown in soil contaminated with fecal material. A sustained increase in HAV among intravenous drug users occurred in the late 1980s, with a substantial decline since then. In HAV infection, most recover with lifelong immunity and no complications. However, in 1%–2%, a fulminant course may ensue, leading to hepatic necrosis and death.

CLINICAL FEATURES

The clinical course of HAV infection is most commonly subclinical especially among children. Adults are more likely to be symptomatic with overt jaundice developing in 40%–70%. The incubation period after exposure is usually 3–4 weeks, with symptoms often occuring 4 weeks after exposure. The prodrome typically consists of low-grade fever, fatigue, nausea, and anorexia; myalgias and malaise are common. Occasionally, pharyngitis, cough, and coryza are associated. On examination, jaundice and hepatomegaly may be noted, with rare splenomegaly. Later, symptoms of dark urine, light stools, right upper quadrant discomfort, and jaundice coincide with markedly decreased infectivity and viral shedding. Symptoms are generally mild and last for a few weeks and are often indistinguishable from other types of viral hepatitis.

Although IgM anti-HAV is diagnostic of acute infection, symptoms often present with associated characteristic laboratory abnormalities. Prior to the onset of jaundice, aminotransferase levels begin to rise, with ALT characteristically exceeding AST. Peak transaminase levels, ranging from several hundred to thousands, are reached with the onset of jaundice, with values returning to nearly normal in several weeks. Cholestatic hepatitis may ensue, with elevated total bilirubin and alkaline phosphatase levels. The cholestatic form is the rarest variant of HAV infection, with protracted jaundice, pruritus, and acholic stools. This is, however, followed by complete clinical improvement, with normalization of laboratory values. HAV infection does not lead to a chronic carrier state, nor does it progress to chronic liver disease. Occasionally, a protracted course of clinical and virologic relapses, lasting for several months, may occur, followed by complete recovery. Fulminant liver failure is uncommon, with HAV infection accounting for less than 10% of all cases of fulminant hepatitis.

MANAGEMENT

The management of HAV infection is generally supportive. In almost all cases, the immune system can eliminate intrahepatic replication of virus. Prevention of HAV infection should be emphasized, with commonsense hygiene precautions, minimizing fecal–oral spread. There is no specific antiviral treatment available for HAV. Steroids have no role in the treatment of this condition, although some studies suggest efficacy in promoting resolution of severe cholestatic HAV. Immune globulin, if administered within 2 weeks of exposure, can be used to protect against illness; however, it does not produce long-lasting immunity. Because peak infectivity precedes clinical illness, recognition of the infection is often too late to allow timely treatment with immune globulin. HAV vaccine is available for travelers to endemic areas, day-care center workers, sewage workers, institutional custodial staff, homosexual men, illicit drug users, food handlers, and individuals with chronic liver disease. Additionally, the U.S. Public Health Service recommends the routine immunization of children living in areas where HAV rates are twice the national average. Universal vaccination has not been recommended at this time.

CASE STUDY: CONTINUED

M.S. admitted to eating raw seafood, a recognized risk factor for HAV. However, the chronic nature of her symptoms, extending over several months, was not consistent with the typical course for HAV, and her anti-HAV test was negative.

Hepatitis B

Hepatitis B virus (HBV) is a double-stranded DNA virus belonging to the Hepadnaviridae family. It was originally discovered in the serum of an Australian aborigine in the form hepatitis B surface antigen (HBsAg). It has thus been called the Australia antigen. HBV can be detected in all body fluids and in the hepatocyte cytoplasm. A brief discussion of the viral structure is helpful for understanding the host response to infection. The inner shell of HBV is the nucleocapsid core. On its outer surface is the external nucleocapsid antigen known

Hygienic precautions minimize oral–fecal spread of HAV.

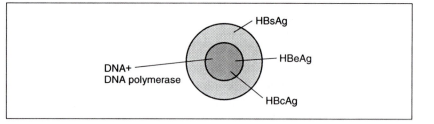

Fig. 18-2. Structure of the HBV

HBsAg = hepatitis B surface antigen; HBeAg = hepatitis B e antigen;
HBcAg = hepatitis B core antigen.

as hepatitis B core antigen (HBcAg), which cannot be detected in the circulation (Figure 18-2). It can be found, however, in the hepatocyte. The nucleocapsid contains HBV DNA, DNA polymerase, protein kinase, and hepatitis B e antigen (HBeAg). It is estimated that as many as 350 million people worldwide are carriers of HBV and that 200,000–300,000 people are infected with HBV each year in the United States. Of all the hepatotrophic viruses, HBV has been associated most often with morbidity and mortality worldwide.

DISTRIBUTION AND TRANSMISSION

There are approximately 1 million HBsAg carriers in the United States (0.1% of adults). Globally, however, the incidence is much higher, with 5%–20% of the population of sub-Saharan Africa and the Far East being HBsAg-positive. Five percent of the Earth's population is thought to be HBsAg-positive. The primary modes of transmission are via body fluids. Common examples are mucous membrane penetration, percutaneous exposure, perinatal spread, and primary sexual contact. In endemic areas, the primary mode is transmission from HBsAg-positive mothers to fetuses. Unlike HAV, the fecal–oral route is not a mode of HBV transmission. In the developed world and low-prevalence areas, most infections occur during early adulthood through sexual behavior and intravenous drug use. Other high-risk groups are hemophiliacs, hemodialysis patients, health care workers, sexually promiscuous individuals, and residents of institutions.

Developing areas experience high numbers of perinatal HBsAg transmission. It is perhaps the most prevalent means of transmission globally. Almost all cases of maternal–fetal transmission occur at the time of delivery by maternal–fetal transfusion or exposure of the fetus to maternal blood during passage through the birth canal. Intrauterine transmission is uncommon. Breastfeeding has not been shown to have an impact on transmission rate, although HbsAg can be detected in breast milk. Maternal–fetal transmission is greatly dependent on the HBeAg status of the mother. Infants born to HBsAg-positive mothers with HBeAg positivity have a 90% chance of being HBsAg-positive. Infants born to HBsAg-positive mothers with HBeAg negativity have a less than 30% chance of becoming HBsAg-positive carriers.

MARKERS

After HBV infection, the first viral serum marker is HBsAg after a 4–6-week incubation period. Symptom onset is often insidious and follows HBsAg positivity. HBsAg is present during the clinical illness and usually clears 6–8 weeks after symptom onset, although HBsAg positivity can last up to 6 months after the acute illness. If the HBsAg remains positive for longer than 6 months after the acute infection, the patient is considered to have chronic HBV, and this indicates a carrier state. Antibody to HBsAg, anti-HBs, appears after HBsAg has cleared, but this may lag for several weeks. Anti-HBs is a marker for subsequent immunity to reinfection with HBV (Figure 18-3).

HBeAg correlates with ongoing viral replication and infectivity. All acute HBV-infected patients with HBsAg positivity develop HBeAg. Persistence of HBeAg positivity suggests chronicity. In most patients, development of anti-HBe is associated with the disappearance of HBV DNA in serum.

HBcAg is not a clinically useful marker because it does not circulate freely in the blood. However, the antibodies to HBcAg, anti-HBc, are easily detected in blood and are a useful tool in the diagnosis of acute HBV infection. Anti-HBc occurs in every case of HBV infection and is detected within 1–2 weeks after HBsAg, long before anti-HBs is demonstrated. High titers of IgM anti-HBc are indicative of acute HBV infection. Persistence of IgM anti-HBc implies ongoing HBV disease, usually chronic active hepatitis. Low-titer IgG anti-HBc with anti-HBs indicates past HBV infection. In a small proportion of patients (< 5%), IgM anti-HBc may be the only detectable marker of acute HBV infection. This occurs during the period between the disappearance of HBsAg and the appearance of anti-HBs.

Notes

Detection of HBsAg denotes active infection.

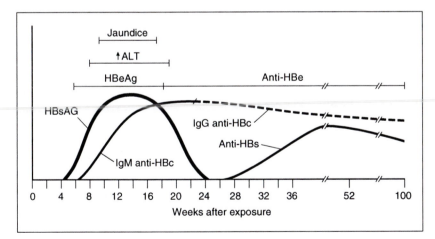

Fig. 18-3. Clinical Course of HBV Infection

ALT = alanine aminotransferase; HBeAg = hepatitis B e antigen; anti-HBe = hepatitis B e antibody; HBsAg = hepatitis B surface antigen; IgM anti-HBc = immunoglobulin M against hepatitis B core antigen; IgG anti-HBc = immunoglobulin G against hepatitis B core antigen; anti-HBs = hepatitis B surface antibody.

CLINICAL FEATURES

HBV infection can present with a wide spectrum of symptoms. Acute HBV may range from an asymptomatic, anicteric, self-limited illness to fatal fulminant hepatitis. Chronic infection ranges from a silent HBV carrier state to chronic hepatitis, cirrhosis, and hepatocellular carcinoma. With acute HBV, a prodromal phase may occur 1–2 weeks prior to an icteric phase. Fever, arthralgias, rash, altered taste sensation, malaise, arthritis, and angioedema secondary to immune complex deposition in tissues, nausea, vomiting, headache, abdominal pain, and weight loss have all been reported. An icteric phase lasting 2–10 weeks can follow, with resolution of most constitutional symptoms except anorexia and malaise, icteric sclerae, jaundiced skin, and hepatic tenderness.

Laboratory abnormalities characteristic of HBV infection are AST and ALT elevations ranging from the high hundreds to low thousands (ALT higher than AST). Less striking changes may be found in elevated levels of alkaline phosphatase and bilirubin, with a fall in albumin. An elevated prothrombin time and hypoglycemia are indicative of severe liver damage.

Ninety percent of immunocompetent adults with acute HBV infection have complete recovery and resolution of hepatocellular injury. Clearance of HBV from the liver and blood is complete, with development of anti-HBs and anti-HBc immunity. In 0.1%–0.5%, fulminant hepatitis may develop, with severe liver injury and a mortality rate of 80%, unless transplantation occurs. In the 20% who survive, most recover with no progressive chronic liver disease. Ten percent of patients with acute icteric HBV continue to have HBsAg positivity 6 months after the acute illness. Of these, half will clear their infections slowly over the next few years, but the remaining half will remain chronic carriers.

The precise factors leading to progression to chronic HBV remain unclear. However, certain features are predictive. Infection during early childhood, immunosuppression, and male gender appear to be the greatest predictors of progression. The sequelae of HBV infection are cirrhosis with portal hypertension, leading to esophageal varices, ascites, edema, splenomegaly, coagulopathy, weight loss, hepatic encephalopathy, and hepatocellular carcinoma.

HBV-infected patients are at great risk for the development of hepatocellular carcinoma (HCC), and HBV is generally considered to be oncogenic, although the exact mechanism remains unclear. Hepatocellular carcinoma rarely occurs in adult-acquired chronic infection but is frequently seen in those with chronic infection with HBV acquired in infancy. In fact, the lifetime risk of hepatocellular carcinoma in HBsAg-positive Asians, a population in which perinatal transmission is high, approaches 50%. Although HCC is more common among patients with cirrhosis, 30%–50% of HCC cases occur in the absence of cirrhosis.

It appears that HBV does not injure hepatocytes directly. Hepatocellular injury results, however, from the host's immune response to the viral antigen expressed on the infected hepatocyte. There is also evidence that cytotoxic T cells are directed toward HBcAg on the hepatocyte, secondarily leading to cellular injury.

MANAGEMENT

Treatment for acute HBV infection has not been found to be effective. The cornerstone of treatment is prevention of HBV infection by vaccination. The vaccine is relatively free of side effects and can produce protective anti-HBs in more than 95% of immunocompetent adults. It has recently been advocated for all children and is recommended for health care workers exposed to blood, hemodialysis patients and staff, intravenous drug users, young sexually active adults, hemophiliacs, developmentally handicapped individuals, and household and sexual contacts of HBsAg carriers.

In individuals with known HBsAg, excess ingestion of alcohol or hepatically metabolized drugs should be discouraged; however, dietary restrictions are not necessary. For patients with chronic, active HBV, the use of corticosteroids and other immunosuppressive therapies are no longer recommended. Controlled trials have not proven their effectiveness and have shown enhanced viral replication with their use. Treated patients appear to do less well than nontreated patients.

Interferon-α (IFN-α) has shown the greatest promise for the treatment of chronic HBV infection. About 30% of patients with chronic HBV who are treated with IFN achieve sustained loss of viral replication markers. Successful therapy usually requires treatment for at least 4 months.

The goal of HBV treatment is to suppress viral replication and avert irreversible liver injury. IFN-α and lamivudine are currently the most frequently used treatments; however, several new antiviral drugs such as adefovir have recently emerged and show significant promise. IFN-α has several advantages, including the absence of resistant mutants and a finite duration of treatment. Lamivudine is less expensive and better tolerated; however, the presence of resistant mutants and long-term response rates need to be considered. Adefovir, a nucleotide analog, can inhibit reverse transcriptase and DNA polymerase. It is effective at suppressing both wild-type and lamivudine-resistant mutants, but long-term follow-up of the drug is not yet available.

CASE STUDY: CONTINUED

M.S. had several risk factors for HBV. She used intravenous drugs, had received blood transfusions, and had had unprotected sex. Her HBsAg, anti-HBs, and anti-HBc reports were all negative.

Notes

Excessive intake of alcohol or drugs metabolized in the liver is contraindicated in individuals with known HBsAg.

HDV occurs only in the presence of HBV.

Hepatitis D

Hepatitis D virus (HDV) is often discussed with HBV, because HDV requires the helper function of HBV to become pathogenic. Thus, HDV is discussed prior to hepatitis C virus. HDV is a unique RNA virus in that it is defective and highly infectious. Identified in 1977, the family to which this unusual virus belongs has yet to be determined. HDV contains a circular single-stranded RNA genome and expresses a specific core antigen named the delta antigen (HDAg). This virus occurs as either a coinfection or a superinfection in an HBV-infected individual, and the duration of the delta infection is solely determined by the duration of the HBV infection. To be expressed or to replicate in humans, HDV requires HBsAg to constitute its outer shell. HDV superinfection of a host with HBV can lead to a reduction in markers of HBV replication secondary to a reliance on the same replicative processes.

TRANSMISSION

Transmission occurs via sexual contact, percutaneous exposure, and blood transfusions. The clinical features of HBV and HDV coinfection do not differ from those of HBV alone. However, superinfection with HDV can present with symptoms of an acute hepatitis exacerbation with a peak in aminotransferase levels on an otherwise stable HBV infection. Coinfection may be diagnosed by the detection of anti-HD in serum and intrahepatic HDAg. HDV superinfection tends to cause a more severe illness than acute or chronic HBV infection alone. HDV superinfection can transform acute or chronic HBV into a fulminant hepatitis, which can cause destruction and necrosis of liver parenchyma.

MANAGEMENT

Treatment of HBV appears to be the most prudent mode of HDV therapy, as HDV depends on HBV for its survival. IFN-α has shown to be of beneficial effect in up to 50% of treated individuals. Corticosteroids and other immunosuppressive agents have not been shown to be of any value.

CASE STUDY: *CONTINUED*

M.S. did not have HBV, and therefore she could not have HDV.

Hepatitis C

The hepatitis C virus (HCV) is a RNA virus of the Flaviviridae family with at least six different genotypes. Only within the past 15 years has the virus been identified, and insight into this fascinating virus is constantly developing. Prior to 1989, HCV was considered part of non-A, non-B hepatitis; it is now known that 85%–90% diagnosed cases of non-A, non-B hepatitis were in fact HCV. Currently about

4 million individuals in the United States and over 100 million worldwide are infected.

TRANSMISSION

The transmission of HCV is elusive. Exposure to contaminated blood and, less frequently, other human secretions are known modes of infection. During 1990–93, the Sentinel Counties Study evaluated risk factors among HCV patients, wherein 36% reported intravenous drug use, 13% had known sexual or household exposure, 5% had received a blood transfusion, 3% were health care workers, and 1% were undergoing dialysis. Forty-two percent had no known risk factors. As direct percutaneous blood exposure clearly carries the highest risk, a number of researchers feel that more in-depth history-taking could eliminate the unknown risks in these patients (e.g., unreported sexual experiences, presence of tattoos). Of considerable interest is the very high percentage of alcoholics who are infected with HCV. The reason for this is unclear; however, numbers of up to 50% have been reported. The risk of transmission from mother to fetus has been estimated at less than 10%. In women coinfected with HIV, however, the risk of transmission is higher, approximately 14%–19%.

As opposed to HBV, once HCV is contracted, patients carry an 80% risk of persistent infection. The amazing ability of HCV to persist in the host has been recognized recently with the use of polymerase chain reaction (PCR) technique, which is able to detect very small quantities of virus in serum or liver. Antibodies to HCV are detected in most of these patients; however, their presence plays a minimal role in viral clearance. With the high mutation rate of HCV and its ability to escape the body's immune system, it appears unlikely that a vaccine will be developed in the near future.

CLINICAL FEATURES

Most acute infections with HCV go unnoticed. From studies following transfusion-related cases, the incubation period lasts about 50 days (2–20 weeks). Over two-thirds of patients are asymptomatic or have only mild fatigue, so early diagnosis is usually made incidentally by investigating abnormal results on routine biochemistry profiles. Laboratory tests often reveal elevations in ALT and AST, which may fluctuate over time. Diagnosis is confirmed by detecting antibodies to HCV by ELISA and recombinant immunoblot assay (RIBA). Viral load is quantified by HCV-RNA level, which is measured using PCR. The pattern of injury on liver biopsy of patients with chronic infection reveals portal tract lymphoid aggregates or follicles, steatosis, and bile duct damage. Extrahepatic syndromes are common and include type II cryoglobulinemia, porphyria cutanea tarda, aplastic anemia, and membranoproliferative glomerulonephritis. These diseases often abate with resolution of the HCV during treatment.

The greatest danger of contracting HCV is the possible consequences of persistent infection. Clinically significant hepatitis arises

Acute HCV infections often go unnoticed.

HEV is the major cause of enteric non-A, non-B hepatitis in the developing areas.

after 10 years on average, and cirrhosis, which affects about 20% of those infected, presents after several decades. Most adults who are infected after the age of 50 will succumb to other causes of death or old age before the sequelae of HCV become clinically apparent. Of greater concern are those infected from infancy through young adulthood and those with more rapid progression to end-stage liver disease, such as HIV-infected individuals with low CD4+ counts. One of the most common reasons for liver transplantation in HCV-infected patients is hepatic failure. The risk of developing HCC increases in cirrhotic livers, presenting about 10 years after cirrhosis has developed.

MANAGEMENT

Eradication of chronic HCV infection is now possible in over 50% of treated patients. The most efficacious current treatment is a combination of IFN-α and ribavirin. Studies have shown that the long-acting pegylated IFNs yield twice the response rates of standard IFN preparations. The pegylated IFNs have a much longer half-life and a significant decrease in clearance. Sustained virologic response rates vary depending on viral genotype, the presence of bridging fibrosis or cirrhosis, and the presence of HIV-coinfection.

CASE STUDY: *CONTINUED*

The same risk factors M.S. had for HBV also apply for HCV. In addition, alcoholism, to which she admitted, has been associated with HCV infection. Her HCV antibody test was positive. The physician decided to confirm this with an HCV-RNA titer.

Hepatitis E

DISTRIBUTION AND TRANSMISSION

The hepatitis E virus (HEV) was first identified in 1983 as an enteric cause of non-A, non-B hepatitis, and the cloning and sequencing of its genome was completed in 1993. It is an RNA virus similar to but not a member of the Caliciviridae family. HEV is the major cause of enteric non-A, non-B hepatitis, with notably large outbreaks occurring in parts of Africa, the Far East, the Middle East, and Central America. Transmission is believed to occur mainly via fecally contaminated drinking water, and the extent of past exposure in endemic areas approaches 40% by adulthood.

CLINICAL FEATURES

After an incubation period of 2–10 weeks, complaints of malaise, anorexia, nausea, vomiting, and abdominal pain are common. Physical examination may reveal fever, jaundice, and hepatomegaly. Laboratory abnormalities include elevation of aminotransferases (similar to the other acute hepatitides), as well as elevation of serum bilirubin, alkaline phosphatase, and γ-glutamyltransferase (GGT). The diagnosis is confirmed in most cases by the detection of serum antibodies to HEV antigen (HEVAg), and ELISA and PCR techniques are also available. Liver biopsies, not ordinarily of clinical use in hepatitis, have revealed cholestatic hepatitis and the characteristic patterns of acute hepatitis, with focal intralobular necrosis. Symptoms and signs generally resolve within 6 weeks, and liver enzymes return to normal within 3 months. Pregnant women are more frequently affected by HEV and have a worse outcome, particularly in the second and third trimester. Fulminant hepatitis can occur and mortality rates range from 5% to 25%.

MANAGEMENT

Because of the self-limited course of HEV and the lack of chronic sequelae, treatment is supportive. Pregnant patients may require special attention. The role of immunoglobulin for prophylaxis either before or after exposure has been examined but has not been shown to alter disease rates.

CASE STUDY: CONTINUED

Although M.S. was from Pakistan, an endemic region for HEV, she had not been there in 10 years, making this diagnosis very unlikely. Her clinical course was also too protracted for HEV. The physician decided not to send blood for serology tests for this virus.

Hepatitis F

The relevance and existence of hepatitis F virus (HFV) is in considerable doubt. In 1994, an enteric virus was recovered from the feces of a patient with hepatitis and was found to be transferable to rhesus monkeys. However, no subsequent data have confirmed this work.

Hepatitis G

Recent isolates in separate laboratories have confirmed the presence of a virus found in some patients with non-A, non-B hepatitis, designated the hepatitis G virus (HGV). It is an RNA virus related to HCV in that it appears to belong to the Flaviviridae family. About 10% of cases of chronic non-A–E hepatitis (serologically negative for hepatitis A, B, C, D, and E) test positive for HGV; however, HGV appears to be present in the general population (people with no clinical or chemical hepatitis). HGV is found in 1%–2% of blood donors (probably an underestimation of the prevalence in the population at large), and it more often coexists with HCV or HBV. HGV is most often associated with intravenous drug users and patients who have received blood transfusions, suggesting similar routes of transmission. It appears to be persistent, but it is not clear whether HGV alone actually causes any liver disease. It has been referred to by some as a possible innocent bystander.

CASE STUDY: *RESOLUTION*

Knowing that HGV is most likely nonpathogenic, the physician correctly decided not to send blood samples for serology tests for this virus. M.S.'s HCV-RNA titer returned, confirming the diagnosis of HCV.

IFN was delayed until after the delivery of M.S.'s healthy HCV-negative infant. She was treated with IFN therapy for 1 year, resulting in normalization of her transaminases. She now lives happily in southern California with her child.

REVIEW QUESTIONS

Directions: For each of the following questions, choose the one best answer.

1 The major risk of transmission of HAV occurs during which point in time within the human host?

A When it is shed in the feces when symptoms are present, just after the incubation period

B During the 6–8-week incubation period in the feces

C During the 3–4-week incubation period through all body secretions

D During the 3–4-week period before symptoms arise

2 HAV infection has which of the following characteristics?

A It usually goes unnoticed.

B It most commonly presents with jaundice, nausea, and vomiting.

C It is transmitted via the fecal–oral route and through sexual contact.

D It usually resolves years after infection.

3 Which of the hepatitis viruses is associated with the greatest worldwide morbidity and mortality?

A HCV   **C** HDV

B HBV   **D** HAV

4 Active infection in HBV is identified by

A hepatitis B core antigen (HBcAg) 26 weeks after exposure.

B IgG hepatitis B core antibody (anti-HBc) 26 weeks after exposure.

C hepatitis B surface antigen (HBsAg) 4–6 weeks after exposure.

D HBsAg immediately on exposure.

5 Which virus requires the helper function of HBV?

A HCV   **C** HFV
B HDV   **D** HGV

6 HCV is a persistent infection in humans as a result of

A the high rate of viral mutation.
B the inability to make antibodies against the virus.
C the integration of the virus into the host genome.
D extrahepatic viral replication.

7 Correct statements regarding the treatment of HGV with IFN include which of the following?

A It decreases the reservoir in the community.
B It prevents progression to end-stage liver disease.
C It decreases the risk of HCC.
D It is not recommended currently.

8 Fulminant hepatitis is of considerable concern in pregnant women infected with hepatitis

A B.   **C** E.
B C.   **D** G.

References

Alter MJ, Gallagher M, Morris TT, et al: Acute non-A–E hepatitis in the United States and the role of hepatitis G virus infection. *N Engl J Med* 336:741–746, 1997.

Alter MJ, Mast EE: The epidemiology of viral hepatitis in the United States. *Gastroenterol Clin North Am* 23:437–455, 1994.

Alter HJ, Nakatsuji Y, Melpolder J, et al: The incidence of transfusion-associated hepatitis G virus infection and its relation to liver disease. *N Engl J Med* 336:747–754, 1997.

Balayan MS, Andjaparidze AG, Savinskaya SS, et al: Evidence for a virus in non-A, non-B hepatitis transmitted via the fecal-oral route. *Intervirology* 20:23–31, 1983.

Bonino F, Smedile A: Delta agent (type D) hepatitis. *Semin Liver Dis* 6:28–33, 1986.

Craig AS. Clinical Practice. Prevention of hepatitis A with the hepatitis A vaccine. *N Engl J Med* 350(5):476–81, 2004.

De Franchis R, Meucci G, Vecchi M, et al: The natural history of asymptomatic hepatitis B surface antigen carrier. *Ann Intern Med* 118:191–194, 1993.

Ganem D. Hepatitis B virus infection-natural history and clinical consequences. *N Engl J Med* 350(11):1118–29, 2004.

Gibas A, Dienstag J: Viral hepatitis. In *Pathophysiology of Gastrointestinal Diseases*. Edited by Chopra S, May RJ. Boston, MA: Little, Brown, 1989, pp 327–356.

Gish RG. Treating hepatitis C: the state of the art. *Gastroenterol Clinics of North America* 33(1 Suppl):S1–9, 2004.

Hoofnagle JH, di Bisceglie AM: The treatment of chronic viral hepatitis. *N Engl J Med* 336:347–356, 1997.

Lemon SM, Thomas, DL: Vaccines to prevent viral hepatitis. *N Engl J Med* 336:196–204, 1997.

Levinthal G, Ray M: Hepatitis A: from epidemic jaundice to a vaccine-preventable disease. *Gastroenterologist* 4:107–117, 1996.

Perrillo RP: The management of chronic hepatitis B. *Am J Med* 96: 34S–39S, 1994.

Perrillo RP, Mason AL: Therapy for hepatitis B virus infection. *Gastroenterol Clin North Am* 23:581–601, 1994.

Schiff L, Schiff ER: Diseases of the Liver, 9th ed. Philadelphia, PA: J. B. Lipincott, 2003.

Sherara AI, Hunt CM, Hamilton JD: Hepatitis C. *Ann Intern Med* 125:658–668, 1996.

19

Hereditary Liver Disease

■ LEARNING OBJECTIVES ■

At the completion of this chapter, the reader should be able to:
- Discuss the pathogenesis, clinical features, classification, and management of the main metabolic liver diseases in adults.
- Describe how iron and copper overload can lead to liver injury.
- Discuss the recent advances in the genetic aspects of these diseases.

CASE STUDY 1: *INTRODUCTION*

A 35-year-old man presented to the physician for evaluation of elevated iron values in studies that were obtained on a routine blood panel for an executive physical examination. The patient felt well and had no medical problems. He had never been hospitalized. The family history was significant for the fact that his father died at a young age from an accident, but his paternal grandfather died from liver disease of unknown etiology. His mother was healthy, and both of her parents perished in World War II before the age of 50.

Introduction

Liver damage resulting from an inherited disease can present at any age. Certain disorders are more likely to manifest during infancy and others during adulthood. In children, some of the most common hereditary diseases are α_1-antitrypsin deficiency, familial intrahepatic cholestatic syndromes, Wilson's disease, cystic fibrosis, and perinatal hemochromatosis. In adults, the order of frequency is slightly different and includes hemochromatosis as the most prevalent disorder, followed by α_1-antitrypsin deficiency, Wilson's disease, cystic fibrosis, and familial intrahepatic cholestatic syndromes, among others (Table 19-1). Here we focus on hemochromatosis and Wilson's disease and briefly discuss α_1-antitrypsin deficiency as the most representative examples of inherited liver disorders that affect adults, with a brief discussion of the prospects for gene therapy.

Hemochromatosis

INTRODUCTION

Hereditary hemochromatosis (HH) is an autosomal recessive disorder of iron metabolism that leads to excessive iron deposition in several organs, including the liver. One of the most common inherited

Table 19-1. Hereditary Liver Disease

DISEASE (ALL ARE AUTOSOMAL RECESSIVE)	FREQUENCY		CHROMOSOME	DEFECT
	HETEROZYGOUS	HOMOZYGOUS		
Hemochromatosis	1/12	1/400	6 (HLA-A3, -B7, -B14)	Unknown; high iron absorption?
α_1-Antitrypsin deficiency	1/30	1/2000	14	Lack of excretion of abnormal protein
Wilson's disease	1/90	1/30,000	13	P-type ATPase inserts copper into protein; transports copper across canalicular membrane
Cystic fibrosis	1/25	1/2500	7	Abnormal chloride transport

disorders among Caucasians, HH is thought to arise secondary to increased intestinal absorption of iron with subsequent storage in parenchymal cells. An increase in the duodenal expression of the iron transporters, DMT-1 and ferroportin 1, is most likely responsible for increased absorption.

Approximately 10–20 mg of iron are ingested each day in the diet. The intestinal mucosa forms an effective barrier to iron, and only one-tenth of ingested iron (1–2 mg) is absorbed from the duodenum and upper jejunum into the portal blood. Once iron is absorbed, there are few routes for excreting it; 1–2 mg a day is shed via excretion in bile; some is lost by cells sloughed from the skin and GI tract; and the rest is lost in the urine. Women lose approximately 30 mg iron during a menstrual cycle. Iron is transported from its site of absorption to the liver bound to transferrin, which carries only two atoms of iron per molecule. In the liver, it is taken up by ferritin, a strorage form of iron capable of holding thousands of atoms per molecule. The normal total body pool of iron is approximately 4 g. Hemoglobin in red blood cells makes up half of total body iron stores. One unit of blood (500 ml) contains 250 mg iron. Iron is also found in myoglobin and in heme-containing enzymes in the liver and elsewhere. The remainder of the body iron is in storage form as ferritin or hemosiderin in the liver and the reticuloendothelial cells.

There are two mutations of the HFE gene responsible for HFE-related HH. Both mutations of the HFE protein result in a change of cysteine to tyrosine at amino acid 282 (C282Y) and histidine to aspartic acid at amino acid 63 (H63D). The vast majority of individuals with phenotypic hemochromatosis are C282Y homozygous.

DIAGNOSIS

Until recently, phenotypic tests for iron overload (serum Fe, transferrin, total iron-binding capacity, transferrin saturation, and ferritin) were used for diagnosis. A number of pitfalls exist with regard to the sensitivity and specificity of these tests. For instance, false-positive elevated transferrin saturation occurs in nonfasting states, and serum ferritin can be increased during acute inflammation. Nevertheless, normal levels for iron and saturation have a negative predictive value of 97%. The combination of a saturation greater than 61% and a ferritin greater than 165 μg/L has shown to be 90% sensitive and 99% specific but has only a 30% positive predictive value in diagnosing hemochromatosis.

In patients with equivocal testing, the diagnosis can be elucidated by HFE mutation analysis. For example, in a patient with abnormal iron studies, normal liver function tests, and a serum ferritin < 1000 ng/ml, C282Y homozygosity or C282Y/H63D heterozygosity confirms the diagnosis of hemochromatosis and no further work-up is necessary. Currently, liver biopsies are rarely needed to confirm the diagnosis of hemochromatosis. Indeed the clinical features of HH and iron overload do not develop in many individuals who are homozygous for C282Y, suggesting that the mutation may have incomplete penetrance. In

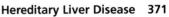

Table 19-2. Iron Studies in Patients with Hemochromatosis

STUDY	NORMAL	HEMOCHROMATOSIS
Serum iron (μg/dl)	60–180	180–300
Serum transferrin (μg/dl)	220–410	200–300
Transferrin saturation (%)	20–50	80–100
Serum ferritin (ng/ml)		
Men	20–200	500–6000
Women	15–50	500–6000
Hepatic iron concentration (HIC)		
(μg/g dry weight)	300–1200	10,000–30,000
(μmol/g dry weight)	5–21	175–550
Hepatic iron index (HII)		
(μmol/g dry weight $\div$ age in years)	< 1.5	> 1.9

several studies, an HII (hepatic iron index) of 1.9 is correlated with severe iron overload. Despite this, about 15% of C282Y homozygous patients have an HII below 1.9.

Symptoms in hemochromatosis usually develop only after sufficient tissue storage has occurred. Patients with symptomatic hemochromatosis tend to have hepatic iron concentrations exceeding 10,000 μg/g dry weight and, in some circumstances, as high as 40,000 μg/g dry weight (normal: < 1500 μg/g dry weight). Symptoms may include fatigue, malaise, abdominal pain, impotence, and arthralgias. Many patients, however, are asymptomatic. The degree of hepatic fibrosis depends on a number of factors, including the hepatic iron concentration (usually > 22,000 μg/g) (Table 19-2).

PATHOGENESIS: INSIGHTS FROM LIVER TRANSPLANTATION

The liver is the main recipient of excess body iron. Several mechanisms for the resulting fibrosis and cirrhosis have been postulated. Peroxidative damage by chronic iron overload to phospholipids of organelle membranes is probably the most unifying hypothesis. Hepatic lysosomes isolated from patients with various types of iron excess show an increase in in vitro membrane fragility that is proportional to the hemosiderin content. This abnormality can be reversed in patients with hemochromatosis who have been adequately treated. Iron initiates a peroxidation on lysosomal membranes that is facilitated by reducing agents, such as ascorbate. However, if intralysosomal pH falls significantly, iron is able to exert this damage without the need for exogenous reducing agents. The iron-induced lysosomal membrane fragility leads to leakage of enzymes ultimately responsible for cellular injury. Other organelles (such as mitochondria and microsomes) are also affected. In the mitochondria, impaired respiratory control caused by an irreversible defect in electron transport has been shown. In the microsomes, there is a reduction in the concentration of cytochromes P-450 and b_5. Additionally, excess iron may result in stellate cell activation and fibrogenesis, as well as hepatic DNA damage.

The biochemical forms of iron responsible for these manifestations are unknown. The formation of alkyl radicals and peroxyl radicals can stimulate lipid peroxidation. Hydroxyl radicals can also initiate this reaction. Regardless of the initiating radical species, peroxidative decomposition of the polyunsaturated fatty acids of membrane phospholipids can result in organelle dysfunction. The role of antioxidants such as vitamin E and vitamin C in the peroxidation produced by iron is under investigation. Finally, the pathophysiologic significance of these abnormalities in initiating and perpetuating the chronic organ damage in hemochromatosis remains to be firmly established.

The basic metabolic defect in hemochromatosis is still unknown. Experimental liver transplantation suggests that the hepatic iron content affects the intestinal absorption of iron by some unknown humoral factor. Transplantation of iron-loaded intestinal grafts into iron-deficient rats has indicated the possible role of a humoral factor in regulating iron transfer from the intestine to other organs. If confirmed, this factor could still be present in patients with hemochromatosis after orthotopic liver transplantation (OLTx), making the recurrence of the disease possible.

The experience with OLTx in hemochromatosis has provided two types of situations. The first occurs in patients with hemochromatosis who received livers from healthy donors. The second occurs in patients who had liver failure as a result of diseases other than hemochromatosis and inadvertently received livers from donors with undiagnosed hemochromatosis. In the first group, the survival rate after OLTx has been poor. Unequivocal evidence of disease recurrence is lacking. In the second group, the first patient with inadvertent transplantation of a liver with hemochromatosis was well at 24 months, with normal ferritin but high iron saturation. In two additional cases with known HII pre- and post-OLTx, there was a significant reduction in the hepatic iron concentration (HIC), with no evidence of disease recurrence. Considered together, these results provide some evidence against a primary hepatic defect in hemochromatosis (perhaps due to the persistence of an intestinal defect) but do not answer the question of cure of the disease by OLTx. Redistribution of the excess iron present in the livers with hemochromatosis in the recipient organs could be the explanation for the initial decrease in HII seen in some of these cases. The observation of a HII below the diagnostic level for hemochromatosis seen at 30 months post-OLTx in one patient suggests lack of disease recurrence. However, it takes decades for the iron deposition in the liver to cause end-organ damage, and therefore, additional information in more hemochromatosis patients with longer follow-up periods is required to answer this important question.

TREATMENT

The goal of treatment in hemochromatosis is to initiate therapy prior to the development of end-stage complications. This means initiating phlebotomy before the development of hepatic fibrosis or cirrhosis.

Therapy for hemochromatosis should be undertaken before irreversible complications occur.

Homozygotes who have 10–30 g of excess storage iron require extended phlebotomy regimens. Symptoms and hematocrit are monitored weekly and dictate the speed of the phlebotomy regimen. Most patients can tolerate weekly phlebotomy of 450–500 ml of whole blood, and some younger patients may be able to tolerate removal of 2 U blood (1000 ml)/wk. In contrast, some older patients may only tolerate a 250 ml phlebotomy (0.5 U) every other week. Every 6–8 weeks, the transferrin saturation and ferritin level can be determined. Some suggest maintaining the ferritin level at less than 50 ng/ml and the transferrin saturation at less than 50%. Liver enzyme abnormalities usually normalize with treatment. The degree of fibrosis is sometimes reduced by iron removal; however, established cirrhosis is not reversible. The use of iron-chelating drugs, such as deferoxamine, is only necessary in those patients who present with cardiac symptoms or those who cannot undergo phlebotomy.

Family screening is necessary for probands with HH. Individuals should be evaluated for C282Y homozygosity or C2828Y/H63D compound heterozygosity. If the mutations and iron overload are present, therapeutic phlebotomy should be initiated.

CASE STUDY 1: *RESOLUTION*

The diagnosis was confirmed by HFE mutation analysis. The patient was treated with phlebotomy, and his siblings and children were referred for further evaluation.

Wilson's Disease

CASE STUDY 2: *INTRODUCTION*

An 18-year-old adolescent with a 2-year history of an unclassified psychiatric disorder was admitted to the hospital with neurologic symptoms, including Parkinson-like rigidity, tremor, and personality changes. Liver enzymes were noted to be elevated.

INTRODUCTION

Wilson's disease is an autosomal recessive disorder of copper metabolism with excessive accumulation of copper in several tissues (i.e., liver, brain, eye, skeleton, kidney). Copper overload can be either primary (Wilson's disease) or secondary, which is seen as an epiphenomenon in any disorder with prolonged cholestasis that results in a decreased biliary excretion of this metal. Copper is ingested in the diet. Many foods are rich in copper (e.g., shellfish, chocolate, nuts, mushrooms). The absorption takes place in the upper intestine and travels to the liver via the portal vein (Figure 19-1). The hepatocyte takes copper from the sinusoid, and a portion is used in the production of copper-containing proteins. The bulk of copper is transported across

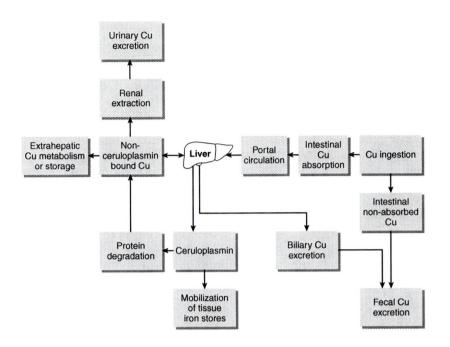

Fig. 19-1. Copper Metabolism

Dietary copper may be absorbed in small intestine, bound to albumin in the portal circulation, and extracted in the liver, where it is bound to ligands and may be used for metabolic needs, transferred to endogenous chelators, incorporated into ceruloplasmin, or excreted into bile. *Source:* Modified from Schiff 2003, vol. 2, p. 1172.

the hepatocyte and into the bile canaliculi through a vesicular pathway dependent on ATP7B function. The absence or diminished function of ATP7B results in decreased biliary copper excretion and increased hepatic copper accumulation.

Once copper is in bile, it is bound to proteins that prevent its reabsorption and favor its excretion in the stool. Very little copper circulates in a free state, and very little is present in the urine. In contrast to iron homeostasis, as much as 50% of ingested copper is absorbed, even though this is in excess of daily requirements, underscoring the importance of maintaining an adequate excretion to achieve a normal balance. Total body copper equals 100 mg/70 kg in humans. In fetal life, almost all of the body's copper is in the liver, whereas the adult liver contains only 8% of the total stores. About 95% of plasma copper circulates bound to ceruloplasmin, and 5% plasma copper is bound to albumin or amino acids. About 1.5 mg of copper is needed daily to maintain a normal balance. Liver copper is always increased in Wilson's disease. Although amounts above 250 μg/g liver suggest Wilson's disease, levels this high can occur in other causes of cholestasis, as previously mentioned. Hepatocellular carcinoma can occur infrequently. Motor system (basal ganglia) and psychiatric disturbances are common, whereas the sensory system is never involved.

The genetic defect is located in the long arm of chromosome 13, and the gene has recently been cloned. The estimated frequency of

Notes

The precise mechanism of pathogenesis in Wilson's disease is unknown.

heterozygote carriers is 1/200 to 1/400. The incidence of homozygotes is approximately 1/30,000. This frequency holds for whites and Asians, the only populations studied so far.

In individuals with a genetic defect in ATP7B, hepatic copper accumulation begins during infancy and gradually increases over time. Clinical evidence of hepatic dysfunction has not been observed before the age of 6 years. One-half of affected patients will have symptoms of Wilson's disease by 15 years of age (42% present with hepatic, 34% with neurologic, and 10% with psychiatric problems). All patients with neurologic disease have preexisting chronic liver disease (steatosis, chronic active hepatitis, cirrhosis, or fulminant hepatic failure). All cases of neurologic Wilson's disease have Kayser-Fleischer rings. In asymptomatic liver disease, serum ceruloplasmin concentration, 24-hour urinary copper excretion, hepatic histology, and quantitative copper studies may suggest the diagnosis. One of the earliest hepatocellular lesions is hepatic steatosis with increased glycogen deposits in enlarged nuclei. Mallory bodies are also seen. The finding of a normal hepatic copper concentration may exclude the diagnosis of untreated Wilson's disease in adults. A hepatic copper index has not been developed and is probably not necessary because clinical, biochemical, and histologic features allow discrimination among the various disorders considered in hepatic copper overload.

The serum free copper (in μmol/L) is equal to total serum copper (in μmol/L) minus the copper bound to ceruloplasmin (there are 0.047 μmol copper per mg ceruloplasmin). Serum free copper is useful for diagnostic and therapeutic purposes. The most discriminating biochemical test to diagnose Wilson's disease in children with liver disease is a 24-hour urinary copper excretion result less than 25 μmol after D-penicillamine challenge. See Table 19-3 for other copper parameters.

PATHOGENESIS: INSIGHTS FROM LIVER TRANSPLANTATION

OLTx in Wilson's disease has provided valuable insights into the pathogenesis of this condition. The apparent reversal of abnormal copper metabolism following OLTx supported the concept that the primary defect is located in the liver. However, the precise mechanism is still unknown.

Table 19-3. Copper Studies in Patients with Wilson's Disease

STUDY	NORMAL	WILSON'S DISEASE
Serum free copper (μg/dl)	8–12	> 25
Urine copper (μg/24 hr)	< 40	> 100
Serum ceruloplasmin (mg/dl)	20–40	< 20
Hepatic copper concentration (μg/g dry weight)	15–50	250–3000

Ceruloplasmin is the main protein involved in the transport of copper. Although it is possible that the incorporation of copper into ceruloplasmin is abnormal, the primary defect in Wilson's disease is not related to this protein for the following reasons: (1) The gene for ceruloplasmin is on chromosome 3—not on 13. (2) Some patients with Wilson's disease ($< 5\%$) have normal ceruloplasmin. (3) Heterozygous patients may have low ceruloplasmin levels without signs or symptoms of the disease. (4) There is no correlation between the plasma levels of ceruloplasmin and the severity of the disease. (5) Administration of ceruloplasmin does not ameliorate the severity of the disease.

As mentioned previously, the primary defect in Wilson's disease appears to be an abnormality on the Wilson's disease gene, which codes for ATP7B. This enzyme inserts copper into the ceruloplasmin molecule, and because it is required to assemble a completely active and three-dimensionally correct ceruloplasmin protein, the low serum ceruloplasmin exhibited by many Wilson's disease patients results from absent or diminished activity of ATP7B. In addition, this ATPase appears to be critical for transport of copper across the canalicular membrane, and this may help explain why biliary copper excretion is very low in Wilson's disease patients.

Interestingly, the copper profile of the normal neonate is very similar to that of patients with Wilson's disease (low serum copper and ceruloplasmin and high hepatic copper), and it has been suggested that the repression of normal copper metabolism in the fetus and its induction during the neonatal period are regulated by a controller gene that switches the positive copper balance (accumulation) of the fetus to the normal of the adult. Such a switch would result in activation of biliary excretion and export of ceruloplasmin out of the liver. Mutations in this controller gene would result in the disease. Implantation of a normal liver (in which the change has taken place) in a patient with Wilson's disease would then restore normal copper metabolism, because this gene would not be structural.

Several mechanisms appear to be responsible for the subcellular injury of copper toxicity. The membrane permeability and diffusion of small molecules and ions can be altered by the introduction of positive charges at normally uncharged or negatively charged sites. In the mitochondria, this effect could explain in part the changes that are characteristic in the early stages of hepatocyte damage. It has also been suggested that sulfur (S) may promote the polymerization of copper-rich proteins through S-Cu-S links formed by interactions with thiol groups, polymerization of tubulin (with resulting steatosis and possibly deposition of Mallory bodies), destabilization of nuclear DNA, and leakage of lysosomal enzymes with stimulation of fibrogenesis. Copper, as well as other metals, also catalyzes the formation of reactive oxygen radicals, which result in membrane damage. The Long-Evans cinnamon (LEC) rat has been found to have a gene with high homology to the human gene for Wilson's disease. Because of its phenotypic

Treatment with oral D-penicillamine improves clinical symptoms in most patients with Wilson's disease.

α_1-Antitrypsin deficiency is an autosomal recessive disorder of serum protease.

features, the LEC rat may represent the ideal animal model in which to characterize the pathogenic abnormalities of Wilson's disease.

TREATMENT

Treatment options for Wilson's disease include pharmacologic treatment and OLTx. Pharmacologic treatments include chelating agents (such as D-penicillamine, trientene, and tetrathiomolybdate) and zinc salts. Oral D-penicillamine (600–1800 mg/d) effectively reduces excess copper stores and improves clinical symptoms in most patients with Wilson's disease. Signs and symptoms resulting from end-organ damage are not reversible. Side effects of this therapy include hypersensitivity reactions, essential trace metal deficiencies (e.g., zinc), and altered collagen metabolism. The success of therapy can be assessed by clinical improvement and by normalization of liver function tests and copper metabolism. As mentioned, OLTx offers a cure for end-stage liver damage in Wilson's disease.

CASE STUDY 2: RESOLUTION

Kayser-Fleischer rings were noted on examination of the patient. The ceruloplasmin was low, a 24-hour urine collection showed elevated copper excretion, and liver biopsy confirmed the diagnosis of Wilson's disease. The patient was treated with D-penicillamine, and this resulted in improvement of liver chemistry values and a reduction in the neurologic symptoms.

α_1-Antitrypsin Deficiency

CASE STUDY 3: INTRODUCTION

A 47-year-old man presented to the physician with abnormal liver chemistry tests. He was in excellent health and had no previous medical problems. The family history was significant for coronary artery disease and chronic obstructive pulmonary disease. Viral serology results were negative, and iron studies were normal.

α_1-Antitrypsin deficiency is an autosomal recessive inherited condition that is the most common genetic cause of liver disease in children. It results in about 85%–90% reduction in plasma α_1-antitrypsin, a glycoprotein that inhibits destructive neutrophil proteases, elastase, cathepsin G, and proteinase 3.

The gene for α_1-antitrypsin is located on chromosome 14. This gene encodes a single-chain polypeptide of 394 amino acids. The liver disease is related to the intracellular accumulation of the abnormally folded mutant protein. Point mutations in the gene alter the amino acid composition of the protein, modify protein glycosylation, and limit the secretion of the glycoprotein from the cell. The alleles for α_1-antitrypsin are named using letters of the alphabet to describe their migratory speed during protein electrophoresis. In general, fast-moving alleles are labeled with earlier letters, M, and slow-moving proteins with later ones, Z. The frequency of α_1-antitrypsin phenotypes (or Pi types) is variable (PiM = 0.95, PiS = 0.03; PiZ = 0.01). Hence, PiZZ will occur in about 1/3500–4000. PiSZ occurs in 1/800.

Although the most profoundly deficient levels of α_1-antitrypsin are found in individuals who are homozygous for the Z allele (ZZ), only a subpopulation of deficient individuals develops liver injury. Only 20% of ZZ neonates demonstrate neonatal cholestasis, and about 10% of ZZ adults have clinically overt liver disease. Therefore, the Pi type correlates poorly with the severity of the liver disease, and other genetic and environmental factors have been implicated. The mutant stored protein is subject to a polymerization process that can be blocked by synthetic peptides. A specific receptor mediates a feed-forward up-regulation of α_1-antitrypsin synthesis, which in turn leads to greater accumulation of the abnormal α_1-antitrypsin molecule that is hepatotoxic. The blockage or manipulation of this receptor could theoretically provide the basis for protein or gene therapy. Abnormally folded proteins are retained by specific protein–protein interactions in the endoplasmic reticulum. A better understanding of the requirements for such protein–protein interactions could allow for specific biochemical inhibition and release of the abnormal protein by default (the abnormal protein has 85% of the functional activity of the normal protein).

TREATMENT

The diagnosis of α_1-antitrypsin is made by phenotype determination in isoelectric focusing or by means of gel electrophoresis. There is no specific therapy for liver disease in α_1-antitrypsin deficiency, but attempts to modify the disease by manipulating the defective gene are in progress. Protease inhibitor therapy for the associated lung disease has been attempted. Because α_1-antitrypsin is primarily synthesized in the liver, OLTx offers a cure for this disorder.

Prospects for Gene Therapy

The principle of somatic gene therapy is that genes can be introduced into selected cells to treat genetic or acquired diseases. As presently conceived, it does *not* involve repairing or replacing mutant genes and, therefore, is not likely to play a role in diseases such as hemochromatosis or Wilson's disease. Replacement of α_1-antitrypsin has been looked at but is not currently an option. Gene therapy may provide an approach to the treatment of various other inherited

No specific therapy exists for liver disease in α_1-antitrypsin deficiency.

disorders of hepatic function, such as familial hypercholesterolemia resulting from low-density-lipoprotein receptor deficiency, phenylketonuria resulting from phenylalanine hydroxylase deficiency, or hyperammonemia resulting from inherited defects in the urea cycle. Such diseases might be treated by introducing a normal gene into hepatic cells to provide the function of the absent or deficient gene.

Gene therapy may also be an approach for treating acquired diseases by altering the course of a pathologic process. Multifactorial hypercholesterolemia, infectious hepatitis, and cirrhosis may be targets for gene therapy in the future. The liver may also be an important target for therapies that use hepatocytes as bioreactors to secrete therapeutic proteins into the blood (hemophilia?). The large size of the liver, its ability to secrete large amounts of protein into the blood, and its ability to perform various posttranslational modifications required for the activity of certain gene products make it a potentially important target for such therapies.

In summary, there have been significant advances made over the past several years in an understanding of the genetic aspects of hemochromatosis, Wilson's disease, and α_1-antitrypsin deficiency. These advances are likely to change some of the current diagnostic and therapeutic strategies currently in practice.

CASE STUDY 3: RESOLUTION

A serum α_1-antitrypsin level was obtained for this patient, and it was low. Phenotyping revealed PiZZ. A liver biopsy showed globules in the periportal hepatocytes with periodic acid–Schiff staining after disease. The patient was followed closely, and family members were evaluated.

REVIEW QUESTIONS

Directions: For each of the following questions, choose the one best answer.

1 A 37-year-old man was evaluated by a liver specialist because of elevated liver enzymes. He had never had blood transfusions. He had abnormal iron studies, a serum ferritin < 1000 ng/ml, and was C282Y homozygous. Which of the following statements about this case is *true*?

    A His disease is likely to be the result of a chronically impaired ability to excrete iron.

    B The low serum ferritin means he cannot have hemochromatosis.

    C He should be educated about this nontreatable disorder and about the ultimate progression toward liver transplantation.

    D Other members of his family should also be studied.

2 A 22-year-old woman had an episode of jaundice. She developed neurologic symptoms that responded to treatment with D-penicillamine. Which of the following statements about this woman's condition is *true*?

A This genetic disorder is inherited as autosomal dominant.
B The gene for her disease has been cloned to chromosome 14, and the defect results in an abnormal binding of copper by proteins in the bile.
C Ceruloplasmin levels are high.
D Lowering the total copper body stores is beneficial.

3 Hemochromatosis, Wilson's disease, and α_1-antitrypsin deficiency all share the same pattern of inheritance. Assuming both parents of a child are heterozygous for one of these same disorders, what is the chance that the child will inherit the disease?

A 100%
B 50%
C 25%
D 10%

4 Which of the following statements regarding iron metabolism is *true*?

A Approximately 50% of ingested iron is absorbed from the GI tract.
B Iron is absorbed in the distal small bowel.
C Iron is transported from the site of absorption bound to transferrin.
D Ferritin is a storage form of iron and can hold two atoms of iron per molecule.

5 Which of the following statements regarding copper metabolism is *true*?

A Copper is absorbed in the distal small bowel.
B As much as 60% of ingested copper is absorbed.
C Copper usually circulates in the free state.
D The adult liver contains about 50% of copper stores.

6 Which of the following statements about α_1-antitrypsin deficiency is *true*?

A There is no specific therapy for the liver disease in α_1-antitrypsin deficiency.
B The α_1-antitrypsin gene is located on chromosome 13.
C The Pi type correlates well with the severity of liver disease.
D Liver transplant is of no benefit in these patients as the disease usually returns.

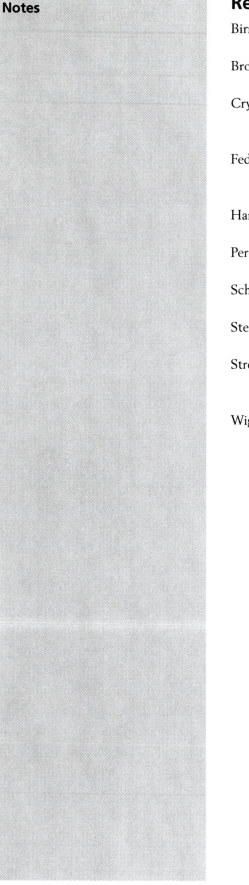

References

Birrer P, McElvaney NG, Chang-Stroman LM: α_1-Antitrypsin deficiency and liver disease. *J Inherit Metab Dis* 14:512–525, 1991.

Brook JH, Halliday JW, Pippard MJ, et al: *Iron Metabolism in Health and Disease.* Philadelphia, PA: W. B. Saunders, 1994.

Crystal RG: α_1-Antitrypsin deficiency, emphysema, and liver disease. Genetic basis and strategies for therapy. *J Clin Invest* 85:1343–1352, 1990.

Feder JN, Gnirke A, Thomas W, et al: A novel MHC class I-like gene is mutated in patients with hereditary hemochromatosis. *Nat Genet* 13:399–408, 1996.

Harrison SA, Bacon BR. Hereditary hemochromatosis: update for 2003. *Journal of Hepatology* 38:S14–S23, 2003.

Perenci P, et al: An international symposium on Wilson's and Menkes' diseases. *Hepatology* 24:952–958, 1996.

Schiff L, Schiff ER: Diseases of the Liver, 9th ed. Philadelphia, PA: J.B. Lipincott, 2003.

Sternlieb I: Perspectives on Wilson's disease. *Hepatology* 12:1234–1239, 1990.

Stremmel W, Meyerrose KW, Niederau C, et al: Wilson's disease: clinical presentation, treatment, and survival. *Ann Intern Med* 115:720–726, 1991.

Wiggers P, Dalhoj J, Hyltoft Petersen P, et al: Screening for haemochromatosis: influence of analytical imprecision, diagnostic limit and prevalence on test validity. *Scand J Clin Lab Invest* 51:143–148, 1991.

20

Autoimmune Liver Disease

■ CHAPTER OUTLINE ■

■ LEARNING OBJECTIVES ■

At the completion of this chapter, the reader should be able to:

- Identify the theories on the pathogenesis of autoimmune liver diseases.
- Differentiate autoimmune from other diseases of the liver.
- Distinguish the clinical characteristics of the three main types of autoimmune liver diseases: autoimmune hepatitis, primary biliary cirrhosis, and primary sclerosing cholangitis.
- Evaluate the unique complications that can result from autoimmune liver diseases.
- Outline the treatment options for these diseases.

CASE STUDY: *INTRODUCTION*

The patient, a 23-year-old Caucasian woman, presented with a 3-month history of right upper quadrant pain. The patient stated that about 3 months ago she developed a vague right-sided abdominal pain. The pain was intermittent initially but gradually became more persistent and nagging. It was not associated with meals or exertion and was relieved only when lying on her back or on her left side. The patient stated that she also had symptoms of anorexia but no vomiting and as a result had lost 15 lbs over the last 2 months. She has also experienced significant fatigue. Over the previous 2 weeks, she noted pain in her wrist and ankle joints. She has had no change in her bowel habits. She has no dysuria. She denied fever, chills, or pruritus. She noted the intermittent appearance of "a yellow color to her eyes" over the past 3 months.

She has not taken any medications regularly prior to this episode; however, for the last month, she has occasionally taken ibuprofen for the abdominal and joint pains. She denied any use of acetaminophen.

Her medical history was insignificant. She has no history of liver disease or blood transfusions. She has never traveled outside the United States. She was concerned, however, because her roommate has a history of hepatitis B (HBV). She denied any sexual contact with this individual. She stated that she has one sexual partner and uses barrier methods to prevent pregnancy. She is a clerk for a record store. She admitted to drinking about one beer a week and smoking one pack of cigarettes a day. She occasionally smoked marijuana but denied intravenous drug use.

Her physical examination was remarkable for icteric sclera. She had no spider angioma, palmar erythema, caput medusa, or asterixis. Her cardiovascular and respiratory examinations were normal. Her abdominal examination revealed a mildly tender liver of about 12 cm by palpation. Her spleen was not palpable. She did not have costovertebral angle tenderness. Her extremity examination showed no evidence of tenderness, swelling, or erythema of any of her joints.

Laboratory results were as follows: a normal white count, normal hemoglobin, normal hematocrit, and normal platelets. Her electrolytes, blood urea nitrogen (BUN), and creatinine were normal. Her liver function tests were grossly abnormal with a serum aspartate aminotransferase (AST, SGOT) of 1022 IU/L, serum alanine aminotransferase (ALT, SGPT) of 800 IU/L, alkaline phosphatase of 173 IU/L, and bilirubin of 11.9 mg/dl (8.2 mg/dl conjugated). Her prothrombin time was normal. Her total protein was elevated at 9.4 mg/24 hr with a normal albumin of 3.8 μg/d.

Autoimmune Liver Disease

Autoimmune liver diseases, like other diseases of autoimmunity, occur because of the inability of the immune system to differentiate "self" from "nonself." Because of this lack of self-tolerance, immune cells target autologous cells for destruction. In the liver, the three most common autoimmune diseases are autoimmune hepatitis (AIH), primary biliary cirrhosis (PBC), and primary sclerosing cholangitis (PSC). Despite a presumed common pathogenic pathway and the finding of syndromes where characteristics of all of these diseases are manifested, AIH, PBC, and PSC vary widely. They differ in clinical manifestations and responses to treatment. In AIH, the target for destruction appears to be the hepatocyte itself, whereas in PBC and PSC, the primary targets of the destruction are the cells that make up the bile ducts.

MECHANISMS OF INJURY

Association with Human Leukocyte Antigen (HLA) Genotype

The pathogenesis of autoimmune liver disease is unknown, although it is suspected that the combination of a genetic predisposition with some unknown environmental trigger causes an immune response generated against a liver antigen. This in turn results in inflammation, which causes cell destruction, fibrosis, and ultimately cirrhosis. The strongest evidence for a genetic predisposition is found in AIH, where there is a strong association with certain HLA genotypes. The HLA loci are the human equivalent of the major histocompatibility complex (MHC), a highly polymorphic genetic region found in all mammals, whose products are cell surface antigens expressed on a variety of cells. The MHC molecules are cell surface antigens, which can associate with proteins and peptides. Antigen-specific T cells can only react to antigens that are presented in association with MHC antigens and not to the antigens in a free and soluble form. The MHC molecule therefore plays a critical role in the presentation of antigens to T cells. Because of the polymorphism of the MHC and differences in the ability of different MHC molecules to bind to different foreign antigens, immune responses to different antigens potentially can be influenced by the expression of particular MHC molecules. In addition, the MHC also can influence the immune responsiveness to particular antigens by shaping the repertoire of mature T cells. This is because the repertoire of antigens that can be recognized by the mature T cells is determined by the positive and negative selection processes that occur in the thymus. In the thymus, the T cells that respond to foreign antigens are positively selected, and those responding to self-antigens are negatively selected. Thus the avidity with which a specific MHC phenotype binds to specific self antigens theoretically determines the ability of the thymus to select that self-reacting T cell.

In AIH, the target for destruction appears to be the hepatocyte itself, whereas in PBC and PSC, the primary targets of the destruction are the cells that make up the bile ducts.

HLA typing of patients with AIH reveals a strong association with the presence of HLA-A1, B8, DR3, and DR4 genotypes. Interestingly, the DR3, DR4, and DR3/DR4 genotypes are also associated with a number of other autoimmune diseases. The role that the HLA genotype plays in the pathogenesis of autoimmune hepatitis is currently unknown. It may play a direct role because the MHC molecule can influence the development of autoimmunity by controlling T cell selection and activation. However, the association of autoimmune diseases with certain HLA types may just be passive. It may be that the gene for autoimmunity may be linked in distance to the HLA antigens, and thus the HLA may be a marker for an as yet unidentified gene.

In PBC and PSC, some HLA associations have been noted. In PSC, there is an association with HLA DR2 and A1. There is also an association with HLA B8 and DR3, just as in AIH and other autoimmune disease. Although the HLA-B8/DR3 phenotype is not increased in patients with inflammatory bowel disease (IBD), patients with this haplotype who contract ulcerative colitis have a tenfold increased risk of developing PSC.

Autoantibodies

Autoantibodies play a major role in the clinical diagnosis of all these diseases, but their role in the pathogenesis is less well defined (Table 20-1). The strongest association with an autoantibody is in PBC, where the antimitochondrial antibody (AMA) is found in 95% of the cases. Further analysis of this antibody reveals that the specific antigen recognized in most PBC patients is the M2 epitope. The M2 epitope is found within the E2 subunit of 2-oxoacid dehydrogenase enzymes. This is a family of enzymes that includes pyruvate dehydrogenase (PDH), 2-oxoglutaric acid dehydrogenase, and branched chain 2-oxoacid dehydrogenase. All of these enzymes have similar overlapping subunit components. Most of the AMAs found in primary biliary cirrhosis react to the E2 subunit of PDH, although some also cross-react with the E2 subunit of

Table 20-1. Summary of Common Autoantibodies Found in Autoimmune Liver Disease

AUTOANTIBODIES	EPITOPE	LIVER DISEASE ASSOCIATIONS
Antimitochondrial antibody (AMA)	E2 subunit of 2-oxoacid dehydrogenase enzyme (found on the inner membrane of the mitochondria)	Primary biliary cirrhosis
Antinuclear antibody (ANA)	Cell nucleus	Autoimmune hepatitis
Anti–smooth muscle antibody (ASMA)	Smooth muscle actin	Autoimmune hepatitis
Anti–liver kidney microsomal antibody-1 (LKM-1)	Cytochrome P-4502D6 (involved in metabolism of drugs such as debrisoquin)	Autoimmune hepatitis
Anti–liver kidney microsomal antibody-2 (LKM-2)	Cytochrome P-4502C9	Drug-induced hepatitis caused by ticrynafen
Anti–neutrophil antibody (ANCA)	Neutrophil	Primary sclerosing cholangitis

2-oxoglutaric acid dehydrogenase and the E2 subunit of the branched-chain 2-oxoacid dehydrogenase. Interestingly, this enzyme system is highly conserved in nature, and the structure of mammalian PDH resembles that of bacterial and yeast PDH, leading investigators to speculate that molecular mimicry may play a role as a potential pathogenic mechanism. They theorize that somehow infection with a bacteria or yeast may lead to the formation of antibodies to bacterial or yeast PDH-E2, which can then cross-react with the host mammalian PDH-E2 and lead to PBC. Convincing data for this theory are still lacking, although an increased incidence of gram-negative urinary tract infections in patients with PBC has been reported.

The question of how AMAs cause a pathologic lesion remains unanswered. The epitope of this antibody, PDH-E2, is normally localized to the inner membrane of the mitochondria, and therefore access to it by a serum antibody is limited. Arguments against the idea that the AMA is pathogenic are as follows: (1) the AMA does not affect mitochondrial function in vivo; (2) the titer of the antibody bears no relationship to the severity of disease; and (3) although one can induce the production of AMAs by immunization with a PDH-E2 fusion protein, immunized laboratory animals do not have liver damage despite the presence of this antibody. One theory is that PDH-E2-specific antibodies bind and remove specific mitochondrial autoantigens from the cytosol as an immune complex, thus initiating an immune response. Alternatively, AMA may be an epiphenomen. Possibly, destruction of bile ducts and hepatocytes cause disruption of the cellular and mitochondrial membrane, which in turn causes exposure of PDH-E2. For some unexplained reason, the process of PBC causes the specific expression of this particular autoantibody rather than another. Autoantibodies also are found in AIH, and again, their role in the pathogenesis is unclear. AIH is characterized by the presence of several autoantibodies, including antinuclear antibody (ANA), anti–smooth muscle antibody (ASMA), anti–liver kidney microsomal (LKM) antibody, and other less defined antibodies like antisoluble liver antigen. For the ANA, there is no defined pattern. In addition, ANAs are very nonspecific and can be found in many other rheumatologic disorders, such as systemic lupus erythematosus. For both the ANA and ASMA, which constitute the majority of autoantibodies found in patients with AIH in the United States, it is unclear how antibodies to these universal antigens (i.e., to nucleus and smooth muscle actin, respectively) can cause organ-specific damage.

A small group of patients with AIH has LKM antibodies, which appear to react to the cytochrome P-450 enzymes. These enzymes play a prominent role in drug metabolism by hepatocytes. LKM-1 antibodies have been found to react to the microsomal P-450 enzyme, which is involved in the metabolism of debrisoquin, cytochrome P-4502D6 (CYP2D6). Again, this enzyme is found in an intracellular location, not on the surface of hepatocytes. Interestingly, however, the LKM-1 antibodies can inhibit the action of CYP2D6 in drug metabolism in

Notes

vitro, but in vivo, patients with the LKM-1 antibodies have no change in their ability to metabolize drugs with CYP2D6. Thus the functional role of LKM-1 antibodies remains unclear. Another antibody, LKM-2, is found in cases of a rare drug-induced hepatitis caused by ticrynafen. LKM-2 is directed against another P-450 enzyme, cytochrome P-4502C9. Although the finding of LKM-2 in drug-induced hepatitis brings up interesting possibilities for the role of drugs and toxic injuries in the evolution of AIH, direct evidence is lacking.

In 80% of patients with PSC, perinuclear antineutrophil cytoplasmic antibodies (p-ANCAs) can be found; however, these can also be associated with AIH and PBC, undermining their specificity. Antibodies to the colon are found more commonly in patients with sclerosing cholangitis and ulcerative colitis than in patients with ulcerative colitis alone. Although a common epitope to the epithelium of the colon and bile duct has been found, disease-specific autoantibodies to this epitope have not.

Although the presence of these autoantibodies characterize these diseases, there is much cross-reactivity in the different diagnoses, and the presence of a particular antoantibody is truly nonspecific. For example, the presence of ASMAs, although common in AIH, can certainly be found in small groups of patients with both PBC and PSC; thus, these autoantibodies are merely markers of the disease rather than the causative factors.

CASE STUDY: *CONTINUED*

The differential diagnosis includes hepatitis, gallstone disease, and tumors. The patient's laboratory studies showed significant elevations of transaminases, consistent with a picture of hepatitis. The relative lack of elevation in the alkaline phosphatase in the face of a very abnormal bilirubin argues against a cholestatic picture. An ultrasound showed no abnormalities, including no evidence of gallstones or biliary dilation. At this point, the differential would include causes of hepatitis in a young woman. More common diseases, such as viral hepatitis and hepatitis A and B, should be considered. Although hepatitis C is a consideration, the degree of transaminase elevation demonstrated by this patient would be unusual. The differential also should include drug toxicities, including acetaminophen, even though the patient denied its use. Although ibuprofen may cause liver dysfunction, it was not begun until after the onset of the illness. Another possibility in this young patient would be Wilson's disease, but a significantly elevated ceruloplasmin, which was found on laboratory testing, is not consistent with this diagnosis. A significantly elevated ceruloplasmin is not an unusual finding in AIH because it is an acute phase reactant and as such increases states of inflammation. Of particular interest is the high total protein level but normal albumin level, suggesting the presence of hypergammaglobulinemia. A quantitation of gammaglobulins would be useful to confirm this. The differential also should include autoimmune liver diseases, such as AIH, which is a disease characterized by hepatocellular injury, and PBC and PSC, diseases characterized by a predominantly biliary injury.

Three Most Common Autoimmune Diseases

AIH

AIH is a disease characterized by chronic hepatitis of unknown etiology. It has a female predominance and can occur at all ages, although it commonly presents between the ages 10 and 30 and after age 50. It is associated with hypergammaglobulinemia (predominantly of immunoglobulin G [IgG] type), the presence of autoantibodies (particularly ANAs, ASMAs, and, in a small group of patients, LKM antibodies), and the presence of other autoimmune diseases and phenomena. There is an association with the HLA-A1, B8, DR3, and DR4 haplotypes. About 80% of patients with AIH respond to immunosuppressive therapy. The differential diagnosis of chronic hepatitis should include viral hepatitis and Wilson's disease, which are usually excluded by serologic testing and clinical presentation (Table 20-2).

Most patients present with symptoms of hepatitis, including fatigue and jaundice. The liver function tests show evidence of

Table 20-2. Summary of the Clinical Features and Treatment of the Three Most Common Autoimmune Liver Diseases

DIAGNOSIS	CLINICAL FEATURES	DIAGNOSTIC TESTS	THERAPY
Autoimmune hepatitis	Female predominance Presence of other autoimmune diseases Fatigue, right abdominal pain, and anorexia	Liver function tests with predominantly transaminase elevation Hypergammaglobulinemia (IgG predominant) Antinuclear antibody, ASMA-positive, anti-LKM antibody-positive HLA-A1, B8, DR3, and DR4 positive	Steroids Immunosuppressive therapy Liver transplantation for end-stage disease or fulminant hepatic failure
Primary biliary cirrhosis	Pruritus and fatigue Female predominance and middle age Presence of xanthelasma	AMA positive Liver function tests with cholestatic picture Liver biopsy with bile duct injury	Supportive therapy Ursodeoxycholic acid in early disease Liver transplantation for end-stage disease
Primary sclerosing cholangitis	Association with ulcerative colitis Association with cholangiocarcinoma	Liver function tests with cholestatic picture Endoscopic retrograde pancreatography picture of stenosis and stricturing	Supportive therapy Biliary stenting if possible Liver transplantation for end-stage disease or recurrent cholangitis

hepatocellular injury with marked elevations of serum transaminases and bilirubin. Alkaline phosphatase tends to be relatively unaffected compared to the transaminases. The disease can present acutely with evidence of liver failure, or it can present as a chronic hepatitis with periods of acute flare. Hypergammaglobulinemia is often present and is predominantly of the IgG type.

Attempts have been made to subdivide AIH based on the panel of expressed autoantibodies, but its clinical relevance is still unclear because all patients with AIH should be given a trial of immunosuppressive therapy, regardless of the subtype. Type 1 AIH is the most common form and is characterized by the presence of ANAs and ASMAs. Type 2 AIH is characterized by the presence of LKM-1 antibodies. About 50% of these patients present at childhood. Antisoluble liver antigen was previously thought to represent a third type of AIH; however, it is now thought to be associated with Type 1 AIH and is identified in 20% of such patients.

Although the physician may suspect AIH following physical examination and serum diagnostic testing, a liver biopsy is usually needed to confirm the diagnosis. On liver biopsy, the pathologic picture is that of infiltration of the portal and periportal area with lymphocytes. Evidence for destruction of the hepatocytes is seen with ballooning and lytic necrosis of the hepatocyte that is often accompained by the collapse and derangement of the liver lobular architecture. Plasma cells can often be seen in this lymphocytic infiltrate but do not necessarily have to be present for the diagnosis (Figure 20-1).

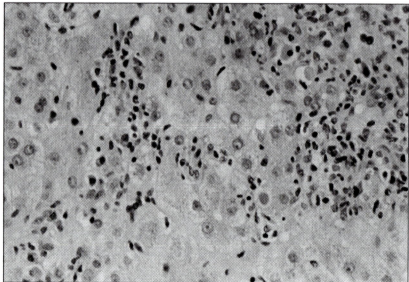

Fig. 20-1.

Liver biopsy slide of a patient with autoimmune hepatitis (H&E 200×). Note the inflammatory infiltration of both the portal tract and lobule composed of lymphocytes, plasma cells, and eosinophils.

In an attempt to make the diagnosis of AIH more uniform, criteria that score the various characteristics in this condition were recently revised by the International Autoimmune Group, a panel of international experts on AIH, and published in 1999 (Tables 20-3 and 20-4). The efficacy of this criteria has yet to be tested clinically.

PBC

PBC is a disease characterized by cholestasis, which results from the immunologically mediated destruction of small intrahepatic bile ducts. This disease affects women more commonly than men in a ratio that has been reported to be as high as 10:1. Patients usually present between the ages of 35 and 65, although the disease has been reported infrequently in individuals younger than 20 years of age and older than 75 years of age. Patients may present with vague symptoms of fatigue and right upper quadrant pain. They often have pruritus. Because jaundice tends to be a symptom of advanced disease, patients classically present with pruritus without jaundice. With the advent of frequent laboratory testing, asymptomatic patients are now diagnosed as a result of elevations of liver enzymes. Typically, the elevations are cholestatic in nature with marked increases in alkaline phosphatase

Notes

PBC is a disease characterized by cholestasis, which results because of the immunologically mediated destruction of small intrahepatic bile ducts.

Table 20-3. Revised Scoring System for Diagnosis of AIH: Minimum Required Parameters

FEATURES	SCORE	FEATURES	SCORE
Female sex	+2	Liver histology	
ALP:AST (or ALT) ratio		Interface hepatitis	+3
<1.5	+2	Predominantly lymphoplasmacytic	+1
1.5–3.0	0	infiltrate	
>3.0	−2	Rosetting of liver cells	+1
Serum globulins *or* IgG above normal		None of the above	−5
>2.0	+3	Biliary changes	−3
1.5–2.0	+2	Other changes	−3
1.0–1.5	+1	Other autoimmune disease(s)	+2
<1.0	0	Optional additional parameters	
ANA, SMA, or anti-LKM-1		Seropositivity for other *defined*	+2
>1:80	+3	autoantibodies	
1:80	+2	HLA-DR3 or -DR4	+1
1:40	+1	Response to therapy	
<1:40	0	Complete	+2
AMA-positive	−4	Relapse	+3
Markers of viral hepatitis		Interpretation of aggregate scores	
Positive	−3	Pretreatment	
Negative	+3	Definite AIH	>15
Drug history		Probable AIH	10–15
Positive	−4	Posttreatment	
Negative	+1	Definite AIH	>17
Average alcohol intake		Probable AIH	12–17
<25 g/d	+2		
>60 g/d	−2		

Source: Reprinted with permission from the European Association for the Study of the Liver 1999, p. 934.

Table 20-4. Explanatory Notes for Table 20-3, the Revised Scoring System for AIH

The ALP:AST (or ALT) ratio relates to the degree of *elevation above upper normal limits* (unl) of these enzymes; for example, (IU/L ALP ÷ unl ALP) ÷ (IU/L AST ÷ unl AST).

Titers determined by indirect immunofluorescence on rodent tissues or, for ANA, on Hep-2 cells. Lower titers (especially of anti-LKM-1) are significant in children and should be scored at least +1.

Score for markers of hepatitis A, B, and C viruses (i.e., positive/negative for IgM anti-HAV, HBsAg, IgM anti-HBc, anti-HCV, and HCV RNA). If a viral cause is suspected despite seronegativity for these markers, tests for other potentially hepatotropic viruses, such as CMV and Epstein-Barr virus, may be relevant.

History of recent or current use of known or suspected hepatotoxic drugs.

Biliary changes are bile duct changes typical of primary biliary cirrhosis or primary sclerosing cholangitis (i.e., granulomatous cholangitis or severe concentric, periductal fibrosis with ductopenia, established in an *adequate* biopsy specimen) and/or a substantial periportal ductular reaction (so-called marginal bile duct proliferation with a cholangiolitis) with an accumulation of copper/copper-associated protein.

Any other *prominent* feature or combination of features suggestive of a different cause.

Score for history of any other autoimmune disorder(s) in patient or first-degree relatives.

The additional points for other defined autoantibodies and HLA-DR3 or HLA-DR4 (if results are available) should be allocated *only* in patients who are seronegative for ANA, SMA, and anti-LKM-1.

Other "defined" autoantibodies are typical pANCA, anti-LC-1, anti-SLA/LP, anti-ASGP-R, and antisulfatide.

HLA-DR3 and HLA-DR4 are mainly of relevance in northern European Caucasoid and Japanese populations. One point may be allocated for other HLA class II antigens if evidence of their association with AIH in other populations has been published.

Assessment of response to therapy may be made at any time. Points should be added to those accrued for features *at initial presentation*.

Response and relapse.

Source: Reprinted with permission from the European Association for the Study of the Liver 1999, p. 934.

and γ-glutamyltranspeptidase and minimal increases in aminotranferases. Other laboratory abnormalities found in patients with PBC are increased cholesterol levels and elevated immunoglobulin M (IgM) levels. The most important serum test to diagnose PBC is the AMA, which is positive in about 95% of cases and is sufficient to establish the diagnosis.

An ultrasound of the liver should be performed to rule out abnormalities of the large bile ducts. A liver biopsy may be helpful to confirm the diagnosis, rule out other causes of cholestatic disease, and assess the stage of the disease. PBC is a slow, progressive disease that has a long asymptomatic phase followed by a symptomatic phase, ultimately resulting in cirrhosis and end-stage liver disease. The stages that have been described on pathology follow the clinical course.

Stage 1 is characterized by infiltration of the portal tract with inflammatory cells. Stage 2 is characterized by spilling of the inflammatory infiltrate into the hepatic lobule, formation of granulomas, and proliferation of small ductules. The proliferation of the small ductules is thought to be a response of the liver, which replaces the loss of the mature bile ducts with these small physiologically ineffective ductules. Stage 3 is characterized by the formation of fibrosis, which links portal tracts. Stage 4 is characterized by the presence of cirrhosis. In all of these stages, there is evidence of inflammatory destruction of intralobular bile ducts. In the later stages, the only evidence of this destruction may be the marked depletion of intralobular bile ducts, defined as ductopenia.

Associated Diseases

The autoimmune nature of PBC is demonstrated by its common association with other autoimmune diseases. The most common association is with Sjögren's syndrome, which is a complex of dry eyes and dry mouth. Other common autoimmune associations are thyroid disease, rheumatoid arthritis, and scleroderma.

Complications

As with other autoimmune diseases, portal hypertensive complications resulting from cirrhosis can occur late in the disease course. Early complications include pruritus, which is often an early symptom in PBC. The cause of the pruritus is unknown. It has been postulated that pruritus may be caused by skin bile acid accumulation. This theory is supported by the improvement in symptoms that occurs with treatment with a bile acid–binding resin or with ursodeoxycholic acid. However, it has been found that skin bile acid levels do not necessarily correlate with the degree of pruritus, and often the bile acid–binding resins and ursodeoxycholic acid afford only minimal relief.

Another common and difficult to treat complication of PBC is osteoporosis, the cause of which is unknown, although these patients have an accelerated rate of bone loss due to decreased formation of bone. It has been suggested that elevated levels of serum bilirubin may contribute to this bone loss by inhibiting osteoblast proliferation. The mechanism of action is unknown. Another potential contributing factor to osteoporosis may be vitamin D malabsorption.

Vitamin D, as well as other fat-soluble vitamins such as vitamin K, may be malabsorbed due to decreased bile acid concentrations in the small intestine. Therefore, patients with PBC and other cholestatic diseases who present with an increased prothrombin time should have a trial of parenteral vitamin K to eliminate vitamin K deficiency as a cause of the malabsorption independent of the degree of liver dysfunction. Other fat-soluble vitamin deficiencies are vitamin E deficiency, which causes a neurologic abnormality affecting the posterior columns that manifests as ataxia and loss of proprioception, and vitamin A deficiency, which causes night blindness.

Hypercholesterolemia, which can be associated clinically with xanthelasma, is characteristically found in patients with PBC as well as those with long-standing cholestasis. In the early stages of PBC, high-density lipoprotein (HDL) predominates, and in later disease, low-density lipoprotein (LDL) exists. Despite the presence of hyperlipidemia, patients with PBC do not have a high risk of developing atherosclerotic disease, and lipid-lowering agents generally are not recommended. The elevations in HDL may be due to a decrease in hepatic lipase activity and an increase in lipoprotein X levels. The increase in lipoprotein X may be a result of a lecithin:cholesterol acyltransferase deficiency, and the decrease in hepatic lipase activity may be due to a circulating plasma inhibitor in some cases.

PSC

Unlike AIH, PSC is a disease that usually presents in men younger than 45 years of age. It is characterized by the presence of inflammation, fibrosis, and obliteration of the intrahepatic and extrahepatic biliary system. There is a strong association with IBD, especially ulcerative colitis, with about 70% of PSC patients having IBD on microscopic examination. However, the activity of one disease is unrelated to the other. Many patients with PSC might not have symptoms of colitis, and alternatively, patients with active ulcerative colitis may not show evidence or symptoms of PSC. The onset of IBD may precede the onset or may occur after the onset of PSC. Prior colectomy does not alter the outcome or clinical course of the liver disease.

Patients may present in a variety of ways. They may present with abnormal liver function tests particularly those of a cholestatic nature with elevations in the alkaline phosphatase and γ-glutamyltransferase. The serum bilirubin level also may be elevated, but in this situation, it is more likely to be a reflection of the degree of biliary obstruction rather than a manifestation of liver dysfunction. Patients may present with evidence of cholangitis, such as fever, chills, and jaundice. The diagnostic test of choice to confirm the diagnosis is endoscopic retrograde cholangiopancreatography (ERCP) (Figure 20-2). The cholangiographic picture is that of diffuse and irregular narrowing and dilatation of the intra- and extrahepatic bile ducts, resulting in a characteristic beaded appearance. The extent of biliary involvement can vary widely, with some patients having only segmental involvement whereas others have diffuse involvement of either the intrahepatic or extrahepatic ducts or both.

Although the diagnosis of PSC is ideally made with an ERCP, a liver biopsy may be obtained to rule out other diseases. On liver biopsy, a characteristic lesion resembling onion skin may be seen in medium-sized portal tracts of 10% of individuals. The appearance is that of a bile duct surrounded by concentric fibrosis. Often there is evidence of bile duct loss in the smaller portal tracts with scattered inflammatory cells and associated ductular proliferation at the periphery of the portal tract.

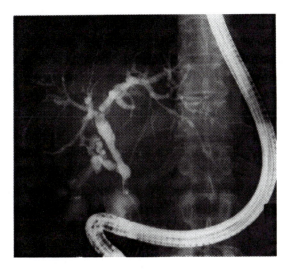

Fig. 20-2.

Typical picture of an ERCP of an individual with PSC.

Complications

In addition to the complications associated with cholestasis discussed previously (i.e., pruritus, fat malabsorption), two other complications of PSC must be mentioned: cholangiocarcinoma and infectious cholangitis.

Although a strong association of cholangiocarcinoma with PSC exists, the actual frequency is difficult to calculate because it is very difficult to differentiate benign from malignant strictures, the hallmark of both diseases. The annual incidence is approximately 0.5%–1%. The pathogenesis of cholangiocarcinoma in PSC may involve immune stimulation, which results in biliary cell dysplasia, leading to malignant transformation. Regardless of the cause, cholangiocarcinoma is a devastating complication and is associated with very poor survival.

Another common complication is the advent of infectious cholangitis. Because of the presence of biliary obstruction, which is inherent to this disease, patients can develop bacterial cholangitis, which usually presents with the onset of fever, chills, and right upper quadrant pain sometimes accompanied by worsening jaundice. This may occur spontaneously or occasionally following manipulation of the biliary tract, such as after an ERCP. Treatment with antibiotics is warranted. Recurrent and refractory cases may be considered for liver transplantation.

Treatment

Steroids and immunosuppressive therapy have been tried for all types of autoimmune liver disease, and although improvement is reflected in the liver injury tests, prolonged survival has only been shown for AIH. In AIH, a response to steroid therapy has been shown in about

The natural history of long-term autoimmune liver disease results in the development of cirrhosis.

80% of patients, and treatment with either steroids alone or steroids with immunosuppressive therapy is clearly indicated. In PBC and PSC, the response to therapy is not as clear; generally, it is felt that given the profound side effects of steroids and other immunosuppressive agents, these therapies should be given only in the context of an experimental protocol.

Ursodeoxycholic acid, which is a nonhepatotoxic hydrophobic bile acid, has been used in both PBC and PSC. In PBC, ursodeoxycholic acid has been shown to improve liver injury tests significantly, particularly in early stage disease. However, its long-term effect on survival is more questionable. Because it has few detrimental side effects, it is used frequently for PSC as well, typically at a higher dose of 20–30 mg/kg per day. The mechanism of action of ursodeoxycholic acid is not entirely clear, but it may compete for absorption and substitute for the more toxic bile acids. It appears to have a less toxic effect on the cell membrane than the more abundant type of bile acids. In addition, it may have immunologic properties that decrease the HLA class 1 antigen expression on hepatocytes and HLA class 2 antigen expression on bile duct epithelium.

In PSC, ERCP can be very useful both for the diagnosis of discrete strictures and for therapy. Some strictures are amenable to endoscopic stenting, which can relieve significant obstruction. Unfortunately, many areas of stricturing are not conducive to stenting because they are diffuse and located in small intrahepatic bile ducts.

The natural history of long-term autoimmune liver disease results in cirrhosis. In selected patients, liver transplantation is the optimal therapy and has been shown to prolong survival in end-stage disease. Liver transplantation should be considered for patients with cirrhosis who either have had complications of portal hypertension or who have extremely limited quality of life due to severe, incapacitating fatigue or pruritus. In patients with PBC, special consideration must be given to a rising bilirubin because this is often a sign of progressive decline.

CASE STUDY: *RESOLUTION*

In the young woman of the case study, serologic findings for HAV, HBV, and HCV were negative. The level of serum IgG was 2.5 times normal. An ASMA was positive at 1:80, and an ANA was 1:6240. AMA was negative. HLA phenotyping was not performed because of the prohibitive cost. A liver biopsy was consistent with an intense portal and periportal inflammatory infiltrate with a predominance of plasma cells and no evidence of significant bile duct damage. A diagnosis of AIH was made. Steroid therapy, in combination with an immunosuppressive therapy, azathioprine, was initiated with significant improvement in clinical symptoms, including the arthralgia. The patient's liver injury tests normalized after 1 month of therapy.

REVIEW QUESTIONS

Directions: For each of the following questions, choose the one best answer.

1 A 50-year-old woman is referred from dermatology to the internal medicine clinic with significant generalized pruritus. The pruritus is worse on the palms and soles and at night. No significant lesions are seen other than scratches. The patient's liver function tests show a fivefold increase in the alkaline phosphatase with nearly normal transaminases and bilirubin. The γ-glutamyltransferase was also elevated. What is the next diagnostic test to obtain?

A Hepatitis B (HBV) serology
B Antimitochondrial antibodies
C Ceruloplasmin
D ERCP
E CT scan of the abdomen to rule out metastatic disease

2 A 50-year-old woman with PBC comes to the physician's office complaining of problems driving at night because she cannot see well. What would be an appropriate next step?

A Do a Rorshach test
B Check vitamin E levels
C Do a Schirmer test
D Do a slit lamp examination
E Check vitamin A levels

3 A 20-year-old woman presents with anorexia and fatigue for 3 months. Liver injury tests show a tenfold increase in the transaminase level and mildly elevated alkaline phosphatase. What would be an appropriate next step?

A Do a laparoscopic cholecystectomy
B Obtain an ERCP
C Refer the patient to an eating disorder clinic
D Obtain an AMA
E Obtain an ASMA

4 A young woman presents to clinic with a 6-month history of fatigue, jaundice, anorexia, and right upper quadrant pain. Liver function tests show an 8-fold increase in transaminase levels and 1.5-fold increase in the alkaline phosphatase. What would be the appropriate next step?

A Admission to the ICU
B Liver transplantation
C Obtain viral hepatitis serologies, antinuclear antibodies, and ceruloplasmin. Perform liver biopsy
D Liver and spleen scan
E ERCP

5 A 40-year-old man with a history of ulcerative colitis who has had a colectomy for his disease complains of recurrent jaundice associated with chills and fevers. Workup for his illness should include

A blood cultures and liver function tests.

B slit lamp examination.

C small bowel follow-through.

D cholecystectomy.

E VDRL testing.

References

European Association for the Study of the Liver: International Autoimmune Hepatitis Group report: review of criteria for diagnosis of autoimmune hepatitis. *J Hepatology* 31:934, 1999.

Johnson PJ, McFarlane IG (Convenors on behalf of the panel): Meeting report: International Autoimmune Hepatitis Group. *Hepatology* 18:998–1005, 1993.

Krawitt EL: Autoimmune hepatitis. *N Engl J Med* 334:897–903, 1996.

LaRusso NF, Wiesner RH, Ludwig J, et al: Current concepts: primary sclerosing cholangitis. *N Engl J Med* 310:899–903, 1984.

Laurin JM, Lindor KD: Primary biliary cirrhosis. *Dig Dis* 12:331–350, 1994.

Martins EB, Chapman RW: Sclerosing cholangitis. *Curr Opin Gastroenterol* 11:452–456, 1995.

Prochazka EJ, Tera Saki PI, Park MS, et al: Association of primary sclerosing cholangitis with HLA DRw52a. *N Engl J Med* 322:1842–1844, 1990.

Schiff L, Schiff ER: *Diseases of the Liver*, 9th ed. Philadelphia, PA: J. B. Lipincott, 2003.

Sherlock S: Primary biliary cirrhosis: clarifying the issues. *Am J Med* 96:27S–33S, 1994.

Vergani D, Mieli-Vergani G: Autoimmune Hepatitis. *Autoimmunity Revs* 2:241–247, 2003.

21

Pathogenesis and Consequences of Portal Hypertension

◼ CHAPTER OUTLINE ◼

◼ LEARNING OBJECTIVES ◼

At the completion of this chapter, the reader should be able to:
- Analyze how portal blood flow and resistance to portal blood flow affect the development of portal hypertension.
- Identify the potential sites of increased resistance in portal hypertension.
- Explain the mechanisms leading to the complications of portal hypertension, notably the development of esophageal varices, ascites, and hepatic encephalopathy.
- Summarize the nature of the neurohumoral responses associated with ascites development.
- Examine the role of ammonia in the pathogenesis of hepatic encephalopathy.

CASE STUDY: *INTRODUCTION*

A 45-year-old man with a long history of alcoholism was brought to the emergency room by his wife because of increased confusion and agitation over the past week. He had been in good health until 2 months previously, when he complained of increased abdominal girth and swelling of his lower extremities. His mental confusion was first noted a day after he had attended a steak cookout where he had eaten heartily but had not consumed any alcohol. His wife had also noted a yellow discoloration in his eyes over the past 3 months. He had no history of trauma, medication, or illicit drug use. He did not have fever, chills, cough, dysuria, or abdominal pain while at home. He did note a 30-lb weight gain over the previous 2 months.

His medical history was remarkable for multiple admissions for alcoholic detoxification. He had abstained from alcohol for the previous 4 months after completing his most recent rehabilitation program. He did not have a history of blood transfusions or intravenous drug use. He had been drinking two to three six-packs of beer a day for the past 20 years.

On examination, he was an agitated, mumbling, disheveled man who was not following commands. His vital signs were recorded as: blood pressure, 160/100 mm Hg; heart rate, 95 beats/min; respiratory rate, 18 breaths/min; and temperature, 99°F.

Head and neck examination revealed no icteric sclera, and no jugular venous distention was noted. Cardiovascular examination revealed a regular rate and rhythm. Lungs were clear to auscultation. Abdominal examination revealed tense ascites, without tenderness, guarding, or rebound. A caput medusae was appreciated along with prominent superficial veins on his abdominal wall. Rectal examination revealed hemoccult-negative brown stool. Extremity examination was notable for 3+ pitting edema of his thighs. Skin examination was notable for multiple spider angiomata on his back. Neurologic examination revealed an alert but agitated man who was mumbling incoherently and did not follow commands. He was moving all extremities and withdrew to painful stimuli. Asterixis was also noted, but other motor reflexes were all intact.

Laboratory tests were ordered. A coagulation profile revealed the following data: prothrombin time (PT), 17 seconds (prolonged); and international normalized ratio, 2.2. A hematologic profile revealed the following data: WBC count, 8000/mm^3; hemoglobin, 12 g/dl; hematocrit, 38 mg/100 ml; and platelets, 74,000/mm^3 (low). Liver function revealed the following data: AST, 100 U/L (increased); ALT, 85 U/L (increased); albumin, 2.3 g/dl (low); and total bilirubin, 6.0 mg/dl (elevated). Electrolyte values were as follows: sodium (Na$^+$), 128 mEq/L (low); chloride (Cl$^-$), 105 mEq/L; BUN, 20 mg/dl; potassium (K$^+$), 3.7 mEq/L; bicarbonate (HCO$_3^-$), 20 mEq/L; and creatinine, 1.1 mg/dl.

Pathophysiology of Portal Hypertension

Portal hypertension is a hemodynamic abnormality that occurs most commonly as a consequence of severe liver disease. Portal vein pressures greater than normal (5–10 mm Hg) define portal hypertension. The three most important clinical consequences of portal hypertension are hemorrhage from gastroesophageal varices, ascites, and hepatic encephalopathy.

ANATOMY

A brief review of anatomy will facilitate understanding of the pathophysiology of portal hypertension. The portal vein carries blood to the liver from the veins that drain the major splanchnic organs. This includes venous drainage from the small and large intestines, the spleen, the pancreas, and the gallbladder. The portal vein is formed by the convergence of the superior mesenteric and splenic veins (Figure 21-1). The superior mesenteric vein drains the capillary beds of the right colon, small intestine, and pancreas. The splenic vein drains the capillary beds of the spleen as well as the inferior mesenteric vein, which drains the left colon and rectum. The portal vein flows into the liver at the porta hepatis, where it divides into the right and left branches and continues to divide progressively until it reaches the level of the hepatic sinusoids, which are uniquely interconnected. The hepatic sinusoids drain into the central vein, which flows into the hepatic veins and finally into the inferior vena cava.

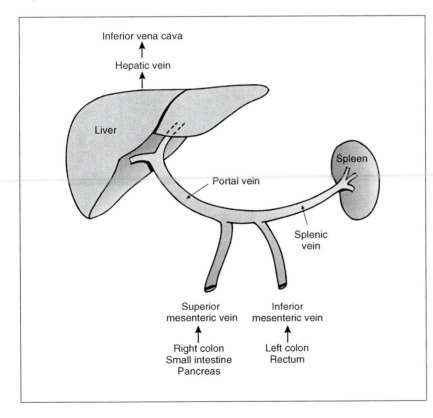

Fig. 21-1. Anatomy of the Portal Venous System

The unique feature of the portal vein is its location between two capillary beds, the splanchnic capillaries and the hepatic sinusoids. Hepatic sinusoids differ widely from other capillaries because they are extensively interconnected and highly permeable. High permeability is due to endothelial cells that line the sinusoids; these endothelial cells have large gaps called fenestrae, which allow diffusion of even high-molecular-weight proteins. Given the extensive interconnections and high permeability, the resistance of the hepatic sinusoids is generally very low (Figure 21-2).

DEVELOPMENT OF PORTAL HYPERTENSION

As with any vascular system, portal venous blood flow (Q) is dependent on the portal pressure gradient (P) and vascular resistance (R). The relationship is a modification of Ohm's law that applies to fluids.

Portal vein pressure is affected by blood flow and vascular resistance as described by Ohm's law:

$$Q \text{ (flow)} = \frac{P \text{ (perfusion gradient along the portal vein)}}{R \text{ (resistance to the flow of fluid)}}$$

The relationship can be restated as:

Portal venous pressure = Q (blood flow) × R (vascular resistance)

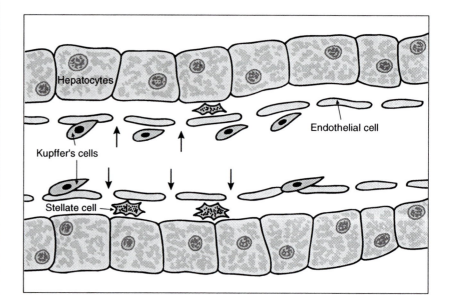

Fig. 21-2. Diagrammatic Drawing of Hepatic Sinusoids

Hepatic sinusoids are highly permeable because the endothelial cells that line the sinusoids have large gaps called fenestrae (arrows), which allow diffusion of high-molecular-weight proteins between the sinusoidal space and the hepatocytes. As demonstrated here, hepatic sinusoids are made up of hepatocytes and nonparenchymal cells including Kupffer's cells, stellate cells, and endothelial cells. The proximity of these cells and the presence of fenestrae allow for interaction of both hepatocytes and nonparenchymal cells with the portal blood flow that traverses the sinusoids.

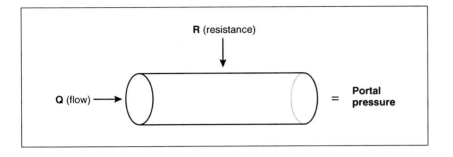

Fig. 21-3. Resistance

Resistance to the flow of blood is expressed by Poiseuille's law: $R = 8nL/\pi r^4$, where n = coefficient of viscosity, π = 3.14, L = length of vessel, and r = radius.

Therefore, portal venous pressure rises if either blood flow (Q) or vascular resistance (R) increases independently, or if both increase together (Figure 21-3).

Resistance

Poiseuille's law states that $R = 8nL/\pi r^4$. Because the length of a vessel (L) generally does not change, the viscosity (n) of blood remains about the same at a stable hematocrit, and π is a constant 3.14; the most important variable is the radius (r). The radius is factored to the fourth power in Poiseuille's law; therefore small changes in the radius can cause large changes in the resistance.

The radius of a blood vessel is affected by the compliance of the vessel. An elastic blood vessel distends as the internal pressure increases, thus increasing the radius and decreasing resistance. The relationship between the change in volume of a blood vessel for a given change in pressure is defined as *compliance.*

Under physiologic conditions, the liver is the main site of resistance to portal blood flow. Because of the unique anatomy of the sinusoids, vascular resistance in the normal liver is very low and can accommodate large changes in portal blood flow without significant changes in portal pressure.

Portal Blood Flow

The other variable in the determination of portal pressure is portal blood flow. Blood flow into the portal veins is determined by the splanchnic arterioles. Unlike the systemic venous system, the portal venous system appears incapable of autoregulation. It passively accepts the venous system that drains into it. Therefore, constriction or dilation of the splanchnic arterioles is the main factor in determining the quantity of blood that drains into the portal venous system.

When the splanchnic arterioles are dilated, there is an increase in the portal venous inflow, and when the splanchnic arterioles are constricted there is a decrease in portal blood flow. Physiologically, portal flow markedly increases after a meal because of a marked increase in splanchnic arterial blood flow. However, with a normal liver, the

The liver has the capacity to accommodate large changes in blood flow.

One way of classifying portal hypertension is by defining the site of increased resistance:
1. Prehepatic
2. Hepatic (presinusoidal, sinusoidal, or postsinusoidal)
3. Posthepatic

portal pressure remains relatively stable because the liver sinusoidal resistance is low while compliance is high, because intra- and extra-hepatic veins dilate as flow is increased.

CAUSES OF PORTAL HYPERTENSION

Increase in Portal Vein Inflow

Portal hypertension may be initiated by an increase in portal venous inflow. A rare cause is an arteriovenous fistula. However, even in this case, it is not just an increase in blood flow that results in portal hypertension. As mentioned earlier, the liver has the capacity to accommodate to large changes in blood flow. In fact, in cases of chronically increased portal venous inflow, the change in blood flow leads to intravascular changes that will alter resistance. This situation is analogous to what occurs in the lungs in patients with left-to-right intraventricular shunts. Although an increase in portal venous inflow exists in portal hypertension, it often is unclear if it is the initiating factor.

The splanchnic circulation in portal hypertension is indeed hyperdynamic and is characterized by low arteriolar resistance. The vasodilation is accompanied by an increased cardiac index and an increased blood flow to splanchnic and systemic organs.

The vasodilation appears to be mediated by the combined effect of circulating vasodilators (e.g., glucagon) and by decreased vascular reactivity to vasoconstrictors (e.g., norepinephrine). The hyperkinetic circulation elevates portal pressure and is a factor in maintaining portal hypertension.

Increases in Resistance

By far the most common causes of portal hypertension are conditions that increase resistance to portal flow. The causes of increased resistance can be intravascular (e.g., thrombi) or extravascular (e.g., fibrosis, tumors, granulomas).

Prehepatic portal hypertensive disorders (e.g., splenic and portal vein thromboses) and posthepatic disorders (e.g., inferior vena caval webs, congestive heart failure) have well-defined sites of increased resistance. The hepatic lesions are more complex and often evolve as the disease progresses. For example, in hepatic schistosomiasis, the disease initially leads to presinusoidal impairment in portal flow as granulomas develop in response to egg deposition, but as the disease progresses, hepatic sinusoids also display increased resistance to flow. Alcoholic liver disease has features of both sinusoidal and postsinusoidal obstruction to flow.

As liver disease progresses and approaches cirrhosis, the intrahepatic resistance is known to increase. The exact mechanism of increased resistance is not clear, but both fixed and dynamic obstructive lesions have been observed. The fixed lesions include deposition of collagen in the spaces of Disse and terminal hepatic vein fibrosis.

The more dynamic lesions include hepatocyte ballooning with compression of the sinusoids, as seen in early alcoholic liver disease.

These ballooning changes can regress with abstinence and reverse the portal hypertension. Myofibroblasts also surround the sinusoids and hepatic venules and can contract, increasing vascular resistance. The contractile myofibroblasts have been shown to be responsive to vasodilators, suggesting that portal hypertension may be treated medically.

Consequences of Portal Hypertension

Regardless of the cause of portal hypertension, the consequences of this hemodynamic change, including variceal bleeding, ascites, and hepatic encephalopathy, account for the morbidity and mortality.

Variceal Bleeding

In portal hypertension, the increased portal pressure leads to the formation of portosystemic collaterals. Chronic elevation in portal pressure leads to dilation of preexisting vessels. Active angiogenesis may also be involved in the formation of collaterals. These collaterals are then responsible for the shunting of blood from the portal vein to the systemic circulation, bypassing the liver. The sites of these shunts at naturally occurring areas of portosystemic contact result in the formation of varices. In the gastroesophageal area, these collaterals result in gastroesophageal varices; in the rectal area, rectal varices are formed; and in the umbilical area, dilated superficial veins form around the umbilicus, creating a venous network known as *caput medusae*. A unique area for formation of varices is peristomal and may be seen as an example in patients who had a colectomy and ileostomy for inflammatory bowel disease and suffer with associated primary sclerosing cholangitis with cirrhosis.

All of these varices can burst and cause bleeding, but the most common site of rupture is the esophagus. As portal pressure increases, the likelihood of esophageal variceal rupture increases and dramatically escalates the rate of mortality from cirrhosis.

A number of treatment modalities have been developed to provide acute hemostasis and prevent rebleeding, including endoscopic, pharmacologic, mechanical, radiologic, and surgical approaches. For acute esophageal variceal bleeding, rubber band ligation is currently the treatment of choice. Another option is injection sclerotherapy, wherein a caustic sclerosant is injected directly into the region of the varices through a flexible endoscope. The two methods are roughly equivalent in terms of control of acute bleeding; however, sclerotherapy carries a greater potential for complications. Prior to endoscopic therapy, pharmacologic therapy should be initiated with either somatostatin (and its analog octreotide) or vasopressin (and its analog terlipressin). The latter option has been associated with serious risks and therefore somatostatin analog is the treatment of choice with its mechanism of action in this scenario of decreasing splanchnic blood flow.

Mechanical treatment has been used with the Sengstaken-Blakemore tube or a similar device. This tube resembles a nasogastric tube but has inflatable gastric and esophageal balloons, which are inflated to tamponade the variceal bleeding temporarily. Because of the high incidence of adverse effects and the temporary nature of the treatment, mechanical treatment is usually not used unless the endoscopic sclerotherapy and pharmacologic therapy have failed or are not available. For a more permanent solution, a portosystemic shunt can be created and is often effective in preventing further bleeding. This can be performed radiologically using a transjugular approach or surgically. The former procedure, known as TIPS (transjugular intrahepatic portosystemic shunt) may increase the risk of encephalopathy but is particularly useful in the setting of treating a serious bleed while awaiting transplantation. Surgical creation of portosystemic shunts is most effective in patients with preserved liver function. In selected patients with poor liver function, liver transplantation is sometimes the best long-term option.

ASCITES

Ascites is most commonly associated with cirrhosis but may also occur as a result of many other disease states, including neoplasm, tuberculosis, and protein deficiency states including nephrotic syndromes and protein-losing enteropathies. Ascites is a sign of decompensation in liver disease and is associated with a mortality rate of up to 50% within 2 years of its initial presentation.

The pathophysiology of ascites formation in cirrhosis is complex and involves the combined effect of portal hypertension, volume overload, and mechanical factors.

Role of Portal Hypertension in the Development of Ascites

Intrahepatic portal hypertension with high sinusoidal pressures is necessary for ascites to develop. Ascites is rare in patients with prehepatic portal hypertension.

Increased hepatic sinusoidal pressure drives fluid across the sinusoidal endothelium into the spaces of Disse, from which it is removed by the hepatic lymphatics. The rate of fluid efflux is directly related to the sinusoidal pressure. When sinusoidal pressure increases to the level where the rate of fluid efflux exceeds the capacity of the hepatic lymphatics to drain it, there is a net seepage of fluid from the hepatic surface to the peritoneal cavity. This fluid accumulates as ascites.

Pathophysiology of Ascites

Ascites is associated with a state of both intravascular and extravascular volume overload. However, the neurohumoral response associated with ascites is that of a volume-depleted state. This is characterized by Na$^+$ and water retention with increased sympathetic activity. Various theories, which are discussed next, explain this apparent paradox by attempting to identify the initial event in ascites formation.

Underfill Theory.   In the underfill theory, the primary event in ascites formation is the spillover of fluid into the peritoneal cavity. The resulting intravascular depletion triggers Na^+ retention, which leads to volume retention and further spillover into the peritoneal cavity. This vicious cycle repeats itself, resulting in accumulation of ascites.

Overfill Theory.   In the overfill theory, renal Na^+ retention is believed to be the primary event, and fluid spillover into the peritoneal cavity is a consequence of the increased intravascular volume.

Peripheral Arterial Vasodilatation Hypothesis.   Neither the overfill or the underfill theory has proved satisfactory. Recently, a hypothesis was proposed that incorporates both the underfill and overflow theories into the development of ascites by evaluating the hemodynamic changes in early and late cirrhosis.

In the early stage before ascites develops, impaired hepatocellular functioning or portosystemic shunting yields to an increase in endogenous vasodilators, which lead to splanchnic arterial vasodilation. The vasodilation results in a decrease in effective arterial blood volume and in intravascular hypovolemia. Transient renal Na^+ and water retention occur to maintain intravascular volume. In the early stages, there is no significant increase in plasma renin, aldosterone, norepinephrine, or antidiuretic hormone (ADH) levels, as a result of the transient nature of the hemodynamic compensations. As the liver disease progresses and ascites develops, the transient Na^+ and water retention are not sufficient to maintain intravascular volume. The renin-angiotensin-aldosterone system is then activated more consistently by afferent baroreceptors in the kidney to maintain intravascular homeostasis. ADH and catecholamines are also released to maintain intravascular volume.

As vasodilatation worsens, renal failure may develop. This state is referred to as hepatorenal syndrome and is characterized by intravascular hypovolemia; elevated renin, aldosterone, and catecholamine levels; and marked renal vasoconstriction and hyponatremia resulting from increased ADH levels.

However, the peripheral arterial vasodilatation theory does not explain some of the experimental findings in ascites development. Experimental models show that Na^+ retention precedes the increase in plasma volume and ascites formation; therefore, this theory needs modification.

Management of Ascites

Ascites is managed by regulating the total body water content using various modalities. Moderate dietary restriction of Na^+ (90 mmol/day) and fluid intake is the simplest intervention and effectively decreases intravascular fluid content. Diuretics, such as aldactone and furosemide, are added when dietary changes alone are ineffective. Abdominal paracentesis is performed to remove fluid actively from

Hepatorenal syndrome is usually irreversible and is associated with a high mortality.

the peritoneal cavity in patients refractory to dietary and pharmacologic intervention. For individuals who require large volumes of fluid to be removed, intravenous albumin should be administered. Large-volume paracentesis without plasma volume expansion frequently impairs circulatory function, which can adversely influence the patient's clinical course. Various peritoneal venous shunts have been used to avoid the need for repeated paracentesis; however, these shunts have been plagued with a high rate of complications and shunt occlusion. Recently, TIPS, which can be performed radiologically, has been used to treat refractory ascites with some promising results. Selected patients with refractory ascites should be considered for liver transplantation.

Spontaneous infection of ascitic fluid, or spontaneous bacterial peritonitis (SBP), occurs in 10%–30% of patients admitted to the hospital with ascites. The most predictive factor for the development of SBP is a low ascitic fluid protein concentration (< 10 g/L). The pathogenesis of SBP is multifactorial and includes (1) colonization of ascitic fluid from an episode of bacteremia, (2) translocation of bacteria from the intestinal lumen into the circulation, (3) impaired reticuloendothelial function, and (4) decreased antibacterial ability of ascitic fluid. The diagnosis of SBP is determined by diagnostic paracentesis and the concentration of polymorphonuclear cells (PMNs) in ascitic fluid. Patients with a PMN concentration of > 250 cells/μl should be started on antibiotics, typically a third-generation cephalosporin. Although the prognosis of SBP has improved with earlier diagnosis and improved antibiotic coverage, the mortality rate still remains high (30%). Moreover, life expectancy after an episode of SBP is poor, so patients recovering from an episode should be considered for transplantation.

HEPATIC ENCEPHALOPATHY

Hepatic encephalopathy is a syndrome encompassing impaired mental functioning, diminished consciousness, and neuromuscular abnormalities associated with liver disease. The clinical presentation of patients may range from subtle changes in intellectual functioning to deep coma.

Pathophysiology of Hepatic Encephalopathy

Hepatic encephalopathy is most commonly associated with portal hypertension and portosystemic shunting. It has also been referred to as portosystemic encephalopathy resulting from the peripheral accumulation of many neurotoxins from the splanchnic circulation that are not extracted by the cirrhotic liver (Table 21-1).

There are various theories that attempt to identify the neurotoxins involved in the pathogenesis of hepatic encephalopathy. These theories are discussed next.

Ammonia Hypothesis.   Many syndromes associated with increased serum ammonia levels, such as Reye's syndrome, urea cycle enzyme

Table 21-1. Common Precipitating Causes of Hepatic Encephalopathy

Increased protein load: dietary or GI bleeding
Hypokalemia from overdiuresis
Drugs, particularly benzodiazepines or other sedatives
Infection (e.g., spontaneous bacterial peritonitis [SBP])
Iatrogenic worsening of portosystemic shunting

deficiencies, and portal hypertension with portosystemic shunting, have clinical features of hepatic encephalopathy. This observation has led to the identification of ammonia as the primary neurotoxin in hepatic encephalopathy.

Ammonia is the key metabolite in nitrogen metabolism and is produced largely in the GI tract through the degradation of luminal protein by bacteria. The ammonia is absorbed into the portal venous system and transported to the liver, where it is first detoxified to glutamine, and then to urea, prior to being excreted in the urine and stool. In the presence of portal hypertension, portosystemic shunting ensues and exposes the systemic circulation to toxic ammonia concentrations.

High arterial and cerebrospinal fluid ammonia levels correlate with hepatic encephalopathy, and measures that decrease serum ammonia are associated with clinical improvement. However, the clinical correlations are not absolute, and a great deal of variability is found in ammonia levels from person to person.

The exact mechanism of ammonia-induced encephalopathy is unknown. Theories include ammonia-induced impairment in synaptic neurotransmission and altered neuron–astrocyte interaction. Histologically, astrocytes containing large vacuolated nuclei with chromatin displaced to the side, referred to as Alzheimer type II astrocytes, are often seen in hepatic encephalopathy. These cells may develop as a consequence of glutamine synthetase activity, which is localized mainly in astrocytes and metabolizes ammonia to the less toxic glutamine. The level of brain glutamine—the product of ammonia metabolism—seems to be more directly related to hepatic encephalopathy than blood ammonia levels.

Multifactorial Hypothesis. This hypothesis predicts a synergistic effect of ammonia, mercaptans, and short-chain fatty acids in the production of hepatic encephalopathy. These substances are all increased in hepatic encephalopathy, and experimental animal models have shown that each substance can increase the encephalopathogenic potential of the others.

False Neurotransmitter Hypothesis. Hepatic encephalopathy is associated with a depletion of the neurotransmitter dopamine. This hypothesis proposes that the depletion of the true neurotransmitter dopamine is compensated for by less effective, false neurotransmitters

Notes

When hepatic encephalopathy is suspected, a thorough search for precipitating causes must be undertaken.

like octopamine. Unfortunately, contrary to this hypothesis, clinical studies that have attempted to restore dopamine levels within the brain by using dopaminergic drugs like bromocriptine have not been successful in improving hepatic encephalopathy.

GABA Hypothesis. γ-Aminobutyric acid (GABA) is the principal inhibitory neurotransmitter in the brain, and its concentrations may be increased in hepatic encephalopathy. Increased GABA may result from increased ammonia levels by means of a pathway in which glutamate, formed from ammonia, may be converted to GABA by neuronal cells. Alternatively, GABA may be gut-derived and may accumulate as a result of lack of clearance by the liver in cirrhosis. The increased GABA concentrations could promote the neural inhibition seen in hepatic encephalopathy. Alternatively, the GABA receptor may be involved in hepatic encephalopathy via the GABA–benzodiazepine complex receptor. GABA can bind to at least two types of receptors, one of which is intimately involved with the benzodiazepine receptor. This complex receptor has distinct binding sites for GABA, benzodiazepines, and barbiturates. Binding of GABA to this complex results in Cl^- conductance and neuroinhibition. It has been found that benzodiazepines and barbiturates can potentiate the neuroinhibition of GABA by binding to this receptor and lowering the concentration of GABA needed to open the Cl^- channel (Figure 21-4). Some studies have found evidence for increases of endogenous benzodiazepines, which can cause hepatic encephalopathy via this mechanism. The use of benzodiazepine antagonists has been shown to be effective in improving hepatic encephalopathy in some patients. Despite some promising results, the role of GABA and of the GABA–benzodiazepine receptor in hepatic encephalopathy is still not firmly established.

Treatment of Encephalopathy

Although the pathophysiology of hepatic encephalopathy is not fully understood, certain empiric treatments have evolved, which appear to be effective in improving mental status. The mainstay of therapy is the use of an osmotic cathartic agent, lactulose. The mechanism by which lactulose works is unclear, but it seems to interact with enteric flora to decrease production of nitrogenous compounds. Dietary restriction of protein may also be effective in improving hepatic encephalopathy, perhaps by reducing the production of ammonia from the breakdown of nitrogenous compounds. Dietary restrictions, however, must be tailored to the needs of patients with cirrhosis who need to maintain adequate nutrition.

In a patient who develops hepatic encephalopathy, one should also focus on the search for an underlying aggravating cause. Some common causes of worsening encephalopathy include increased protein load, either dietary or as a result of GI bleeding; hypokalemia; drugs, especially benzodiazepines; infection; and the iatrogenic worsening of portosystemic shunting with the introduction of either a TIPS or a surgical shunt.

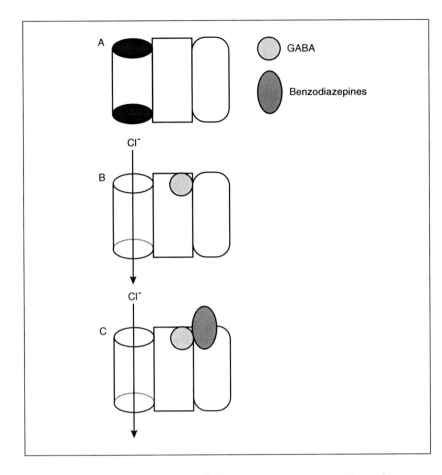

Fig. 21-4. Illustration of the GABA Receptor Complex

(A) Without binding of GABA, the chloride (Cl⁻) channel is closed. (B) With the binding of GABA to the receptor complex, the Cl⁻ channel is open and an influx of Cl⁻ occurs and inhibits further neurotransmission. (C) Binding of the GABA complex by benzodiazepines allows for a lower concentration of GABA needed to open the Cl⁻ channel.

CASE STUDY: *RESOLUTION*

This is a classic presentation of a patient with acute hepatic encephalopathy in the context of established cirrhosis. The patient had a long history of significant alcohol abuse, which placed him at risk for alcoholic cirrhosis. The patient's confusion and agitation, which developed after a large protein meal, often is a sign of hepatic encephalopathy.

The cirrhosis had been well compensated until the recent development of ascites. Other signs of hepatic decompensation included increased prothrombin time and decreased albumin, both suggesting impaired hepatic synthetic function of albumin and coagulation factors.

The presence of portal hypertension was illustrated by the patient's tense ascites and low platelet count. The ascites developed

as a result of the increasing intrahepatic resistance with progressive cirrhosis. The low platelet count was a more subtle clue, suggesting the sequestration of platelets in an enlarged spleen, which develops as a result of increased portal pressure.

The skin findings of a caput medusae suggested increased umbilical vein pressure due to portal hypertension. The spider angiomata were telangiectasias caused by dilation of superficial arteries, often seen in chronic liver disease. Asterixis is a flapping tremor, consisting of involuntary jerking movements, best elicited by having the patient dorsiflex his wrists. It is a clinical sign often seen in hepatic encephalopathy.

The patient was admitted to the hospital, and a paracentesis was performed, which did not show signs of SBP. He was diagnosed with hepatic encephalopathy induced by his high-protein meal. He improved with lactulose treatment and was discharged home after 2 days.

*R*EVIEW *Q*UESTIONS

Directions: For each of the following questions, choose the one best answer. Questions 1–4 are based on the case study below.

A 56-year-old woman with a history of chronic alcoholism and hepatitis C is brought to the emergency room for the evaluation of increasing confusion and agitation. She has had increasing ascites over the past 2 months associated with a 30-lb weight gain. Her physical examination is notable for agitation and confusion without focal neurologic findings, tense ascites, a caput medusae, multiple spider angiomata on her back, and asterixis. Laboratory abnormalities include a prolonged prothrombin time and an international normalized ratio of 2.5. Platelets were decreased (60,000/mm^3); transaminases were increased (AST, 150 U/L; ALT, 50 U/L); albumin was decreased (2.2 g/dl); bilirubin was increased (4.0 mg/dl); and hyponatremia was present (sodium, 128 mEq/L).

1 If this patient presented to the physician's office complaining of increasing swelling in her lower extremities and weight gain, which drug would be the first-line agent to manage excess total body water if therapy was aimed at reversing the underlying mechanism that contributes to ascites formation?

A β-blocker
B Carbonic anhydrase inhibitor
C Aldosterone antagonist
D Thiazide diuretic

2 β-Adrenergic blockers are useful in the management of portal hypertension primarily because of their effect on

   A decreasing the vasodilation of the portal vasculature by their effect on the β_2 receptors.
   B minimizing the effect of the hyperdynamic state associated with portal hypertension.
   C promoting relaxation of the afferent arterioles in the renal vasculature, facilitating renal excretion of excess fluid.
   D promoting relaxation of the contractile myofibroblasts surrounding hepatic sinusoids and venules, reducing intrahepatic resistance.

3 The patient's agitation should be managed with

   A sedative drugs, such as benzodiazepines.
   B aggressive diuresis to decrease portal pressure.
   C nonabsorbable osmotic cathartic agents.
   D dietary protein restriction.

4 Abstinence from alcohol can reverse the portal hypertension associated with alcoholic liver disease by

   A reducing the portal flow as a result of the decreased intake of fluid.
   B reducing the intrahepatic resistance as a result of the regression of collagen deposition in the spaces of Disse.
   C reducing the intrahepatic resistance by the reversal of hepatocyte ballooning.
   D reversing the portal vein thrombosis associated with liver disease.

5 A 50-year-old woman with cirrhosis secondary to hepatitis C presents to the clinic with new symptoms of lethargy, abdominal pain, and mild confusion. On physical examination, she is noted to have asterixis and worsening ascites. What is the most appropriate next step?

   A Admittance to the hospital for more aggressive diuretic therapy
   B Diagnostic paracentesis, electrolyte analysis, rectal examination, CBC, and careful history of any recent drug ingestion
   C Ultrasound of the abdomen
   D Lumbar puncture and EEG

References

Blei AT: Portal hypertension. *Curr Opin Gastroenterol* 10:295, 1994.
DeFranchis R: Developing consensus in portal hypertension. *J Hepatol* 25:390–394, 1996.
Dudley FJ: Pathophysiology of ascites formation. *Gastroenterol Clin North Am* 21:215–235, 1992.

Notes

Jones EA, Skolnick P, Gammal SH, et al.: The γ-aminobutyric acid A receptor complex and hepatic encephalopathy. *Ann Intern Med* 110:532–546, 1989.

Mousseau DD, Butterworth RF: Current theories on the pathogenesis of hepatic encephalopathy. *Proc Soc Exp Biol Med* 206:329, 1994.

Mullen KD, Jones EA: Natural benzodiazepines and hepatic encephalopathy. *Semin Liver Dis* 16:255–264, 1996.

Rocco VK, Ware AJ: Cirrhotic ascites: pathophysiology, diagnosis, and management. *Ann Intern Med* 105:573–585, 1986.

Terblanche J, Burroughs AK, Hobbs KEF: Current controversies in the management of bleeding esophageal varices (pt 1). *N Engl J Med* 320:1393–1398, 1989.

Terblanche J, Burroughs AK, Hobbs KEF: Current controversies in the management of bleeding esophageal varices (pt 2). *N Engl J Med* 320:1469–1475, 1989.

Villanueva C, Balanzo J, Novella MT, et al: Nadolol plus isosorbide mononitrate compared with sclerotherapy for the prevention of variceal rebleeding. *N Engl J Med* 334:1624–1629, 1996.

22

Disorders of Cholestasis, Bilirubin Metabolism, and Jaundice

■ CHAPTER OUTLINE ■

■ LEARNING OBJECTIVES ■

At the completion of this chapter, the reader should be able to:
• Define cholestasis, jaundice, and pruritus.
• Review bile synthesis and secretion and explain the consequences of
  alterations of bile secretion.
• Classify extrahepatic and intrahepatic cholestasis and explain their causes.
• Explain disorders of bilirubin metabolism and excretion.

Cholestasis is a syndrome resulting from impaired delivery of bile from the hepatocyte to the duodenum and is characterized by specific changes in certain biochemical markers in serum.

Jaundice refers to a yellow pigmentation of the skin, sclerae, and mucous membranes, resulting from deposition of bilirubin in these tissues.

CASE STUDY: *INTRODUCTION*

A 7-day-old male infant was brought to the clinic by his mother because she noticed that he appeared to have a yellow tinge to his skin. The infant was born 3 weeks prior to his expected due date and weighed 2790 g. The pregnancy, the mother's first, was uncomplicated except for prolonged morning sickness; labor and the vaginal delivery were normal. The infant's Apgar score was 8. The mother was a 33-year-old graduate student with no significant medical history other than having a body weight about 10%–15% above normal for most of her adult life and severe seasonal allergies. Mother and child were discharged when the baby was 2 days old. He appeared to have a good appetite and was drinking 2–3 oz of a standard cows' milk–based infant formula every 3 hours. He showed no signs of GI distress. However, he had lost 175 g since birth. Stools were regular and yellow, with no apparent diarrhea.

The physical examination revealed moderate jaundice, but otherwise the infant appeared to be healthy with no other significant physical findings.

The initial laboratory screening showed: total bilirubin, 9.5 mg/dl; direct (conjugated) bilirubin, less than 1 mg/dl; and hemoglobin, 13.5 g/dl.

Introduction

Cholestasis is a syndrome of characteristic serum (biochemical) and hepatic (morphologic) findings that result from impaired bile delivery from the hepatocyte to the duodenum. Cholestasis is a descriptive term, not a diagnosis per se. Cholestasis can arise from diseases that affect hepatocytes, the biliary system, or the pancreas and may include genetic and acquired diseases. Disruption of bile flow for *any* reason eventually interferes with excretion of bile components, resulting in the cardinal features of cholestasis: jaundice (bilirubin pigmentation), pruritus (bile acid–associated itching), xanthomas (cholesterol deposits), and impaired emulsification of dietary fat leading to steatorrhea (fatty stool).

Jaundice (or icterus) refers to a yellow (or sometimes yellow-greenish) pigmentation of the skin, sclerae, and mucous membranes. This coloration results from excess levels of serum *bilirubin*, the end product of heme degradation, which deposits in these tissues; these tissues are particularly affected because they contain high concentrations of elastin, an extracellular matrix protein for which bilirubin has a high affinity. Jaundice is most likely to occur when bilirubin values are 2–4 mg/dl (normal, < 1); however, the visualization of jaundice depends on several factors, such as the natural skin color of the patient, the type of light, and the rapidity of rise in bilirubin levels.

Jaundice can result from disorders that affect overall bile flow or may develop as a consequence of abnormal bilirubin metabolism with normal bile flow.

Pruritus is the itching (often quite severe) that frequently accompanies cholestasis. Sometimes this is the presenting symptom in cholestasis. It was originally postulated to be caused by the increased bile acids in serum, but several lines of evidence now suggest that the causative agents are other substances that are associated with bile acids but are not the acids themselves. Pruritus may be treated with histamine (H_1) blockers, ursodeoxycholic acid, and in recent trials, naloxone (opiate antagonist) and its derivatives. The pruritus may become so severe that it adversely affects quality of life and may be relieved only by drastic measures, such as liver transplantation.

Bile Synthesis and Secretion: Consequences of Impaired Secretion

The process of bile synthesis and secretion involves several critical physiologic functions. Bile adds emulsifying agents (bile acids) to the contents of the duodenum, which allows efficient digestion of dietary lipids and absorption of fat-soluble vitamins.

Bile also allows excretion of several critical materials from the body. Bilirubin, a waste product of heme catabolism, is very toxic and insoluble when present in abnormal amounts. Excretion of cholesterol in bile represents the only significant mechanism of ridding the body of cholesterol, which is also insoluble. In addition, excretion of lipophilic substances (drugs, toxins, xenobiotics), which are metabolized by the liver, occurs via bile. Thus, disruption of these processes can result in a broad spectrum of biochemical and physiologic abnormalities.

NORMAL BILE SYNTHESIS AND SECRETION

Hepatocytes contain *bile acids*, which result from two sources: primary synthesis within the hepatocyte from cholesterol and from the enterohepatic circulation via the portal vein. The latter are mainly secondary bile acids resulting from bacterial action on primary bile acids during digestion. The hepatocyte plasma membrane (basolateral) has two important high-affinity anion carrier systems: one is for *bile acids* (bile acid–sodium transporter), which uses Na^+-K^+-ATPase. This system is very efficient and removes 99% of the bile acids from the blood in one pass. The second is an active *anion transport system*, which takes up bilirubin (transported from the reticuloendothelial system via binding to albumin) as well as a number of other organic anions. This transport system solubilizes the bilirubin and prevents its reflux back into plasma. The anion transport system can be used as a measure of *liver function;* when anions such as bromosulfophthalein or indocyanine green are administered, the rate of clearance can be measured. Impairment of hepatocyte function is characterized by a slower-than-normal clearance of these injected substances from the blood.

Once the bile acids and the bilirubin enter the hepatocyte, they are individually transported to the endoplasmic reticulum via specific transport proteins (bile acid–binding proteins and ligandin, respectively), where each substance undergoes conjugation and bile components are assembled. Bilirubin, because of its toxicity and insolubility, undergoes conjugation with glucuronic acid to form mono- and diglucuronides by the enzyme bilirubin uridine diphosphate–glucuronosyltransferase (UDPGT).

Bile flow into the canaliculus is promoted by bile acids (*bile acid–dependent flow*), carrying along bilirubin and organic anions and promoting secretion of water as a response to the osmolality of the bile acids. This flow is enhanced by secretin. *Bile acid–independent flow* is poorly understood but accounts for 30%–50% of flow. Ductular flow is unidirectional because of secretory pressure. As ducts become larger, flow is enhanced by secretin. In the ducts, bicarbonate (HCO_3^-) is added and water is removed along with sodium chloride (NaCl), thus concentrating the bile. Once bile reaches the gallbladder, further concentration occurs. Contraction of the gallbladder is regulated by meal-induced release of cholecystokinin (CCK).

Because of this complex process of excretion, problems may occur at any step, leading to jaundice (hyperbilirubinemia). If the disruption occurs *prior to conjugation*, increased levels of unconjugated or "indirect-reacting" bilirubin appear in the blood and tissues. If conjugation occurs (but not excretion), conjugated hyperbilirubinemia or "direct-reacting" bilirubin results. The terms *direct* and *indirect* refer to the original diazo laboratory method for detecting bilirubin; the water-soluble conjugated bilirubin reacted directly, whereas the insoluble unconjugated bilirubin bound to albumin reacted indirectly. Cholestasis is one of the causes of *conjugated* hyperbilirubinemia.

CELLULAR ALTERATIONS IN CHOLESTASIS

Cholestasis results in a number of changes in liver cells. Certain relatively nonspecific changes can occur because of the detergent action of the bile acids and the tendency of bilirubin to bind to proteins. Alterations in liver plasma membranes can occur, resulting in changes in membrane structure, function, and activity of membrane-associated enzymes, receptors, and transport proteins, as noted in Table 22-1.

Table 22-1. Cellular Alterations in Cholestasis

OBSERVED CHANGES	CONSEQUENCE	EXAMPLE OF CAUSE
Decreased membrane fluidity	Decreased bile flow	Ethinyl estradiol
Decreased plasma membrane Na⁺-K⁺-ATPase	Reduced anion transport	Chlorpromazine
Dysfunction of microfilaments or microtubules	Reduced cellular and membrane motility	Norethandrolone (anabolic steroid)
Changes in canalicular permeability	Decreased bile flow	Several estrogens
Solubilization of membrane enzymes via detergent action of bile salts	Increased serum levels of alkaline phosphatase 5′-nucleotidase, γ-glutamyltransferase	Drugs, hormones, inherited disorders

CONSEQUENCES OF IMPAIRED BILE DELIVERY

Impaired bile flow has a number of consequences. Among them are maldigestion and malabsorption of dietary fats in the absence of bile salts, resulting in loss of energy or calories, steatorrhea, and possibly a fat-soluble vitamin deficiency. Cholesterol excretion may also be decreased, leading to the appearance of xanthomas. Membrane changes may also occur because of increased cholesterol. Alternative mechanisms of bile acid excretion may be induced, for example, an increase in sulfation and glucuronidation of bile acids to promote renal excretion. As a result of reflux of bile contents back into the liver and into the circulation, enzymes that are components of the cell membranes, particularly the canalicular membranes, may be released into the circulation. These enzymes include alkaline phosphatase (ALP), γ-glutamyl transpeptidase (GGT), and 5'-nucleotidase, which serve as markers for the excretory capacity of the liver and, with other tests, as an indication of cholestatic disease.

Mechanisms of Extrahepatic and Intrahepatic Cholestasis

Cholestasis is commonly classified as intrahepatic or extrahepatic. Intrahepatic refers to cholestasis resulting from a defect within the hepatocyte or the microscopic ducts within the liver. Extrahepatic cholestasis typically results from some mechanical obstruction of the main bile ducts. Table 22-2 reviews a number of causes of each. Common clinical findings are increased bile components in serum, with bilirubin the most common and easiest to measure. Although results of all liver tests are likely to be abnormal, a first step in diagnosis is to determine whether hepatocellular tests (ALT, AST) or cholestatic tests (ALP, GGT, 5'-nucleotidase) are more abnormal. If the latter tests are more abnormal, this finding suggests cholestasis, and the next step is to determine whether the origin of the cholestasis is intrahepatic or extrahepatic. An ultrasound examination can predict extrahepatic obstruction if dilated canaliculi or bile ducts are observed.

Table 22-2. Causes of Intrahepatic and Extrahepatic Cholestasis

INTRAHEPATIC CHOLESTASIS	EXTRAHEPATIC CHOLESTASIS
Viral and alcoholic hepatitis	Biliary disease
Hepatotoxicity: environmental agents	Primary biliary cirrhosis (90% female)
Steroid hormones: oral contraceptives and anabolic steroids	Primary sclerosing cholangitis (65% male, associated with IBD)
Pregnancy (especially third trimester)	Stones in common bile duct (choledocholithiasis)
Drugs: antithyroids, chlorpromazine, phenobarbital, NSAIDs, and others	Pancreatic disease
Extrahepatic bacterial infection	Pancreatic carcinoma
Prolonged total parenteral nutrition	Pancreatitis, acute and chronic
Congenital abnormalities: Byler's disease (a canalicular membrane defect) and Zellweger's syndrome (defective peroxisomes, which help metabolize bile acids)	Gallbladder carcinoma
	Surgical trauma
	Parasitic obstruction

Endoscopic retrograde cholangiopancreatography (ERCP) can permit mechanical obstructions to be visualized and removed. If only bilirubin is elevated, disorders of bilirubin metabolism should be suspected.

The treatment of cholestasis, of course, depends on the original cause. In some cases, nutritional support with a low-fat (< 40 g/d) diet is useful. Additional fat calories may be supplied via medium-chain fatty acids, which are absorbed in the absence of bile acids. In chronic cases, fat-soluble vitamins may be administered parenterally. Alcohol should be avoided. The pruritus should be relieved, as noted earlier, because this is a very common symptom and a source of distress for many patients that severely affects their quality of life.

Disorders of Bilirubin Metabolism and Excretion

Bilirubin is a pigment derived from heme catabolism, most of which is produced as a result of red blood cell (RBC) senescence. Bilirubin is produced in the spleen, transported to the liver bound to serum albumin, transported through the aqueous cytoplasm of the hepatocyte bound to ligandin, conjugated with one or two molecules of glucuronic acid, then excreted into bile. A malfunction in any of these steps can lead to hyperbilirubinemia and cholestasis. The laboratory values that define hyperbilirubinemia are: total bilirubin level greater than 1.5 mg/dl, an unconjugated level above 1 mg/dl, or a conjugated level greater than 0.3 mg/dl.

The causes of hyperbilirubinemia fall into two categories: excessive production and abnormal clearance. Any process that either impairs uptake of bilirubin into the liver, conjugation, or excretion will result in hyperbilirubinemia. Excessive production stems from ineffective erythropoiesis or from increased hemolysis of RBCs. Abnormal clearance occurs in a variety of conditions, as described next.

Hyperbilirubinemia is further characterized as conjugated and unconjugated bilirubin excess. Most hyperbilirubinemias fall into this category. Overproduction of bilirubin results in unconjugated bilirubin. Table 22-3 outlines a number of causes of both types of hyperbilirubinemia. Several of these are described in more detail in the text.

Unconjugated Hyperbilirubinemias

Hyperbilirubinemias related to an increased hemolysis are most often caused by an inherited disorder, glucose 6-phosphate deficiency, and certain drugs. Discontinuation of the drug usually reverses the hyperbilirubinemia. Long-term use of total parenteral nutrition is also a common cause of hyperbilirubinemia.

Very commonly, unconjugated hyperbilirubinemias result from impaired ability of the enzyme UDPGT. *Neonatal jaundice*, sometimes referred to as physiologic jaundice, is very common in infants because of retarded induction of UDPGT. In general, this jaundice is noted about 5 days after birth and several days later in premature infants. The bilirubin may rise for several more days and usually

Table 22-3. Causes of Hyperbilirubinemia

UNCONJUGATED BILIRUBIN

Hemolysis	Glucose-6-phosphate deficiency and drugs
Neonatal occurrence	Retarded induction of UDPGT and breast milk jaundice
UDPGT deficiency	Gilbert's syndrome and Crigler-Najjar syndromes 1 and 2
Other causes	Fasting, drugs, and hypothyroidism

CONJUGATED BILIRUBIN

Congenital syndromes	Rotor's syndrome and Dubin-Johnson syndrome
Familial syndromes	Cholestasis of pregnancy and benign recurrent intrahepatic cholestasis
Neonatal problems	Neonatal hepatitis, idiopathic, biliary atresia, choledochal cyst, Alagille's syndrome, and Zellweger's syndrome
Cholestatic defects	Biliary obstruction, pancreatic diseases, primary biliary cirrhosis, and primary sclerosing cholangitis
Other causes	Renal disease, infection, surgical complications, and carcinomas

Notes

Neonatal jaundice occurs because of retarded induction of UDPGT and is more frequently seen in breastfed infants.

normalizes within 2 weeks, but it may remain elevated for a month or more in premature infants. Because it is important to prevent the complication of hyperbilirubinemia known as kernicterus (bilirubin encephalopathy), which may result in cerebral palsy or mental retardation, infants with jaundice should be carefully monitored. Neonatal jaundice is commonly treated with phototherapy or phenobarbital, a drug that induces UDPGT. Infants who are breastfed are more susceptible to neonatal jaundice, because maternal milk appears to contain an inhibitor of UDPGT. Cessation of breastfeeding usually results in prompt normalization of bilirubin levels.

Inherited disorders affecting UDPGT expression and activity also lead to unconjugated hyperbilirubinemia. Gilbert's disease is a benign disorder characterized by mild unconjugated hyperbilirubinemia as a result of reduced (~50%) activity of UDPGT. This condition affects 3%–8% of the population and is inherited in an autosomal dominant manner. The age of presentation is usually 18 years or older. Most patients are asymptomatic. Increased jaundice is associated with fasting, fatigue, alcohol use, stress, illness, and, in women, the premenstrual period. In general, no treatment is required.

A much more severe syndrome, Crigler-Najjar syndrome type 1, is characterized by a complete lack of UDPGT activity. The resultant severe hyperbilirubinema proceeds to kernicterus and death within 18 months without aggressive management. Treatment in the early neonatal period is critical and consists of phototherapy, plasmapheresis, or orthotopic liver transplantation. Phenobarbital treatment cannot induce the enzyme in these patients.

Crigler-Najjar syndrome type 2, also known as Arias' disease, results in somewhat less severe hyperbilirubinemia, and patients appear to have low levels of UDPGT activity ($\sim$10%) that can respond partially to phenobarbital induction of enzyme activity. This syndrome is apparent in some patients at 1 year of age but may be later in others. The exact genetics of this disorder remain unclear, and it is thought by some to be the homozygous form of Gilbert's disease. Patients usually survive, although jaundice is a constant problem.

CONJUGATED HYPERBILIRUBINEMIAS

Conjugated hyperbilirubinemia is defined as having a conjugated bilirubin level greater than 30% of total bilirubin. Several different causes have been identified, both congenital and acquired, and may be identified as intrahepatic or extrahepatic.

Congenital forms include Dubin Johnson syndrome, a rare, relatively benign, autosomal recessive condition in which mixed hyperbilirubinemia develops as a result of impaired storage or impaired excretion of bilirubin (and other organic anions) from the hepatocyte through the canalicular membrane. Overall liver function is well preserved. Phenobarbital may reduce bilirubin levels. Rotor's syndrome is also a rare, relatively benign autosomal recessive condition in which mixed hyperbilirubinemia develops as a result of impaired intracellular storage of organic anions, possibly because of a deficiency of glutathione S-transferase. Bile acid excretion is normal. Like Dubin Johnson, overall liver function is not affected, and no treatment is required. Progressive familial intrahepatic cholestasis, or Byler's disease, a disease of neonatal cholestasis named for the Amish kindred in which the disease was first noted, appears to be a defect in secretion of conjugated bile acids across the canalicular membrane. Thus, a characteristic of this disease is elevated levels of bile acids in the hepatocyte and low levels in bile. The mode of inheritance is thought to be autosomal recessive. These patients present with severe pruritus, failure to grow, severe watery diarrhea, and cholestasis. Death from liver failure usually occurs during childhood or early adolescence.

Familial forms include benign recurrent intrahepatic cholestasis and cholestasis of pregnancy. In the former, patients often present with severe pruritus and elevated ALP levels. The onset of the symptoms and their duration differ among patients, and attacks may persist for weeks or months and may occur months or years apart, with complete resolution between attacks. The defect may involve altered bile acid transport and enterohepatic circulation. Women with this defect should avoid estrogen-containing therapies. Women with cholestasis of pregnancy have onset during the last trimester and usually present with pruritus, which may be treated with oral cholestyramine resin therapy to adsorb bile acids in the intestine. Both cholestasis and pruritus disappear spontaneously after delivery; however, cholestasis frequently recurs in subsequent pregnancies.

Acquired hyperbilirubinemias include both intrahepatic and extrahepatic cholestasis, as noted in Table 22-2, and make up the majority of cases of hyperbilirubinemia. Extrahepatic cholestasis usually results from a physical blockage of the bile duct lumen by gallstones, scarring or stricture, pancreatic disease, or tumor. Intrahepatic causes may include drug interactions, chronic liver diseases, and infections. Liver diseases that commonly result in hyperbilirubinemia are alcoholic liver disease and viral hepatitides. Two progressive cholestatic diseases, primary biliary cirrhosis and primary sclerosing cholangitis, result in hyperbilirubinemia in the later stages of disease. Many drugs also can result in hyperbilirubinemia of all types. Agents include many common drugs, such as oral contraceptives, aspirin, acetaminophen, antidepressants, NSAIDs, and even the vitamin niacin. Total parenteral nutrition, most likely as a result of the type of fat used, may result in hyperbilirubinemia when used for more than 3 weeks.

Given the large number of potential causes of hyperbilirubinemia, evaluation of a patient with jaundice must be systematic. The patient's history, family history, and physical examination are all critical in identifying the cause of hyperbilirubinemia. Laboratory tests, including total and conjugated bilirubin and tests for both hepatocellular injury (AST, ALT) and cholestasis (ALP, GGT, and 5'-nucleotidase), along with viral hepatitis screening, aid in identifying the causes of hyperbilirubinemia. Other useful tests include ultrasonography, radionuclide imaging, ERCP, and liver biopsy.

CASE STUDY: *RESOLUTION*

A day after the first visit, the infant appeared to be alert, with a good appetite, and otherwise well. The bilirubin had risen to 12.2 mg/dl, with conjugated bilirubin less than 1 mg/dl. Phototherapy treatment was begun. After a week, total bilirubin dropped to 5.5 mg/dl. At 4 weeks, the total bilirubin was within the normal range.

In a full-term infant, jaundice may be apparent about 5 days after birth. This infant showed a slight delay, perhaps as a result of not being full-term. Because infants are usually released from the hospital before 2 days of age, it is important that the parents are aware of the possibility of neonatal jaundice. Phototherapy, consisting of light at 450 nm, is helpful in altering the chemical isomeric structure of bilirubin and speeding its excretion. Had this infant been breastfed, he may have had a more pronounced jaundice. However, cessation of breastfeeding would have helped resolve the jaundice. If the mother had preferred breastfeeding, she would have been encouraged to resume once the jaundice was resolved. Once the UDPGT was induced to appropriate levels, the infant had no further problems.

*R*EVIEW *Q*UESTIONS

Directions: For each of the following questions, choose the one best answer.

1 A common cause of extrahepatic cholestasis is

A excessive use of acetaminophen.
B Byler's disease.
C stones in the common bile duct.
D bacterial infections.

2 Crigler-Najjar syndrome type 1 is caused by the complete lack of which of the following enzymes?

A ALP
B UDPGT
C Canalicular Na$^+$-K$^+$-ATPase
D 5'-Nucleotidase

3 A 77-year-old man presents with jaundice. He has a history of cholecystectomy 20 years ago. Which of the following statements about this man's condition is *true*?

A Stone disease can be ruled out because the patient does not have a gallbladder.
B An ultrasound examination showing a normal common bile duct absolutely rules out a stone.
C The physician should ask him about medications because they may cause a cholestatic problem.
D A liver biopsy must be done as soon as possible.

References

Merriman RB, Peters MG: Approach to the patient with jaundice. In: *Textbook of Gastroenterology*, 4th ed., edited by Yamada T. Philadelphia, PA: Lippincott, Williams, & Wilkins, 2003.

Schiff ER, Sorrell MF, Maddrey WC: *Diseases of the Liver*, 9th ed. Philadelphia, PA: J. B. Lippincott, 1993.

23

Orthotopic Liver Transplantation

▓ CHAPTER OUTLINE ▓

▓ LEARNING OBJECTIVES ▓

At the completion of this chapter, the reader should be able to:
- Recognize the cellular mechanisms and pathophysiology of liver allograft rejection.
- Identify the various types of rejection and know their clinical relevance.
- Evaluate the role of immune tolerance in the outcome of liver transplantation.
- Summarize the mechanisms of action of immunosuppressive agents used in organ transplantation.
- Explain the phenomenon of microchimerism and its effect on immune tolerance.

CASE STUDY: *INTRODUCTION*

A 24-year-old woman was admitted with the complaints of jaundice, abdominal pain, vomiting, and confusion. Four days earlier she had ingested 30 tablets of acetaminophen, 500 mg each, along with some alcohol after having an argument with her boyfriend. Her medical history was unremarkable, and she was not taking any medications regularly. She consumed on average about 10 alcoholic drinks a week. She was a nonsmoker and had no history of intravenous drug usage or blood transfusions. She lived with her parents and worked as a bank clerk.

On admission, she was confused and somnolent but easily arousable. Her vital signs were as follows: temperature, 36.4°C (97.5°F); pulse, 110/min; and blood pressure, 100/68 mm Hg. She had scleral icterus, her tongue was dry, and there was no peripheral edema. Her chest was clear to auscultation, and both heart sounds were normal. Her abdomen was soft with no distention or tenderness. Liver and spleen were both nonpalpable, and there was no shifting dullness. There were no focal neurologic signs, but she had generalized muscular hypotonia. Blood studies showed the following: sodium (Na^+), 132 mmol/L; potassium (K^+), 4.8 mmol/L; chloride (Cl^-), 102 mmol/L; bicarbonate (HCO_3^-), 16 mmol/L; BUN, 38 mg/dl; creatinine, 3.1 mg/dl; bilirubin, 14.4 mg/dl; ALT, 620 IU/L; AST, 480 IU/L; ALP, 135 IU/L; albumin, 3.5 mg/dl; total protein, 6.8 mg/dl; prothrombin time, more than 46 seconds; hemoglobin, 15.4 g/dl; WBC count, 5.4×10^9/ml; and platelets, 180×10^9/ml. Hepatitis A, B, and C serologic and antinuclear antibody values were negative. Her blood group was O positive. A chest x-ray revealed no abnormalities. An abdominal ultrasound scan revealed hyperechoic liver parenchyma without any focal lesions, normal spleen, and patent hepatic vasculature.

Within 24 hours, she was comatose and was placed on mechanical ventilation. A transjugular liver biopsy revealed massive hepatic necrosis with no viable hepatocytes. She was enlisted for liver transplantation, and because of her rapidly deteriorating condition and the lack of an ABO-compatible donor, she received a blood group A hepatic allograft. Immediately afterward, immunosuppressive therapy was instituted with intravenous tacrolimus and methylprednisolone. The hepatic allograft initially produced bile, but after 24 hours, bile production declined, and the patient developed a temperature of 40°C (104°F). Her serum bilirubin, AST, and ALT levels remained markedly elevated. A Doppler ultrasound scan showed patent hepatic vasculature and an absence of bile duct dilatation. A liver biopsy revealed thrombosis within the hepatic arterioles, massive hepatocyte necrosis, and cholestasis. She was placed on plasmapheresis, and tacrolimus and methylprednisolone were continued. Her condition remained unchanged during the subsequent 48 hours. She was therefore retransplanted with an ABO-compatible liver, which resulted in gradual improvement in her general condition and in her liver tests. However, 10 days later, bile production declined, and serum transaminases and bilirubin levels started to rise. An allograft biopsy revealed portal tract inflammation, lymphocytic infiltration of the bile ducts, and portal and hepatic venular endothelitis. She received increased doses of tacrolimus and corticosteroids, to which she responded, and was discharged home.

She had two similar episodes over the subsequent 6 months, which were successfully treated. Eighteen months after the second transplant, she developed itching, progressive jaundice, dark urine, and fatigue. Blood studies revealed the following: bilirubin, 12 mg/dl; ALP, 670 IU/L; γ-glutamyl transferase, 1200 IU/L; ALT, 90 IU/L; AST, 54 IU/L; albumin, 2.1 g/dl; and prothrombin time, 18.8 seconds. Serologic tests for hepatitis B and C were negative, and the hepatic artery was patent on Doppler flow studies. A liver biopsy showed mild portal tract inflammation, extensive fibrosis, bile duct paucity, and cholestasis.

Introduction

The development of liver transplantation as a therapeutic modality has had a major impact on the outlook of patients with end-stage liver disease. The first long-term survivor of orthotopic liver transplantation was reported by Thomas Starzl in Denver, Colorado, in 1967. However, the general application of this procedure did not begin until the National Institutes of Health consensus conference in 1983, which recognized liver transplantation as an accepted therapy for advanced liver disease. Orthotopic liver transplantation involves the removal of the native liver (complete hepatectomy) and its replacement by a donor hepatic allograft at its natural site, whereas heterotopic liver transplantation involves the placement of the allograft at an alternative site. The term *allograft* refers to transplantation between genetically different individuals within the same species, and the molecules in the allograft recognized as foreign by the recipient's immune system are termed *alloantigens*. In the United States, more than 3000 liver transplants are performed annually.

The common indications for transplantation include fulminant hepatic failure and life-threatening complications of cirrhosis, such as advanced hepatic encephalopathy, ascites refractory to medical therapy, repeated episodes of spontaneous bacterial peritonitis, and the development of small hepatocellular carcinoma. In addition, liver transplantation is now often performed for problems that mainly affect the quality of life, such as excessive fatigue resulting in the inability to perform activities of daily living. Certain inherited metabolic conditions, such as primary hyperoxaluria, hyperlipidemias, and variant transthyretin amyloidosis, are also cured by liver transplantation, which acts as a form of gene therapy. Eligible patients are listed based on the severity of illness. The MELD score is used to prioritize cases and is calculated from a patient's creatinine, bilirubin, and INR. The contraindications for liver transplantation include sepsis, uncontrolled HIV infection (HIV unresponsive to Highly Active Anti-Retroviral Therapy (HAART)), severe cardiorespiratory disease, large hepatocellular carcinoma, extrahepatic malignancy, and active substance abuse. To meet the increasing demand for liver transplantation, alternatives to cadaveric transplantation have been developed, including split liver and living-related transplants.

The success of liver transplantation has been largely due to advances in surgical techniques, developments in organ procurement, and the discovery of effective immunosuppressive agents. Some of the major achievements include the use of veno-venous bypass, the development of UW (University of Wisconsin) solution, and the discovery of cyclosporine. The technique of veno-venous bypass allows blood to be diverted from the liver during hepatectomy, which results in relatively stable hemodynamics. The development of UW solution increased the cold preservation time of the allograft from 4–6 hours to about 16 hours. The use of cyclosporine-based immunosuppression significantly improved graft survival by controlling rejection and led to a dramatic rise in the application of organ transplantation during the 1980s.

A better understanding of the pathophysiology of transplantation has been crucial in the realization of these goals. Two phenomena that play a key role in the management of patients with organ transplantation are rejection and immune tolerance.

Rejection

Liver allograft rejection is a common occurrence following transplantation and can cause considerable morbidity resulting from graft dysfunction or occasionally can lead to graft loss. Rejection is defined as the response of the recipient's immune system to the donor allograft, leading to graft damage. The main elements of liver allograft targeted by the immune system are biliary epithelial and vascular endothelial cells and, to a much lesser extent, hepatocytes.

CELLULAR MECHANISMS OF REJECTION

The immune system is the body's natural defense against invasion. The recognition and memorization of the body's own structure as self by the immune system occurs early in human development and ensures self-tolerance. A failure of these mechanisms leads to the development of autoimmune diseases. More often, the immune system acts to control infections when the body is invaded by microorganisms that are quickly recognized as foreign. In a similar fashion, when a donor organ is grafted in the human body, the immune system quickly recognizes it as foreign or nonself and mounts a response.

The immunologic responses can be broadly classified as antibody-mediated (humoral) or cell-mediated. To initiate a response, the immune system first recognizes the alloantigens that are proteins expressed on the surface of hepatic parenchymal cells. This recognition of transplanted tissues is mediated by alloreactive T cells (so called because they react against alloantigens) that express certain markers called CD4 and CD8. The CD8-positive cells function as cytolytic T lymphocytes (CTLs) and have receptors that recognize donor class I major histocompatibility complex (MHC) molecules, such as human lymphocyte antigens (HLAs). There are several class I HLA molecules, classified as A, B, or C, which in the liver are expressed predominantly on biliary epithelial and vascular endothelial cells. Each CTL binds to a particular HLA. The cell damage that follows is mediated by factors such as perforins, which produce perforations in the target cell wall, and the *Fas* ligand, which binds to a *Fas* receptor on the cell membrane that triggers target cell death, or apoptosis. The CD8-positive cells, therefore, cause direct graft damage. The CD4-positive cells function as helper T cells. They are activated by class II MHC molecules, such as HLA-DR, -DP, or -DQ, expressed on the donor parenchymal cells. The recognition of HLA molecules by helper T cells causes the release of certain cytokines, such as interleukin-1 and -2 (IL-1, IL-2), which initiate chemotaxis. There is recruitment and activation of macrophages, as well as of other T cells, which results in delayed graft damage. The action of CD4- and CD8-positive cells is specific for the particular class I and II molecules and is therefore called MHC-restricted. However, the action of certain other cells, called natural killer cells, is not MHC-restricted, and they can cause graft damage without the involvement of specific HLA molecules. The role of B cells in rejection is limited. Some recipients have preformed alloantibodies that bind to donor antigens, particularly blood group antigens expressed on vascular endothelium. This causes activation of the complement system, which results in vascular damage and graft failure.

Rejection has been classified into hyperacute (humoral), acute (cellular), and chronic (ductopenic) types. This classification is based on the timing of rejection as well as the clinical and histopathologic features of rejection (Table 23-1).

HYPERACUTE REJECTION

Relatively uncommon, hyperacute rejection occurs in less than 1% of liver allografts, usually within 1–2 days after transplantation. The pathogenesis involves the presence of preformed antibodies in the recipient, directed against donor antigens. It is particularly common in patients who have received ABO-incompatible grafts or in those who had previous blood transfusions that caused antibody formation

Graft recognition is mediated by alloreactive T cells expressing CD4 or CD8 markers.

Hyperacute rejection is caused by preformed cytolytic alloantibodies in the recipient.

against the blood group antigens. The incidence of hyperacute rejection remains low because recipient and donor are almost always matched for the blood group antigens. HLA mismatching does not appear to play a significant role.

The preformed antibodies bind to alloantigens expressed on the surface of donor cells, mainly vascular endothelial cells, which leads to the activation of the complement cascade. Proinflammatory cytokines are released and promote chemotaxis of inflammatory cells and macrophages. The endothelial cells are activated to secrete von Willebrand's factor, which causes platelet aggregation and adhesion. These phenomena result in rapid vascular thrombosis and inflammation and in the subsequent destruction of the hepatic allograft. Clinically, the patient has marked elevation of the serum transaminase levels and prolonged prothrombin time. Grossly, the graft becomes swollen and dusky in color with a decline in bile production. Liver histology shows lymphocytic infiltration of portal and lobular areas, bile-ductular inflammation, and endotheliitis affecting the terminal hepatic venule, portal vein, and hepatic artery branches. These changes are associated with marked cholestasis and massive ischemic necrosis of the allograft. Hepatic artery thrombosis and preservation injury should be excluded. Hyperacute rejection is usually irreversible and unresponsive to immunosuppressive agents, and it leads to rapid failure of the graft, requiring retransplantation.

ACUTE (CELLULAR) REJECTION

The most common type of liver allograft rejection, acute cellular rejection, has been reported in 50%–100% of cases. It usually occurs within the first 3 weeks of transplantation; however, later episodes may occur. Younger recipients (< 40 years of age) are more at risk, probably because of better immune responsiveness. Other risk factors include complete donor recipient HLA-DR mismatch and the recipient's Rh-positive blood type.

Table 23-1. Clinical and Histologic Features of Hepatic Allograft Rejection

TYPE	FREQUENCY	ONSET FOLLOWING TRANSPLANTATION	HISTOLOGIC FEATURES	THERAPY AND OUTCOME
Hyperacute (humoral)	< 1%	1–2 days	Ischemic necrosis, portal and lobular hepatitis, cholangitis, and endotheliitis	Plasmapheresis; usually irreversible
Acute (cellular)	50%–100%	Usually within 3 weeks	Lymphocytic portal and periportal hepatitis, nonsuppurative cholangitis, and portal and hepatic vein endotheliitis	High-dose corticosteroids, OKT3, tacrolimus rescue; often responds to therapy
Chronic (ductopenic)	3%–17%	Few weeks to several months	Loss of small bile ducts, cholestasis, and foam cell arteriopathy	Usually irreversible; requires retransplantation

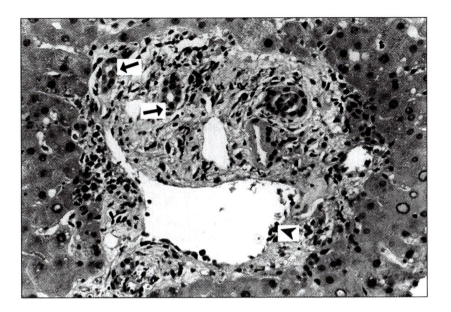

Fig. 23-1. Acute Cellular Rejection

Liver biopsy shows portal and periportal hepatitis, nonsuppurative cholangitis, and endotheliitis. The portal vein endothelium is denuded and infiltrated with lymphocytes (arrowhead). The bile ducts are also infiltrated with lymphocytes (arrows).

Clinically, acute rejection is characterized by malaise, fever, jaundice, and reduction in bile production or a lightening of bile color. The change in bile is observed if there is external biliary drainage. Serum transaminase and bilirubin levels rise, and later is followed by prolonged prothrombin time and a decline in serum albumin level. The transplant recipients are also prone to develop infections, and the described features often do not distinguish infection from rejection. The diagnosis of acute rejection is therefore based mainly on liver histology (Figure 23-1). This typically shows portal and periportal lymphocytic infiltration, nonsuppurative cholangitis, and endotheliitis affecting portal and hepatic vein branches. Arteritis (without the presence of foamy macrophages) and centrilobular (zone 3) necrosis may also be noted.

Several different mechanisms are involved in the production of acute cellular rejection. Cytotoxic T lymphocytes (CTLs), activated macrophages, and natural killer cells all participate in graft destruction. The most important mechanism, however, is the recognition of graft antigens by alloreactive CD8-positive CTLs. The graft class I MHC molecules are recognized by CTLs as if they were self–class I MHC molecules presenting an endogenously synthesized foreign peptide. Acute cellular rejection responds to treatment with high doses of corticosteroids, but sometimes polyclonal or monoclonal antibodies against lymphocytes, such as antilymphocyte globulin and OKT3, have to be used. If therapy fails, severe ductopenic rejection sets in, requiring retransplantation.

Acute cellular rejection is characterized by the triad of portal and periportal hepatitis, nonsuppurative cholangitis, and vascular endotheliitis.

Notes

The **hallmarks of chronic ductopenic rejection** are small bile duct loss and foam cell arteriopathy.

CHRONIC (DUCTOPENIC) REJECTION

Chronic rejection has been reported to occur in 3%–17% of liver allograft recipients. It has a progressive, irreversible course that leads to graft loss. Depending on the rapidity of its onset, it is classified as *early*, *delayed*, or *late*. Chronic rejection is called early if it occurs within the first 6 weeks of transplantation. If it occurs between 6 weeks and 6 months or later than 6 months, it is termed delayed and late-onset, respectively. The primary targets in this type of rejection are the bile ducts and hepatic artery branches. Most patients initially present with symptoms of acute cellular rejection, mainly malaise, fever, jaundice, and elevated serum transaminase and bilirubin levels. Serum transaminase levels eventually decline, but serum bilirubin, alkaline phosphatase, and γ-glutamyl transpeptidase levels remain elevated. The disease continues to progress despite aggressive immunosuppressive therapy and ultimately leads to irreversible graft damage. Delayed ductopenic rejection is the most common type of chronic rejection. It occurs after one or more episodes of acute cellular rejection and progresses to severe cholestasis and irreversible graft dysfunction. Late-onset chronic rejection is less frequent and develops insidiously. There are usually no preceding episodes of acute cellular rejection. The patient develops progressive cholestasis and graft failure over a period of months or years.

The typical histologic features of chronic rejection include the progressive loss of small bile ducts, cholestasis, and foam cell arteriopathy (Figure 23-2). At least 20 portal areas should be available for

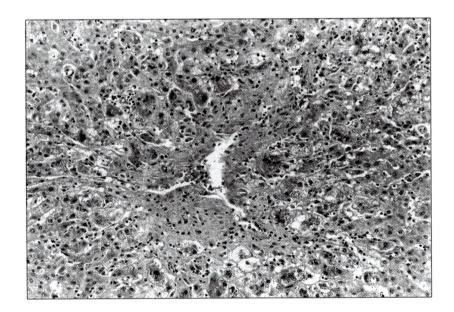

Fig. 23-2. Chronic Ductopenic Rejection

Liver allograft biopsy shows severe fibrosis of the portal area. Note complete absence of bile ducts, feathery degeneration of periportal hepatocytes, and cholestasis.

examination, and the loss of bile ducts should be demonstrated in at least 50% of them. This may be achieved over a period of time as several liver biopsies may be performed during management of this condition. Normally, bile ducts are present in at least 80% of the portal areas containing a hepatic artery branch. Foam cell arteriopathy has been recognized as a hallmark of chronic rejection; however, it is found only in a minority of cases. It is characterized by the infiltration of arterial endothelium with foam-laden macrophages, myointimal cells, or both, accompanied by myofibroblast proliferation and collagen deposition. This process eventually leads to arterial narrowing and thrombosis.

The graft loss in chronic ductopenic rejection is primarily the result of direct lymphocytotoxic damage of the biliary epithelium mediated through the MHC antigens. Arterial endothelium is also targeted, causing arteritis and vascular thrombosis, which leads to obliterative vasculopathy and ischemic bile duct damage. Chronic rejection occurs more frequently in patients transplanted for primary sclerosing cholangitis, in those who had poorly treated acute rejection episodes, and among those who develop cytomegalovirus infections. In addition, there is a high recurrence rate of chronic rejection following retransplantation.

Immune Tolerance

For the liver allograft to survive in the recipient, a state of immune tolerance is essential. The induction of immune tolerance avoids or delays graft rejection. This can be achieved either by selecting a graft that is likely to be well tolerated by the recipient or by suppressing the recipient's immune system. Removal of immune effectors, such as alloantibodies, may also be helpful. Another phenomenon is leukocyte chimerism, in which the leukocyte population represents both donor and recipient, thus contributing to immune tolerance.

Graft Selection

It is apparent that immune tolerance of a graft is achieved if the donor and recipient have the same antigens. This occurs if transplantation is performed between identical twins. However, in practice this is a rare situation, as almost always liver transplants are performed between genetically different individuals (allotransplantation). In such situations, immune tolerance can be facilitated by matching the donor and recipient for the major alloantigens, such as the ABO blood group antigens and HLA. In the early days of transplantation, the use ABO-incompatible grafts was associated with severe hyperacute rejection. This phenomenon is rarely observed now, as hepatic allografts are almost always matched for the ABO blood groups. Grafts are, however, seldom matched for the HLA because of limited organ supply and the relatively short time of preservation. Fortunately, this has not led to an unacceptably high rate of graft rejection. Thus, in liver transplantation,

Notes

The most widely used drugs for the induction and maintenance of immunosuppression are cyclosporine and tacrolimus.

ABO blood group matching is essential; however, adequate immune tolerance is possible despite HLA mismatching.

SUPPRESSION OF THE IMMUNE SYSTEM

The suppression of the immune system can be achieved by the use of immunosuppressive agents. A number of drugs have immunosuppressive effects, principally corticosteroids, azathioprine, antilymphocyte globulin, calcineurin inhibitors such as cyclosporine, and tacrolimus, sirolimus, and mycophenolate mofetil. Additionally, monoclonal antibodies (e.g., OKT3) are used for induction and to treat acute cellular rejection (Table 23-2).

Corticosteroids

Prednisone, prednisolone, and methylprednisolone are widely used to induce remission in the early posttransplantation period and are typically withdrawn after 3 months. They are also used in high doses to treat episodes of acute cellular rejection. Corticosteroids suppress the immune system by blocking the release of cytokines, such as IL-1, IL-6, and tumor necrosis factor-α, from activated macrophages and lymphocytes. These cytokines cause chemotaxis and promote inflammatory reactions. Corticosteroids also cause lysis of immature T cells within the thymus but do not lyse mature T cells in the peripheral blood or lymphoid organs.

Table 23-2. Mechanisms of Action and Adverse Effects of Immunosuppressants

IMMUNOSUPPRESSANT	MECHANISM OF ACTION	ADVERSE EFFECTS
Corticosteroids	Block release of proinflammatory cytokines (IL-1, IL-6, tumor necrosis factor-α) from activated macrophages and lymphocytes	Weight gain, hypertension, hypokalemia, hyperglycemia, myopathy, osteopenia, acne, hirsutism, mood swings, and cataracts
Azathioprine	Nucleoside analog that blocks synthesis of cellular DNA	Leukopenia, thrombocytopenia, macrocytic anemia, vomiting, pancreatitis, hepatotoxicity, and infections
Antilymphocyte globulin	Polyclonal antibodies directed against T lymphocytes	Fever, leukopenia, anaphylaxis, serum sickness, infections, and hypertension
OKT3	Monoclonal antibody directed against lymphocyte CD3-receptor complex	Fever, chills, vomiting, diarrhea, infections, pulmonary edema, and lymphoproliferative disease
Cyclosporine	Inhibits synthesis and release of IL-2	Renal dysfunction, hypertension, tremor, gingival hyperplasia, hypertrichosis, hyperglycemia, and seizures
Tacrolimus	Inhibits synthesis and release of IL-2	Renal dysfunction, headache, tremor, hypertension, hyperkalemia, hyperglycemia, and seizures
Mycophenolate mofetil	Inhibitor of purine synthesis	Diarrhea, vomiting, leukopenia, sepsis, and neutropenia
Sirolimus	mTOR inhibitor	Thrombocytopenia, mouth ulcers, and hyperlipidemia

Azathioprine

A nucleoside analog, azathioprine is metabolized to 6-mercaptopurine once it is absorbed. It blocks the synthesis of cellular DNA and thus interferes with the proliferation and differentiation of lymphocytes. Its major posttransplant use is for steroid-sparing as well as to treat underlying autoimmune conditions. It is also useful as a calcineurin-sparing agent because it does not have the nephrotoxicity associated with cyclosporine and tacrolimus.

Antilymphocyte Globulin

This contains polyclonal antibodies, which are directed against T lymphocytes, resulting in their inhibition and destruction. It has been used for induction of immunosuppression and for treatment of acute rejection.

OKT3

A mouse monoclonal antibody, OKT3 is directed against the CD3-receptor complex expressed on the surface of T lymphocytes. The binding of this antibody prevents T cell activation and induces cell lysis. It is used mainly to treat acute rejection episodes that have failed to respond to corticosteroids. However, its use is associated with a higher incidence of bacterial and viral infections and with the development of lymphoproliferative disorders. Most patients quickly develop anti-mouse immunoglobulin antibodies, which render OKT3 ineffective for repeated use.

Cyclosporine

The discovery of cyclosporine is one of the most significant achievements in the history of organ transplantation. It is a cyclic peptide that occurs naturally in the fungus *Tolypocladium inflatum Gams.* Cyclosporine binds and blocks a small cellular protein, cyclophillin, which is involved in the transcription of certain genes, in particular the IL-2 gene. IL-2 is essential for T cell proliferation and activation; failure of its release therefore results in profound inhibition of cell-mediated immunity. Cyclosporine also inhibits certain other genes, such as *c-myc* and interferon-γ, which are also involved in the immune effector responses. Cyclosporine does not appear to have a direct effect on B cells. It is currently the most widely used drug for maintenance immunosuppression; however, it has a narrow therapeutic window, requiring the monitoring of serum levels. Side effects include renal dysfunction, hypertension, tremor, seizures, gingival hyperplasia, hypertrichosis, and hyperglycemia.

Tacrolimus

Also known as FK506, tacrolimus is a macrolide antibiotic derived from the fungus *Streptomyces tsukubaensis.* Structurally, it differs from cyclosporine, and within the cell, it binds to tacrolimus-binding protein. However, like cyclosporine, it is a calcineurin inhibitor and causes the inactivation of several genes involved in T cell activation and proliferation, in particular the IL-2 gene. Tacrolimus is more potent than cyclosporine and appears to be less toxic. It is used for maintenance immunosuppression as well as rescue therapy for acute cellular and chronic rejection episodes that fail to respond to corticosteroids and OKT3. Side effects include renal dysfunction, headache, tremor, seizures, hypertension, hyperkalemia, and hyperglycemia.

Mycophenolate Mofetil

This is a recently introduced drug that acts as an inhibitor of purine synthesis, which results in decreased lymphocyte response. It is better tolerated than other immunosuppressants, and side effects are limited to GI disturbance. It is useful as a steroid- or calcineurin-sparing agent.

Sirolimus

Also known as rapamycin, sirolimus has potent antifungal, antiproliferative, and immunosuppressive effects. It is used as both a steroid- and calcineurin-sparing agent and can be administered with either cyclosporine or tacrolimus without the concomitant use of steroids. Dose-related side effects include mouth ulcers and thrombocytopenia.

PLASMAPHERESIS

Certain recipients have preformed cytotoxic antibodies directed against alloantigens, which may result in hyperacute rejection. Immunosuppressants are usually ineffective in such situations; however, removing the alloantibodies by plasmapheresis may confer immune tolerance.

MICROCHIMERISM

Immunosuppressants can be gradually withdrawn in some patients who have received a hepatic allograft. Several of these patients continue to maintain good graft function several years later. They have therefore developed complete immune tolerance to the graft. The leukocyte population in these patients is often of both donor and recipient origin. This phenomenon is called *cellular microchimerism*, and it plays an important role in the development of immune tolerance.

The transplanted liver is rich in hematopoietic stem cells. The leukocytes that evolve from such stem cells migrate and populate the recipient; similarly, the recipient's leukocytes populate the allograft. This two-way migration and coexistence of cells from the donor and the recipient lead to graft acceptance and the development of immune tolerance. The underlying mechanisms of this bidirectional tolerance are not well understood. Augmentation of the chimerism by infusion of donor bone marrow cells has also been attempted to enhance immune tolerance.

CASE STUDY: *RESOLUTION*

The patient developed acute liver failure and massive hepatic necrosis as a result of acetaminophen toxicity. She was unlikely to survive without liver transplantation, and because an ABO-compatible graft was not immediately available, she was transplanted with an ABO-incompatible graft. This led to the development of hyperacute rejection and failure of the graft. She was retransplanted with an ABO-compatible graft, which initially worked well; however, she soon developed acute cellular rejection, which was successfully treated with corticosteroid boluses and an increased dosage of tacrolimus. Subsequently, she had two further episodes of acute rejection that responded to therapy. Several months later she presented with progressive graft failure resulting from chronic ductopenic rejection. She eventually underwent retransplantation and retained a good functioning hepatic allograft.

REVIEW QUESTIONS

Directions: For each of the following questions, choose the one best answer.

1 A 50-year-old man received a hepatic allograft because of advanced alcoholic cirrhosis. Despite the use of maintenance immunosuppression with tacrolimus and prednisone, he developed acute cellular rejection. The acute rejection should be treated with

A bolus corticosteroids.
B mycophenolate mofetil.
C cyclosporine.
D azathioprine.

2 The histologic hallmarks of chronic rejection include

A portal and periportal hepatitis.
B loss of bile ducts in 25% of the portal areas.
C hepatic vein endotheliitis.
D foam cell arteriopathy.

3 Acute cellular rejection is characterized by

A extensive hepatocyte necrosis.
B nonsuppurative cholangitis and portal phlebitis.
C arteritis with the presence of foam cells.
D polymorphonuclear infiltration of the hepatic lobules.

4 The recognition of an allograft by the recipient's immune system involves

A B cells expressing IgM immunoglobulins.
B CD4-positive T cells that recognize the recipient's class I MHC molecules.
C cytolytic T cells expressing CD8 markers.
D MHC restricted natural killer cells.

5 Cyclosporine suppresses immune effector response principally by

A blocking expression of the IL-2 gene.
B combining with cyclophillin, which results in the lysis of T cells.
C inhibiting B cell proliferation.
D reducing T cell purine synthesis.

References

Demetris AJ, Murase N, Delaney CP, et al: The liver allograft, chronic (ductopenic) rejection, and microchimerism: what can they teach us? *Transplant Proc* 27:67–70, 1995.

Hubscher SG: Pathology of liver allograft rejection. *Transplant Immunol* 2:118–123, 1994.

Krams SM, Ascher NL, Martinez OM: New immunologic insights into mechanisms of allograft rejection. *Gastroenterol Clin North Am* 22: 381–400, 1993.

Schiff L, Schiff ER: *Diseases of the Liver*, 9th ed. Philadelphia, PA: J. B. Lipincott, 2003.

Starzl TE, Demetris AJ, Murase N, et al: Cell migration, chimerism, and graft acceptance. *Lancet* 339:1579–1582, 1992.

Weisner RH: Advances in diagnosis, prevention, and management of hepatic allograft rejection. *Clin Chem* 40:2174–2185, 1994.

24

Alcohol and the GI Tract

■ CHAPTER OUTLINE ■

■ LEARNING OBJECTIVES ■

At the completion of this chapter, the reader should be able to:

- Discuss the incidence of alcohol use and abuse in the U.S. population.
- Describe alcohol (ethanol) metabolism.
- Review the role of alcohol in the pathogenesis of GI, liver, and pancreatic disease.
- Review the effects of alcohol on other organs.
- Discuss nutritional deficiencies in patients who abuse alcohol.

CASE STUDY: *INTRODUCTION*

B.K., a 53-year-old man, was referred to the university gastroenterology practice. He was employed as an organic chemist for a pharmaceutical company. He stated that for 3–4 weeks he had felt very tired, had frequent headaches, often felt slightly nauseated, and had little or no appetite. He had tried to eat more, at his wife's insistence, but he often missed meals. He felt that he had lost weight, which was verified by consulting his medical record. On examination, B.K. was thin, had a mild fever (38.2°C), tender hepatomegaly, and icterus. He admitted to drinking alcohol almost daily but claimed that he was really only a social drinker and had a few drinks after work with his friends to relax. When asked whether he had been drinking more in the recent past, he stated that he had been under a lot of pressure at work and he had not been getting along with his wife; because of these problems, he thought he might have increased his intake somewhat. After more questioning, he described his intake as about five or six double martinis a day. He denied drinking in the morning or during work or driving while under the influence of alcohol. He had no history of viral hepatitis and denied using any drugs other than alcohol or having other risk factors for hepatitis. He had been taking acetaminophen for his headaches, because he believed that this drug would not upset his stomach further.

B.K. was sent for liver function tests. His laboratory values were: ALT, 170 U/L (normal: 0–35 U/L); AST, 210 U/L (normal: 0–35 U/L); albumin, 3.2 g/dl (normal: 3.5–5.5 g/dl); bilirubin, 4.5 mg/dl (normal: < 1 mg/dl); and prothrombin time, 16 seconds (normal: 9–11 seconds). He was negative for hepatitis A, B, and C. A review of the record indicated that he had abnormal liver enzymes 6 months ago with normal prothombin time and bilirubin.

A liver biopsy was performed, and the histologic examination demonstrated the presence of fatty infiltration, Mallory bodies, hepatocellular necrosis, ballooning degeneration, inflammation with polymorphonuclear leukocytes, and a slight degree of fibrosis. No evidence of cirrhosis existed.

Alcohol Abuse in the U.S. Population

Alcohol is a major health issue in the United States and worldwide. Over two-thirds of Americans drink moderately, and over 18 million actively abuse alcohol. *Alcohol abuse* defines patterns of alcohol use that result in adverse consequences to health, social and family structures, and the ability to fulfill obligations at work or school. *Alcohol dependence*, often called alcoholism, includes physical dependence and the inability to control alcohol intake in addition to the characteristics of alcohol abuse.

Alcohol use differs among groups. Men use more alcohol than women, both in quantity and frequency, and use is most prevalent in the 18–29-year age group. Alcohol use is more common for whites than nonwhites. Younger people drink more than their elders; abstinence increases with age. Alcohol use also increases with income and education levels. Alcohol abuse tends to follow the same demographics as usage.

The effect of alcohol on health and mortality is considerable. Alcohol-associated mortality accounts for about 5% of all deaths in this country. Furthermore, alcohol abuse is associated with premature mortality; estimates of potential life lost from alcohol abuse far exceed those from cancer or heart disease. Alcohol is a contributing factor in half of all fatal traffic accidents, although the number of deaths from accidents is declining, most likely as a result of prevention programs, public awareness, and societal pressure. It has been estimated that up to 25% of the patients at Veterans Administration hospitals have alcohol-related morbidity. Thus, alcohol abuse and alcoholism have a profound effect on the health of Americans, and the cost of treatment of these individuals to health care delivery systems is considerable.

Alcohol Metabolism

Alcohol is absorbed from the stomach and intestinal tract, primarily the duodenum, and is transported via the blood to the liver. The rate of absorption of alcohol can be influenced by the presence or absence of food in the stomach, the composition of the meal, the concentration of alcohol, and the type of beverage consumed. Gastric mucosa appears to contain an isoenzyme of alcohol dehydrogenase (ADH), and this enzyme may contribute to the "first-pass" metabolism of alcohol. Some evidence suggests that this isoenzyme may be more prevalent in men than in women.

Most alcohol (ethanol) metabolism takes place in the hepatocyte, and metabolism of ethanol is obligatory in that there is no storage form. The ethanol metabolism capacity in a healthy adult can dispose of about 0.5–1.0 oz of pure ethanol (200 proof) per hour without raising the blood level above legal limits. However, as noted, absorption and metabolism depend on a number of factors, such as food intake, body size, age, sex, race, and the presence of liver disease. In general, a given amount of alcohol generates a higher blood alcohol concentration in a woman than in a man. The reasons for this finding are not completely understood but may include sex differences in absorption, gastric metabolism, body water or volume of distribution, body size, and clearance kinetics.

In the liver, ethanol is completely metabolized to acetate by the action of two enzymes, *alcohol dehydrogenase (ADH)* and *acetaldehyde dehydrogenase (ALDH)* in sequential reactions, as shown in Figure 24-1. Both of these enzymes require the oxidized form of

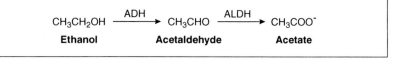

Fig. 24-1. Metabolism of Alcohol

The two major enzymes involved in metabolism of relatively low levels of alcohol are ADH and ALDH.

nicotinamide adenine dinucleotide (NAD^+) as a cofactor in the reaction, which is reduced to NADH in the process. In addition, zinc ion (Zn^{2+}) is an essential cofactor. It should be noted that alcoholics are frequently deficient in zinc.

ADH

Class 1 ADH is actually a family of cytosolic isoenzymes in the liver and accounts for about 80% of the hepatic metabolism of ethanol under conditions of light to moderate drinking. These isoenzymes have relatively low K_m for ethanol, but the affinity for ethanol varies greatly with the alleles expressed by an individual. Three genetic loci for ADH have been identified (*ADH1, ADH2, and ADH3*), and allelic polymorphisms have been demonstrated in the latter two. Each allele encodes a single subunit of the dimeric ADH enzyme: *ADH2* encodes for β_1-, β_2-, and β_3-subunits, and *ADH3* encodes for γ_1- and γ_2-subunits. These subunits are expressed differently in Asian, Caucasian, and African American populations and may account for the observed differences in alcohol metabolism among these groups, because the subunits differ in kinetic properties and therefore in activity. For example, the K_m for alcohol ranges from a low of 0.05 mmol for the $\beta_1\beta_1$ isoenzyme to a high of 36 mmol for the $\beta_3\beta_3$ isoenzyme. These polymorphisms may result in significant physiologic and pathologic responses to alcohol.

Liver also contains another enzyme that contributes to the metabolism of alcohol. The microsomal enzyme cytochrome P-450IIE1 (CYPIIE1) accounts for about 20% of hepatic alcohol metabolism. It has a higher K_m for alcohol than do most of the class 1 ADHs. Thus, this enzyme becomes more important during periods of high blood alcohol concentration and is induced in chronic drinkers. CYPIIE1 has a broad substrate specificity, metabolizing not only alcohol but also acetone (as in diabetics), acetaminophen, solvents such as carbon tetrachloride, and pyrazole, among others. The enzyme can be induced by these substances and, in fact, significantly higher CYPIIE1 activity is present in alcoholics. This increased activity results in these individuals being more susceptible to acetaminophen toxicity, because the product resulting from CYPIIE1 metabolism of acetaminophen is a highly toxic intermediate. Even relatively low doses of acetaminophen can be hepatotoxic in chronic alcoholics.

ALDH

ALDH is a family of isoenzymes that catalyze the second step in the complete metabolism of alcohol, the conversion of acetaldehyde to acetate. Acetate is a two-carbon metabolic product common to several pathways and may proceed to further metabolism through the Krebs (tricarboxylic acid) cycle or may be activated to enter the pathway for fatty acid synthesis. ALDH also requires NAD^+ and Zn^{2+} as cofactors. There are two major isoenzymes that metabolize alcohol. ALDH1 is a cytosolic enzyme that has a low K_m for acetaldehyde (30 μmol), and the ALDH2 isoenzyme is a mitochondrial enzyme with a K_m of 3 μmol. The latter enzyme appears to be the major enzyme involved in acetaldehyde metabolism. Although ALDH1 variants occur with relatively low frequency, variants of ALDH2 are common. About 50% of Chinese and Japanese people have a variant that differs in a single amino acid and exhibits very low or no metabolizing activity. The consequence of this variant is a significant elevation of acetaldehyde in these individuals after consuming alcoholic beverages. Facial flushing after drinking is correlated with ALDH2 deficiency and with acetaldehyde levels. The symptoms may be mild to severe and involve flushing, particularly of the face and upper chest, severe headaches, profuse sweating, tachycardia, and nasal congestion. More severe symptoms may occur, such as asthma, hypotension, or vascular collapse. In many Asians, these symptoms provide a strong reason to avoid alcoholic beverages. These symptoms mirror those exhibited by individuals who take disulfiram (trade name Antabuse) as a deterrent to drinking but ingest alcohol nonetheless. Disulfiram is a potent, irreversible inhibitor of ALDH activity.

Because acetaldehyde is a highly reactive molecule, it is critical that its metabolism be rapid. Acetaldehyde has been shown to form adducts with proteins, which then may become immunogenic. Furthermore, it may promote membrane damage by generation of free radicals.

Effects of Alcohol on the GI Tract

LIVER

The liver is the organ most affected by alcohol ingestion, and virtually all its normal functions can be disrupted by alcohol. In fact, chronic excessive use of this substance is the single most important cause of liver disease and death from liver disease in this country and ranks fourth as a cause of death in people from 20–70 years of age. Thus, the treatment costs and social costs of chronic alcoholism are immense.

Liver damage resulting from alcohol abuse was previously thought to result solely from nutritional deficiencies in the alcoholic. However, more recent research has determined that a number of factors may influence liver damage. One major factor is lipid peroxidation, which is consequence of free radicals generated during alcohol metabolism and results in membrane damage. Another factor that may contribute

Alcohol can disrupt all normal liver functions.

to liver damage is immunologic reaction to altered proteins resulting from acetaldehyde action.

The obligatory alcohol metabolism results in an enhanced NADH:NAD$^+$ ratio and ratios between the reduced form of nicotinamide adenine dinucleotide phosphate (NADPH) and NADP$^+$ within the liver cell; this altered redox capacity affects both carbohydrate and lipid metabolism, as well as metabolism of some xenobiotics. For example, the altered redox homeostasis promotes enhanced production of lactate, which contributes to the acidosis frequently observed in alcoholics. Also, lipogenesis is increased, and fatty acid beta oxidation is depressed; both factors enhance fat storage in the liver. The activity of the Krebs cycle is reduced, which in turn decreases the availability of ATP. Protein secretion is impaired, possibly as a result of low ATP and disordered cellular membranes and microfilaments. Serum levels of ammonia are elevated as a result of a depressed urea cycle. The biochemical consequences of alcohol abuse are reviewed in Table 24-1.

Alcoholics also display increased liver injury from such drugs as acetaminophen, tolbutamide, barbiturates, warfarin, cimetidine, propranolol, and others, as well as from organic and industrial chemicals, anesthetics, and environmental toxins. As reviewed in Table 24-2, chronic alcohol ingestion results in altered metabolism and clearance of a wide variety of drugs affecting many organ systems.

Three types of liver damage frequently encountered as a result of alcohol ingestion are fatty liver, alcoholic hepatitis, and cirrhosis. An alcoholic patient may have only one of these conditions or two or three

Table 24-1. Metabolic Changes in Livers of Chronic Alcoholics

OBSERVATION	CONSEQUENCE
Changes in activity of CYP450s	Altered clearance of drugs and xenobiotics Decreased clearance of carcinogens (?)
Decreased glutathione content	Decreased conjugation of excretory products
Decreased protein secretion	Decreased clotting factors Decreased albumin Decreased lipoproteins
Increased conversion of acetate to fatty acids	Increased storage of fats (steatosis)
Increased NADH, decreased NAD$^+$ (ethanol metabolism)	Loss of redox homeostasis
Decreased urea cycle efficiency in zone 3 (perivenular and centrilobular)	Increased blood ammonia
Altered sex hormone homeostasis	"Feminization" (gynecomastia), spider angiomata, and palmar erythema in males

Note: NAD$^+$ = oxidized form of nicotinamide adenine dinucleotide; NADH = reduced form of nicotinamide adenine dinucleotide.

Table 24-2. Drug–Alcohol Interactions

CLASS OF DRUG	SPECIFIC EXAMPLES
Antibiotics and antimalarials	Furazolidone, griseofulvin, quinacrine, isoniazid, and metronidazole
Ulcer medications	Cimetidine
Antihistamines	Diphenhydramine
Antidiabetic medications	Tolbutamide
Antiseizure drugs	Phenytoin
Antipsychotics	Chlorpromazine
Antidepressants	Tricyclics, such as amitriptyline
Cardiovascular medications	Nitroglycerin, reserpine, methyldopa, hydralazine, guanethidine, and propranolol
Narcotics	Morphine, codeine, propoxyphene, and meperidine
Sedatives and hypnotics	Benzodiazepines (diazepam and lorazepam) and barbiturates
Pain relievers	Acetaminophen and aspirin
Anesthetics	Propofol, enflurane, and halothane

simultaneously. Previously, it was thought that these conditions were sequential, beginning with fatty liver, then progressing to hepatitis, then to cirrhosis, but recent evidence suggests that alcoholic hepatitis is not necessarily an intermediate stage in the progression. Only about 10% of alcoholics who exhibit fatty liver progress to cirrhosis, because adequate nutrition plays a major role in preventing cirrhosis. The morphologic spectrum of liver damage is reviewed in Table 24-3.

Fatty Liver

Fatty liver, or hepatic steatosis, can be induced by even short-term excessive intake of alcohol and is usually a benign condition that reverses completely after a period of abstinence from alcohol. It may be seen in moderate drinkers as well as in alcoholics. However, it is important to note that fatty liver is not caused exclusively by alcohol;

Table 24-3. Morphologic Effects on Liver by Chronic Alcohol Ingestion

OBSERVATION	CAUSE
Ballooning hepatocytes	Cellular and membrane damage
Membrane lipid peroxidation	Free radical formation
Megamitochondria	Increased oxygen demand of liver
Proliferation of microsomal membranes	Reduced ability to secrete protein
Fatty liver (mild damage)	Reduced ability to mobilize lipids
Fibrosis (deposition of collagen)	Not understood; may be altered growth-factor regulation
Mallory's bodies (random microfilament deposits)	Not understood

other causes include hepatotoxins, drugs, obesity, hyperlipidemia, diabetes, malnutrition, and systemic disease. The most common cause of nonalcoholic fatty liver disease (NAFLD) in the United States is insulin resistance (which is not necessarily associated with diabetes mellitus) and obesity. Both clinically and histologically NAFLD is indistinguishable from alcoholic hepatitis. Thus the diagnosis of NAFLD requires the exclusion of significant alcohol intake (< 20–40 g/day). The data on the management of NAFLD remains limited. In patients with mild steatosis, there is less likelihood of progression to cirrhosis and no specific therapy is indicated, other than glycemic control and gradual weight loss, if applicable. Other potential treatment options include diabetic medications (e.g., metformin), antioxidants (e.g., vitamin E), and cytoprotective agents (e.g., ursodeoxycholic acid).

The accumulation of lipid in the liver probably results from an imbalance between the arrival of fatty acids from peripheral adipose tissue, fatty acid oxidation, and the ability of the liver to secrete very low-density lipoproteins to mobilize the triglycerides. In the early stages, the fat accumulates mostly in the relatively hypoxic perivenular zone 3 and is macrovesicular; the fat accumulation may progress to a more diffuse distribution with chronic disease. Fatty liver is frequently asymptomatic, but when it is severe, it may be associated with nausea, anorexia, malaise, and jaundice and may lead, in extreme cases, to portal hypertension and esophageal varices. Treatment of fatty liver involves complete abstention from alcohol and good nutrition; resolution may take up to 6 weeks.

Alcoholic Hepatitis

Alcoholic hepatitis occurs as an *acute* clinical consequence of abuse. It typically occurs in malnourished patients and may be precipitated by a period of binge drinking. To make the diagnosis, patients should have a significant history of alcohol consumption (≥ 80 g/day). A prodrome, usually of 2–3 weeks, consists of anorexia, nausea, fatigue, and weight loss. The patient often presents with tender hepatomegaly, a mild fever, and jaundice. More severe cases may display higher fever, significant jaundice, and other complications, such as ascites and encephalopathy. Serum aminotransferases are typically elevated, although they are rarely elevated more than 10 times above normal values; the elevations in AST and ALT do not correlate with the extent of liver damage, and AST is characteristically higher than ALT. The commonly used markers of hepatic synthetic capacity—serum albumin and prothrombin time—are affected, with a depressed albumin content and a prolonged prothrombin time typical. Histologically, the disease is characterized by both inflammation and necrosis, and after staining with hematoxylin and eosin, Mallory bodies or alcoholic hyaline are evident. Mallory bodies are cytoplasmic inclusions consisting of aggregates of microfilaments. Varying degrees of fibrosis may be observed. Treatment of alcoholic hepatitis involves complete abstinence from alcohol, bed rest, and a nutritionally adequate diet or possibly a high-protein diet if encephalopathy is not present, because obtaining a positive nitrogen balance is critical in these patients. Several additional therapies have been tested, such as branched-chain amino acids, corticosteroids, propylthiouracil, pentoxifylline, and others, but to date none of these have proven to be ideal.

Patients such as B.K. in the case study have a relatively good prognosis. Findings that predict a poor prognosis include encephalopathy, bilirubin above 20 mg/dl, and a prolonged prothrombin time of 8 seconds or more above control values. Abstaining from alcohol is critical to recovery, and virtually all patients need the support of some type of cessation therapy to achieve lifelong sobriety.

Cirrhosis

Cirrhosis is typically a disease of midlife following a history of chronic, heavy drinking for many years, but it may also occur in well-nourished heavy social drinkers. The disease is often insidious and is accompanied by nonspecific symptoms, such as those noted for alcoholic hepatitis. For reasons that are not well understood, women are at particular risk of developing cirrhosis. Signs of liver failure become evident as the disease progresses; hepatic encephalopathy, esophageal variceal bleeding, infection, and malnutrition are often present. Treatment is complete abstinence from alcohol and a diet adequate in protein (1 g/kg/d) but low in salt. Administration of branched-chain amino acids has shown benefit in some studies. Colchicine, which interferes with collagen synthesis, has also shown some promise when used for long-term treatment. Liver transplantation has become an important option in cirrhotic patients who have achieved sobriety for at least 6 months. The 5-year survival rate of such patients after transplantation is comparable to that of patients who received transplants for other conditions.

OTHER ORGANS OF THE GI TRACT

Although the liver is the organ most affected by alcohol abuse, virtually all the organs of the GI tract are affected, as reviewed in Table 24-4.

The salivary glands may be fibrotic, and there may be decreased salivary flow and a decreased salivary concentration of sodium, bicarbonate, and protein. When this occurs, chewing and swallowing become more difficult, and the risk of choking is increased.

The esophagus may exhibit damage as a result of esophageal reflux, because alcohol increases acid secretion and reduces lower esophageal sphincter pressure. Esophageal varices are common in patients with alcoholic hepatitis and cirrhosis and rare in patients with fatty liver; ruptured varices can be a life-threatening condition. Mallory-Wiess tears from vomiting may be present in the lower esophagus. Alcoholics are at increased risk for esophageal stricture as well as malignant neoplasms of the upper GI tract; alcohol abusers who smoke are at significantly higher risk for oral cancers.

Table 24-4. Major Effects of Chronic Alcohol Ingestion on the GI Tract

ORGAN	CONSEQUENCE
Esophagus	Esophageal reflux
	Esophageal varices
	Increased cancer of upper GI tract, including oral cancer
	Mallory-Weiss tears from vomiting (lower esophagus)
Stomach	Mucosal injury
	Gastritis
	Stimulation of gastric secretion
	Increased ulcer bleeding (decrease in clotting factors)
	Decreased gastric emptying
Small bowel and colon	Decreased motility
	Malabsorption
	Diarrhea
	Villus flattening and loss of disaccharidases
	Decreased amino acid absorption
	Decreased intraluminal bile acids
Pancreas	Chronic pancreatitis
	Acute pancreatitis, sometimes with chornic pancreatitis
	Fibrosis of gland, which can result in loss of both endocrine and exocrine function

Alcoholics experience stomach problems, including acute gastritis, as a result of a decreased gastric mucosal barrier and mucosal injury. Alcohol stimulates gastric secretions and decreases the rate of gastric emptying, which may partly contribute to the reduced appetite in these patients. They are at risk for increased ulcer bleeding, as a result of a decrease in clotting factors produced by the liver. It is important to note that alcoholics should not use cimetidine because this drug suppresses CYPIIE1 metabolism of alcohol and thus may lead to higher blood alcohol concentrations.

The small bowel and colon of alcoholics are also abnormal. In general, there is decreased motility and malabsorption of several classes of nutrients. An important change in the morphology of the small intestine is a decrease in villus height (flattening) and a concomitant loss of disaccharidases including lactase, which may lead to lactose intolerance. Diarrhea is common and occurs in at least 25% of chronic alcoholics. Absorption of amino acids and carbohydrates is reduced because of the reduction of enzyme activity as a result of villus atrophy. Chronic alcohol ingestion also reduces hepatic synthesis of cholic acid and alters the bile acid pool in the intestine, which reduces fat emulsification and digestion, resulting in steatorrhea.

After the liver, the organ of the GI tract that is most severely affected by alcohol abuse is the pancreas. Chronic pancreatitis is

Table 24-5. Effects of Chronic Alcohol Ingestion on Body Systems Other Than GI

SYSTEMS	EFFECT
Immune	Lowered resistance
	Depressed production and adherence of polymorphonuclear neutrophils
	Depressed natural killer cells
	Antibodies formed against acetaldehyde-protein adducts
Brain	Hepatic encephalopathy (due to increased NH_3)
	Alcohol withdrawal syndromes, including delirium tremens
	Wernicke's encephalopathy (thiamine deficiency)
	Korsakoff's psychosis
Endocrine	
Adrenals	Increased output of adrenal cortex hormones
Gonads	
Male	Hypogonadism
	Testicular atrophy
	Reduction in serum testosterone (biosynthesis impaired)
	Reduced sperm count; azospermia
	Reduced libido, impotence (temporary or permanent)
Female	Decrease in ovulation; thus, a decrease in progesterone
Neurologic	Damage may depend on timing of alcohol ingestion by mother
Fetal alcohol syndrome (FAS)	Growth deficiencies: short stature
	Mental retardation; behavioral problems
	Neurologic deficiencies
	Delayed puberty

Chronic pancreatitis is common in alcoholics.

common in alcoholics, and they may incur attacks of acute pancreatitis, particularly after binge drinking. The fibrosis induced in the pancreas can result in loss of both endocrine and exocrine function, thus precipitating diabetes as well as the inability of the GI tract to digest critical nutrients.

In addition to affecting the GI tract, alcohol abuse impacts on virtually all systems of the body, as outlined in Table 24-5.

Nutritional Consequences of Alcohol Abuse

Individuals who drink moderately usually consume about 5%–10% of their calories as alcoholic beverages, whereas alcoholics may consume over 50% of their total caloric intake as ethanol. A "standard drink" is considered to be 12 oz of beer, 5 oz of wine, or 1.5 oz of 80-proof distilled spirits, each of which contains roughly the same amount of absolute alcohol, approximately 0.5 oz or 12 g. A moderate drinker is generally defined as one for whom alcohol does not cause problems, either for the drinker or for society. However, a safe limit for alcohol intake depends on many factors, and recent research has indicated that intake of as low as 80 g/d for men and 40 g/d for women are associated with an increased risk for development of cirrhosis.

Alcohol has a relatively high caloric value, 7.1 kcal/g, as compared to protein and carbohydrate at 4.5 kcal/g or fat at 9 kcal/g. These values relate to the alcohol content and do not consider the contribution of any carbohydrate that may be present in alcoholic beverages (particularly wine and beer). In theory, then, the caloric content of alcohol is more like fat than carbohydrate.

However, the effects of alcohol metabolism on body weight are complex. Although alcohol has a high relative caloric value, alcohol consumption may not necessarily result in increased body weight. Data collected from the first National Health and Nutrition Examination Survey show that although drinkers had significantly higher caloric intakes than nondrinkers, they were not more obese than nondrinkers. In particular, women drinkers had significantly lower body weight than nondrinkers. When chronic heavy drinkers substitute alcohol for carbohydrates in their diets, they tend to lose weight and weigh less than nondrinkers. Furthermore, when chronic heavy drinkers add alcohol to an otherwise normal diet, they do not gain weight. Thus it appears that alcohol has a low biologic value, that is, "empty calories." There is evidence that alcohol consumption increases basal metabolic rate and diet-induced thermogenesis, an increase in heat production without ATP production.

The nutritional status of alcoholics varies widely and reflects the content of their diets apart from alcohol. Those alcoholics and heavy drinkers who consume more than 30% of their total calories as alcohol are likely to have diets deficient in a number of critical elements, such as protein, carbohydrates, and fats, as well as vitamins and minerals. Many deficiencies reflect inadequate intake, but reduced absorption or altered excretion may also contribute. Table 24-6 shows deficiencies that are common in chronic alcoholics.

In general, the goals of nutrition management of alcoholics are repletion of deficient nutrients and prevention of complications. Standard hospital diets are adequate in required nutrients and serve to replenish many of the deficiencies. However, several nutrients deserve special mention. A thiamine deficiency may contribute to Wernicke-Korsakoff syndrome, an alcohol-induced psychosis, and should be treated promptly. Zinc deficiency is almost universal in alcoholics. Vitamin A repletion should be modest and reserved for those with confirmed clinical deficiency, because vitamin A is not stored well in the livers of chronic alcoholics. Similarly, iron repletion should be used only in those with confirmed deficiencies because of the potential for iron overload toxicity. In patients with ascites, fluid and sodium management is important; sodium should be restricted to no more than 2 g and fluid to 1.2–1.5 L/d.

Table 24-6. Effects of Chronic Alcohol Ingestion on Nutrients

NUTRIENT	DECREASED INTAKE	DECREASED ABSORPTION
Macronutrients	Protein	Amino acids
	Fat	Fat
	Carbohydrate	Mono- and disaccharides
Water-soluble vitamins	Thiamine (B$_1$)	
	Riboflavin (B$_2$)	
	Pyridoxine (B$_6$)	
	Folic acid	Folic acid
	Vitamin C	
Fat-soluble vitamins	Vitamin A	Vitamin A
	Vitamin D	Vitamin K
Trace elements	Iron[a]	Iron[a]
	Zinc	
	Magnesium[b]	
	Calcium	

[a]Deficiency or overload may be present.
[b]Excretion is increased.

Good nutrition and abstinence from alcohol, along with careful management, can increase the length and quality of life of many alcoholics, even when significant liver disease is present.

CASE STUDY: *RESOLUTION*

B.K. was admitted to the hospital and received a nutritionally sound diet, supplemented with branched-chain amino acids, zinc, and vitamin A. He felt better after a few weeks, but his laboratory values remained somewhat abnormal with the exception of albumin, which rose to 3.8 g/dl. He was counseled to abstain from alcohol for the rest of his life and was recruited into a rehabilitation program. Follow-up visits were scheduled to assess his liver function and his compliance with the program.

R EVIEW Q UESTIONS

Directions: For each of the following questions, choose the one best answer.

1 Alcoholics frequently display

A fatty liver.
B diabetes mellitus.
C increased absorption of water-soluble vitamins.
D strikingly increased (> 10 times normal) ALT and AST.

Notes

2 Alcohol is metabolized primarily using the liver enzyme ADH. This enzyme uses which of the following important nutrients as cofactors?

A Ca^{2+} and Mn^{2+}
B Thiamine and Fe^{2+}
C Zn^{2+} and pantothenic acid
D Niacin as NAD^+ and Zn^{2+}

3 Alcoholics who display fatty liver (steatosis) early in their disease and continue to drink will

A almost always become cirrhotic.
B develop alcoholic hepatitis.
C have about a 10% chance of developing cirrhosis.
D develop cirrhosis if male.

4 A life-threatening complication of chronic alcoholism may be

A ruptured esophageal varices.
B decreased prothrombin times.
C thyroid storm.
D vitamin and mineral deficiencies.

5 Which factor listed below is commonly associated with chronic alcohol abuse?

A Pancreatitis
B Excess body fat
C Gastric carcinoma
D Blood clots in extremities

6 Chronic alcohol ingestion results in ultrastructural damage to the liver, including

A membrane changes as a result of vitamin deficiencies.
B micromitochondria as a result of nucleotide metabolism alterations.
C peroxidation of membrane lipids.
D reduction of the smooth endoplasmic reticulum.

References

An overview of many aspects of alcoholism and important references may be found online at www.niaaa.nih.gov.

The Eighth Special Report to the US Congress on Alcohol and Health. U.S. Department of Health and Human Services, National Institutes of Health Institute on Alcohol Abuse and Alcoholism. EEI, Alexandria, VA, 1993.

Feinman L, Lieber CS: Nutrition and diet in alcoholism. In *Modern Nutrition in Health and Disease*. Edited by Shils ME, Olson JA, Shike M. Philadelphia, PA: Lea & Febiger, 1994, pp 1081–1101.

Haber PS, Warner R, Seth D, Gorrell MD, McCaughan GW: Pathogenesis and management of alcoholic hepatitis. *J Gastroenterol Hepatol* 18(12):1332–1344, 2003.

Holeski CJ, DeLeve LD: Drug- and toxin-induced liver disease. In *Consultations in Gastroenterology*. Edited by Snape WJ. Philadelphia, PA: W. B. Saunders, 1996, pp 643–653.

Mezey E: Interaction between alcohol and nutrition in the pathogenesis of alcoholic liver disease. *Semin Liver Dis* 11:340–348, 1991.

Munoz SJ: Nutritional therapies in liver disease. *Semin Liver Dis* 11:278–291, 1991.

Thomasson, HR: Gender differences in alcohol metabolism: physiological responses to ethanol. In *Recent Developments in Alcoholism 12: Women and Alcoholism*. Edited by Galanter M. New York, NY: Plenum Press, 1995, pp 163–179.

Wong F, Blendis L: Alcoholic liver disease. In *Consultations in Gastroenterology*. Edited by Snape WJ. Philadelphia, PA: W. B. Saunders, 1996, pp 707–714.

Notes

25

Pathophysiology of Abdominal Pain and Pain Syndromes

■ **CHAPTER OUTLINE** ■

■ **LEARNING OBJECTIVES** ■

At the completion of this chapter, the reader should be able to:

• Discover some of the underlying conditions that can manifest as chronic abdominal pain.

• Integrate the anatomic, physiologic, and functional differences of the autonomic and somatic components of the nervous system, with clinical correlation.

• Develop an overview for evaluation and treatment of chronic abdominal pain based on physiology, pharmacology, and an appreciation of clinical limitations.

• Recognize that abdominal pain can be a nonspecific symptom that can arise from many different anatomic, physiologic, or psychosocial causes.

• Realize that diagnosis and treatment for similar presenting symptoms can be quite varied.

CASE STUDY 1: *INTRODUCTION*

A 58-year-old man with a 30-year history of heavy alcohol ingestion presented with chronic mid-upper abdominal burning and unrelenting, diffuse abdominal pain of several years' duration. The pain radiated toward his back and had been gradually increasing in severity over time. It seemed to be slightly worse after ingestion of fatty foods but was otherwise constant. The patient had not had an alcoholic drink and had not smoked for several years. His social situation was stable, with a supportive spouse who accompanied him on health care visits.

The patient's history was remarkable for surgical renal stone extraction 25 years previously, known chronic pancreatitis, and mild hypertension. There were no recent changes in bowel habits or diet, and a recent stool occult blood test was negative. He had no known allergies and was prescribed a diuretic and pancreatic replacement enzyme.

Physical examination demonstrated a well-developed man experiencing mild upper abdominal distress on movement. He was 5 feet, 7 inches (165 cm) tall, weighed 160 lbs (73 kg), and appeared well nourished. His vital signs were as follows: blood pressure, 150/90 mm Hg; pulse, 80 beats/min; respiratory rate, 18 breaths/min; and temperature, 36.8°C (98.2°F). Sclera were nonicteric; there was no demonstrated lymphadenopathy, jugular vein distention, tracheal deviation, or bruits. There was full cervical range of motion and bilateral symmetry.

Breath sounds were present throughout without rales, rhonchi, or wheezes. There was no retraction, splinting, or point tenderness. Heart sounds revealed a normal S1, S2 without S3, S4, or murmur. The abdomen was nondistended, symmetrical, with normal bowel sounds throughout. There was no point tenderness or rigidity. Initially, there was some minor guarding over the mid-upper area, but that was voluntary and resolved during the examination. Normal male genitalia were present.

Back examination was remarkable for a right posterolateral subcostal well-healed incision. There was no point or subcostal tenderness or skin lesion. Rectal examination was unremarkable, with normal sphincter tone and a slightly enlarged, nontender prostate.

The patient's extremities were well developed, bilaterally symmetrical without varicosities, and he had normal sensorimotor function. He was alert and responsive, with normal neurologic function.

CBC and coagulation profiles were normal for the laboratory; bilirubin and amylase were also low normal. Liver enzymes were not elevated, and urinalysis did not demonstrate any protein, sugar, or cells. ECG was normal sinus rhythm, borderline left ventricular hypertrophy with no evidence of ischemic changes.

Chest x-ray was normal, with symmetric diaphragmatic position, and an abdominal flat plate was remarkable only for some diffuse calcifications slightly to the left of midline in the upper abdomen. Some gas-filled loops of bowel were also noted.

CASE STUDY 2: *INTRODUCTION*

A 38-year-old woman who was referred by her surgeon presented with a 1-year history of chronic abdominal pain. She stated that the pain began several weeks before upper abdominal surgery (for repair of an incisional hernia). Initially, her surgeon thought that the hernia was causing her discomfort, but the same pain pattern persisted after the repair. On initial interview, she expressed a strong desire for interventional therapy and seemed extremely knowledgeable about her history, treatments, and various future options. However, there were several notable factual differences between her recollection and the chart history concerning past medication (narcotic) usage, legal proceedings against previous medical caregivers, and current psychiatric history.

The pain was described as having several separate and distinct components. First, she described a chronic, burning, poorly localized discomfort in the mid-upper abdomen unrelated to food intake. Then there was a sharper, more pronounced pain over the hernia repair site. This was associated with reproducible point tenderness and was also aggravated by certain types of movement. Finally, there was an occasional intermittent, very distinct midepigastric discomfort that was relieved by eating.

The patient's surgical history was significant for an emergency laparotomy 1 year previously for treatment of a perforated duodenal ulcer. Several weeks after the first procedure, she experienced a leak at the duodenal repair site, which required a second abdominal operation. Afterward, there was a small incisional hernia at the site of the surgical incisions, which had been repaired 11 months ago.

According to both the patient and surgeon, her pain symptoms were consistent over the past year and of unclear etiology. Initially, the surgeon thought that repair of the incisional hernia and lysis of several small adhesions would relieve the symptoms; however, they remained similar to the preoperative baseline.

Medical history was significant for her past duodenal ulcer history. Pancreatitis and cholelithiasis had previously been ruled out, and there was no evidence of infection. Current medications included acetaminophen with codeine and antidepressants. She stated that the narcotic's effects were short-lived, and this was supported by the observation that she consumed many times her prescribed daily dose of pain medication as evidenced by the shorter than expected intervals between prescription refill requests. (It was discovered later that she was seeing several clinicians at the same time and that each clinician was unaware of the involvement of others and was prescribing narcotics for her.)

Psychosocially, the patient was divorced and had lived for several years in another country. Immediately prior to the initial surgical procedure, she had moved back to her parents' home. Their relationship was not ideal, and she was eager to move out of the area. However, she was currently unemployed and had no immediate job prospects. She was under the care of a psychiatrist, who in conjunction with her surgeon prescribed the antidepressants and analgesic with codeine. She was referred to an anesthesiologist for global management of her pain symptoms, because her surgeon and psychiatrist felt that her needs were outside their areas of expertise. They hoped that a coordinated pain management plan would benefit the patient.

On initial physical examination, she appeared well developed and well nourished and was resting comfortably while reading a book in the waiting area. Her vital signs were normal, and the only remarkable findings were a 15-cm midline vertical midabdominal healed surgical incision with some diffuse midline subcostal and xyphoid point tenderness.

The laboratory studies and x-rays were unremarkable with the exception of several radiopaque objects (surgical staples) in the upper abdomen, noted on both abdominal and chest x-rays.

CASE STUDY 3: *INTRODUCTION*

A 72-year-old woman was referred by her internist for palliation of chronic, increasingly severe upper midabdominal pain radiating toward her back. She was recently admitted after being found on the floor of her home by a friend.

She enjoyed her usual good state of health until very recently, and it was noted that she had lost 10 lbs (4.5 kg) over the 2 weeks immediately prior to admission. There was no other significant medical history. She did not smoke, drink alcohol, or take any medication. In the hospital, she was administered intermittent intramuscular meperidine with good pain relief. However, she did not like the fuzzy feeling with which it left her, and the severe pain was breaking through between medication doses.

On physical examination, the patient was responsive but somewhat drowsy and in moderate discomfort. She appeared thin, but not cachectic, with evidence of recent rapid weight loss (5 feet, 3 inches [161 cm] tall, weighing 95 lbs [43kg]). Her vital signs were normal, and fluid was infusing via an intravenous line. Physical examination was also notable for icteric sclera, and a 10 × 10-cm fixed, nonpulsatile mid-upper abdominal mass. There was no clinical evidence of coagulopathy or bleeding at recent injection sites. Aneurysm had been previously ruled out, and tissue for biopsy had been obtained at the time of an endoscopic evaluation. Bilirubin was slightly elevated, as were several other liver enzymes. The patient had undergone endoscopic biliary stent placement to bypass the obstruction the day before and had tolerated the procedure well, with minimal use of intravenous sedation (midazolam).

Introduction

Abdominal pain in one form or another is probably the most common complaint of humankind. In its chronic form, varying in magnitude from barely noticeable to debilitating, it has many possible roots. Though they may be unrelated, these various underlying causes often manifest with similar clinical symptoms. Severity of discomfort in itself has little correlation with the pain's etiology, prognosis, and ultimate outcome.

Chronic abdominal pain, possible etiologies, the mechanism of neural transmission and sensory perception, and some modes of therapy are the focus of this chapter. Emphasis will be on the correlation of basic physiology and pharmacology in relation to symptoms. Some evaluation and treatment methods are emphasized. More detailed discussions of therapy can be found in surgical, anesthesiology, and internal medicine texts. Symptoms associated with upper abdominal neoplasm and chronic pancreatitis are presented. General clinical interventions and associated decision-making processes are highlighted. It must be stressed that because there are many causes of chronic abdominal pain, evaluation and intervention for seemingly similar symptoms can be quite varied, as seen in the three clinical cases in this chapter. These cases provide a summary, help in identifying key concepts, and form the background for the review questions.

At times, a chronic pain state can provide some degree of secondary gain or perceived benefit. Often the sufferer has a psychosocial component to his or her symptoms that must be appreciated as part of a comprehensive evaluation and therapy plan. Chronic pain states are frequently associated with complex interdependent relationships between the sufferers, those around them, and society in general. These complicated interactions can be considered part of a cycle that is interrelated with symptoms. Determining exact temporal order of pain and psychosocial effects can be likened to the question of which came first, the chicken or the egg? It is often a frustrating exercise in futility.

However, some types of chronic abdominal pain have specific physiologic or anatomic etiologies. The pain associated with pancreatic disease (e.g., chronic pancreatitis, pancreatic cancer) is an example. It is estimated that approximately 30,000 patients die each year of pancreatic cancer in the United States. Several times this number of patients suffering from chronic pancreatitis are also diagnosed. Survival rates for pancreatic cancer are poor, whereas those who suffer from pancreatitis, colitis, and irritable bowel syndrome (IBS) may experience symptoms lasting over several years.

Definition of Pain

Physical pain can be defined as a sensation of hurting, or strong discomfort, in some part of the body, caused by an injury, disease, or functional disorder and transmitted through the nervous system. Pain is individual in perception, effect, and expression and is highly subjective. Several measuring systems attempt to quantify it in a consistent, reproducible manner with variable results. Variations of "happy faces," linear scales, and comfort indexes adorn the walls of postanesthesia care units (recovery rooms) and pain centers throughout the country. Intensity, severity, and effect on the ability to function can vary with time of day, outlook, presence or absence of distraction, as well as with a host of other factors.

Mechanism of Pain: Pathways

Table 25-1 presents the various pain pathways classified by nerve fibers.

SENSORY PATHWAY

Pain, temperature, and touch are transmitted along the small myelinated somatic A δ fibers, which are the nerve fibers that are smallest in diameter (1–3 μm in diameter) of the A group.

AUTONOMIC PATHWAY

Preganglionic sympathetic myelinated B fibers (1–3 μm in diameter) constitute the celiac plexus. Even though they are myelinated, B

Notes

Acute pain, which is sudden or has specific onset over a short time, is differentiated from **chronic pain,** which is more insidious in onset and can take a longer time to become clinically significant. Pain associated with upper abdominal processes is often a combination of acute and chronic, with significant psychosocial overlay.

Table 25-1. Classification of Nerve Fibers

TYPE	DIAMETER (μm)	MYELIN	LOCATION AND FUNCTION
A α	10–22	Yes	Afferent and efferent; muscles and joints; motor and proprioception
A β	5–12	Yes	Afferent and efferent; muscles and joints; touch and pressure
A γ	5–12	Yes	Muscle spindles; muscle tone and proprioception
A δ	1–3	Yes	Pain, temperature, and touch
B	1–3	Yes	Preganglionic sympathetic vasomotor and viceromotor
C	0.4–1.2	No	Postganglionic sympathetic vasomotor and viceromotor; pain, temperature, and touch

Notes

fibers are more susceptible to local anesthetic blockade than A and postganglionic sympathetic nonmyelinated C fibers (0.4–1.2 μm in diameter). This explains why spinal and epidural sympathetic blockade extends several levels beyond that of the observed sensory and motor blockade. Conduction time increases with decreasing diameter and lack of myelination.

Clinicians are mainly concerned with the preganglionic myelinated B fibers when considering celiac plexus sympathetic blockade. All sympathetic and afferent pain fibers from upper abdominal viscera are contained in the splanchnic nerves, which form the celiac (splanchnic) plexus.

Characteristics of Pain

Pain can be classified as *visceral* or *somatic*. The characteristics of both types are summarized in Table 25-2.

SOMATIC PAIN

With somatic pain, sensation is precisely localized, discrete, and definite. It is localized to stimulus and usually associated with external factors. One usually is aware of the exact location and intensity of somatic pain. It is mediated at cortical levels, and an increase in intensity is directly related to an increase in stimulus.

VISCERAL PAIN

Visceral pain tends to be poorly localized and vague in quality. It is often referred or attributed to other areas of the body, and is usually associated with internal stimuli. Visceral pain is mediated at the reflex or cord level. As compared with somatic pain, in which both the intensity and quality of the stimulus directly affect the resultant sensation of pain, visceral pain is more diffuse or less localized for a given stimulus.

A specific characteristic of visceral pain is the sensation of pain or discomfort that is referred or localized to an area of the body removed from the actual stimulus. Examples of referred pain include shoulder pain from intra-abdominal or diaphragmatic processes. As pointed out in Chapter 14, the leading hypothesis for symptoms in IBS is visceral hyperalgesia.

Table 25-2. Characteristics of Pain

ATTRIBUTE	VISCERAL SENSATION	SOMATIC SENSATION
Localization	Poor	Good
Quality	Vague	Sharp, definite
Association	Internal	External
Referred	Often	No
Level	Reflex or spinal cord	Cortical levels

460 Chapter 25

Evaluation of Chronic Abdominal Pain

HISTORY

Evaluation of chronic abdominal pain consists of a history and physical examination, a psychosocial history, and consideration of possible secondary gains. Obtaining a thorough history is key in evaluating abdominal pain. Onset, duration, associated activities, and relief patterns all help in the differential diagnosis. Association with specific types of food, temporal relation to food intake or hunger, travel history, medication (prescription and nonprescription), alcohol and tobacco use, and bowel patterns all offer clues toward diagnosis.

General physical condition, including changes in body habitus and psychosocial status, should be considered. Upper abdominal neoplasms can occur throughout the general population, and chronic pancreatitis is often associated with long-term alcohol use or biliary obstruction. Examples of several different pain evaluation scales distributed by the U.S. Department of Health and Human Services are reproduced in Figures 25-1 and 25-2.

PHYSICAL EXAMINATION

A complete physical examination should be performed, with emphasis on the abdomen, and with attention to signs of adenopathy, venous congestion, ascites, and thoracic effusion or infiltrate. Laboratory studies, including coagulation tests and chest and abdominal x-rays, are useful, especially if an invasive procedure is contemplated.

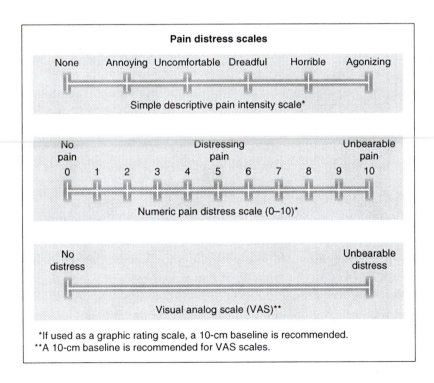

Fig. 25-1. Pain Distress Scales

The **ability to cope** with pain varies widely from person to person.

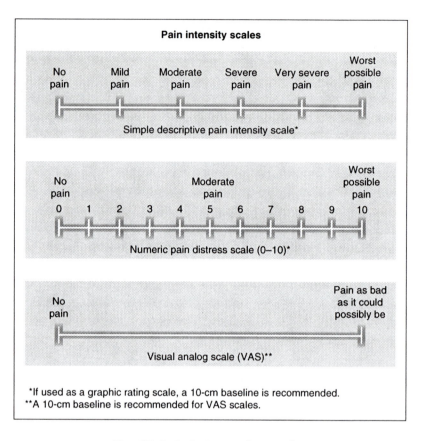

Fig. 25-2. Pain Intensity Scales

PSYCHOSOCIAL HISTORY

The examiner should ascertain recent changes in mental status, normal routine, social or work situation, and the patient's ability to cope with chronic abdominal pain. The evaluation should include current and past pharmaceutical and street drug, alcohol, and tobacco histories. The key questions are those that reveal the interaction between symptoms and lifestyle and how they affect each other.

The McGill Pain Questionnaire and the Minnesota Multiphasic Personality Inventory (MMPI) are useful in assessing pain states and the individual's ability to deal with it. Higher scores on three scales, *hypochondriasis*, *hysteria*, and *depression*, also known as the neurotic triad, are common with chronic pain patients.

The ability to cope or deal with pain states and alteration of physical status varies widely from person to person and is often affected by external influences. Depression, anxiety, or feelings of hopelessness have been shown to affect pain perception. Several pain evaluation scales have been developed and are in clinical use. Although they are similar, each has a slight difference in focus or approach. Techniques have to be adjusted for children and patients who may not be able to cooperate fully for various reasons.

One commonly held misconception is that the elderly have a different pain threshold or greater tolerance for pain. This is not true, and it only emphasizes the importance of evaluation and treating every patient as an individual, no matter what their age or physical state may be.

SECONDARY GAIN

The advantage of a pain state to the sufferer may not be immediately obvious; therefore, it cannot be discounted as a contributing factor. GI dysfunction and neoplastic processes have powerful effects on interpersonal relationships. IBS symptoms can be affected by external events, and it is often difficult to separate cause and effect when dealing with autonomically mediated conditions. When pain symptoms occur, there are complicated changes in perceived roles with regard to relationships, dependence, and demonstration of affection, possibly leading to changes in, for example, attention and affection. It may not be intentional on the part of any of the involved parties, but it evolves as part of the complex interaction with chronic pain. These and other complicated and sometimes unpredictable changes in relationships are among the rewards, or secondary gain, that result from maintenance of a chronic pain state.

Examples of secondary gain include increased attention from family and loved ones or health care professionals during times of symptoms, compensation or disability benefits tied to the pain condition, access to a health care support system otherwise not so available, and access to potentially habit-forming or addictive medications. Not all secondary gain behavior is antisocial or undesirable. However, its role in chronic pain states cannot be ignored.

Therapy

Therapy for chronic abdominal pain is pursued through one or several modes: pharmacologic, psychosocial, anesthetic, and autonomic. Table 25-3 lists the options available in these general cagegories. The case studies illustrate the practical applications.

Notes

Motivation to achieve relief from chronic pain states is sometimes mixed or altogether lacking.

Table 25-3. Therapeutic Modes

MODE	CLASS	EXAMPLES
Pharmacologic	Antispasmodic	Donnatal
	Narcotic	Morphine, codeine
	Phenothiazine	Hydroxyzine
	Antidepressant	Amitryptyline
Psychosocial	Pain scales	McGill Pain Questionnaire, U.S. Dept. of Health and Human Services
	Personality inventory	Minnesota Multiphasic Personality
	Support therapy	Inventory
Anesthetic	Celiac plexus block	
	Diagnostic and therapeutic	Bupivacaine with or without steroids
	Ablative	Ethyl alcohol and phenol
Surgical	Autonomic	Sympathectomy

Tachyphylaxis, or rapid development of tolerance to the clinical effect of an agent, is often seen with chronic narcotic usage.

CASE STUDY 1: CONTINUED

After the history, physical examination, and workup, it was felt that the best approach for the patient's chronic pancreatitis would be a celiac plexus block. He had a good quality of life and did not want to depend on oral medications for symptomatic relief because their side effects were unpleasant for him. In addition, their effectiveness diminishes over time (tachyphylaxis). If the initial block using local anesthetic agents was satisfactory, a longer-lasting block with alcohol would be considered.

CASE STUDY 2: CONTINUED

Because of the confusing history and findings, the patient's surgeon, psychiatrist, and anesthesiologist met to review her history and outline several possible treatment plans. Her surgeon felt that there were no probable reasons for further surgical intervention. Coordination assumed greater importance because all the physicians needed to have a consistent goal and means of approaching it. The patient had been extremely manipulative when there was no communication between the several care providers.

It was decided that all narcotic medications were to be coordinated and that the patient would continue with the tricyclic antidepressants. The overall effect on reported symptoms was to be evaluated by both the anesthesiologist and psychiatrist. Attempts were to be made to isolate and characterize the several different types of pain symptoms over the following 2-week period.

It was also agreed that a diagnostic sympathetic block be placed to help differentiate her symptoms. Supportive counseling (including her family) was to continue throughout this period. Behavior modification was in progress, and her other health care providers were contacted (with her permission) for coordination of care.

CASE STUDY 3: CONTINUED

The patient's history, examination, and biopsy were consistent with pancreatic carcinoma. She wanted continued pain relief without excessive sedation and needed some quality time for personal needs. After consultation with the patient and her family, a celiac plexus block was selected as the initial treatment of choice.

PHARMACOLOGIC THERAPY

Anticholinergics are often employed to reduce spasms, narcotics for analgesia, and pancreatic enzymes and hypoglycemic agents for pancreatic hypofunction. Laxatives and bulking agents may be used to offset some of the constipating effects of narcotics. Antidepressants have been shown to be beneficial for increasing overall effectiveness of a pain relief regimen. Phenothiazines and other antiemetics also help potentiate analgesic states and offer some sedation as well as easing the nausea and vomiting associated with both the disease state and narcotic usage. With chronic narcotic use, ever greater doses of more potent narcotics are required to achieve a baseline level of relief. Narcotic side effects, such as urinary retention, constipation, and pruritus, may not decrease at the same rate as the clinical effectiveness, leading to a need for change in therapeutic approach.

Patients suffering from abdominal neoplastic processes or pancreatic lesions often progress from acetaminophen and codeine combinations, through morphine and hydromorphone hydrochloride to methadone, with decreasing pain relief. Some clinicians feel that there is little advantage in switching from morphine to other narcotics. The addition of antidepressants can sometimes slow but not arrest this progression.

Dosing needs to be individualized for each patient and stage of symptoms. Availability of medication may need to be continuous, such as with patient-controlled analgesia (PCA) pumps. PCA pumps can be individually programmed to provide continuous baseline medication infusions as well as peak or breakthrough supplements of pain relief medication. Otherwise, arrangements for around-the-clock access to oral medications may be required. The patient must have a mechanism for obtaining interval or additional doses when required for acute exacerbations or breakthrough pain at unpredictable times. Transdermal application of some medications promotes sustained delivery over time.

PHYSICAL INTERVENTION

Anesthetic Block. Celiac plexus (sympathetic autonomic) blockade is a classically accepted treatment tool for the pain associated with upper abdominal neoplasms, autonomic conditions, and chronic pancreatitis that is transmitted via the splanchnic nerves. Its effect can be either temporary or permanent and its purpose either diagnostic or therapeutic, depending on whether an anesthetic or neurolytic agent is chosen, the overall severity of symptoms, and the patient's life expectancy.

Approach to the celiac plexus can be made from either anterior or posterior aspects. The plexus is anterior to the spinal column and adjacent to both the aorta and vena cava. Because of its relatively well-protected position, it can be difficult to position a needle in the proper location within the plexus. Proximity of the dural membrane, vena cava, and aorta make inadvertent damage or injection into these structures a possibility.

Retroperitoneal bleeding and intravascular or subarachnoid injection of medication have all been reported. The most common side effect associated with this block is transient hypotension, with an occurrence rate of about 30%. However, this is usually avoidable with adequate prehydration prior to the procedure.

Although often performed without radiologic guidance in the past, celiac plexus blocks are now often placed under CT or fluoroscopic guidance. This also allows documentation of needle and medication placement, as well as positioning in relationship to adjacent structures. Figures 25-3 to 25-6 demonstrate a celiac plexus block under CT guidance.

Temporary Block. Diagnostic and therapeutic blocks are placed with local anesthetics, such as 0.25% bupivacaine. Steroids can be added if an inflammatory component is suspected. Duration of action is for up to several months. Axonal uptake of the local anesthetic and greater susceptibility of B preganglionic fibers are factors in the prolonged duration of the pain relief. Interruption of the pain cycle may in itself be a factor contributing to prolonged pain relief.

Patients with upper abdominal neoplasms often require only one or two block treatments because of the time course of their disease. Those with chronic pancreatitis usually have a local anesthetic block placed first, to evaluate its effectiveness for their particular condition. In either case, a permanent block can be placed if prolonged relief is required and if the local anesthetic block has demonstrated that celiac plexus blockade is beneficial.

Permanent Block. Ethyl alcohol (ET-OH) is most commonly used for neurolytic blocks. Phenol is used to a lesser degree, but because of its possible destructive effect on adjacent blood vessels, it is not

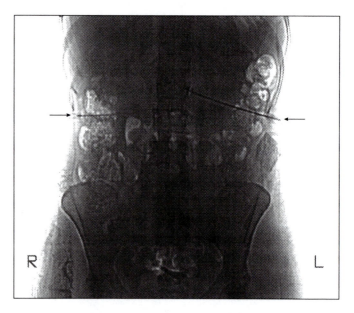

Fig. 25-3. Celiac Block under CT Guidance

Initial scout film with line drawn along projected needle path from left posterior flank to body of L2.

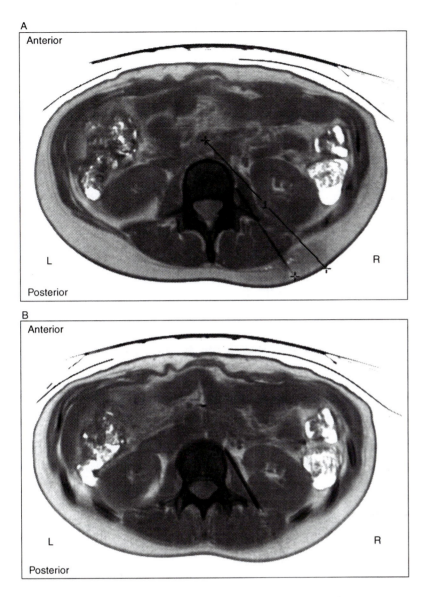

Fig. 25-4. Celiac Plexus Block under CT Guidance

Films show actual needle placement just lateral (A) with superimposed
computer-generated line, then final position of needle tip anterior (B) to
the body of L1 and posterior–lateral to the aorta from a posterior approach
immediately prior to the injection of local anesthetic.

considered for this specific use. Chemical destruction of the celiac
plexus is considered only after it has been demonstrated that the treatment would be effective by use of a local anesthetic test block, and the
clinical benefits are to outweigh side effects of sympathectomy.

ET-OH works by myelin sheath disruption, intracellular edema,
and eventual Wallerian degeneration. It tends to be extremely painful
on injection and is often administered in combination with a local
anesthetic, such as lidocaine or bupivacaine.

Phenol tends to be less painful on injection and works by the
mechanism of protein denaturation. It is not as destructive as ET-OH

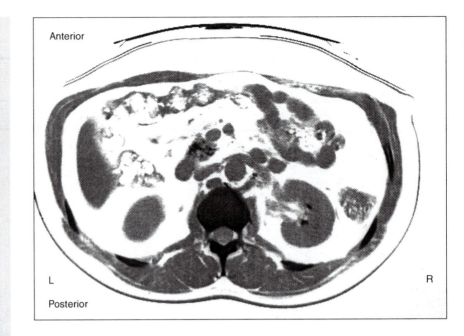

Fig. 25-5. Celiac Plexus Block under CT Guidance

Taken during injection and showing separation of the aorta, vena cava, and L1 body as a result of displacement of tissue planes by injected volume of local anesthetic.

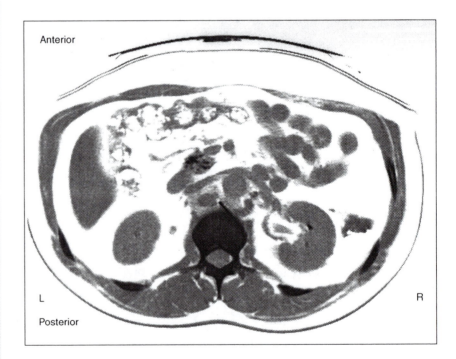

Fig. 25-6. Celiac Plexus Block under CT Guidance

Taken after injection to reconfirm needle tip placement. Contrast has been added to demonstrate spread of injected solution.

on posterior root ganglia, although this characteristic is not as well demonstrated with higher concentrations.

Electrical Intervention

In theory, it is possible that electrical stimulation such as transcutaneous electrical stimulation (TENS) may provide some measure of relief for the skeletal muscle component of chronic abdominal pain. Which component of pain is responsible in overall discomfort and the overall effect of this therapy, if any, have yet to be studied in depth. Several theories for its effect—such as gating and inhibition of afferent pathways—are postulated; however, the exact mechanism of sensory alteration with such therapy is uncertain. It does work for some people, but its effect and duration of effectiveness are unpredictable at best.

Surgery

Sympathectomy, or physical interruption of the lumbar sympathetic plexus, is sometimes considered for those patients with intractable pain in whom other therapies have failed. It is usually reserved for terminally ill cancer patients, because long-term side effects such as orthostatic hypotension, GI and sexual dysfunction, and general parasympathetic predominance can be debilitating in their own right.

Psychosocial Therapy

Chronic pain patients tend to require a great deal of trust in their caregivers. Close working relationships often develop, and a great deal of support is frequently required on the part of the caregiver. Collaboration with a social worker or therapist in dealing with the patient as a complex entity is probably more important than the act of administering medication itself in caring for the chronic pain sufferer.

Summary

Pain may present in a variety of ways and may be due to many different causes. It can be classified as chronic or acute, somatic or visceral. No matter how it is labeled, its interpretation and effect on a person is individual and quite varied. Psychological makeup, coping ability, depression, and optimism all affect how pain is perceived. Support is for the person as a whole, not just a disease entity.

Treatment is as varied as the pain state. Pharmacologic intervention treats pain, associated symptoms, and other medication side effects. Anesthetic and surgical intervention are part of a continuous progression of therapy for patients who will benefit from them. Side effects are significant and must be weighed against possible benefits. As a general rule, working in cooperation with the whole patient and, if appropriate, in an integrated team setting results in the most satisfactory therapy.

CASE STUDY 1: *RESOLUTION*

Immediately after placement of the celiac plexus block, there was a transitory drop in blood pressure. The blood pressure rapidly returned to baseline, and the patient reported rapid diminution of symptoms. On follow-up the next day, he reported some slight discomfort at the injection site and a mild, dull midabdominal aching, which was not nearly as severe as his preblock pain.

The patient returned 7 months later because the pain was starting to return. However, he had gained 8 kg (17.5 lbs) in the interim because he felt so well. A repeat local anesthetic celiac plexus block was performed, and he remained symptom-free for another 10 months.

CASE STUDY 2: *RESOLUTION*

Most of the acute and sharp pain diminished on medication therapy. However, the patient continued to complain of nonspecific midabdominal burning pain. After endoscopy to rule out mucosal disease, she had a lumbar sympathetic block placed.

She reported immediate relief of symptoms, but symptoms returned after 24 hours. At this time, her psychiatrist suggested that she no longer share living quarters with her parents and that she reassume control over her circumstances.

After several months more of continued therapy, she was found to be consuming large quantities of narcotic analgesics obtained from another source. After another physician team meeting, her psychiatrist confronted her with this information. Subsequently, she moved out of the area and was lost to follow-up.

CASE STUDY 3: *RESOLUTION*

A celiac plexus block was placed the following morning. Relief was immediate even though some slight but noticeable discomfort remained. The patient was able to leave the hospital a few days later and did not require additional oral pain medication. She fully understood the ultimate outcome of her illness and was willing to have a repeat block procedure if the symptoms returned and she was physically able.

REVIEW QUESTIONS

Directions: For each of the following questions, choose the one best answer.

1 A 42-year-old man presents with a 6-month history of occasional nausea and severe, sharp, mid-upper abdominal pain radiating to his back. What is the first thing the physician should do?

A Upper GI endoscopy
B Abdominal CT scan
C Barium swallow
D Obtain a comprehensive history and physical examination
E Electrocardiogram

2 Diffuse, poorly localized, burning pain is mediated at the level of the

A spinal cord.
B limbic system.
C cerebellum.
D celiac plexus.
E cerebral cortex.

3 Secondary gain in chronic pain states is best described as

A a win-win situation for all involved.
B making the best of a situation.
C using one set of circumstances to receive other benefits.
D the second most needed item according to a hierarchy of needs.

4 Treatment of chronic abdominal pain states can include

A biofeedback.
B muscle relaxants.
C appetite stimulants.
D antidepressants.
E antipsychotics.

5 Which of the following criteria is considered *most* important in determining a patient's maximum safe local anesthetic dosage?

A Local anesthetic drug class (amide or ester)
B Body weight
C Concentration of local anesthetic in a preparation
D Gender
E Site of planned anesthetic action

References

Abram SE, Haddox JD, Lynch NT: Chronic pain management. In *Clinical Anesthesia*, 3rd ed. Edited by Barash PG, Cullen BF, Stoelting RK. Philadelphia, PA: Lippincott-Raven, 1997.

Carr DB, Jacox AK, Chapman CR, et al: *Acute Pain Management: Operative or Medical Procedures and Trauma. Clinical Practice Guideline No. 1* (AHCPR pub. no. 92-0032). Rockville, MD: Agency for Health Care Policy and Research, Public Health Service, U.S. Department of Health and Human Services, 1992.

Collins VJ: Autonomic nervous system. In *Physiologic and Pharmacologic Basis of Anesthesiology*. Edited by Collins VJ. Baltimore, MD: Williams & Wilkins, 1996.

Raj PP: Guidelines for regional anesthetic techniques. In *Regional Anesthesia: An Atlas of Anatomy and Techniques*. Edited by Hahn MB, McQuillan PM, Sheplock GJ. St. Louis, MO: C. V. Mosby, 1996.

Thompson GE, Moore DC, Bridenbough LD, et al: Abdominal pain and alcohol celiac plexus nerve block. *Anesth Analg* 56:1, 1977.

Williams MJ: Pharmacology for regional anesthetic techniques. In *Regional Anesthesia: An Atlas of Anatomy and Techniques*. Edited by Hahn MB, McQuillan PM, Sheplock GJ. St. Louis, MO: C. V. Mosby, 1996.

26

GI Disorders in Pregnancy

■ CHAPTER OUTLINE ■

■ LEARNING OBJECTIVES ■

At the completion of this chapter, the reader should be able to:

- Explore physiologic, biochemical, and morphologic changes in pregnancy.
- Discuss motility disorders in pregnancy.
- Identify effects of inflammatory bowel disease (IBD) on pregnancy and of pregnancy on IBD.
- Differentiate diseases unique to pregnancy from chronic liver diseases in pregnancy and intercurrent liver diseases during pregnancy.

CASE STUDY: *INTRODUCTION*

The patient is a 24-year-old female medical student who was well until 4 weeks prior to presentation. At that time, she developed nausea and vomiting. She denied having a fever or abdominal pain.

Introduction

Although pregnancy is a normal state, special attention should be considered for the changes associated with alterations in the hormonal environment, especially with the presentation of new signs or symptoms. It is common knowledge that pregnant women experience frequent GI symptoms, such as nausea, vomiting, and constipation. Table 26-1 lists the normal physiologic changes that occur during pregnancy.

Table 26-1. Physiologic, Biochemical, and Morphologic Changes in Pregnancy

INCREASED	DECREASED	UNCHANGED
Physiologic changes		
Total blood volume	Hepatic blood flow/	Hepatic blood flow
Total plasma volume	cardiac output	
Total body water		
Cardiac output		
Total renal blood flow		
Biochemical changes		
Serum alkaline phosphatase	Serum total protein	Aspartate aminotransferase (AST)
Serum α- and β-globulins	Serum albumin	Alanine aminotransferase (ALT)
Serum cholesterol and triglycerides	Serum γ-globulin	γ-Glutamyl transpeptidase
Conjugated fraction of bilirubin	Hemoglobin and	5'-Nucleotidase
Erythrocyte sedimentation rate	hematocrit	Lactate dehydrogenase isoenzyme V
Leukocyte count	Blood urea nitrogen	Total bilirubin
Coagulation factors VII–X	Uric acid	Prothrombin time
Fibrinogen	Serum ferritin	
α_1-Antitrypsin		
Ceruloplasmin and serum copper		
Transferrin		
Leucine aminopeptidase		
Ornithine carbamyltransferase		
Morphologic changes		
Spider nevi		Liver volume and histology[a]
Palmar erythema		
Upward displacement		

[a]Minimally changed.

CASE STUDY: CONTINUED

It is important to consider pregnancy in any woman of childbearing age. Many young women present to the gastroenterologist with GI complaints, and the diagnosis of pregnancy may reveal the origin of those symptoms. Pregnancy was confirmed in the 24-year-old patient. Continuing to experience nausea and vomiting, she presented to the emergency room with these complaints and was found to be dehydrated and tachycardic and to have orthostatic hypotension.

Nausea and Vomiting

Nausea, the most common GI symptom during pregnancy, may occur in 50%–90% of pregnant women, and vomiting may occur in 25%–55%. There appears to be no correlation between the presence of nausea and vomiting and complications of pregnancy, such as hypertension, diabetes, or preeclampsia. The cause of nausea and vomiting is unknown and may be related to hormonal factors, motility, or even psychologic factors. Patients should be advised to eat multiple small meals that are high in carbohydrates and low in fats. Controlled human data are not available regarding the use of antiemetics during pregnancy. Studies suggest that pyridoxine (vitamin B_6) may be a therapeutic alternative.

HYPEREMESIS GRAVIDARUM

Hyperemesis gravidarum is a syndrome of intractable vomiting during pregnancy associated with fluid and electrolyte imbalance. The pathogenesis of this condition is unknown but may involve endocrine and psychologic factors. It is uncommon and occurs in 3.5/1000 pregnancies. There appears to be increased prevalence in obese patients, multiple gestations, and molar pregnancies. Social and psychologic factors have also been implicated. Table 26-2 lists treatment options.

Hyperemesis gravidarum may become a liver disease that is unique to pregnancy. Hepatic complications may include jaundice, hepatomegaly secondary to macrovesicular steatosis, loss of glycogen stores, and elevated liver enzymes.

Table 26-2. Treatment of Hyperemesis Gravidarum

Bed rest
Intravenous therapy
Hydration
Correction of electrolyte abnormalities
Peripheral hyperalimentation
Total parenteral nutrition
Sedation, only when necessary
Phenothiazines (best avoided)
Behavior modification

CASE STUDY: *CONTINUED*

The patient was diagnosed with hyperemesis gravidarum. She was found to have electrolyte abnormalities, which were corrected with repletion and hydration. Further discussion revealed that she had mixed emotions about the pregnancy because she was anxious about completing her education and beginning her training.

After treatment with intravenous hydration, she was able to leave the hospital in 2 days on an oral diet. She was told to drink plenty of fluids to maintain adequate hydration. In 2 weeks, she entered her second trimester, and her symptoms resolved. She was left with only nocturnal reflux symptoms.

Gastroesophageal Reflux Disease

The pathogenesis of gastroesophageal reflux disease (GERD) in pregnancy involves both mechanical and intrinsic factors. Heartburn and regurgitation are very common symptoms. Progesterone is a mediator of lower esophageal sphincter relaxation, and estrogen may be a possible primer for this to occur.

Treatment consists of lifestyle modification with antireflux precautions, avoiding foods that tend to decrease lower esophageal sphincter pressure (e.g., chocolate, peppermint) and foods that may irritate the esophageal mucosa, eating smaller meals, and not eating before lying down. Head-of-bed elevation should be recommended. Nonsystemic therapy with antacids appears to be both safe and effective in pregnancy. Antacids may, however, interfere with iron absorption. Surcralfate, which is not systemically absorbed, has been shown to be more effective than placebo in treating symptoms of heartburn in pregnant patients. The safety of histamine (H_2)-blockers in pregnancy has not been studied in a prospective manner, but clinical experience, especially for cimetidine and ranitidine, suggests that pregnant women and their infants are not at increased risk with their use. Animal studies of famotidine (high doses) have revealed sporadic abortions, and nizatidine in high doses has been associated with fetal anomalies in rabbits. Omeprazole is Category C, but the other proton pump inhibitors are classified as Category B (see Table 26-3).

Pregnant patients who require anesthesia during delivery are at high risk for aspiration of gastric contents. Gastric acidity is a major factor in determining the severity of aspiration pneumonitis, and prevention should therefore include increasing the gastric pH. Antacids, H_2 blockers, or a proton pump inhibitor may be used in this acute setting.

Peptic ulcer disease (PUD) and its complications are rare during pregnancy, perhaps because of gestational changes in gastric acidity. PUD may actually improve during pregnancy. Factors in the development of GI mucosal disease, such as NSAIDs and aspirin, may be reduced because pregnant women avoid these medications. *Helicobacter*

Table 26-3. FDA Drug Categories in Pregnancy

Class A	No risk in controlled human studies.
Class B	No risk in controlled animal studies, no studies in pregnant women.
	Animal studies show risk, but adequate studies in pregnant women show no risk.
Class C	Small risk in controlled animal studies.
	No adequate studies in humans.
Class D	Strong evidence of risk to the human fetus.
Class X	Very high risk in the human fetus.
	Never to be used in pregnancy.

Notes

Causes of Constipation

Multiple hypotheses have been proposed for the cause of constipation, including hormonal effects on GI smooth muscle, decreased motilin, increased absorption of water and sodium, iron supplementation, and mechanical pressure on the rectosigmoid by the gravid uterus.

pylori in pregnancy has not been evaluated. Any treatment considerations must take the pregnancy into account.

Irritable Bowel Syndrome

Irritable bowel syndrome (IBS) is a very common problem and has been reported in 15% or more of the general population. There are no specific studies of IBS during pregnancy. The effect of the menstrual cycle on GI transit has been studied, with findings showing that transit is significantly prolonged in the luteal phase of the cycle, a time when progesterone levels are increased. It is possible that progesterone may act as a smooth muscle relaxant and may result in intestinal hypomotility in pregnancy. In a pregnant patient with symptoms suggestive of IBS, serious conditions such as IBD and even systemic disorders such as thyroid disease should be eliminated. A careful history should be elicited to rule out other sources of symptoms, including lactose, sorbitol, or fructose intolerance. Because of the possible teratogenic effects of anticholinergics, antispasmodics, antidepressants, and anxiolytics, these should be avoided in pregnancy, and treatment of IBS symptoms should be conservative. Elimination of exacerbating foods and treatment with a high-fiber diet or fiber supplements can be considered.

Constipation

Constipation is a very common symptom during pregnancy. Patients should be educated to pay attention to rectal sensations, which may be most evident after eating, and to avoid delay of defecation once they sense the urge to have bowel movement. A noninvasive, safe option for treatment includes Kegel exercises, isometric exercises for strengthening pelvic floor muscles. Kegel exercises have been used to treat constipation and to promote an increased number of bowel movements with prolonged benefit. Conservative treatment with dietary modification including high-fiber foods may be initiated. Bulking agents may be recommended; these are safe during pregnancy. Emollient laxatives such as docusate sodium appear to be safe in pregnancy; however, they have not been extensively studied, although they are prescribed quite

often. These agents theoretically may make it easier to pass stool and may result in less straining.

Lubricants such as mineral oil should be avoided for routine use because decreased absorption of fat-soluble vitamins may result. Hyperosmotic agents, such as lactulose, sorbitol, and saline, work by increasing the osmotic tension with increased intraluminal water and subsequent peristalsis. The saline hyperosmotics may cause sodium retention. Castor oil should be avoided in pregnancy because it may initiate uterine contractions. Cascara sagrada has been reported to result in loose stools in the newborn. Other stimulant laxatives are apparently safe but should not be employed routinely because they may lead to dependency. Severe and persistent constipation in the pregnant woman may cause back pain, fecal impaction, and hemorrhoids.

Hemorrhoids

Hemorrhoids, another common problem in pregnancy, may first appear during pregnancy and worsen with each subsequent pregnancy. They very likely result from increased intra-abdominal pressure and venous stasis related to the gravid uterus. Straining for a bowel movement, constipation, and bearing down during delivery may exacerbate hemorrhoids. Symptoms may include bright-red blood per rectum, anal discomfort, pruritus, pain, protrusion of a mass, or a sense of fullness. Conservative measures are very often successful and include increasing dietary fiber or taking fiber supplements, promotion of regular bowel movements, sitz baths, topical ointments, and suppositories. Other treatments (injection of sclerosant, banding, infrared photocoagulation, direct current electrotherapy, heater probe coagulation) have not been extensively investigated in pregnant patients and should be considered only for severe cases.

Diarrhea

Diarrhea in the pregnant patient is usually caused by an infectious pathogen. Relaxin, which is a substance released by the placenta to decrease smooth muscle contractions in preterm labor, may also affect GI smooth muscle. Treatment of diarrhea in pregnancy must take the fetus into consideration as well as the mother. Volume depletion may not be as evident in pregnancy because of the increased intravascular volume, and as always, fluid resuscitation and electrolyte repletion should be undertaken.

Acute diarrhea usually improves with conservative management. If diarrhea persists, evaluation of stool specimens may be necessary. Flexible sigmoidoscopy may be indicated if IBD is considered; results of this study may determine management options. Endoscopic procedures in a stable pregnant patient are infrequently associated with complications for the mother or the fetus, but as always, the risk of the procedure must be weighed against potential benefits.

Treatment of diarrhea should be tailored to the underlying cause; systemic pharmacologic treatments are limited because of possible effects on the fetus. Deleterious effects should be determined, especially in pregnant patients, prior to initiating drug therapy. Metronidazole, which may be used to treat *Giardia lamblia* and *Entamoeba*, should be avoided in the first trimester because it has been shown to have a teratogenic effect. Antidiarrheal agents kaolin and pectin absorb water and reduce the frequency of stools and may be considered. Opiates, which may promote bacterial overgrowth, should be avoided. Loperamide studied in laboratory animals produced no harm to the fetus in up to 30 times the human dose, but higher doses resulted in impaired maternal and fetal survival. Human data with limited follow-up include pregnancies resulting in congenital malformations, spontaneous abortions, and one infant with Erb's palsy. Diphenoxylate with atropine has been shown to produce teratogenic effects in animals, and malformations have occurred in several human infants exposed to this medication in the first trimester. Bismuth subsalicylate should also be avoided because salicylates are teratogenic in animals and may cause neonatal hemorrhage in humans.

IBD

IBD often presents during or before the childbearing years. The major concerns of the patients and their physicians are fertility, the effect of IBD on pregnancy, and the effect of pregnancy on IBD. Table 26-4 addresses these issues for both ulcerative colitis and Crohn's disease.

Female fertility in ulcerative colitis does not appear to be reduced; however, some data suggest that fertility may be reduced in women with Crohn's disease. This may be multifactorial and could be due to structural disease from Crohn's, such as occlusion of the fallopian tubes, but it may also be due to generalized debility and lack of libido. Male fertility may be reduced when sulfasalazine is administered for either form of IBD. When sulfasalazine therapy is discontinued, the reduced sperm density and impaired sperm motility and forms of sperm reverse, and all parameters return to normal. It does appear that

Table 26-4. IBD and Pregnancy

	ABILITY TO CONCEIVE	INFLUENCE OF DISEASE ON THE PREGNANCY	INFLUENCE OF THE PREGNANCY ON THE DISEASE
Ulcerative colitis	No evidence that fertility is diminished[a]	No detrimental effect on pregnancy outcome[b]	Approximately 34% relapse, which is similar to nonpregnant rate; highest risk for relapse is in first trimester
Crohn's disease	Inability to conceive correlates with disease activity[a] Other factors: decreased libido, nutrition, adnexal disease, and perineal disease	No detrimental effect on pregnancy outcome[b]	Approximately 27% relapse, which is similar to nonpregnant rate; relapse occurs most commonly in first trimester and puerperium

[a] Male fertility decreased with sulfasalazine therapy.
[b] Except with increased disease activity.

Notes

Appendicitis is the most common surgical problem during pregnancy requiring emergent intervention.

men with Crohn's have fewer children, but this may be a result of a voluntary decision.

Most women who have IBD and become pregnant have normal, full-term pregnancies. Those women with active colitis have a smaller chance of a successful outcome. The risk of congenital abnormalities, spontaneous abortions, and stillbirths is similar to that seen in the general population, except in increased disease activity in both ulcerative colitis and Crohn's.

In terms of the effect of pregnancy on IBD, about 34% of ulcerative colitis patients relapse during pregnancy, which is similar to the rate in nonpregnant patients. In cases where the colitis is active when the pregnancy occurs, there is a 45% chance the disease will worsen and 26% chance the degree of activity will continue. In Crohn's disease, the relapse rate is reported at 27%. If Crohn's disease is active at the time of conception, it will worsen in a third of cases, stay the same in a third, and regress in a third.

In general it is recommended that patients with IBD be in the best possible condition prior to conceiving. Preconception counseling is important, and a multidisciplinary approach with the gastroenterologist and obstetrician is encouraged.

Appendicitis

The incidence of acute appendicitis in pregnant women has been reported as 1/1400 or 1500. Appendicitis has been reported to occur more commonly in the second trimester. The symptoms of appendicitis, including nausea, anorexia, and abdominal discomfort, are the same as those that may occur simply as a result of pregnancy, but a high index of suspicion must be maintained, especially for the patient with increasing complaints and localization of pain. The location of the pain may be displaced toward the upper quadrant.

Fecal Incontinence

It is now widely recognized that anal sphincter disruption may occur as a result of mechanical or neurologic injury to the sphincter during vaginal delivery. A third-degree or fourth-degree tear is reported to occur in about 0.7% of deliveries associated with posterolateral episiotomies. Vaginal delivery is frequently associated with mechanical disruption of both the internal and external anal sphincter, and there appears to be a relationship between the presence of defects of the sphincter, anal pressures, and bowel symptoms. Idiopathic fecal incontinence in middle-aged women may be associated with prolonged pudendal latencies, resulting from childbirth injury.

Liver Disorders

Liver disorders in pregnancy can be classified into one of three categories: diseases unique to pregnancy, chronic liver diseases and pregnancy, and liver disease complicating pregnancy.

DISEASES UNIQUE TO PREGNANCY

There are several liver disorders that are unique to pregnancy. These include intrahepatic cholestasis of pregnancy, preeclampsia and eclampsia, acute fatty liver of pregnancy, and HELLP syndrome (hemolysis, elevated liver enzymes, and low platelets).

Intrahepatic Cholestasis of Pregnancy

Genetic factors may play a role in the development of intrahepatic cholestasis of pregnancy. The clinical presentation usually occurs in the third trimester. Symptoms include pruritus, dark urine, light stools, and jaundice. The pruritus may be severe. Steatorrhea may occur and is thought to be due to decreased intraluminal bile acids. This may affect the nutritional status. Fetal distress, stillbirths, and prematurity have been reported to occur. The pathogenesis is likely multifactorial and is probably related to estrogen, bile acid levels in serum, and other factors.

Preeclampsia and Eclampsia

Although liver involvement is not an initial concern at the onset of preeclampsia and eclampsia, it may occur in the advanced stages of the condition.

Preeclampsia is defined as hypertension occurring in the second or third trimester associated with rapid weight gain, edema, and proteinuria. This may progress to severe preeclampsia or eclampsia, which is manifested by organ damage with headache, visual disturbances, epigastric or right upper quadrant pain, congestive heart failure, seizures, azotemia, oliguria, or pulmonary edema.

Liver complications associated with eclampsia account for 10%–15% of eclampsia-related deaths. Right upper quadrant or epigastric pain may be present. The hepatocellular enzymes may be elevated. High elevations of bilirubin may be seen in severe involvement, such as subcapsular or intrahepatic hematoma, free intraperitoneal hemorrhage, or infarction. Spontaneous rupture of the liver may result in a devastating outcome for the mother and fetus.

The histopathologic changes in eclampsia include occlusion of the hepatic sinusoids with fibrin deposition, resulting in perisinusoidal hemorrhage. Local injury of the liver cells with subsequent necrosis follows.

The pathogenesis is uncertain. Predisposing factors may include diet, diabetes, obesity, hypertension, renal disease, sodium overload,

Notes

hydramnios, fetal hydrops, age extremes, family history, plural gestations, and molar pregnancies.

Preeclampsia and eclampsia are the leading causes of maternal death in pregnancy. These conditions also carry increased morbidity for the fetus. Treatment involves early recognition and management of preeclampsia. The definitive treatment of eclampsia is delivery or termination of the pregnancy.

Acute Fatty Liver of Pregnancy

Acute fatty liver of pregnancy (AFLP) may have a fulminant course. The true incidence is not known, but one report estimated 1/13,000 pregnancies. Symptoms include anorexia, nausea, vomiting, malaise, epigastric pain, headache, and progressive jaundice. In severe cases, oliguria, GI bleeding, somnolence, or coma ensue. On physical examination, jaundice may be noted. In addition, there may be right upper quadrant or epigastric tenderness, and signs of encephalopathy may be seen. The pathology of AFLP is a microvesicular fatty change of the liver occurring in a panacinar or zonal distribution involving zones 2 and 3 or just zone 3. There is little hepatocellular necrosis.

The pathogenesis of AFLP is not well understood. A defect in mitochondrial function may be involved. Pregnancy-associated carnitine deficiency may also play a role. Studies suggest that some cases of AFLP may be due to deficiency in long-chain 3-hydroxyacyl coenzyme A dehydrogenase.

Preeclampsia is associated with 20%–40% of cases of AFLP. Complications may include liver failure with coagulopathy and encephalopathy, disseminated intravascular coagulation (DIC), upper GI bleeding, azotemia, renal failure, hypoglycemia, postpartum hemorrhage, pancreatitis, seizures, shock, and fluid and electrolyte abnormalities.

Treatment consists of supportive care with a view toward early delivery by cesarean section. Recent mortality reports are estimated at 8%–33% for the mother and 14%–66% for the infant. Survivors have no long-term sequelae. There does not appear to be a high risk for recurrence in subsequent pregnancies, but there are a few reported cases, and many women with a history of AFLP do not attempt subsequent pregnancies because of their fear of recurrence.

CASE STUDY: *CONTINUED*

Preeclampsia was suspected in this patient, and she was monitored very closely. Three weeks later the patient presented to the emergency room with epigastric pain, nausea, and vomiting. Her blood pressure was 160/112 mm Hg, and there was peripheral edema. A blood smear showed burr cells and schistocytes, and the haptoglobin was low.

Hemolysis, Elevated Liver Enzymes, and Low Platelets (HELLP)

Approximately 4%–12% of patients with preeclampsia develop HELLP. HELLP is defined as a manifestation of preeclampsia involving hemolysis, elevated liver enzymes, and a low platelet count. Symptoms may include epigastric or right upper quadrant pain, headache, nausea, or vomiting. The physical examination may reveal a diastolic blood pressure greater than 110 mm Hg and peripheral edema.

Laboratory studies typically show low haptoglobin, burr cells and schistocytes on smear, increased lactate dehydrogenase and indirect bilirubin, elevated transaminases, thrombocytopenia, proteinuria, increased BUN and creatinine levels, and normal prothrombin time, partial thromboplastin time, and fibrinogen.

Maternal complications may include DIC, placental abruption, acute renal failure, or liver rupture. The following fetal complications have been described: increased incidence of intrauterine growth retardation, prematurity, thrombocytopenia, and DIC.

The pathogenesis may involve microemboli in the hepatic vasculature with resulting ischemia and tissue damage, among other possibilities. It has been hypothesized that segmental vasospasm may lead to vasculopathy by exposing subendothelial collagen, thus initiating platelet aggregation and local fibrin deposition. Treatment includes supportive care and prompt delivery of the infant by cesarean section.

CASE STUDY: *CONTINUED*

The patient was diagnosed with HELLP syndrome. She was taken to the delivery room, and a 6 lb, 1 oz healthy boy was delivered by cesarean section. The mother recovered, and she and the infant were discharged to home in excellent condition.

CHRONIC LIVER DISEASE

Preexisting chronic liver disease may be present in women who become pregnant. It should be noted that pregnancy in the setting of cirrhosis is unusual, because amenorrhea and anovulation are common in women with advanced liver problems.

LIVER DISEASES COMPLICATING PREGNANCY

Many types of liver disease may occur as intercurrent liver disease during pregnancy. These include viral and toxic hepatitis, biliary tract disorders, Budd-Chiari syndrome, and nonviral hepatic infections.

Viral Hepatitis

Viral hepatitis may be a preexisting condition or may occur during pregnancy. Management of acute viral hepatitis is the same as in the nonpregnant patient. Hepatitis B virus (HBV) does not cross the placenta, but vertical transmission is common. The exposed infant

Viral hepatitis is the most common cause of jaundice in pregnancy.

Evaluation and treatment of GI disorders in pregnancy must take into consideration a number of factors affecting both the mother and the fetus.

Table 26-5. Factors Associated with Lithogenic Environment during Pregnancy

Increased bile acid pool size
Decreased enterohepatic circulation
Decreased percentage of chenodeoxycholic acid
Increased percentage of cholic acid
Increased secretion of cholesterol
Stasis of bile

should be treated immediately postpartum with HBV hyperimmune globulin and simultaneously begin the HBV vaccination series.

Herpes simplex hepatitis has been associated with fulminant hepatic failure in pregnancy. Epidemic non-A, non-B hepatitis (HEV) has been observed in Southeast Asia, Africa, and Mexico. The morbidity and mortality of this form of hepatitis are higher in the pregnant patient, and it appears that a pregnant patient is at greater risk of acquiring this disease during epidemics than are men and nonpregnant women.

GALLSTONES

Pregnancy certainly promotes the development of cholesterol gallstones. The factors associated with a lithogenic environment are listed in Table 26-5. The treatment of gallstone disease during pregnancy is conservative if the clinical situation allows. Pancreatitis and cholecystitis are rare during pregnancy. Acute cholecystitis will usually resolve, and surgical intervention is required in about one-third of cases. Patients are generally treated medically in the first trimester, but if symptoms persist, surgery can be performed electively in the second trimester. Laparoscopic cholecystectomies have been performed in pregnant patients.

Summary

Although pregnancy is a common and normal state, special attention must be paid to symptoms and problems in the pregnant woman. Many GI illnesses and syndromes may be present in the pregnant patient. It is important first of all to recognize the normal physiologic changes that occur in pregnancy as outlined in Table 26-1 and to apply these changes to a specific clinical scenario.

CASE STUDY: *RESOLUTION*

The patient presented to the physician with a GI complaint that was in effect due to pregnancy. This patient went on to develop hyperemesis gravidarum but recovered. She did well until late in her pregnancy, when she developed preeclampsia and then HELLP syndrome. The patient and her infant had an excellent clinical outcome because her problem was recognized early and the infant was delivered promptly.

REVIEW QUESTIONS

Directions: For each of the following questions, choose the one best answer.

Questions 1–3 refer to the following case study.

I.M. Fertel is a 33-year-old woman who presents to the physician's office with nausea and vomiting and lower abdominal pain of 2 weeks duration. She has no known medical history. The physical examination is normal. Laboratories show a white blood cell count of 10,500/μl (normal: $\leq$10,000/μl) and an alkaline phosphatase of 135 U/L (normal: 130 U/L). The physician sends the patient for an ultrasound of the right upper quadrant, which shows gallstones. The ultrasound technician was in training, and with the patient's informed consent and permission, an examination of the pelvis was also performed, which shows a viable pregnancy of approximately 10 weeks gestation. The physician tells the patient of the findings.

1 Which one of the following physiologic changes is *true* of this patient?

   A Total blood volume is decreased.
   B Total plasma volume is unchanged.
   C Hepatic blood flow is increased.
   D Hepatic blood flow is unchanged.
   E Total renal blood flow is unchanged.

2 The patient is thrilled with the news. She does extremely well throughout her pregnancy, but at 27 weeks gestation she presents with increased blood pressure, peripheral edema, and proteinuria. The patient is most likely to have

   A nothing serious; this occurs in almost all pregnancies.
   B intrahepatic cholestasis of pregnancy.
   C preeclampsia.
   D essential hypertension.

3 Three weeks later, the patient presents to the emergency room with epigastric pain, nausea, and vomiting. Her blood pressure is 180/118 mm Hg. There is right upper quadrant tenderness on examination, and peripheral edema is noted. A blood smear shows burr cells and schistocytes, and the haptoglobin is low. The patient has now most likely developed

   A intrahepatic cholestasis of pregnancy.
   B acute fatty liver of pregnancy.
   C HELLP syndrome.
   D viral hepatitis.

4 Which of the following may promote a lithogenic environment for the formation of gallstones in pregnancy?

A Decreased bile acid pool size
B Increased enterohepatic circulation
C Stasis of bile
D Decreased percentage of cholic acid

5 What is the most common cause of acute diarrhea in the pregnant patient?

A Ulcerative colitis
B Crohn's disease
C Infectious pathogen
D Cholecystitis

6 What is the most common cause of jaundice in pregnancy?

A Viral hepatitis
B Acute cholecystitis
C Autoimmune liver disease
D Alcoholic liver disease

7 Which of the following statements about GERD is *true*?

A Progesterone is a mediator of lower esophageal sphincter contraction.
B Gastric acidity helps to prevent severe aspiration pneumonitis.
C Antacids may interfere with iron absorption.
D Patients should be treated aggressively with H_2 blockers with the onset of symptoms.

8 Treatment of constipation in the pregnant patient may include

A fiber.
B mineral oil.
C castor oil.
D cascara sagrada.

References

Baron TH, Ramirez B, Richter JE: Gastrointestinal motility disorders during pregnancy. *Ann Intern Med* 118:366–375, 1993.

Crawford LA, Quint EH, Pearl ML, et al: Incontinence following rupture of the anal sphincter during delivery. *Obstet Gynecol* 82:527–531, 1993.

Doshi S: Liver emergencies during pregnancy. *Gastroenterol Clin North Am* 32(4):1213–1227, 2003.

Hasler WL: The irritable bowel syndrome during pregnancy. *Gastroenterol Clin North Am* 32(1):385–406, 2003.

Kane S: Inflammatory bowel disease in pregnancy. *Gastroenterol Clin North Am* 32(1):323–340, 2003.

Karlstadt RG, Surawicz CM, Croitoru R (eds): *Gastrointestinal Disorders during Pregnancy*. Arlington, VA: American College of Gastroenterology, 1994.

Knox TA, Olans LB: Liver disease in pregnancy. *N Engl J Med* 335:569–576, 1996.

Koch KL: Nausea and vomiting during pregnancy. *Gastroenterol Clin North Am* 32(1):201–234, 2003.

Richter JE: Gastroesophageal reflux disease during pregnancy. *Gastroenterol Clin North Am* 32(1):235–261, 2003.

Sandhu BS: Pregnancy and liver disease. *Gastroenterol Clin North Am* 32(1):407–436, 2003.

Singer AJ, Brandt LJ: Pathophysiology of the gastrointestinal tract during pregnancy. *Am J Gastroenterol* 86:1695–1712, 1991.

Sultan AH, Kamm MA, Hudson CN, et al: Anal-sphincter disruption during vaginal delivery. *N Engl J Med* 329:1905–1911, 1993.

Wald A: Constipation, diarrhea, and symptomatic hemorrhoids during pregnancy. *Gastroenterol Clin North Am* 32(1):309–322, 2003.

27

Molecular Biology of GI Malignancies and Overview of Neoplasms of the GI Tract

---

■ **CHAPTER OUTLINE** ■

■ **LEARNING OBJECTIVES** ■

At the completion of this chapter, the reader should be able to:

- Discuss the progression of the normal cell through the cell cycle and the mechanisms by which cell growth is regulated.
- Discuss the molecular biology of cellular transformation.
- Identify the principles of oncogenesis, including multistep tumor formation and clonal expansion.
- Distinguish the two categories of oncogenes.
- Apply the principles of molecular biology to the genetic model of colorectal tumorigenesis.

Introduction

Cancers of the GI tract represent a major international health problem. In the United States, colon cancer is the second leading cause of death due to malignancy in both males and females. Approximately 5% of Americans will be diagnosed with colon cancer, and 40% of this population will succumb to the disease. The most common site for GI cancer is the colorectum, with tumors of the esophagus, stomach, liver, and pancreas accounting for the remainder. Exciting new advances in experimental molecular technology have helped elucidate the role of genetics and molecular biology in the pathogenesis of these cancers.

It is important to understand that cancer is a disease of somatic genes. The evidence for this is as follows: First, cancer cells produce other cancer cells, and this trend is generally irreversible. Second, most mutagens are carcinogens, and most carcinogens are mutagens; that is, agents that cause genetic mutations may cause cancers and vice versa. Third, cancer-prone strains of animals develop malignant neoplasms at a significantly higher rate than non–cancer-prone strains, presumably as a result of genetic predisposition. Similarly, there are many hereditary syndromes that predispose humans to cancers. Fourth, both DNA and RNA viruses may cause tumors in animals. Finally, chromosomal alterations are found in tumors.

Although the genetic nature of cancer has been well established, it has only been possible in the past 15 years or so to determine the molecular alterations present in the DNA of cancer cells. The GI cancers that have been studied most extensively are colorectal cancer and gastric cancer because these types are common in the regions from which these studies emerge—that is, colorectal cancer in the United States and Europe and gastric cancer in Japan. The genetic

model for colorectal tumorigenesis is the prototypical model for the development of multiple genetic alterations in all solid cancers.

This chapter first reviews the mechanisms by which proliferation and differentiation are regulated in GI epithelium and then discusses the basic principles of molecular biology as they apply to carcinogenesis. Finally, a discussion of the molecular biology of two GI cancers (colorectal cancer and esophageal adenocarcinoma) and their precursor lesions (colonic polyps and Barrett's esophagus, respectively) follows.

Cell Replication Cycle

The entire luminal GI tract is lined with columnar-type mucosa except for the esophagus and anus, which are lined with a squamous type. In the squamous lining, the proliferative region is in the basal layer, and daughter cells migrate to the surface, where they differentiate. The columnar lining of the stomach and intestines is different in that there are numerous specialized cells that are absorptive, secretory, or endocrine in nature. The proliferative zone tends to be in the mid to lower portion of the glands.

The cell replication cycle can be broken down into five phases (Figure 27-1). The duration of each of these phases varies among different cell types. Resting cells enter the G0 phase. The duration of this phase is the most variable among different cell types. From here,

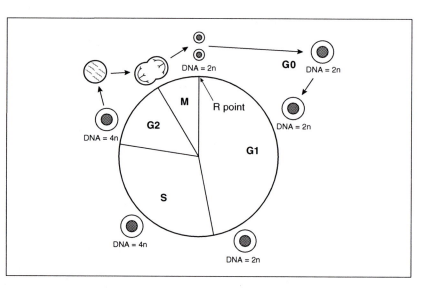

Fig. 27-1. Normal Cell Cycle

The cell cycle consists of five phases. During G0, the cell is resting. When it enters the postmitotic phase, G1, the cell prepares for DNA synthesis. After the cell receives the signal to divide, it enters the S phase, in which replication of DNA occurs. During the G2 phase, the cell is tetraploid and prepares for cell division. Cell division occurs during the M phase. The two daughter cells can then undergo another round of division by entering the G1 phase at the start or restriction (R) point, or enter the G0 phase.

the cell enters a G1 phase, which is the postmitotic phase. In this phase, the cell prepares for DNA synthesis. After the signal to divide is received, the cell enters the S phase, which is the period during which DNA synthesis occurs. After the entire genome is duplicated, the cell is tetraploid and briefly enters the G2 phase, where preparation for cell division occurs. Finally, the cell divides during the M phase. After cell division, the cell is either committed to another round of replication and cell division during G1 at the start or R (restriction) point, or it enters the G0 phase before the R point. Cells can subsequently reenter the cell cycle from the G0 phase.

Regulation of Normal Cell Growth

Cellular proliferation is achieved when the cell enters the cell cycle. The progression through the cell cycle is modulated by the regulatory proteins intrinsic to the process; however, these events are also controlled by conditions and stimuli external to the cell. These external stimuli include a variety of proteins that bind to specific receptors on the cell surface. The proteins may include peptide growth factors, which are recognized for their growth-modulating effects, or other growth-modifying proteins, such as cytokines or hormones, which modulate other cellular responses that occur after interaction with their receptors. Both protein types are distinguished by their ability to alter cell proliferation through interaction with specific receptors, which typically bind a specific ligand. Several exceptions to the specificity of the ligand–receptor relationship exist where closely related ligands can bind to the same receptor. For example, epidermal growth factor receptor can bind both epidermal growth factor and transforming growth factor-α.

The interaction of ligands with their receptors at the cell surface must be translated into an intracellular signal and ultimately leads to alterations in gene transcription in the nucleus. There are at least four distinct pathways by which these ligand–receptor interactions effect a cellular response (Table 27-1). These include tyrosine phosphorylation, serine and threonine phosphorylation, cyclic nucleotide generation, and calcium-phosphoinositol production.

The binding of a growth factor at the cell surface leads to the transduction of a signal, resulting in alterations in a variety of cellular functions that influence growth. These functions include ion transport (most notably of sodium [Na^+] and hydrogen [H^+]), nutrient

---

Table 27-1. Intracellular Pathways Induced by Ligand–Receptor Binding to Effect Cell Response

Tyrosine phosphorylation, that is, intrinsic tyrosine kinase activity
Serine and threonine phosphorylation
Cyclic nucleotide generation, that is, GTP-binding proteins or G proteins
Calcium-phosphoinositol production, that is, phospholipase C alterations

uptake, and protein synthesis. However, the ligand–receptor interaction must ultimately modify gene expression with the nucleus.

Gene Expression

Genes consist of specific DNA nucleotide sequences that encode a gene product (protein) as well as regulatory elements in the promoter that control transcription (Figure 27-2). RNA polymerase positions itself at a specific site on the gene with a specific sequence (TATA) and produces RNA by a process known as *transcription*. Nuclear RNA is composed of exons (DNA sequences that result in a specific messenger RNA [mRNA] message) and intervening introns (intervening segments of DNA that are not incorporated into the mRNA). After cleavage of introns and splicing of exons into mRNA, translation of the mRNA produces a protein, which then undergoes posttranslational modifications. The regulation of gene expression through the modification of transcriptional factors represents the final stage in the pathway connecting an external stimulus to an alteration in cell proliferation or differentiation.

In addition to these ligand–receptor interactions, constituents of the extracellular matrix or adjacent cells may interact with distinctive

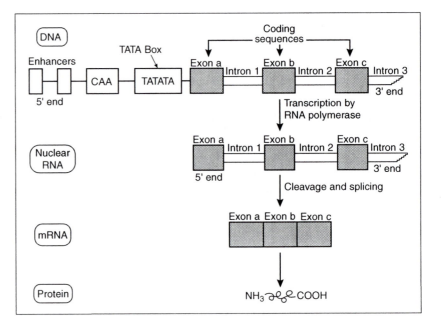

Fig. 27-2. Overview of Gene Transcription

Genes consist of specific DNA nucleotide sequences, which encode a particular protein, and regulatory elements in the promoter region. RNA polymerase positions itself at a specific site on the gene with a specific sequence (TATA box) and produces nuclear RNA by transcription. Nuclear RNA consists of exons, which are specific DNA sequences that result in a particular mRNA message, and introns, which are intervening DNA sequences that are not incorporated into the resultant mRNA. After cleavage of introns and splicing of exons, mRNA is produced. Translation of mRNA produces a protein, which then undergoes posttranslational modifications.

molecules present on the cell surface. These encompass many classes of adhesion molecules, including integrins, cadherins, selectins, and proteoglycans, which lead to changes in the cell cytoskeleton and indirectly modulate external growth stimuli. These matrix or cell–cell interactions are particularly important in contributing to the phenotypic changes characteristic of malignant cells.

Characteristics of Malignant Cells

Malignant cells have several biologic characteristics that distinguish them from normal cells. These characteristics have been identified by the in vitro study of cells maintained in cell culture. Distinctive "transformed" phenotypes have been recognized in cultures that share many important parallels with malignant cells in vivo, thereby validating the potential of tissue culture models as a means of providing new insights into oncogenesis.

First, transformed cells (and by analogy malignant cells) are characterized by their propensity for *uncontrolled proliferation*. These cells are not bound by the R point during the G1 phase of the cell cycle as are normal cells; therefore, each cell continually divides. Because the duration of each phase of the cell cycle is unchanged, the total replication time is the same as in the normal cell.

Normal cells obey the law of *density-dependent contact inhibition;* that is, they cease to divide after they have reached sufficient cell density to ensure uniform cell–cell contact. Transformed cells do not follow this law and therefore pile up on each other in multiple layers. Similarly, malignant cells possess the capacity to grow in the absence of cellular matrix or substrate. Normal cells are dependent on anchorage to an underlying surface, whereas malignant cells are *anchorage independent*.

Transformed cells have a reduced need for a variety of growth factors. These cells can grow without serum and the growth-promoting factors that serum provides. This is partly due to the ability of transformed cells to produce essential growth factors that can bind to the cell's own receptors, a process known as *autocrine growth regulation*.

Transformed cells have a property known as *tumorigenicity*. When these cells are injected into a suitable host animal that is incapable of mounting an immune response, they lead to the growth of tumors. Finally, the study of malignant cells has led to the identification of a variety of *biochemical alterations* in neoplastic cells, many of which reflect alterations of specific genes that contribute directly to malignant transformation. Other biochemical alterations have been noted in association with transforming activity. These functional and structural alterations probably play an important role in determining the biologic characteristics of the transformed cell.

Mechanisms of Oncogenesis

The debate over the relative importance of inherited or environmental factors in oncogenesis has raged for many years. It has become

Notes

Key Features of Malignant Cells
Uncontrolled proliferation
No density-dependent contact inhibition
Anchorage independence
Autocrine growth regulation
Tumorigenicity
Biochemical alterations

Multistep (Multiple-Hit) Formation Theory
Malignancy develops as a result of a series of events, possibly related to alterations in a cell's behavior, thereby eventually producing the malignant phenotype.

An **oncogene** may be (1) a gene encoding inappropriately high levels of a normal cellular protein or (2) a mutant gene producing an altered protein with inappropriate function.

increasingly evident that both factors are important, because both ultimately lead to either the expression of abnormal genes or the inappropriate expression of normal genes. Genetic mutation is the common denominator of the mechanisms by which these factors lead to the development of neoplasia.

Genetic mutations may be inherited (germline), or they may be acquired through the actions of environmental factors or the failure of intrinsic cellular mechanisms of DNA replication or transcription (somatic). The mutations may take several forms: (1) point mutations or mutations of a single nucleotide; (2) DNA rearrangement or translocation; (3) DNA amplification, that is, the duplication of a gene or cluster of genes; (4) DNA deletion, that is, the loss of a specific gene; or (5) alterations in DNA methylation.

The perceived dichotomy between inherited and environmental factors in neoplasia may be reconciled by two important and closely related concepts of oncogenesis: *multistep formation* and *clonal expansion*. The concept of multistep or "multiple-hit" tumor formation postulates that neoplasia develops as a result of a series of events, possibly related to incremental change in cell behavior through which the cell eventually acquires the malignant phenotype. The clinical correlate of this concept is found in the intermediate alterations that are recognized in premalignant lesions of the GI tract. This is best exemplified by the colorectal tumorigenesis model, in which mutations of several genes have been noted. The progressive accumulation of genetic alterations roughly parallels the sequential change from normal colonic mucosa, to adenomatous polyps, and finally to the development of frank carcinoma.

Clonal expansion occurs when a mutated gene leads to increased growth or proliferation of the cell. Clonal expansion occurs again when another mutation further enhances its growth properties. After a series of mutations, a genetic alteration eventually confers a property that in aggregate with the preceding genetic alterations makes a cell malignant. Clonal expansion of this cell leads to tumor development.

Tumor-Associated Genes

Tumor-associated genes may be of two broad types: *oncogenes*, which confer an active growth-promoting property directly, or *tumor suppressor genes* or *antioncogenes*, whose gene product normally suppresses growth or proliferation. Activation of the former or inactivation of the latter can be important in the development of neoplasia.

ONCOGENES

Oncogenes are typically one of two types of genes: a normal gene that encodes a normal cellular protein that becomes expressed at inappropriately high levels or a mutant gene that produces a structurally altered protein exhibiting inappropriate function. *Proto-oncogenes*, otherwise known as *cellular oncogenes*, are the normal cellular genes from which oncogenes are derived. The conversion of a proto-oncogene to an oncogene may be the result of a variety of mechanisms, including gene transduction or insertion, point mutations, gene rearrangements, and gene amplification.

Oncogene products are of four distinct types: peptide growth factors, protein kinases, signal-transducing proteins, and transcriptional regulatory proteins. Collectively, these four groups represent surrogate proteins for the entire pathway, extending from the cell surface to the nucleus. Therefore, alterations of cell growth can occur at any level along this pathway, and perhaps the accumulation of mutations at each level, as suggested by the multistep formation theory, is necessary for tumor development.

Peptide Growth Factors

Many peptide growth factors encoded by mutated oncogenes have been recognized, such as *sis*, *int-2*, *hst*, and *FGF-5*. In addition, many tumor cells exhibit enhanced expression of normal peptide growth factors without mutations, such as transforming growth factor-α and β (TGF-α and -β), epidermal growth factor (EGF), and insulin-like growth factor I and II (IGF I and II). A characteristic feature of growth factor expression that is intrinsic to neoplastic development is the presence of an autocrine growth-stimulating loop, as previously described.

Protein Kinases

Some oncogenes have been shown to encode proteins with intrinsic kinase activity. These encompass the entire spectrum of protein kinases, including receptor (e.g., *erb B*, *neu*, *met*) and nonreceptor tyrosine kinases (e.g., *src*) and cytoplasmic serine and threonine kinases (e.g., *raf*). As with all oncogenes, some of these oncogenes alter cell growth by increased expression of normal genes or by expression of mutant genes, resulting in a structurally altered protein with abnormal (generally enhanced) enzymatic activity.

Signal-Transducing Proteins

Two factors, growth factors and protein kinases, are external modulators of cellular growth. Ultimately, growth is changed through alterations in the transcription of genes located within the nucleus. Therefore, intermediate steps must effectively translate the cell surface ligand–receptor binding to an intracellular signal that modulates nuclear activity. These intermediate steps are known as signal transduction pathways. Mutations of the genes encoding key proteins involved in signal transduction can therefore lead to cellular transformation. The *ras* oncogenes are the prime examples of this type of oncogene.

Transcriptional Regulatory Proteins

The final class of cellular oncogenes encodes nuclear proteins that appear to act through their ability to alter gene transcription. This class of proteins represents the final mediator of the signal transduction pathways affected by cytoplasmic and membrane-bound oncoproteins. The *myc* gene family best exemplifies this class.

TUMOR SUPPRESSOR GENES OR ANTIONCOGENES

Genes in this class act in an opposite manner to oncogenes; that is, they prevent the acquisition of the transformed phenotype. These genes are normally expressed and function to suppress growth. Inactivation of these tumor suppressor genes results in tumor formation.

Germline mutations of these genes may underlie all known inherited cancer syndromes. In fact, Knudson hypothesized that tumors in familial cancer syndromes were derived from independent mutations in the two alleles of a specific gene (Figure 27-3). He hypothesized that the first mutation was an inherited germline mutation and therefore present in all affected members of the cancer syndrome family. A single somatic mutation of the remaining allele, which might occur in any cell, would cause tumor development, thus explaining the high incidence of cancers in these patients. Although this same gene would

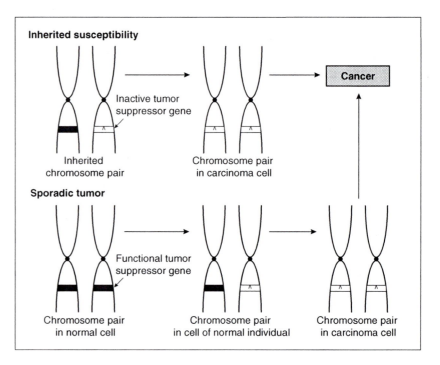

Fig. 27-3. Knudson's Hypothesis

Knudson hypothesized that all familial cancer syndromes occur as a result of independent mutations of both alleles of a specific gene. He hypothesized that the first mutation was an inherited germline mutation affecting one of the alleles; therefore, all affected members of the family would have this mutation and have an inherited susceptibility. A single mutation of the remaining allele, which could occur in any cell, might result in tumor development. Although it is possible that the same gene may play a role in sporadic cancers (those of the general population who have no inherited susceptibility), this would require independent mutations of both alleles of the gene in a single cell. This is a relatively uncommon random event. Therefore, it would help explain why the incidence of cancers in the family cancer syndromes is higher than those in the general population. It was later suggested that the relevant gene in these familial cancer syndromes might be a tumor suppressor gene.

also play a role in the development of sporadic cancers (i.e., those occurring in the general population and not associated with an inherited syndrome), this would require independent somatic mutations of each of the two alleles of the specific gene within a cell, an uncommon random event. It was later suggested that the relevant gene in a cancer family syndrome might be a tumor suppressor gene. Tumors would only arise when both copies of the gene were inactivated.

A host of putative tumor suppressor genes have been identified and partly characterized. Perhaps the most notable example is the *p53* gene. The *p53* gene is located on chromosome 17p. The normal or wild-type allele of the *p53* gene encodes a 53-kDa nuclear phosphoprotein involved in the control of the cell cycle. Both G1 arrest and apoptosis (programmed cell death) are potential mechanisms of growth suppression by *p53*. The importance of this gene in human carcinogenesis is best exemplified by the fact that it is inactivated in up to 50% of all human solid cell cancers. In fact, it has been suggested that more than half of the patients dying of cancer do not do so until and unless their tumor evolves a *p53* mutation. An inherited germline mutation of this tumor suppressor gene is found in the Li-Fraumeni syndrome, in which affected family members are prone to a variety of cancers at an early age.

CASE STUDY: *CONTINUED*

The patient underwent colonoscopy. A 4-cm sessile lesion was seen in the sigmoid colon. There was an 8-mm polyp in the right colon, which was removed; it was a tubulovillous adenoma. The patient was referred for surgery.

Colorectal Cancer

Colorectal carcinoma (CRC) is the second leading cause of cancer death in the United States. There are approximately 150,000 new cases and more than 57,000 deaths from CRC per year. CRC is a disease of aging, with the incidence rising sharply after age 60. Survival of patients with CRC is related to the stage of disease. Because treatment of advanced CRC is limited and because early-stage cancers have a better prognosis, efforts to control CRC have been focused on early detection and prevention.

ADENOMA-CARCINOMA SEQUENCE

Screening for CRC holds great promise because evidence suggests that it develops slowly, progressing from an adenomatous polyp to a malignant stage that is endoscopically or surgically curable, and then to more advanced, incurable disease (Figure 27-4). There is strong circumstantial evidence supporting the adenoma-carcinoma sequence, which includes the following: (1) There is a parallel prevalence of

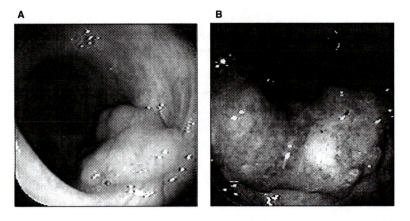

Fig. 27-4. The Adenoma-Carcinoma Sequence

(A) This endoscopic photograph reveals an adenomatous colonic polyp, a premalignant lesion with the potential to evolve into colorectal cancer.
(B) This endoscopic photograph reveals a colon cancer.

adenomas and carcinomas, with adenomas occurring 5–7 years earlier; (2) carcinomas and adenomas are often seen together, sometimes within the same lesion; (3) individuals with the autosomal dominant condition known as familial adenomatous polyposis (FAP) have thousands of adenomas, and all individuals with this condition develop colon cancer unless they undergo a colectomy; and (4) as adenomas grow and advance toward cancer, genetic abnormalities accumulate, with the most frequent abnormalities seen with carcinoma. Several studies now suggest that the excision of adenomatous polyps decreases the subsequent incidence of cancer. For example, in the National Polyp Study, after 6 years of follow-up, the incidence of CRC in the study cohort that underwent periodic colonoscopic screening and polypectomy was 80% less than the expected incidence.

Colon cancer screening is an important preventive practice. Guidelines for screening have been identified by many of the medical societies, and screening for prevention is reimbursable by Medicare and insurance carriers. The use of colonoscopy versus other screening methods has fostered healthy debate. The American College of Gastroenterology recommends colonoscopy for screening in average risk persons every 10 years beginning at age 50. Screening strategies stratify patients by their risk for colon cancer and define the interval for repeat examinations based on findings.

SOMATIC GENETIC ABNORMALITIES

Information on the somatic genetic abnormalities associated with progression to CRC has been enhanced by the ability to sample neoplastic colonic tissue through colonoscopy at a variety of stages, from small adenoma to carcinoma. Progressive accumulations of changes in gene structure, expression, and activity have been identified with transformation from early adenoma to carcinoma (Figure 27-5). The genetic abnormalities characterized thus far include changes in both

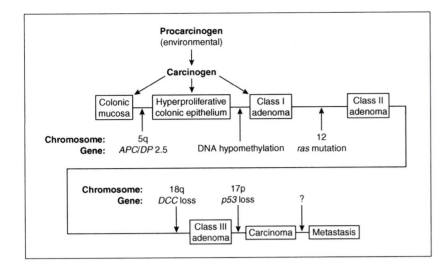

Fig. 27-5. Genetic Model of CRC Tumorigenesis

This prototypic model correlates the increasing aggregate number of genetic mutations with the progression from a benign colon polyp to cancer. Colon polyps were segregated into risk categories, reflected by an analysis of polyps by size (class I < 1 cm without tumor focus, class II > 1 cm without tumor focus, class III > 1 cm with tumor focus). The molecular changes in this original model occurred in a stepwise manner, with the accumulation of alterations ultimately leading to CRC. These molecular changes included mutations of the ras oncogene and allelic deletions of chromosomal segments 5q, 18q, and 17p, later identified as the gene loci for the tumor suppressor genes *APC*, *DCC*, and *p53*, respectively. It is important to note that this model was inferred from in vitro data on the relative frequency of these alterations in polyps at varying stages of development. For example, about 40% of all class II polyps had a mutation of the ras gene, and 43% of all colon cancers had the same mutation. Therefore, it was inferred that *ras* mutations, when they occurred, would occur relatively early in the progression to cancer. Mutations of the *p53* gene, on the other hand, were seen in over 70% of cancers but very rarely in polyps; therefore, it was felt to be a late mutation. Although the molecular changes were not seen in every case, the model provided a useful paradigm for the future study of other malignant neoplasms.

proto-oncogenes, such as K-*ras* and c-*myc*, and tumor suppressor genes, such as the *APC* gene on chromosome 5, the *DCC* gene on chromosome 18, and the *p53* gene on chromosome 17p. Although the progression of genetic abnormalities associated with phenotypic progression to carcinoma was initially presented graphically as an ordered accumulation of changes, it is now believed that it is the accumulation of abnormalities that predicts the evolution of carcinoma, in accordance with the multiple-hit concept.

The understanding of how genetic derangements contribute to the development of carcinoma has also advanced. For example, the *APC* gene mutation, which causes FAP, encodes a huge protein that is 2843 amino acids long. This protein is related to cell adhesion molecules known as cadherins, and abnormalities in these proteins are thought to predispose to malignant transformation.

Notes

HNPCC is a syndrome that includes familial clustering of colon cancer over at least two generations with an onset of disease before 50 years of age.

A practical clinical impact of the characterization of somatic genetic mutations has also emerged. Mutations have been correlated to prognosis in patients with CRC. Allelic loss or deletions of chromosomal segments can identify subsets of patients with worse prognoses for extensive metastasis and death. In studies, allelic loss at 18q, in the region of the *DCC* gene, was correlated with reduced survival. Patients with stage II CRC without 18q loss or the *DCC* protein survived much longer than stage II patients with loss and absence of *DCC*. Molecular markers such as these may supplant the traditional staging classification for predicting survival and outcome with CRC. Furthermore, the results of marker studies may impact decisions regarding adjuvant therapy.

MOLECULAR SCREENING

Molecular screening is an exciting new approach to early detection of CRC, although the technology for such an approach is still maturing. For example, about 40%–70% of CRCs have mutations in K-*ras*. A similar percentage of mutations are found in large adenomas. One study found K-*ras* mutations in the stool of 8 of 9 patients with CRC, and another found K-*ras* mutations in colonic effluent from high-risk patients. Interestingly, in at least one instance, the K-*ras* mutation preceded the development of a CRC. Other researchers have worked on increasing the sensitivity of the assay for K-*ras* to detect mutations in normal mucosa. If perfected, such techniques could add a new approach to screening for CRC, but these assays must be tested in the population at large before wide-scale implementation.

ABNORMALITIES IN MISMATCH REPAIR GENES

Hereditary nonpolyposis colorectal cancer (HNPCC) is a syndrome that includes familial clustering of colon cancer over two or more generations, with early onset of disease before age 50. Families with these conditions also have an elevated incidence of cancers of the endometrium, stomach, and urinary tract. In 1993, investigators described an unusual form of somatic mutation, found in nearly all CRC tumors associated with HNPCC, termed replicative errors (RERs) or microsatellite instability. These are changes in the length of DNA tandem repeat sequences, or microsatellites, scattered about the genome.

Microsatellites

What are microsatellites? Throughout the genome, often located in noncoding regions (introns), are sequences consisting of 1–5 base pairs (bp) that are repeated. The most common of these are single or dinucleotide repeats, such as ACACACACACACAC. These tandem repeat sequences are numerous enough that nearly every gene has one within or close to it.

Why are microsatellites so important? During DNA replication, the length of a tandem repeat can change. Using the example, the repeat can go from 14 bp to 12 bp, from ACACACACACACAC to

ACACACACACAC. Tandem repeat sequences are a rich source of genetic variation among humans and thus are polymorphic. However, the *rate of change* of the length of a given tandem repeat is not as great, so that within a family the length of a tandem repeat is a stable trait. Because of unique flanking sequences, the length of a particular microsatellite can be evaluated via polymerase chain reaction (PCR) and detected via gel electrophoresis. There are now thousands of unique primer sequences for probing microsatellite lengths throughout each of the chromosomes in the genome.

Microsatellites have become an ideal way to perform genetic linkage studies. For example, say there is a family of 36 members, of whom 20 seem to have a disease called hereditary exophthalmos. Using microsatellite markers for each of the chromosomes, the DNA of all members is tested and a genetic linkage map constructed. The relative positions of markers and, by association, genes (because markers are within or near genes) can be specified, with linkage occurring if a marker and a gene are inherited together. In the example of the hereditary exophthalmos family, a microsatellite marker, whose length was the same in the 20 affected members but different in the 16 nonaffected members, would point strongly to linkage between that marker and the gene for hereditary exophthalmos. The region of the chromosome from which the marker came would then become the area on which to focus to discover the gene for hereditary exophthalmos.

In addition to helping with the discovery of new genes, microsatellites are also teaching us about the mechanism of carcinogenesis. In patients with HNPCC, there is generalized microsatellite instability. For example, DNA from CRC tissue of a patient with HNPCC will have a number of microsatellites with different nucleotide lengths in contrast to DNA from normal tissue of the same patient; that is, during DNA replication in tumor development, a given microsatellite may have gone from 14 to 12 nucleotides long or have been the victim of "slippage." This slippage occurred because of an undetected or uncorrected error during DNA replication.

Why did this error in replication occur? Further research has led to discovery of a new genetic mechanism linked to CRC, that of a defect in mismatch repair (MMR) genes. These genes control the fidelity of DNA replication, acting as proofreaders during DNA replication. When mutations in MMR genes occur, microsatellite instability results. Several MMR genes have been cloned and characterized, including *hMSH2* on chromosome 2p, *hMLH1* on chromosome 3p, *hPMS1* on chromosome 2q, *hPMS2* on chromosome 7p, and *GTBP* near the *hMSH2* locus on chromosome 2.

Although studies of MMR gene mutations were primarily focused on explaining HNPCC, these discoveries may have important implications for sporadic CRC. Microsatellite instability has been described in approximately 12%–15% of sporadic CRC tumors. Assays to detect MMR gene mutations are the subject of active investigation.

Microsatellites, DNA tandem repeat sequences, provide an ideal way to perform genetic linkage studies.

One assay is the in vitro synthesized protein assay for detection of a truncated protein product. This technology is already in use to diagnose FAP. With this technique, the subject's genomic DNA for the gene of interest is amplified via PCR and mixed together with the machinery needed for synthesis of RNA and translation to protein, and the diagnostic test is for the presence of normal protein. In theory, if the gene is mutated, a normal-sized protein is not produced. However, there is still considerable technological improvement and epidemiologic testing required before these assays can be applied to the general population.

Barrett's Esophagus

Barrett's esophagus is a precursor lesion for adenocarcinoma of the esophagus. It represents a metaplastic change of the normal stratified squamous epithelium of the esophagus to a simple columnar type. Prevalence data reveal that Barrett's esophagus occurs in 5%–15% of all patients with chronic gastroesophageal reflux disease (GERD) and is associated with a 30- to 125-fold increased risk of developing esophageal adenocarcinoma. The impact of this lesion has recently been emphasized by the finding that the incidence of esophageal adenocarcinoma in the United States has been rising at an alarming rate of 5%–10% per year, a rate virtually higher than that of any other cancer type.

Cancer develops in Barrett's esophagus through the stepwise accumulation of genetic events that lead to progressive loss of growth regulation. This is manifested by increasing grades of dysplasia noted on histopathologic examination. The favored sequence is one in which metaplastic tissue goes through low-grade dysplasia, to high-grade dysplasia, to carcinoma in situ, and finally to invasive cancer. This sequence has formed the basis for endoscopic surveillance programs in which endoscopic biopsies are taken at intervals of 1–2 years and histologically evaluated for dysplasia. If dysplasia is seen, the patient is followed at shorter intervals. When high-grade dysplasia or carcinoma is found, the patient is often referred for a surgical esophagectomy.

The molecular biology of Barrett's esophagus and esophageal adenocarcinoma has only recently been investigated. Cell cycle abnormalities as well as mutations of oncogene and tumor suppressor genes have been found.

DNA CONTENT ABNORMALITIES

DNA content abnormalities, as demonstrated by flow cytometry, have been found in premalignant Barrett's tissue and in esophageal adenocarcinoma. Flow cytometry analyzes the ploidy status of cells. Normal cell populations are predominantly diploid ($2n$) with a small percentage (less than 5%) of tetraploid cells ($4n$ cells in the G2 phase of the cell cycle). Aneuploidy is defined as the presence of cell populations that are not diploid or tetraploid, that is, any population that is not $2n$ or $4n$. In one study, aneuploidy was found in 79% of esophageal adenocarcinoma specimens and even in seven patients with Barrett's esophagus *without* cancer. Investigators from several laboratories in the United States and France have substantiated their hypothesis that significant genetic alterations occur commonly both in cancers and in premalignant tissues at risk for malignant transformation.

An increase in the proportion of cells that are $4n$ (i.e., in the G2 phase) has also been suggested as a predictor of malignant transformation of Barrett's esophagus. The potential for aneuploidy or increased G2-tetraploid populations to predict risk was evaluated in 62 patients prospectively followed for 34 months. Over this relatively short interval, 9 of 13 patients with aneuploidy or increased G2-tetraploid populations in their initial flow cytometry study progressed to high-grade dysplasia or adenocarcinoma. None of the 49 patients without aneuploidy developed either of these end points.

p53 GENE

The high prevalence of 17p allelic deletions in esophageal adenocarcinoma suggests that inactivation of the *p53* gene, a putative tumor suppressor gene, may be an early event in the neoplastic transformation of Barrett's esophagus. Studies of *p53* expression in Barrett's esophagus have revealed overexpression in 0%–9% of nondysplastic tissue, 0%–15% of tissues with low-grade dysplasia, 45%–100% of tissue with high-grade dysplasia, and 53%–87% of tissue with adenocarcinoma of varying degrees of differentiation and invasion.

ONCOGENES

Growth regulatory factors have also been evaluated in Barrett's esophagus. Overexpression of EGF receptor and TGF-α has been found in Barrett's tissue. The coexpression of EGF-R and TGF-α may represent an autocrine growth regulatory loop.

Summary

In this chapter, we have reviewed the proliferation and differentiation of normal cells, including a review of the cell cycle and gene expression. We have provided an overview of the mechanisms of oncogenesis and a description of the types of genes involved in cancer development. Finally, we applied these concepts to the development of CRC and esophageal cancer from their respective premalignant lesions, colon polyps, and Barrett's esophagus.

Dramatic advances in the field of oncology have provided new insights into the pathogenesis and etiology of tumorigenesis. Modern molecular technology has provided novel ways of diagnosing, prognosticating, and even treating malignant neoplasms. An understanding of the molecular and genetic basis of tumorigenesis is essential to keep abreast of the many exciting new developments occurring in this era of molecular biology.

Notes

REVIEW QUESTIONS

Directions: For each of the following questions, choose the one best answer.

1 Which one of the following statements concerning genes and oncogenes is *true?*

 A Mutations of the *ras* oncogene are the earliest alteration in the model.
 B Inactivation of the *p53* gene is a late event in colorectal tumorigenesis.
 C The *APC* gene is involved in FAP syndrome but *not* in sporadic colorectal cancers.
 D The *DCC* gene is an oncogene.

2 The transformed cell has which of the following characteristics?

 A Anchorage dependence
 B Autocrine growth regulation
 C Density-dependent contact inhibition
 D Mutagenicity

3 Which of the following statements regarding oncogenesis is *true?*

 A The concept of multistep tumor formation suggests that multiple tumors develop as a result of independent genetic alterations.
 B Knudson's hypothesis states that the loss of a single allele of a tumor suppressor gene may lead to malignancy.
 C Clonal expansion occurs when a cell develops a series of mutations that confers a growth advantage to that cell and subsequently leads to malignancy.
 D Activation of oncogenes and tumor suppressor genes leads to malignancy.

4 Correct statements regarding the cell cycle include which of the following?

A Entry into the cell cycle determines how a cell will differentiate.

B The longest of the five phases of the cell cycle is the G1 phase in all cell types.

C Intrinsic and extrinsic regulation of the cell cycle determines the rate of proliferation.

D The cell is tetraploid for half of the cell cycle duration.

5 A 50-year-old patient is referred to the gastroenterology clinic for a possible screening flexible sigmoidoscopy. While taking the patient's history, the physician discovers that he has a family history of colon cancer, in his paternal uncle at age 42 and in his father at age 45. Because of this strong history, the physician decides to perform a colonoscopy instead of a sigmoidoscopy. He finds an adenocarcinoma in the ascending colon and four colonic polyps in the transverse colon. This patient likely has a familial form of colorectal cancer known as

A familial adenomatous polyposis (FAP).

B inherited K-*ras* mutation syndrome.

C Li-Fraumeni syndrome.

D hereditary nonpolyposis colorectal cancer (HNPCC).

6 A physician is performing an endoscopy in a patient and incidentally notices that he has Barrett's esophagus. Biopsy specimens of the Barrett's tissue reveal that there is low-grade dysplasia. The patient returns to the physician's office and wants to know what to do. The physician must now advise the patient to

A undergo an esophagectomy because the development of adenocarcinoma of the esophagus is likely.

B have his Barrett's esophagus monitored every 2 years.

C have his Barrett's esophagus monitored closely because of the presence of dysplasia.

D relax because this is a benign condition.

References

AGA: *The Burden of Gastrointestinal Disease*. AGA, 2001.

Beilstein M: Cellular and molecular mechanisms responsible for progression of Barrett's metaplasia to esophageal carcinoma. *Hematol Oncol Clin North Am* 17(2):453, 2003.

Chung DC, Rustgi AK: DNA mismatch repair and cancer. *Gastroenterology* 109:1685–1699, 1995.

Fearon ER, Vogelstein B: A genetic model for colorectal tumorigenesis. *Cell* 61:759–767, 1990.

Itzkowitz SH: Gastrointestinal adenomatous polyps. *Semin Gastrointest Dis* 7(2):105–116, 1996.

Kundson AG: Hereditary cancer oncogenes and anti-oncogenes. *Cancer Res* 45:1437–1443, 1985.

Marra G, Boland CR: Hereditary nonpolyposis colorectal cancer: the syndrome, the genes, and historical perspectives. *J Natl Cancer Inst* 87:1114–1125, 1995.

Nowell P: The clonal evolution of tumor cell populations. *Science* 194: 23–28, 1976.

Rex DK, Johnson DA, Lieberman DA, et al. ACG Recommendations on Colorectal Cancer Screening for Average and Higher Risk Patients in Clinical Practice, April 2000. Online document available at www.acg.gi.org/patientinfo/ccrk/crc2000.pdf.

Robbins DH: The molecular and genetic basis of colon cancer. *Med Clin North Am* 86(6):1467–1495, 2002.

Shibata D, Reale MA, Lavin P, et al: The DCC protein and prognosis in colorectal cancer. *N Engl J Med* 335:1727–1732, 1996.

Spechler SJ: Barrett's esophagus and esophageal adenocarcinoma: pathogenesis, diagnosis, and therapy. *Med Clin North Am* 86(6):1423–1245, vii, 2002.

Weinberg RA: Oncogenes, antioncogenes, and the molecular basis of multistep carcinogenesis. *Cancer Res* 49:3713–3721, 1989.

Notes

28

Pharmacology

■ CHAPTER OUTLINE ■

■ LEARNING OBJECTIVES ■

At the completion of this chapter, the reader should be able to:

- Identify the different actions of histamine receptor (H_2-receptor) antagonists and proton pump inhibitors (PPIs).
- Evaluate the different mechanisms of action and adverse effects of prokinetic agents.
- Assess the physiologic mechanisms of action of the various laxatives.
- Develop a physiologic approach to the pharmacotherapy of nausea and vomiting.

CASE STUDY: *INTRODUCTION*

A 45-year-old woman with a 20-year history of insulin-dependent diabetes mellitus came to the physician because of recurrent nausea and vomiting accompanied by intractable heartburn. The patient had been hospitalized numerous times in the previous year for persistent nausea and vomiting. Each time, she improved during her hospitalization only to relapse on returning home. Currently, she described postprandial bloating, epigastric pain, and constant nausea. Vomiting occurred intermittently. In addition, the patient had chronic substernal chest discomfort that worsened after each meal and at night, which she described as "burning." There was accompanying regurgitation but no dysphagia. The patient did not smoke or drink. She also related that she had been chronically fatigued, had a breast discharge, and had felt "down" for the previous 12 months.

Medications at the time of her visit included sliding-scale insulin injections; cimetidine, 300 mg four times daily; and metoclopramide, 20 mg four times daily. The patient was interested in other therapeutic options for her problem.

The medical history was significant for diabetic neuropathy and retinopathy. There was no history of renal insufficiency. There were no other medical or surgical problems. The family history was unremarkable.

The patient was married and had two teenage children. She was employed as an administrative assistant and had worked on a full-time basis for her entire adult life.

On physical examination, the patient appeared healthy and in no discomfort. Her blood pressure was 120/80 mm Hg, and her pulse was 80 beats/min. The skin examination was normal. Her eyes revealed classic findings of diabetic retinopathy. Her breasts were tender with a milky discharge. Her lungs were clear, and her heart rate was regular with no murmurs, rubs, or gallops. Her abdomen was nontender without hepatomegaly or mass. The neurologic examination revealed decreased sensation to fine touch in her hands and feet only.

Laboratory studies revealed a normal blood count and differential. The glucose was elevated to 165 mg/dl. All other laboratory studies were normal, including blood chemistry and thyroid function studies. A urinalysis revealed trace proteinuria.

Introduction

This chapter will focus on pharmacology for GI issues: acid suppression therapies, prokinetic drugs, laxatives and antiemetics. Other chapters in this book review therapy for clinical disorders such as functional bowel disorders (Chapter 14), IBD (Chapter 16), infectious disorders of the

GI tract (Chapter 17), viral hepatitis (Chapter 18), portal hypertension (Chapter 21), and abdominal pain and pain syndromes (Chapter 25). The focus of this chapter is on pathophysiologic mechanisms related to these therapies that influence choices of treatment.

Acid Suppression

Physiology of Gastric Acid Secretion

Acid secretion is discussed in detail in Chapter 11. Because acid suppression therapy and pharmacology is such an important topic in GI diseases, this chapter will focus on the pharmacology recognizing that an understanding of the pathophysiology is the basis for therapy.

Acid secretion occurs in the parietal cells, which are located in the oxyntic glands of the fundus and body of the stomach. These cells may be stimulated to secrete acid by three different pathways (Figure 28-1). The neurocrine pathway involves the vagal release of acetylcholine (ACh); the paracrine pathway is mediated by the release of histamine from mast cells and enterochromaffin-like cells in the stomach; and the endocrine pathway is mediated by the release of gastrin from antral G cells. Each of these transmitters has a specific receptor located on the basolateral surface of the parietal cell. Stimulation of these receptors leads to activation of intracellular second messenger systems; gastrin and ACh promote the accumulation of intracellular calcium (Ca^{2+}), whereas histamine causes a stimulatory G protein (G_s) to activate adenylate cyclase, which in turn generates cyclic AMP (cAMP). These intracellular messengers then activate protein kinases, which activate the proton pump, the H^+-K^+-ATPase enzyme, which is located at the apical surface of the parietal cell to secrete hydrogen ions (H^+) in exchange for potassium ions (K^+). Prostaglandins and somatostatin inhibit parietal cell function by binding to receptors that act through inhibitory G proteins (G_1) to inhibit adenylate cyclase. Acid is necessary to convert pepsinogen, secreted from gastric chief cells, into pepsin, a proteolytic enzyme that is inactive at a pH greater than 4.

H₂-Receptor Antagonists

Clinical Pharmacology

H₂-receptor antagonists competitively inhibit the binding of histamine to the H₂ receptor of the parietal cell. This causes a decrease in intracellular cAMP and, subsequently, a decrease in gastric acid secretion. There are four different H₂-receptor antagonists: cimetidine, ranitidine, famotidine, and nizatidine (Figure 28-2). All of these compounds act by the same mechanism but have different relative potencies for inhibiting gastric acid secretion that vary from 20-fold to 50-fold: Cimetidine is the least potent, whereas famotidine is the most potent (Table 28-1). With usual doses, the duration of action of these drugs (to inhibit pentagastrin-stimulated gastric acid secretion by 50%) varies from 6 hours for cimetidine to 10 hours for ranitidine, famotidine, and nizatidine. As a consequence of inhibiting gastric acid secretion, gastric

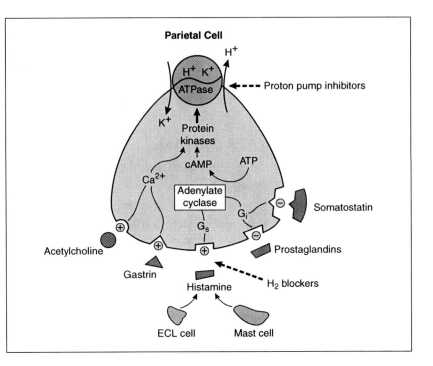

Fig. 28-1. Schematic Representation of Acid Secretion by the Parietal Cell

The neurocrine pathway involves the vagal release of ACh; the paracrine pathway is mediated by the release of histamine from mast cells and ECL cells in the stomach; and the endocrine pathway is mediated by the release of gastrin from antral G cells. Each transmitter has a specific receptor located on the basolateral surface of the parietal cell. Stimulation of these receptors leads to activation of intracellular second messenger systems: gastrin and ACh promote the accumulation of intracellular calcium (Ca^{2+}), and histamine causes a stimulatory G protein (G_2) to activate adenylate cyclase, which in turn generates cAMP. These intracellular messengers then activate protein kinases, which activate the proton pump, the H^+-K^+-ATPase enzyme, located at the apical surface of the parietal cell to secrete hydrogen ions (H^+) in exchange for potassium ions (K^+). Prostaglandins and somatostatin inhibit parietal cell function by binding to receptors that act through inhibitory G proteins (G_1) to inhibit adenylate cyclase. Dotted arrows indicate sites of action of various drugs that inhibit acid secretion.

pH rises, serum gastrin concentration rises 10–20 pg/ml, and pepsin activity decreases because of both a decrease in pepsinogen secretion and impaired activity of pepsin when gastric pH increases above 4. Once therapy with these compounds ceases, gastric acid secretion returns rapidly to pretreatment levels, although there may be a slight increase in acid secretion for several days to weeks.

Pharmacokinetics

Absorption of the H_2-receptor antagonists is rapid. Ranitidine, famotidine, and cimetidine undergo extensive first-pass metabolism in the liver, resulting in 43%–60% bioavailability after oral administration, whereas nizatidine undergoes little (if any) first-pass metabolism, with

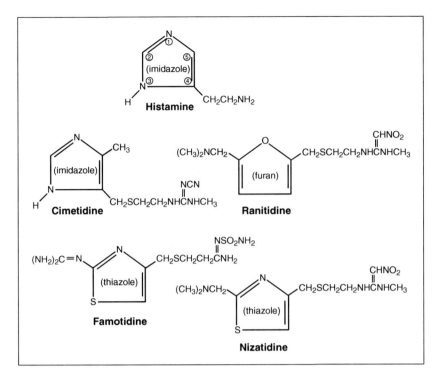

Fig. 28-2. Chemical Structure of Histamine and the Four H₂-Receptor Antagonists

a subsequent bioavailability of close to 100%. Peak concentrations occur within 1–3 hours after oral dosing. All four compounds cross the blood-brain barrier and placenta and may be excreted in breast milk. The serum half-life varies from 1.5 to 4 hours, and elimination occurs by a combination of hepatic metabolism, glomerular filtration, and renal tubular secretion for all of the drugs except for nizatidine, which is excreted primarily by the kidney. Pharmacokinetics of the H₂-receptor antagonists are altered by abnormal renal function, and doses need to be decreased with moderate to severe renal impairment. Hepatic dysfunction does not alter pharmacokinetics substantially.

Adverse Effects

The H₂-receptor antagonists are a remarkably safe class of drugs, with a clinical experience now in excess of 20 years. They are available over the counter in lower-dose formulations than the dose that is

Table 28-1. Comparison of H₂-Receptor Antagonists

DRUGS	RELATIVE POTENCY	AVERAGE BIOAVAILABILITY (%)	SERUM HALF-LIFE (hr)	CLEARANCE OF ORAL DOSE (%)	
				HEPATIC	RENAL
Cimetidine	1	60	1.5–2.3	60	40
Ranitidine	4–10	50	1.6–2.4	73	27
Famotidine	20–50	43	2.5–4.0	50–80	25–30
Nizatidine	4–10	98	1.1–1.6	22	57–65

Source: Modified from Feldman and Burton 1990, p. 1674.

prescribed. Adverse effects are more common in patients if they are elderly, have multiple medical problems, or have hepatic or renal dysfunction. The most common side effects, with a frequency of 1%–2%, are diarrhea, headaches, drowsiness, fatigue, muscle pain, and constipation. All of the compounds may be associated with mental confusion in the critically ill patient, but this is uncommon in outpatients. Cimetidine may cause gynecomastia in men because it increases the serum prolactin concentration. Less common side effects include abnormalities in liver aminotransferases, thrombocytopenia, anemia, leukopenia, and bradycardia.

Drug interactions may occur because of either impaired absorption, caused by a decrease in gastric pH, or altered metabolism. Cimetidine binds to the cytochrome P-450 (CYP450) system of enzymes in the liver, which is especially important in altering the metabolism of warfarin, theophylline, and phenytoin, all of which are drugs with narrow therapeutic windows. The other H$_2$-receptor antagonists have much less interaction with the CYP450 enzymes. Absorption of ketoconazole is impaired by concomitant administration of H$_2$-receptor antagonists because of the increase in gastric pH. Similarly, antacids may impair the absorption of the H$_2$-receptor antagonists. It should be noted that famotidine is excreted primarily by the kidney and can therefore have additional risks for patients with renal disease. The U.S. Food and Drug Administration has placed a warning on the label to reduce the dose and increase the time between doses in patients with kidney failure.

Clinical Indications

Prior to the development of PPIs, H$_2$-receptor antagonists had been the cornerstone of therapy for peptic ulcer disease (PUD) for years. At nocturnal doses of 800 mg for cimetidine, 300 mg for ranitidine, 40 mg for famotidine, and 300 mg for nizatidine, healing rates at 4 and 8 weeks for duodenal ulcers are 78% and 92% and for gastric ulcers, 63% and 88%, respectively. Although the dose can be split into a twice-daily regimen, the single nocturnal dose is simpler for patient compliance. In the past, maintenance therapy with a half-dose of any of the compounds effectively decreased the recurrence rate for ulcers. The emergence of *Helicobacter pylori* as an important factor causing ulcer recurrence means that maintenance therapy is no longer indicated in patients positive for *H. pylori*.

In patients who have duodenal ulcers that heal after bleeding, ranitidine at a nocturnal dose of 150 mg is effective for the prevention of rebleeding. However, cure of *H. pylori* and elimination of the NSAIDs may be more important.

Although H$_2$-receptor antagonists improve the symptoms of gastroesophageal reflux disease (GERD), the efficacy of these agents in the healing of erosive and ulcerative esophagitis is less. In contrast to the uniform benefit of this class of drugs in the healing of PUD, H$_2$-receptor antagonists heal no more than 60% of patients with macroscopic esophagitis. Nevertheless, H_2-receptor antagonists are still used in treating GERD. In contrast to nocturnal dosing for PUD, when used, H_2-receptor antagonists should be used twice daily for 12 weeks at the following doses: cimetidine, 800 mg; ranitidine, 150 mg; famotidine, 20 mg; and nizatidine, 150 mg. Doubling the dose of the H_2-receptor antagonists improves healing of esophagitis. Another usage of H_2 blockers has been to treat nighttime breakthrough of acid for patients on PPIs. However a recent study failed to show additional benefit from this strategy.

PPIs

Clinical Pharmacology

The PPIs—omeprazole, esomeprazole, lansoprazole, rabeprazole, and pantoprazole (Figure 28-3), are substituted benzimidazoles that inhibit the H^+-K^+-ATPase enzyme of the gastric parietal cell, thereby blocking the final step of gastric acid secretion in response to any type of stimulation. This mechanism of action is very different from that of H_2-receptor antagonists that block only the H_2-receptor located on the basolateral membrane of the parietal cell. The PPIs accumulate in the acidic environment of the parietal cell secretory canaliculus, where they are transformed into an active form, the sulfenamide derivative, which reacts with sulfhydryl groups on the H^+-K^+-ATPase enzyme to form an inhibitory complex (Figure 28-4). The PPIs bind irreversibly to the H^+-K^+-ATPase enzyme, resulting in long-lasting inhibition of gastric acid secretion. For gastric secretory activity to be restored, new enzyme needs to be resynthesized.

PPIs inhibit both basal and stimulated acid secretion in a dose-dependent manner. Acid suppression occurs within 1–2 hours after a dose of these compounds. After therapy is discontinued, acid secretion gradually returns to normal in 2–5 days.

Pharmacokinetics

Absorption is rapid, with peak plasma levels at 1–5 hours after oral administration. PPIs are metabolized via the CYP450 enzyme system. Lansoprazole and pantoprazole appear to be less affected by this enzyme system, however, clinically none of the PPIs usually have a significant impact on metabolism of other drugs. However, it is cautious to monitor carefully when PPIs are used with other medications which are metabolized by the liver. PPIs can impair cyanocobalamin absorption. Under normal circumstances, hydrochloric acid (HCl) is required for cyanocobalamin to be released from dietary protein. PPIs result in a profound suppression of gastric acid secretion and therefore may inhibit cyanocobalamin release. This same hypochlorhydria may result in iron malabsorption, especially if these agents are used for prolonged periods. The decrease in intragastric acidity caused by PPIs may also interfere with the absorption of drugs that require intragastric acidity for absorption, such as ketoconazole and iron salts.

PPIs block the final step of gastric acid secretion.

PPIs bind irreversibly to the H^+-K^+-ATPase enzyme, resulting in long-lasting inhibition of gastric acid secretion. For gastric secretory activity to be restored, new enzyme needs to be resynthesized.

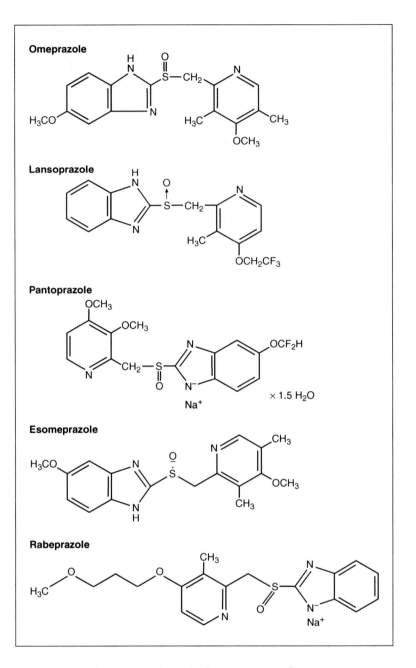

Fig. 28-3. Chemical Structure of PPIs

Drug elimination is rapid, with an elimination half-time of 0.5–2.0 hours. In direct comparisons of lansoprazole, rabeprazole, and pantoprazole with omeprazole, symptom relief and healing rates were similar for both gastric and duodenal ulcers and also for moderate to severe GERD.

Elimination of PPIs is unaffected by impaired renal function. In the elderly, elimination is decreased somewhat, whereas in patients with impaired hepatic function, bioavailability is increased. The clinical significance of this phenomenon is uncertain, and there are no recommendations to alter doses in these patient populations.

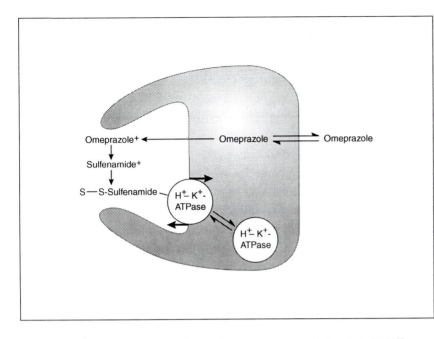

Fig. 28-4. Omeprazole Acting on a Gastric Parietal Cell

Omeprazole enters the cytoplasm freely. It is protonated in the secretor canaliculus of the parietal cell, converted to a sulfenamide, and then bound by disulfide bonds to the H^+-K^+-ATPase enzyme, where acid secretion is inhibited. *Source:* Modified from Maton 1991, p. 966.

Adverse Effects

PPIs are remarkably well tolerated. Adverse effects are uncommon, typically no more common than those experienced with placebo. Minor symptoms, such as nausea, diarrhea, and headaches, have been described most frequently. Omeprazole has been approved for over-the-counter use.

Initial enthusiasm over the potential applications of the PPIs was tempered by the discovery of gastric carcinoid tumors in rats exposed to lifelong high doses of these compounds. Approximately 10% of the male and 40% of the female rats treated with 400 μmol/kg of omeprazole over a 2-year period developed carcinoid tumors in the stomach. However, this dose is far greater than that used to treat acid peptic disorders in humans. The cells in these tumors were enterochromaffin-like (ECL) endocrine cells, and the tumors appeared to represent a progression in a continuum from diffuse ECL-cell hyperplasia to focal hyperplasia to focal carcinoids. The carcinoid tumors in rats appear to be species-specific, as similar results have not been seen in other experimental models, such as mice or dogs.

The development of carcinoid tumors has since been studied extensively. It appears that these tumors are not caused directly by the PPIs but are related to the marked elevation in serum gastrin caused by the inhibition of gastric acid secretion by these compounds. Under normal conditions, gastrin release is inhibited by intragastric acidity. The

Notes

The PPIs are clearly superior to H₂-receptor antagonists in the treatment of erosive or ulcerative esophagitis.

reduction of intragastric acidity caused by PPIs results in the loss of this normal feedback inhibition of gastric acid on gastrin release. In the rat model, elevated gastrin levels caused by the administration of omeprazole and high-dose ranitidine or the exogenous administration of gastrin correlate with an increase in the density of ECL cells in the stomach. This increase in the density of the ECL cells is seen in the setting of an increase in the proliferation rate of these cells, a finding that also correlates with plasma gastrin levels. When omeprazole was administered to rats after antrectomy, thereby eliminating the major endogenous source of gastrin, neither elevations in plasma gastrin nor increased ECL-cell density and proliferation rates were seen when compared to intact animals. The ECL-cell changes were reversible, as ECL-cell density returned to normal 20 weeks after cessation of therapy.

Gastric carcinoids are rare in humans, accounting for only 3%–5% of all GI carcinoids and 0.3% of gastric tumors. These carcinoid tumors have been seen in patients with Zollinger-Ellison syndrome and pernicious anemia, two naturally occurring states of hypergastrinemia. As in the animal model, a relationship is also seen between ECL-cell density and serum gastrin levels in patients with atrophic gastritis, with the highest gastrin levels found in those patients with carcinoid tumors. This has led to further study of the possible influence of omeprazole on the ECL-cell population in humans. In short-term studies, PPIs increase fasting serum gastrin levels and 24-hour gastrin profiles approximately two- to fivefold when compared to pretreatment values. The gastrin levels then return to normal within 2 weeks of completion of therapy. The most profound increase in gastrin level is seen in the first month of treatment and, where examined, correlates with the gastrin level prior to starting treatment. To put the gastrin data in some perspective, in contrast to the almost fivefold increase in 24-hour gastrin profiles seen in duodenal ulcer patients after treatment with omeprazole for 28 days, pernicious anemia patients have a 30-fold increase in the 24-hour gastrin profile.

Long-term therapy with omeprazole is associated with an increase in inflammation of the gastric corpus and with the development of atrophic gastritis and argyrophilic-cell hyperplasia only in patients who are infected with *H. pylori*; these findings are not seen in patients who are not infected.

All of the data suggest that the extent and duration of acid suppression and *H. pylori* infection are the crucial determinants for the development of gastric carcinoids. There have been no reports of gastric carcinoids with PPIs in the treatment of acid peptic diseases. The original black-box FDA warning limiting the duration of use of omeprazole was discontinued some time ago.

Clinical Indications

The FDA-approved indications for PPIs are listed in Table 28-2. PPIs have revolutionized the medical therapy of GERD. They are superior to H₂-receptor antagonists in the treatment of erosive or ulcerative esophagitis. Healing of erosive esophagitis is seen in 80%–90% of patients treated with omeprazole (20 mg daily) or lansoprazole (30 mg daily). Symptoms of GERD, including heartburn, regurgitation, and dysphagia, also improve rapidly with these compounds. Once therapy is stopped, symptoms and inflammation return. However, maintenance therapy with either omeprazole 10 mg daily or lansoprazole 15 mg daily can decrease the relapse rate of GERD symptoms to approximately 31%–38% at 1 year.

The PPIs achieve duodenal ulcer healing rates at 4 weeks that typically are seen at 8 weeks with H_2-receptor antagonists. Omeprazole 20 mg once daily and lansoprazole 15–30 mg daily result in healing rates of 90%–100% at 4 weeks. In addition to accelerating duodenal ulcer healing, the PPIs typically relieve symptoms more rapidly than H_2-receptor antagonists.

In contrast to the dramatic acceleration of healing of duodenal ulcers with PPIs, gastric ulcer healing is essentially comparable to that with H_2-receptor antagonists at 8 weeks. Furthermore, the dose used for gastric ulcers is double that used for duodenal ulcer therapy (omeprazole, 40 mg daily; lansoprazole, 30 mg daily) to achieve comparable healing rates, resulting in much higher drug costs to the patient. Rates of ulcer recurrence within 6 months of therapy are no different in patients treated with omeprazole or ranitidine. As in other indications, treatment has been uniformly well tolerated without reports of any significant adverse effects.

PPI cotherapy with NSAIDs has been shown to be effective in endoscopic and clinical outcome trials. Misoprostol (discussed later)

Table 28-2. FDA-Approved Indications for PPIs

INDICATION	LANSOPRAZOLE	OMEPRAZOLE	ESOMEPRAZOLE	PANTOPRAZOLE	RABEPRAZOLE
Duodenal ulcers	X	X			X
Duodenal ulcer, maintenance	X				
Erosive esophagitis	X	X	X	X*	X
Erosive esophagitis, maintenance	X	X	X		X
Gastric ulcers	X	X			
Helicobacter pylori	X	X	X		
Pathological hypersecretory conditions	X	X			X
Symptomatic GERD	X	X	X		
GERD, short-term treatment				X	X**
Healing of NSAID-associated gastric ulcers	X				
Risk reduction of NSAID-associated gastric ulcers	X				
Zollinger-Ellison syndrome	X	X			X

*Oral pantoprazole is indicated for the short-term (up to 8 weeks) treatment in the healing and symptomatic relief of erosive esophagitis associated with GERD.

**IV pantoprazole is indicated for short-term treatment (7 to 10 days) of GERD in patients unable to take the oral formulation.

has also been shown to be effective, but it requires multiple dosing and may cause side effects. The role of COX-2 inhibitors is discussed in Chapter 11.

Control of gastric acid hypersecretion is central to the management of Zollinger-Ellison syndrome. Although this syndrome was previously managed by total gastrectomy, H_2-receptor antagonists were recognized as effective in the treatment of gastric acid hypersecretion. However, large doses are often needed, dosing intervals are frequent, and drug requirements often increase with time. The PPIs have simplified the treatment of gastric acid hypersecretion in Zollinger-Ellison syndrome. Chronic therapy with PPIs for up to 5 years has uniformly resulted in continued inhibition of acid secretion, good symptom control, complete healing of mucosal lesions, and lack of adverse effects. Treatment of Zollinger-Ellison syndrome with PPIs does not result in further elevation of gastrin levels because of independent gastrin production by the tumor. The initial dose is typically higher than for treatment of ulcers for GERD, 60 mg daily of either omeprazole or lansoprazole, for example. The dose should then be titrated to a basal acid output 24 hours after the last dose of the drug of less than 10 mEq/hr. Symptoms alone are an unreliable guide to assess control of gastric acid secretion in Zollinger-Ellison syndrome, and the presence of GI pathologic conditions correlates with gastric acid secretion rates greater than 10 mEq/hr.

ANTACIDS

Antacids used to be the mainstay of therapy for PUD prior to the development of H_2 blockers and PPIs. They are effective agents for healing ulcers and controlling symptoms. However, from a practical perspective, the inconvenient dosing frequency and the adverse effects of therapy limit the use of antacids to symptom control only. Antacids are frequently used by patients to relieve symptoms of upper abdominal pain or discomfort associated with PUD, GERD, and functional dyspepsia.

Antacids neutralize acid that is already secreted. This increases intragastric pH, which also inactivates pepsin. The greatest buffering capacity is achieved when antacids are given 1 hour after eating. However, antacids may also have other mucosal cytoprotective actions: increasing mucosal prostaglandin levels, binding to epidermal growth factor, stimulating mucus and bicarbonate (HCO_3^-) production, increasing microvascular flow, and binding to bile acids.

Magnesium Hydroxide

Magnesium hydroxide reacts with HCl to form magnesium chloride and water. The magnesium also reacts with phosphates in the diet and pancreatic secretions to form insoluble salts. It is rarely used alone because of its cathartic effect, and it may accumulate in patients with renal failure. Its primary use is in combination with other agents.

Aluminum Hydroxide

Aluminum hydroxide reacts with HCl to form aluminum chloride and water. The aluminum also reacts with phosphates in the diet and pancreatic secretions to form insoluble salts. It is less potent than magnesium hydroxide and has side effects of phosphate depletion and constipation. It is primarily used in combination with magnesium hydroxide. Examples include brand names Alternagel, Amphojel, and Basaljel.

Calcium Carbonate

Calcium carbonate reacts with HCl to form calcium chloride and carbon dioxide. When given in large amounts, it may increase serum calcium levels and cause metabolic alkalosis with renal insufficiency, an entity known as milk alkali syndrome. These often chewable antacids can also increase acid secretion.

Sodium Bicarbonate

Sodium bicarbonate reacts with HCl to produce sodium chloride, water, and carbon dioxide. If used in large amounts, this agent can cause sodium retention and volume overload, a special problem in patients with congestive heart failure. This antacid is available as baking soda.

Combination Antacids

The combination antacids typically combine magnesium hydroxide and aluminum hydroxide. Examples include brand names Maalox, Mylanta, Gaviscon, and Gelusil. Despite the combinations, adverse effects (such as diarrhea) still occur.

SUCRALFATE

Sucralfate is a complex salt of sucrose sulfate and aluminum hydroxide. It is insoluble in water, but in the acid milieu of the stomach, sucralfate is broken down into sucrose sulfate and an aluminum salt. There it becomes a gel-like substance that binds to both defective and normal mucosa in the stomach and the duodenum.

Sucralfate has little or no effect on acid secretion and acts through several different mucosal protective mechanisms. It binds to mucosal surfaces and acts as a physical barrier to the diffusion of acid, pepsin, and bile acids. Sucralfate also increases prostaglandin-mediated HCO_3^- and mucus production, binds to epidermal growth factor, and has many effects on the production, composition, and structure of mucus.

Sucralfate is as effective as H_2-receptor antagonists in the treatment of duodenal ulcer disease. The drug is well tolerated with few adverse effects. The evidence for efficacy in gastric ulcer disease is less compelling, and sucralfate is not FDA-approved for this indication. It also is useful for the prophylaxis of GI bleeding in critically ill patients. The correct dose is 1 g four times daily, which makes it far less convenient than other agents for the treatment of PUD.

Misoprostol

Misoprostol is a prostaglandin E_1 analog that is effective for the prophylaxis of NSAID-induced gastric and duodenal ulcers. It acts by prostaglandin-dependent pathways to decrease gastric acid secretion and enhance mucosal defenses. Misoprostol can prevent acute damage to the gastroduodenal mucosa and decrease the frequency of both gastric and duodenal ulcers in patients requiring long-term therapy with NSAIDs. Lower doses of misoprostol (200 μg twice daily or three times daily) are just as effective as doses given four times daily for prevention of duodenal and gastric ulcers. Adverse effects are no more common than placebo with these lower doses, in contrast to the common reports of diarrhea and abdominal cramps in patients treated with full doses (200 μg four times daily).

Administration of misoprostol 200 μg four times daily can decrease serious GI complications, such as bleeding, perforation, and gastric outlet obstruction associated with NSAID consumption. However, the high cost of routine administration of misoprostol and the fact that NSAID use is so common makes the routine use of this drug unjustifiable. Rather, it should only be used in high-risk individuals: those over age 75 and those with underlying cardiovascular disease, prior PUD, or prior ulcer bleeding.

Prokinetic Agents

Normal Control of GI Motility

Motor events of the GI tract are very different in the fasted and fed periods (refer to Chapter 4). During fasting, electromechanical activity is characterized by a pattern of cyclic changes known as the interdigestive migrating motor complex (IMMC) that typically occur every 90–120 minutes. The IMMC begins in the stomach and migrates down the length of the small bowel. It has four characteristic phases. Phase I is characterized by motor quiescence. During phase II, there is irregular motor activity. Phase III motor activity is a final crescendo of activity, during which contractions occur at the maximum rate of 3 per minute in the stomach and 10–12 per minute in the small bowel. This lasts for about 5 minutes. Phase IV is a short transition period between the constant activity of phase III and the quiescence of phase I. The IMMC is thought to function as a "housekeeper" that sweeps residual material after a meal through the GI tract.

Immediately after a meal is eaten, the motor activity of the stomach and small intestine changes from a fasted to a fed pattern. This is characterized by irregular contractile activity that lasts for a variable period of time, depending on the contents of the meal. Shifting from the fasted to the fed pattern appears to be regulated at least in part by the vagus nerve.

Normal motor activity of the gut requires the functional and structural integrity of intestinal smooth muscle and its neural networks. The intestinal smooth muscle consists of an inner circular layer and an outer longitudinal layer. Located in between these two layers is the myenteric plexus. The enteric nervous system directly modulates intestinal smooth muscle function, but function is also influenced by extrinsic input from the parasympathetic and sympathetic branches of the CNS. Thus, regulatory defects of the GI tract may occur at the level of the smooth muscle contractile apparatus, the myenteric plexus, or the extrinsic nervous system.

PROKINETIC AGENTS

Prokinetic drugs are agents that improve transit of the GI tract (Table 28-3). The four agents in this class are reviewed next.

Metoclopramide

Metoclopramide, a substituted benzamide, has both antiemetic and prokinetic effects (Figure 28-5). Metoclopramide is a dopamine-(D_2-) receptor antagonist that also facilitates the release of ACh from cholinergic nerve terminals in the gut and sensitizes GI smooth muscle to the action of ACh. Metoclopramide inhibits dopamine both centrally and peripherally. Centrally, inhibition results in an antiemetic effect at the chemoreceptor trigger zone (CTZ), whereas peripherally, it blocks the inhibitory effects of dopamine on receptive relaxation of the fundus of the stomach. However, the action of metoclopramide on the GI tract is thought to be related to its cholinergic properties. Cholinergic innvervation is denser in the upper GI tract, thereby explaining the preferential proximal action of metoclopramide.

Metoclopramide enhances esophageal peristalsis, increases the pressure of the lower esophageal sphincter, accelerates gastric emptying by increasing the frequency and amplitude of antral contractions, relaxes the pylorus, and facilitates the propagation of peristaltic motor

Table 28-3. Prokinetic Agents

AGENT	MECHANISM OF ACTION	HALF-LIFE	METABOLISM	ADVERSE EFFECTS
Metoclopramide	Central and peripheral dopamine receptor antagonist Facilitates release of ACh at myenteric plexus	4 hr	80% excreted unchanged in kidneys	Multiple central nervous system Extrapyramidal Galactorrhea Menstrual irregularity
Domperidone	Peripheral dopamine-receptor antagonist	7.5 hr	Hepatic	Galactorrhea Menstrual irregularity
Cisapride	Facilitates ACh release	7–10 hr	Hepatic	Headaches Abdominal cramps Diarrhea Life-threatening cardiac arrythmias
Erythromycin	Motilin agonist	1.5 hr	Hepatic	Nausea Vomiting Abdominal pain

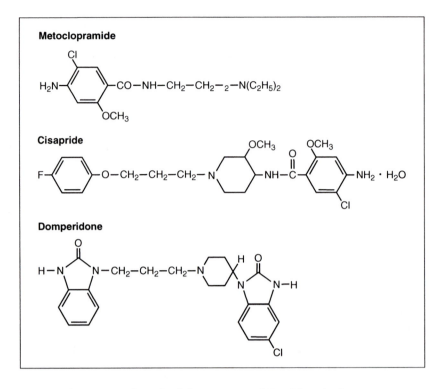

Fig. 28-5. Chemical Structure of Prokinetic Agents

activity from the stomach into the duodenum. It also increases small intestine motor activity.

Metoclopramide is rapidly absorbed and reaches peak plasma levels 40–120 minutes after oral ingestion. The half-life of metoclopramide is 4 hours. Approximately 80% of the drug is excreted unchanged in the urine, and the remainder is conjugated in the liver. Thus, impaired renal function delays drug elimination and necessitates dosage modification.

The efficacy of metoclopramide is inconsistent, and long-term therapy is complicated by adverse effects and the development of tolerance. It has been used in mild GERD, although many other agents with a better safety profile are available. Its primary indications are in diabetic and idiopathic gastroparesis, where it improves symptoms of gastric stasis and increases the rate of emptying of both solids and liquids. However, there is poor correlation between symptom improvement and acceleration of gastric emptying in diabetic gastroparesis. This suggests that central antiemetic effects of metoclopramide may play a role in symptom relief. Metoclopramide also decreases symptoms in postsurgical gastroparesis.

Adverse effects occur in up to 20% of patients. Common effects include drowsiness, anxiety, fatigue, insomnia, restlessness, and agitation. Mood swings in patients on metoclopramide therapy may be confused with primary psychiatric disorders. Extrapyramidal effects occur in 1% of patients and may be quite debilitating. A variety of dystonic reactions, such as torticollis, facial spasms, oculogyric crisis, opisthotonos, and akathisia have been reported, especially in children, renal failure patients, and patients receiving cancer chemotherapy when high doses are used for emesis control. Although most of these effects disappear spontaneously, intramuscular injection of diphenhydramine can reverse them more rapidly. Parkinsonian symptoms, such as tremor, rigidity, and akinesia, may also be provoked. Tardive dyskinesia develops rarely and may be irreversible. Because metoclopramide also is a D_2-receptor antagonist, it can stimulate prolactin secretion. This can result in breast and nipple tenderness, galactorrhea, changes in libido, and menstrual irregularities.

The typical dose is 10 mg 20–30 minutes prior to meals and at bedtime, although doses as high as 80 mg or as low as 20 mg total may be used daily. Although the pill form is usually used, the liquid preparation may allow for more reliable absorption in disorders of gastric emptying, because liquid emptying is generally less severely affected in these states. Dosage can be titrated more easily with the liquid preparation. Other alternatives include subcutaneous injections or suppositories to facilitate absorption.

Domperidone

Domperidone is an investigational drug that has been widely available in Canada and Europe for about 20 years. This agent is unlikely to be approved by the FDA in the United States, where an approval process has languished since the mid-1980s. Domperidone is a benzimidazole derivative that has both prokinetic and antiemetic properties. It is a peripheral D_2-receptor antagonist without cholinergic properties. Unlike metoclopramide, it does not cross the blood-brain barrier. Domperidone inhibits gastric relaxation induced by dopamine and causes an increase in the duration of antral contractions and an increase in the duration and frequency of duodenal contractions. It facilitates propagation of peristaltic waves from the antrum into the duodenum, thereby causing an increase in the rate of gastric emptying of both solids and liquids. It also increases lower esophageal sphincter pressure.

Peak plasma levels occur approximately 30–120 minutes after an oral dose. The half-life of domperidone is about 7.5 hours. Bioavailability is only 13%–17% because of extensive first-pass metabolism in the liver. Because metabolism is almost exclusively by the liver, no dose modifications are necessary in the setting of chronic renal failure.

Domperidone increases the emptying rates of both solids and liquids and improves symptoms in patients with gastroparesis. However, there is a poor correlation between symptom improvement and objective measure, such as radionuclide gastric emptying. Domperidone may also improve esophageal emptying and symptoms of nausea.

Domperidone increases prolactin release, which can cause galactorrhea, breast discomfort, and menstrual abnormalities. Prolongation of the QT interval, life-threatening arrythmias, and cardiac arrest have been reported.

The dose of domperidone is 10–40 mg prior to meals and at bedtime. It is only available in an oral formulation. It has the benefit of both the prokinetic and antiemetic effects of D_2-receptor blockade without the CNS side effects.

Cisapride

Cisapride is a substituted benzamide that facilitates the release of ACh at the myenteric plexus by stimulating 5-hydroxytryptamine (5-HT_4) receptors. It has no direct cholinergic actions and no antidopaminergic actions. Cisapride promotes smooth muscle contraction along the entire GI tract. It increases the amplitude of esophageal contractions, increases lower esophageal sphincter pressure, increases gastric motor activity, and enhances the coordination between antral and duodenal contractions. It also increases salivary flow, which may account in part for its beneficial effect in GERD.

Cisapride is only available in the United States to certain patients meeting eligibility criteria and whose doctor is enrolled in a special prescription program (it is no longer available through retail pharmacies). Cisapride may cause serious irregular heartbeats, which can lead to death. Ventricular tachycardia, ventricular fibrillation, torsades de pointes, and prolongation of the QT interval have been reported when cisapride is administered with other drugs that inhibit the CYP450 system. Drugs to be avoided during the use of cisapride include clarithromycin, ketoconazole, fluconazole, itraconazole, miconazole, and erythromycin.

Cisapride is rapidly absorbed after oral administration, with peak plasma levels after 1–2 hours. The half-life of cisapride is 7–10 hours. There is extensive first-pass metabolism in the liver to inactive metabolites that are excreted equally in urine and stools. In these circumstances, renal dysfunction has no effect on drug accumulation.

Cisapride is well tolerated because of the lack of extra-GI actions. The most frequently reported side effects are headaches, cramping, and diarrhea.

Cisapride is as effective as H_2-receptor antagonists in the treatment of mild to moderate GERD. It consistently accelerates gastric emptying in patients with gastroparesis of various etiologies. In patients with diabetic gastroparesis, cisapride increases the rate of emptying of solids, liquids, and indigestible solids. Cisapride also accelerates gastric emptying in gastroparesis of various other etiologies, including idiopathic etiologies, anorexia nervosa, and progressive systemic sclerosis. It is effective in selected patients with chronic intestinal pseudo-obstruction and functional dyspepsia.

The typical dose is 10–20 mg 15–20 minutes prior to meals and at bedtime. The suspension form may be more useful in gastroparesis because of the typical preservation of liquid emptying in these patients. This drug is not widely in use because of the special access program in place due to serious potential side effects.

Erythromycin

Erythromycin is a macrolide antibiotic that stimulates smooth muscle motilin receptors located at all levels of the GI tract. The prokinetic effect of erythromycin is related to its ability to mimic the effect of the GI peptide motilin on GI motility. Erythromycin binds to motilin receptors, which are preferentially located in the antrum and duodenum, to stimulate smooth muscle contraction.

After intravenous administration, erythromycin typically induces a premature phase III complex of the IMMC. It increases antral contraction amplitude, inhibits pyloric tone, and enhances antroduodenal coordination. These actions account for the acceleration of solid and liquid gastric emptying caused by erythromycin. The effects of erythromycin on GI motility are dose-dependent. When given in lower doses, such as 1–3 mg/kg intravenously, erythromycin induces phase III activity in the stomach that migrates into the small intestine. At higher doses, antral contractions are stimulated, but small intestinal contractions are inhibited. Although erythromycin also increases lower esophageal sphincter pressures, its clinical application is based on its effect on gastric emptying.

After oral administration, erythromycin is concentrated in the liver and secreted in the bile. Less than 5% is excreted unchanged in the urine. The half-life of erythromycin is 90 minutes, and optimal drug levels are obtained by administration when fasting or just prior to ingestion of a meal.

The role of erythromycin as a prokinetic agent is fairly limited. It may have beneficial effects in diabetic gastroparesis, postvagotomy gastric stasis, Roux-en-Y syndrome, and chronic intestinal pseudo-obstruction. It is most useful when administered acutely at an intravenous dose of 1–3 mg/kg every 8 hours. Erythromycin may dramatically improve gastric emptying in patients with severe diabetic gastroparesis when administered in this fashion. Long-term use of the drug at a dose of 250–500 mg orally every 8 hours in patients with gastric stasis is invariably of limited efficacy either because of tachyphylaxis or because of side effects, especially cramping and increased nausea and vomiting. The efficacy of erythromycin is limited to short-term treatment of hospitalized patients at a dose of 1–3 mg/kg intravenously every 8 hours.

Laxatives

Laxatives a most widely used class of drugs. Most are available over the counter, and some are derived from naturally occurring substances. This has led to the assumption by many patients that these drugs are safe and free of side effects. Given the large variety of laxatives available, it is important to become familiar with a certain number of laxative preparations. Laxatives work by promoting mechanisms involved in diarrhea: active electrolyte secretion, decreased fluid and electrolyte absorption, increased luminal osmolarity, increased hydrostatic

Table 28-4. Classification of Laxatives

CLASS	AGENT	EXAMPLES
Bulk	Psyllium	Metamucil
		Konsyl
	Methylcellulose	Citrucel
Hyperosmolar	Lactulose	Chronulac
	Sorbitol	Sorbitol
	Polyethylene glycol	Golytely
		Colyte
		Nulytely
Saline	Magnesium citrate	Evac-Q-Mag (citrate of magnesia)
	Magnesium hydroxide	Phillips milk of magnesia
	Sodium phosphate	Fleet enema
Lubricant	Mineral oil	Agoral
Emollient	Docusate salts	Colace
		Surfak
Stimulant	Bisacodyl	Dulcolax
	Phenolphthalein	Ex-Lax
	Castor oil	Neoloid
	Anthraquinones	
	Cascara	Caroid
	Senna	Senokot
	Danthron	Doxidan
	Casanthranol	Peri-Colace

pressure in the gut, and gut motor activity. Laxatives may be classified into the following general categories: bulking, hyperosmolar, saline, emollient, lubricant, and stimulant (Table 28-4).

CLASSIFICATION OF LAXATIVE AGENTS
Bulk Agents

Bulk agents are high-fiber products that increase fecal bulk and softness by absorbing water and expanding. These are available as derivatives of polysaccharides or methylcellulose. Bulk agents increase the stool frequency of patients with chronic constipation and are the safest agent for chronic use in these patients. Bulk agents may take several days to be effective and should always be taken with at least 8 oz of water, because bowel obstruction may occur if they are taken without adequate fluids. The most common adverse effects are flatulence and distention. Bulk agents should be avoided in patients with mechanical narrowing of the GI tract, as is common in Crohn's disease.

Hyperosmolar Agents

This category includes the nonabsorbable sugars (sorbitol and lactulose) and polyethylene glycol. The osmotic action of these agents causes water retention in the gut lumen, thereby increasing stool volume and stimulating peristalsis. Lactulose is a synthetic disaccharide that is not metabolized by intestinal enzymes. It reaches the colon unchanged, where it is metabolized by colonic bacteria into short-chain fatty acids that increase stool osmolarity and decrease intraluminal pH. Lactulose, at a dose of 30–60 ml daily, increases stool frequency in chronically constipated patients. It is well tolerated, although common side effects include flatulence, cramps, and diarrhea. Sorbitol is another nonabsorbable sugar that acts by a similar mechanism to that of lactulose. It is a low-cost alternative to lactulose with equal efficacy. Polyethylene glycol (trade names Colyte, Golytely, Nulytely, Miralax) is used primarily for bowel preparation prior to surgery or colonscopy. It may be useful in the treatment of selected patients with constipation, although the large volume (4 L) is difficult for most patients to tolerate. Polyethylene glycol is nonabsorbable, thereby increasing luminal osmotic activity and resulting in diarrhea. It is combined with sodium and potassium salts to maintain electrolyte balance. The final hyperosmotic agent is glycerin, which is absorbed if given orally and hence is useful only when given as a suppository. It typically acts within 30 minutes of administration.

Saline Laxatives

Saline laxatives contain poorly absorbable magnesium, citrate, sulfate, and phosphate ions that cause intraluminal water accumulation. This increases intraluminal volume and is a stimulus for intestinal motility. These agents are typically fast-acting and lead to a bowel movement within 3 hours of administration. Saline laxatives may cause mineral imbalances if not used cautiously. Magnesium salts should be given with special caution to patients with renal failure, as magnesium accumulation may lead to toxicity. Phosphate salts may cause an increase in sodium absorption, which may lead to fluid overload in patients with underlying heart failure. Phosphate enemas may (rarely) lead to traumatic injury to the rectosigmoid colon.

Lubricant Laxatives

Mineral oil is the prototypical lubricant laxative. It acts by coating the feces, thereby allowing for easier passage, and by decreasing colonic water absorption. At a dose of 15–45 ml, it may be considered for short-term use only. Significant side effects may be associated with this agent, including lipoid pneumonia if aspirated, pruritus ani from anal leakage, and malabsorption of the fat-soluble vitamins A, D, E, and K with chronic use.

Emollient Laxatives

Emollient laxatives are the docusate salts that are typically thought of as stool softeners. They have detergent properties that facilitate the mixture of aqueous and fatty substances in the stool, thereby softening it. They may also increase fluid and electrolyte secretion by stimulating mucosal cAMP. The docusate salts are generally used in hospitalized patients and should not be used for patients with chronic constipation. It

Notes

Most patients who abuse
laxatives have psychiatric
problems.

should be noted that laxatives were in use before the advent of laws governing the efficacy and safety of medications, therefore there is a general lack of primary literature evaluating the efficacy of these agents or documentation of efficacy. In general emollient laxatives are indicated to promote stool softening and have minimal true laxative effect.

Stimulant Laxatives

Stimulant laxatives include the anthraquinone derivatives, bisacodyl, phenolphthalein, and castor oil. As a group, these agents act by stimulating colonic motor activity, water secretion, and electrolyte transport. Use of stimulant laxatives should be avoided in most settings because of the potential for side effects, including metabolic acidosis or alkalosis, hypokalemia, damage to the myenteric plexus, and pigment deposition and discoloration of the colon known as melanosis coli.

LAXATIVE ABUSE

Surreptitious use of laxatives is the major cause of factitious diarrhea. This is almost exclusively a disorder of women and is characterized by watery diarrhea, abdominal pain, nausea, vomiting, and weight loss. Chronic laxative use results in excessive losses of sodium through stools. This activates the renin-angiotensin-aldosterone system, which subsequently decreases renal sodium losses but increases renal and fecal losses of potassium. This can result in hypokalemia. Myopathy may also be seen in these patients.

Why do patients abuse laxatives? The cause is unknown, but patients may wrongly assume that over-the-counter medications have no adverse effects. However, most patients who abuse laxatives have psychiatric abnormalities, such as personality disturbances, depression, anorexia nervosa, bulimia, or Munchausen syndrome.

Nausea, Vomiting, and Antiemetics

Nausea is a sensation of being sick to the stomach, queasy, and feeling that vomiting is imminent. Although nausea typically precedes vomiting, vomiting may not necessarily ensue. Nausea is often accompanied by signs of sympathetic nervous system activation: diaphoresis, hypersalivation, pallor, and tachycardia.

Retching, or dry heaves, precedes vomiting and involves the contraction of respiratory and abdominal muscles against a closed glottis, forcing gastric contents into the esophagus without expelling them. Vomiting is the forceful expulsion of gastric contents up and through the mouth. This occurs via the sustained contraction of abdominal wall and diaphragmatic muscles, accompanied by relaxation of the upper esophageal sphincter.

A large range of stimuli can cause nausea and vomiting. These include mechanical causes, such as gastric outlet obstruction and intestinal obstruction; motility abnormalities, such as gastroparesis and pseudo-obstruction; diverse CNS causes, such as visceral pain, psychologic distress, labyrinthine stimulation, increased intracranial pressure, and meningeal irritation; and a host of metabolic abnormalities related to ingestion of drugs, especially chemotherapeutic agents, or GI irritants and hormonal changes related to thyroid disease, hypoadrenal states, or pregnancy.

NEUROPHYSIOLOGY OF NAUSEA AND VOMITING

The neurophysiology of nausea and vomiting is complex, reflecting the diverse stimuli that can cause either to occur. The neural pathways that mediate nausea are unknown, although it is thought that nausea may represent a less intense activation of the pathways that result in vomiting. The vomiting reflex is coordinated by a vomiting center located in the lateral reticular formation of the medulla (Figure 28-6). It receives direct input from vagal and sympathetic afferent pathways that may be activated by peripheral chemoreceptors or mechanoreceptors from diverse visceral stimuli, such as GI hollow organ distention, mesenteric vessels, the peritoneum, and the heart. Input is also received from higher cortical centers, which may account for the anticipatory vomiting of chemotherapy.

The vomiting center also receives input from the unique CTZ located in the area postrema at the floor of the fourth ventricle. The CTZ lies outside the blood-brain barrier and acts as an emetic chemoreceptor that is activated by a variety of stimuli, including drugs, toxins, hypoxemia, radiation therapy, uremia, and diabetic ketoacidosis. The CTZ is rich in dopamine receptors but may also be activated by other neurotransmitters, including serotonin, norepinephrine, and opiates.

Finally, the vomiting center receives neural input from the vestibular system, which accounts for the pathway of motion sickness. The final pathways involved in the vomiting reflex involve dopamine, serotonergic 5-HT$_3$, H$_1$, and muscarinic cholinergic receptors. This provides the rationale for antiemetic therapy (Figure 28-7).

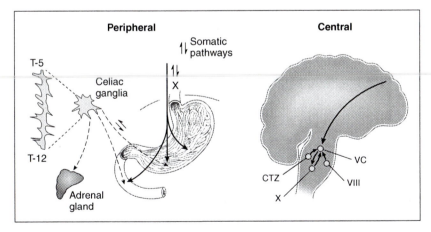

Fig. 28-6. Key Pathways in the Brain (Central) and Abdomen (Peripheral) Involved in the Act of Vomiting

VC = vomiting center; CTZ = chemoreceptor trigger zone; VIII and X = cranial nerves; T-5 to T-12 = sympathetic chain. Arrows indicate somatic pathways.
Source: Modified from Malagelada and Camilleri 1984, p. 213.

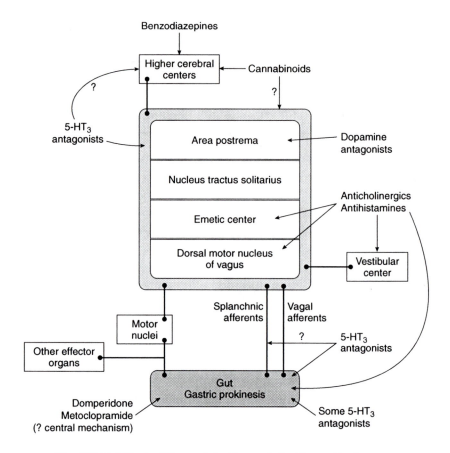

Fig. 28-7. Likely Sites of Action of Antiemetic Agents

Source: Modified from Allan 1992, p. 601.

ANTIEMETIC AGENTS

Prior to commencing therapy with pharmacologic agents, the underlying cause of nausea and vomiting should be sought. If the cause can be treated without medications (for example, if there is gastric outlet obstruction or an underlying metabolic or CNS abnormality), every effort should be made to do so. The complex neural mechanisms involved in nausea and vomiting should make it clear that no single pharmacologic agent will be effective in managing all the emetic stimuli. Dopamine-receptor antagonists are especially useful for stimuli reaching the CTZ, which is richly supplied with dopamine receptors. Agents such as phenothiazines, butyrophenones, and benzamides are especially good for targeting this area. The vestibular apparatus has predominantly H_1 and muscarinic cholinergic receptors. Therefore, anticholinergics and antihistamines are especially good for motion sickness. The various agents, their primary mechanisms of action, and their doses are outlined in Table 28-5.

Phenothiazines

Phenothiazines are excellent first-line agents for nonspecific nausea and vomiting. This class of drugs acts by antagonizing dopamine receptors in the CTZ, although they also have antihistaminergic and anticholinergic properties. Useful applications include radiation sickness, chemotherapy-induced vomiting, and postoperative vomiting. Examples of commonly used phenothiazines include prochlorperazine (trade name Compazine) and promethazine (trade name Phenergan). Sedation is the most common adverse effect, along with anticholinergic effects, such as dry mouth, drowsiness, and urinary retention. Chronic use can lead to adverse extrapyramidal effects, including tardive dyskinesia, dystonia, and akathisia.

Antihistamines

Antihistamines act by blocking H_1 receptors in the vomiting center and in the vestibular pathways. As such, the primary role for these agents is in motion sickness and vestibular disorders such as Ménière's disease. Examples of compounds in this class include diphenhydramine (trade name Benadryl), dimenhydrinate (trade name Dramamine), cyclizine (trade name Marezine), and meclizine (trade name Antivert). Sedation is the main side effect of each of these agents.

Butyrophenones

Blockade of the dopamine receptor is the primary mechanism of action of this class of antiemetics. Droperidol is the prototype compound of this class of antiemetics and is available for injectable delivery only. It is used primarily for postoperative and chemotherapy-induced nausea and vomiting. Side effects are extrapyramidal, which is what one would expect with dopamine-receptor inhibition.

Table 28-5. Pharmacologic Therapy of Nausea and Vomiting

DRUG CLASS	GENERIC NAME	TRADE NAME	RECEPTOR SITES	ADVERSE EFFECTS
Phenothiazines	Chlorpromazine	Thorazine	$D_2 = H_1 > M_1 > S$	Hypotension extrapyramidal
	Prochlorperazine	Compazine	$D_2 = H_1 > M_1 = S$	Hypotension
Benzamides	Metoclopramide	Reglan	$D_2 > S > H_1$	Extrapyramidal and central nervous system
	Cisapride	Propulsid	$S > M_1$	Diarrhea, cramping, and headache
	Domperidone	Motilium	D_2	Prolactinemia
Anticholinergics	Scopolamine	Transderm Scop	M_1	Drowsiness
Antihistamines	Dimenhydrinate	Dramamine	H_1	Drowsiness
	Diphenhyramine	Benadryl	H_1	Drowsiness
	Cyclizine	Marezine	H_1	Drowsiness
	Meclizine	Antivert	H_1	Drowsiness
	Promethazine	Phenergan	H_1	Drowsiness
Serotonin antagonists	Ondansetron	Zofran	S	Increased liver function test values
Other drugs	Erythromycin		Motilin receptor	Abdominal pain
	Bethanechol	Urecholine	M_1	Abdominal pain
	Leuprolide	Lupron	GnRH agonist	Menopausal symptoms

Source: Modified from Koch in Yamada 1995, p. 744.
Note. D_2 = dopamine; H_1 = histamine; M_1 = muscarinic; S = serotonergic.

Anticholinergics

The short duration of action of anticholinergics limits the potential use of this class of antiemetics. However, this problem has been overcome with the transdermal sustained-release delivery system available for scopolamine, which provides a constant release of scopolamine while minimizing adverse effects. This compound blocks muscarinic cholinergic transmission affecting afferent pathways to the vomiting center and in the vestibular apparatus. This class of drugs is especially useful for motion sickness and postoperative vomiting.

5-HT$_3$-Receptor Antagonists

Ondansetron (trade name Zofran) is the first of this class of drugs to become available. It acts by inhibiting 5-HT$_3$ receptors in the CTZ, vagal afferent pathways, and the GI tract mucosa. It is an excellent agent for chemotherapy-induced nausea and vomiting. The drug can be given either as a continuous infusion or at dosing intervals of every 6 hours. It is also available for oral therapy. Adverse effects are minimal, but drowsiness, headache, elevated transaminases, constipation, and diarrhea have been reported.

Prokinetics

The various prokinetic agents can be useful in the treatment of nausea and vomiting. These agents were all discussed in the section on prokinetics.

Tetrahydrocannabinol

Marijuana (active ingredient tetrahydrocannabinol) is an effective treatment option for chemotherapy-induced nausea and vomiting. The mechanism of action of this compound is unclear, but it may act on the cerebral cortex to inhibit cerebral activity. It is available as dronabinol (trade name Marinol). Adverse effects include drowsiness, dysphoria, tachycardia, dry mouth, and orthostatic hypotension.

CASE STUDY: *RESOLUTION*

This patient presented with a complication of diabetes mellitus, specifically, diabetic gastroparesis. Symptoms can be incapacitating and may lead to frequent hospitalizations. The symptoms of diabetic gastroparesis are nausea, vomiting, early satiety, and abdominal discomfort. Furthermore, the delay in gastric emptying may contribute to symptoms of GERD, such as heartburn and regurgitation. Metoclopramide was causing the adverse effects of galactorrhea, fatigue, and feeling down. Thus, this medication should have been discontinued months earlier.

Cimetidine at a dose of 300 mg four times a day heals ulcers but is not very effective for the treatment of heartburn. Heartburn is most efficaciously treated with administration of a PPI. She was switched to a PPI with improvement of her symptoms.

REVIEW QUESTIONS

Directions: For each of the following questions, choose the one best answer.

1 A 43-year-old patient comes to the physician for treatment of severe heartburn characterized by daily symptoms of substernal burning and regurgitation. He is otherwise healthy. Two years ago, the patient had an upper GI endoscopy, which revealed erosive esophagitis involving 50% of the lumen of the esophagus. The best reason for using omeprazole rather than cimetidine is that omeprazole

A inhibits both histamine and ACh receptors of the parietal cell.
B inhibits histamine, ACh, and gastrin receptors.
C stimulates release of somatostatin to decrease acid secretion.
D inhibits the final step of acid secretion at the H^+-K^+-ATPase enzyme.

2 A 65-year-old man with chronic duodenal ulcer disease has been on maintenance therapy with famotidine, 20 mg nightly, for the past 10 years to prevent a recurrence of his duodenal ulcer. He does not smoke or use NSAIDs and has just been told that he can no longer use famotidine because it is no longer covered by his insurance plan (unless he chooses to pay for the prescription or buy the OTC brand and uses the appropriate dose—which can be expensive!). He has no symptoms. The best advice to this patient would be

A switch to cimetidine, 400 mg nightly, because it is covered by the insurance plan.
B test for *H. pylori* and treat if positive because maintenance therapy is no longer required if the bacteria are eradicated.
C switch to omeprazole, 10 mg daily, for increased potency of acid suppression.
D discontinue all therapy because there are no symptoms.

3 A 50-year-old woman with insulin-dependent diabetes mellitus sees a physician because of intractable nausea, early satiety, bloating, and intermittent vomiting. A radionuclide gastric emptying test shows no emptying of a solid meal after 2 hours. A barium study of the esophagus, stomach, and duodenum shows no anatomic abnormality. The physician decides to treat her with metoclopramide. The most likely mechanism of this drug's benefit is

A stimulation of motilin receptors of the antrum and duodenum.
B inhibition of gastric dopamine receptors.
C facilitation of gastric and duodenal ACh release at the myenteric plexus.
D stimulation of receptors of the CTZ.

4 A 45-year-old woman sees a physician because of chronic constipation. She is a vegetarian and consumes large amounts of fiber each day; however, she has only two bowel movements each week and is uncomfortable in between. She is concerned about the long-term consequences of laxative use. The safest agent to use in this patient would be

A sorbitol.

B mineral oil.

C phenolphthalein.

D bisacodyl.

E castor oil.

5 A 35-year-old man comes to see a physician because of recurrent bouts of nausea, vomiting, and dizziness when driving. This problem is particularly vexing because the patient drives a taxi to earn the necessary income to go to night school. The most rational antiemetic to prescribe for this patient would be

A ondansetron.

B metoclopramide.

C prochlorperazine.

D meclizine.

E transdermal scopolamine.

References

Allan SG: Antiemetics. *Gastroenterol Clin North Am* 21:597–611, 1992.

Barbey JT: Spontaneous adverse event reports of serious ventricular arrhythmias, QT prolongation, syncope, and sudden death in patients treated with cisapride. *J Cardiovasc Pharmacol Ther* 7(2):65–76, 2002.

Camilleri M: The current role of erythromycin in the clinical management of gastric emptying disorders (editorial). *Am J Gastroenterol* 88:169–171, 1993.

Del Valle J, Chey WD, Schieman JM: Acid peptic disorders. In: *Textbook of Gastroenterology*. Edited by Yamada T. Philadelphia, PA: Lippincott Williams & Wilkins, 2003.

Feldman M, Burton ME: Histamine₂-receptor antagonists: standard therapy for acid-peptic diseases. *N Engl J Med* 323:1674, 1990.

Hasler WL: Pharmacotherapy for intestinal motor and sensory disorders. *Gastroenterol Clin North Am* 32(2):707–732, viii–ix, 2003.

Koch KL: Approach to the patient with nausea and vomiting. In *Textbook of Gastroenterology*, 2nd ed. Edited by Yamada T, Alpers DH, Owyang C, et al. Philadelphia, PA: J. B. Lippincott, 1995, p. 744.

Malagelada JR, Camilleri M: Unexplained vomiting: a diagnostic challenge. *Ann Intern Med* 101:211–218, 1984.

Maton PN: Omeprazole. *N Engl J Med* 324:965–975, 1991.

Rao SS: Constipation: evaluation and treatment. *Gastroenterol Clin North Am* 32(2):659–683, 2003.

Sekas G: The use and abuse of laxatives. *Practical Gastroenterol* 11:33–39, 1987.

Smith DS: Diagnosis and treatment of chronic gastroparesis and chronic intestinal pseudo-obstruction. *Gastroenterol Clin North Am* 32(2): 619–658, 2003.

Spencer CM, Faulds D: Lansoprazole: a reappraisal of its pharmacodynamic and pharmacokinetic properties and its efficacy in acid-related disorders. *Drugs* 48:404–430, 1994.

Tedesco FJ: Laxative use in constipation. *Am J Gastroenterol* 80:303–309, 1985.

Weber FH, Richards RD, McCallum RW: Erythromycin: a motilin agonist and gastrointestinal prokinetic agent. *Am J Gastroenterol* 88:485–490, 1993.

Welage LS: Pharmacologic features of proton pump inhibitors and their potential relevance to clinical practice. *Gastroenterol Clin North Am* 32(3 Suppl):S25–235, 2003.

Wolfe MM: Managing gastroesophageal reflux disease: from pharmacology to the clinical arena. *Gastroenterol Clin North Am* 32(3 Suppl): S37–S46, 2003.

Wolfe MM, Soll AH: The physiology of gastric acid secretion. *N Engl J Med* 1319:1707–1715, 1988.

29

Principles of Nutritional Support in the GI Patient

▣ CHAPTER OUTLINE ▣

CASE STUDY: *Introduction*

GI Disease and its Effect on Nutrient Absorption

▪ Malnutrition

▪ Nutritional Assessment

▪ Nutritional Requirements

Forms of Nutritional Therapy

▪ Enteral Nutrition

▪ Parenteral Nutrition

Summary

CASE STUDY: *Resolution*

Review Questions

References

▣ LEARNING OBJECTIVES ▣

At the completion of this chapter, the reader should be able to:

• Define the various types of malnutrition.

• Describe nutrient requirements for adults, including caloric needs, protein, carbohydrates, fats, vitamins, and trace elements.

• Evaluate how GI diseases may affect nutrient absorption.

• Assess the indications for parental nutrition (i.e., those conditions that prevent adequate nutrient absorption).

CASE STUDY: *INTRODUCTION*

The patient is a 32-year-old woman with a 10-year history of Crohn's disease. Over the course of her disease, she had undergone laparotomy three times. The first operation was an ileocolic resection for disease in the ileum during which 100 cm of small bowel were removed along with the ileocecal valve. The second operation was for repair of multiple strictures caused by Crohn's. The last operation was an attempted repair of multiple enterocutaneous fistulas that did not respond to medical therapy. The last surgery was unsuccessful, and the patient was left with three enterocutaneous fistulas that drained small-bowel contents continually despite infliximab therapy. Since the final surgery, she had lost weight from her pre-illness weight of 72 kg (158 lbs) to 50 kg (110 lbs). Her serum albumin was now 2.5 mg/dl, transferrin level 150 mg/dl, and cholesterol level 79 mg/dl, all of which are indicative of moderately severe malnutrition. Recently she had become intolerant of any enteral nutrition and had been placed on long-term parenteral nutrition.

GI Disease and Its Effect on Nutrient Absorption

GI diseases may cause malnutrition by many mechanisms. One of the most common is the development of anorexia as a result of the debilitating effects of the underlying disease, which may include nausea, intermittent vomiting, cramping, or diarrhea. In this case, although nutrient absorption is not impaired, the patient's loss of appetite leads to inadequate intake of nutrients, and malnutrition occurs.

In other cases, the underlying condition prevents proper nutrient absorption either by causing partial or complete obstruction or by impairing villous absorption of nutrients. These conditions can include Crohn's disease, celiac disease, or radiation enteritis. In all of these cases, the absorptive function of the intestine can be sufficiently impaired to prevent adequate absorption of nutrients.

Fistulization can also be a complication of many GI conditions. When a patient has an enterocutaneous fistula, two problems causing malnutrition may occur. First, the fistula may cause the enteral contents to exit the small bowel prematurely, either to the skin or colon, producing a functional short bowel syndrome. Second, the chronic inflammation that occurs in the skin of a patient with an enterocutaneous fistula may cause increased protein losses, which cannot be adequately addressed with a regular diet.

Finally, obstruction can cause malnutrition. As with enteric fistulas, the presence of an obstruction prevents nutrients from reaching the small bowel or, in a large bowel obstruction, prevents passage of the contents from the small bowel, thus preventing its normal function.

Malnutrition occurs when there is failure to consume and absorb adequate amounts of calories and protein to maintain lean body mass.

Marasmus and **kwashiorkor** are two clinically recognized kinds of malnutrition.

Table 29-1. Signs and Symptoms of Marasmus

Generalized body wasting	Marked loss of subcutaneous fat and skeletal muscle
GI failure	Diarrhea
Pulmonary failure	Pneumonia
Immune failure	Increased infection rates
Impaired wound healing	Increased incidence of postoperative hernias

MALNUTRITION

Malnutrition is particularly prevalent in hospitalized patients, 50% of whom may develop clinical malnutrition during their hospitalization. Although it may be caused by conditions such as anorexia nervosa or by the unavailability of food, in most cases malnutrition results from the inability of the small bowel to absorb adequate nutrients because of either intrinsic bowel disease or obstruction. Two clinical kinds of malnutrition are commonly recognized. The first, *marasmus*, occurs when the patient lacks adequate amounts of calories and protein to maintain lean body mass. This produces classic starvation caused by the autocatabolism of the patient's visceral and somatic protein stores as well as fat stores (Table 29-1).

The second type of malnutrition, *kwashiorkor*, occurs when the patient takes in adequate overall calories but insufficient protein to maintain the lean body mass. In this case, the signs and symptoms may be less obvious because the subcutaneous fat stores are maintained (Table 29-2). This type of malnutrition is seen less often in hospitalized patients because, normally, once the patient is admitted, he or she is placed on a diet that provides the proper ratio of protein to nonnitrogen calories.

Vitamin and trace element deficiencies may also develop in patients with GI disease. The deficiency states are easily recognizable in their advanced states (Tables 29-3 and 29-4) but may be obscure in patients who have marginal deficiencies. These are prevented by the administration of adequate vitamin supplements on a daily basis. Because adequate amounts of trace elements are present in all enteral diets, supplementation is not needed for patients who are on any kind of enteral diet. The solutions used in parenteral nutrition (amino acids, dextrose, and intralipid) do not contain any trace elements, and therefore, supplementation is required in patients receiving parenteral nutrition.

Table 29-2. Signs and Symptoms of Kwashiorkor

Bloated abdomen	Psychomotor changes
Pale, edematous skin	Peeling skin
Muscle wasting	Purpura
Hepatosplenomegaly	

Table 29-3. Vitamin Deficiency States

VITAMIN	DEFICIENCY STATE
A	Night blindness
D	Osteomalacia
K	Hemorrhage
Thiamine	Beriberi, heart failure, and Korsakoff psychosis
Niacin	Diarrhea, dermatitis, and dementia
Folate	Anemia
B_{12}	Anemia
C	Scurvy

Table 29-4. Trace Element Deficiencies

ELEMENT	DEFICIENCY STATE
Iron	Anemia
Zinc	Rash, hair loss, and loss of taste
Copper	Anemia and leukopenia
Chromium	Hyperglycemia
Selenium	Muscle necrosis and cardiomyopathy

NUTRITIONAL ASSESSMENT

Any patient who presents with a GI problem is at risk for malnutrition. The first step in the workup for malnutrition is the subjective assessment of the patient. This includes obtaining a dietary history, an appraisal of the functional ability of the patient (i.e., exercise capacity, easy fatigability), and questioning about recent episodes of anorexia, dysphagia, weight loss, or other manifestations of GI problems. The workup can then move on to more objective testing. Tests include the measurement of several visceral proteins as well as possible testing for immune incompetence induced by malnutrition (Table 29-5). Newer methods of nutritional assessment are aimed at body composition measurement. In these techniques, attempts are made to determine the lean body mass (i.e., visceral and somatic protein) as differentiated from fat

Table 29-5. Objective Nutritional Assessment

MEASUREMENT	MALNUTRITION
Baseline weight	< 20% of ideal weight for height
Weight loss	< 10% of usual weight over past 6 months or < 5% usual body weight in 1 month
Albumin	< 3.0 mg/dl
Transferrin	< 200 mg/dl
Total lymphocyte count	< 1200/ml
Anergy to standard recall antigens	Anergic to 2 out of 4: moderate malnutrition Anergic to 4 out of 4: severe malnutrition

Harris-Benedict Equations

Equation 1
BEE (males) = 66.47 + 13.75W
              + 5.0H − 6.76A

Equation 2
BEE (females) = 655.1 + 9.56W
                + 1.85H − 4.68A
(W = weight in kg; H = height
in cm; A = age in years)

and bone. Although techniques for measuring body composition, such as underwater weighing and CT scanning, may have use for the stable patient, they may be impractical for the acutely ill patient.

NUTRITIONAL REQUIREMENTS

Calories

The estimation of caloric needs can be one of the most difficult problems in the nutritional therapy of the patient. Inadequate caloric intake can lead to malnutrition, whereas excessive intake can lead to obesity in the healthy patient and hepatic or pulmonary dysfunction in the acutely ill patient. Several methods are available to determine the caloric needs of the acutely ill patient. Estimation of caloric needs is most commonly done by the Harris-Benedict equations (equations 1 and 2). These formulas use the patient's age, height, and weight to determine the resting energy expenditure. This is the amount of energy that an unstressed, healthy adult requires at rest. Because most patients are not considered to be resting or at a basal level of energy expenditure (BEE), an activity factor must be added to account for the additional energy required by the illness. In most cases, this is about 1.5 times the resting energy expenditure or in the range of 30 kcal/kg.

Because the Harris-Benedict equations do not take into account the patient's metabolic state and simply estimate the caloric needs, newer techniques have been developed to obtain a direct measurement of the patient's energy expenditure. The most common of these is called indirect calorimetry, in which oxygen consumption and carbon dioxide production are measured by analysis of expired gases, and this is used to calculate the patient's actual energy expenditure. The utility of this method, however, may be limited by the patient's ability to tolerate the mask necessary for these measurements. Diurnal fluctuations of energy expenditure may also limit the usefulness of this method because any single measurement may not be representative of the actual overall energy expenditure. Although these two methods have technical limitations, they are the most useful ways of determining energy expenditure and are widely used in hospitalized patients.

Protein

The most important factor in adequate nutrition of the stressed patient is the provision of sufficient protein. As already stated, malnutrition can exist even when the patient takes in adequate calories if the protein intake is inadequate. Acute illness requires the synthesis of many acute phase reactants as well as antibodies and new structural proteins. If the patient's protein intake is inadequate, the body will break down its endogenous stores to provide essential amino acids for the required proteins. Because there are no storage forms of protein and proteins must be present for normal body function, this breakdown may lead to multisystem organ failure.

The average healthy adult requires 1.2 g of protein per kilogram of lean body mass to maintain normal protein homeostasis. During periods of stress, protein requirements are increased to about 1.5 g/kg/d. In patients with protein-losing enteropathies or multiple enterocutaneous fistulas, this protein loss can reach the stage where the patient requires over 2 g/kg/d. To determine if the patient is receiving adequate protein, the nitrogen balance can be calculated (equation 3). An unstressed adult should normally be in zero nitrogen balance; that is, the protein intake equals the protein loss. However, for a stressed patient, the goal of nutritional therapy is to place the patient in positive nitrogen balance. These calculations require accurate measurement of protein intake and a complete 24-hour collection of the patient's urine.

Much work has been done in recent years to evaluate the effects of certain amino acids in protein homeostasis. These include branched-chain amino acids (BCAAs) (leucine, isoleucine, valine) and glutamine. BCAA levels fall significantly during periods of stress and in patients with both chronic and acute hepatic failure. Enteral and parenteral feedings with increased levels of BCAAs have been evaluated in these patients to determine if the increase leads to increased nitrogen balance. Studies of acutely stressed patients have failed to show any consistent improvement in nitrogen retention with increased intake of BCAAs. In patients with hepatic failure, the results are more equivocal. Use of a high-BCAA solution for patients with acute hepatic failure has shown increased survival along with a reduction in hepatic encephalopathy. However, in all of these studies, the high-BCAA solutions were compared with a dextrose-only nutrient solution because of the potentially harmful effects of standard protein solutions in the hepatic failure patients. This led to difficulties in interpretation of the results because there is no question that supplying protein to patients with acute hepatic failure is superior to starvation in influencing recovery. There may never be a properly controlled study to answer these questions because most review boards will not approve using standard protein as a control arm in any experiment involving patients with acute hepatic failure.

Glutamine is an amino acid that under normal circumstances is considered nonessential because it can be synthesized from α-ketoglutarate, an intermediate product in aerobic metabolism. During periods of stress, glutamine requirements exceed the synthetic capacity of the patient, and a state of glutamine deficiency ensues. Glutamine is the preferred fuel for the enterocyte, and provision of a glutamine-deficient nutritional product, such as parenteral nutrition, leads to villous atrophy in the small intestine during stress, exacerbating malabsorptive problems and possibly impairing the healing of damaged mucosa. Additionally, luminal glutamine is a preferred energy source for the immune cells of gut-associated lymphoid tissue. It plays an integral role in maintaining the intestinal barrier, preventing bacterial translocation, and potentiating the effect of growth factors. Glutamine-enriched enteral products are readily available and have been shown to prevent villous atrophy during periods of stress. A few

Nitrogen (N) Balance

Equation 3
N balance = N intake − N excretion
N balance = protein intake/6.24
− (24-hr urinary urea N + 4)

The 4 estimates insensible nitrogen loss from stool, skin, and so on, which equals loss of 25 g/d of protein.

studies have also reported decreased protein breakdown with parenteral glutamine supplementation.

Carbohydrates

Carbohydrates, or the products of their intermediate metabolism, provide the energy substrates for many organ systems, including the kidneys, red blood cells, and brain. Under normal circumstances, it is difficult to become carbohydrate-deficient because complex and simple sugars are normally present in more than adequate amounts in all enteral products, and patients on oral intake restriction in a hospital are usually on an intravenous solution containing dextrose. Therefore, most patients who become carbohydrate-deficient are outpatients who either have an enteropathic condition producing carbohydrate malabsorption or a GI obstruction preventing the nutrients from reaching the small bowel.

Storage forms of carbohydrate are limited. During periods of stress starvation, liver glycogen stores are depleted in a few hours, whereas muscle and renal glycogen stores are exhausted within 24 hours. After depletion occurs, the liver begins to increase gluconeogenesis to provide carbohydrate substrates. Because fat cannot be converted into carbohydrate, the only endogenous substrates available for gluconeogenesis are amino acids. This conversion of amino acids to glucose leads to protein breakdown, a negative nitrogen balance, and uremia in the stressed patient.

Carbohydrate requirements for the stressed adult range from 3 to 7.5 g/kg/d. Although inadequate carbohydrate intake can lead to the complications noted, excessive intake is equally harmful. In unstressed adults, carbohydrate overload leads to storage of the excess material in the form of fat. In the stressed adult, the mechanisms to remove this fat from the liver are inhibited by decreased insulin levels and increased glucagon, steroid, and epinephrine levels, leading to retention of the lipids in the hepatocyte (the site of production) and hepatic dysfunction. Normally this dysfunction takes the form of cholestasis with elevation of serum bilirubin and alkaline phosphatase. This process is reversible with reduction of the carbohydrate intake and does not normally cause long-term hepatic dysfunction. Problems with carbohydrate intake can also occur during stress with increasing serum glucagon, steroid, and epinephrine levels causing the patient to become glucose intolerant. In this case, the patient takes on the characteristics of a non–insulin-dependent diabetic condition with elevation of the serum glucose levels without development of ketosis. Treatment for this condition consists of lowering the glucose intake while supplying adequate exogenous insulin to control blood sugar levels.

Fats

Daily fat intake is not required in most adults. Unless the patient is severely malnourished, the average adult has approximately a 30-day supply of essential fatty acids present in the tissues. Because fats make up a large proportion of the normal diet and are present in more than adequate amounts in all enteral products, fatty acid deficiency is a rare event, except in patients with fat malabsorption resulting from pancreatic insufficiency; in patients with other impairments of intestinal absorption of fat, such as bile acid deficiency; or in patients maintained on long-term total parenteral nutrition (TPN) without intravenous sources of fat. In these cases, essential fatty acid deficiencies occur after about a month of starvation. A dry, scaly appearance to the skin is the most visible symptom of this condition, but the significant complications occur secondary to decreased prostaglandin synthesis and decreased absorption of fat-soluble vitamins, such as A and D.

Forms of Nutritional Therapy

ENTERAL NUTRITION

Enteral nutrition is the preferred form of nutritional therapy for all patients. It presents nutrients in the most physiologic form and permits the normal processing of the absorbed nutrients. It also promotes maintenance of the normal structure of the bowel as well as maintaining the integrity of the gut–mucosal barrier. Several types of specialized enteral nutritional products are available to provide nutrition for patients who are not able to tolerate a regular diet.

Elemental Diets

These consist of partially or completely hydrolyzed nutrients. These formulas are used in cases where the absorptive capacity of the small bowel is limited. Essentially, an elemental diet is totally absorbed in the proximal 2 feet of the small intestine and presents little or no residue to the large intestine. It is suitable for patients who have colonic disease or mid to distal small bowel disease or fistulas, such as in Crohn's disease. It can also be used for patients with a proximal small bowel fistula if the end of the feeding tube can be passed distal to the site of the fistula. One problem with the use of elemental diets is that they do not promote the maintenance of normal intestinal integrity, and villous atrophy with loss of absorptive capacity occurs with time.

Defined Formula Diets

These consist of intact proteins, complex carbohydrates, and fats and may contain soluble or insoluble fibers. These diets are used for patients with an essentially intact small and large bowel and normal pancreatic function who cannot swallow a normal diet. They may be delivered by gastrostomy or feeding enterostomy or, in some cases, may be consumed orally as a supplement to a regular diet. Because they present a fiber load to the colon, they are not suitable for patients with ulcerative colitis, Crohn's colitis, enterocutaneous fistula, or any condition where colonic rest is required. They also present a greater metabolic load to the small intestine and may not be absorbed

Enteral nutrition is the preferred form of nutritional therapy for all patients.

Table 29-6. Causes of Diarrhea Induced by Tube Feeding

Lactose intolerance	Fat malabsorption
Hyperosmolar food	Ileus
Cold food	Enteritis

properly if vascular insufficiency exists. Because they require a much larger proportion of functional intestine to be present, they are not normally suitable for patients with severe short gut syndromes.

Complications of Enteral Nutrition

Complications occur when the patient is inadequately monitored. They include aspiration and diarrhea. Aspiration can occur when a patient receives enteral feeding in the supine position. Under these circumstances, reflux of gastric contents occurs and may be aspirated by patients with an impaired gag reflex. This can be prevented by feeding patients with an enteric feeding tube with the tip distal to the ligament of Treitz. Aspiration can then occur only if feeding is continued in the presence of an intestinal ileus. Diarrhea is a much more common occurrence and has many causes (Table 29-6), most of which are correctable by modifying the enteral product used. For example, for patients with lactose intolerance, a lactose-free enteral product may be used.

PARENTERAL NUTRITION

Parenteral nutrition is used only when failure of normal nutrient absorption occurs to the extent that malnutrition ensues and cannot be corrected by medical therapy. The American Society of Parenteral and Enteral Nutrition (ASPEN) has developed a consensus on the indications and contraindications for parenteral nutrition. This was first published in 1986 and was reviewed and updated in 2002 (Table 29-7). To summarize these opinions, any patient who has inadequate functional

Table 29-7. Indications for Specialized Nutrition Support

INDICATIONS FOR SPECIALIZED NUTRITION SUPPORT*

Specialized nutrition support (SNS) should be implemented in patients who cannot meet nutrient requirements by oral intake.

When SNS is indicated, enteral nutrition (EN) should be used preferentially.

When SNS is required, parenteral nutrition (PN) should be used when the GI tract is not functional or cannot be accessed. SNS should be used in patients who cannot be adequately nourished by oral diets or EN.

SNS should be initiated in patients with inadequate oral intake for 7–14 days, or in those patients in whom inadequate oral intake is expected over a 7–14-day period.

*Defined as the provision of nutrients, orally, enterally, or parenterally with therapeutic intent.

Table 29-8. Complications of Parenteral Nutrition

Hyperosmolar coma
Acute hypophosphatemia (refeeding syndrome)
Acute hypokalemia
Hyperglycemia
Line sepsis

small bowel to maintain adequate nutrition status is a candidate for parenteral nutrition. TPN consists of a solution of amino acids, dextrose, and intravenous fats in adequate amounts to supply the patient's nutritional needs. TPN has proven to be a life-saving treatment for patients with severe short bowel syndrome, allowing them to regain their strength and resume a nearly normal lifestyle. Patients have been maintained on home parenteral nutrition for over 15 years without major complications. Because the osmolarity of most parenteral solutions is greater than 1600 mOsm/L, TPN requires that the patient have central venous access. Infusion of a parenteral solution into a peripheral vein would cause immediate phlebitis and occlusion of the vein.

Complications of Parenteral Nutrition

Careful monitoring of electrolytes and serum glucose levels are necessary to prevent complications related to the infusion of a solution high in glucose and other nutrients (Table 29-8). One of the most life-threatening complications is the refeeding syndrome. In this condition, the infusion of a glucose load in a chronically malnourished patient causes a rapid drop in serum phosphorus as the phosphate is absorbed into the cells along with the nutrients. This acute hypophosphatemia can cause life-threatening problems, including respiratory failure and cardiac arrhythmias. Parenteral nutrition should be started at levels adequate to supply the patient's nutritional needs. There is no indication for "a little TPN." The complications of parenteral nutrition are such that if it is considered for use, adequate therapy should be given. With proper monitoring, TPN can be an extremely safe treatment for malnutrition, but its use should never be considered casually.

Summary

GI disease may produce malnutrition by many mechanisms, including malabsorption and obstruction. Such malabsorption is a major cause of increased morbidity in patients with acute and chronic intestinal disease because the sequelae of malnutrition, pulmonary failure, and immune system failure lead to increased complications in these patients. The proper use of nutritional support, either by enteral or parenteral nutrition, can be a life-saving adjunct in patients who have malnutrition from GI disease.

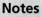
Notes

CASE STUDY: *RESOLUTION*

Since starting the parenteral nutrition, the patient's serum albumin returned to 3.2 mg/dl and her cholesterol to 125 mg/dl. She has regained 15 kg. The drainage from the enterocutaneous fistulas has minimized to less than 50 ml/d and has become controllable. She has adapted well to TPN and will be maintained on this form of nutritional therapy for the foreseeable future.

---

*R*EVIEW *Q*UESTIONS

Directions: For each of the following questions, choose the one best answer.

1 A stressed 60-kg woman requires how many kcal per day for adequate nutrition?

 A 1200
 B 1800
 C 2400
 D 3000

2 Which of the following is *not* an indication for parental nutrition?

 A High-output enterocutanteous fistula
 B Small bowel obstruction from carcinomatosis
 C Crohn's enteritis
 D Refusal to allow insertion of a nasoenteric feeding tube

3 Which of the following is a true statement concerning elemental diets?

 A They are used in cases of short bowel syndrome.
 B They consist of intact proteins.
 C They are tasty and well tolerated.
 D They contain fiber.

4 Kwashiorkor is caused by

 A colonic obstruction.
 B a typical hospital diet.
 C inadequate protein intake with adequate caloric intake.
 D protein overload.

5 Substrates for gluconeogenesis include

    A fat.
    B visceral protein.
    C soluble fiber.
    D trace elements.

6 Indications for enteral nutrition include

    A an intact GI tract.
    B severe enteritis.
    C small bowel obstruction.
    D severe malabsorption.

References

Allard JP, Jeejeebhoy KN: Nutritional support and therapy in the short bowel syndrome. *Gastroenterol Clin North Am* 18:589–601, 1989.

ASPEN Board of Directors: Guidelines for the use of parenteral and enteral nutrition in adult and pediatric patients. *J Parenter Enteral Nutr* 26(Suppl):18SA–20SA, 2002.

Bistrian BR, Blackburn GL, Vitale J, et al: Prevalence of malnutrition in general medical patients. *JAMA* 235:1567–1570, 1976.

Buzby GP: Veterans Affairs Total Parenteral Nutrition Cooperative Study Group: perioperative total parenteral nutrition in surgical patients. *N Engl J Med* 325:525–532, 1991.

Cerra FB, Cheung NK, Fischer JE, et al: Disease-specific amino acid infusion (F080) in hepatic encephalopathy: a prospective, randomized, double-blind controlled trial. *J Parenter Enteral Nutr* 9:288–295, 1985.

Glade MJ. 25th Clinical Congress of the American Society for Parenteral and Enteral Nutrition, January 21–24. Chicago, Illinois, 2001.

Jeejeebhoy KN, Detsky AS, Baker JP: Assessment of nutritional status. *J Parenter Enteral Nutr* 14:193S–196S, 1990.

Kudsk KA: Clinical applications of enteral nutrition. *Nutr Clin Pract* 9:165–171, 1994.

Moore FA, Moore EE, Jones TN, et al: TEN vs. TPN following major abdominal trauma: reduced septic morbidity. *J Trauma* 29:916–923, 1989.

Torosian MH: Stimulation of tumor growth by nutritional support. *J Parenter Enteral Nutr* 16:72S–75S, 1992.

30

GI Bleeding

■ CHAPTER OUTLINE ■

■ LEARNING OBJECTIVES ■

At the completion of this chapter, the reader should be able to:
• Assess the physiologic response to acute blood loss.
• Distinguish between upper GI and lower GI bleeding based on clinical characteristics and physiologic response.
• Delineate the different etiologies in most cases of upper and lower bleeding.
• Generate a rational diagnostic algorithm for GI bleeding.
• Outline the therapeutic options for managing the treatment of patients with upper and lower GI bleeding.

CASE STUDY: *INTRODUCTION*

A 61-year-old man with a history of alcohol abuse presented to the emergency room with syncope and rectal bleeding. Approximately 2 weeks previously, during a binge of heavy drinking, the patient developed midepigastric pain radiating to the back. He did not seek medical attention but started taking over-the-counter NSAIDs in the form of ibuprofen up to 2 g/d. He also continued to drink alcohol in an attempt to relieve the pain, but the pain failed to improve. He denied previous nausea, vomiting, or melena. On the day of admission, he developed an intense urge to move his bowels. When he got up from bed, he immediately felt dizzy and lightheaded. He passed what he described as a "gallon of clotted blood" per rectum. When he tried to arise from the toilet, he grew lightheaded and collapsed. There his wife found him, incontinent with copious amounts of clotted blood and loose, dark stool. On arrival of emergency medical technicians, the patient was pale and diaphoretic. His pulse was 160/min, and systolic blood pressure was 60 mm Hg. Two large-bore intravenous lines were started in his antecubital veins, and lactated Ringer's solution was administered through both lines, wide open.

Introduction

GI hemorrhage is an extraordinarily common phenomenon whose clinical presentation varies according to the site of bleeding, the mechanism of blood loss, and the volume of blood loss. GI bleeding is categorized according to location: upper versus lower. Upper GI bleeding occurs proximal to the ligament of Treitz and includes bleeding from the oropharynx, esophagus, stomach, or duodenum. Lower GI bleeding arises distal to the ligament of Treitz and includes small bowel bleeding, colonic bleeding, and bleeding from the anal canal. The spectrum of clinical syndromes caused by GI bleeding ranges from a hemoccult-positive stool in an asymptomatic individual to shock from exsanguination as demonstrated in the clinical case. Small amounts of GI blood loss may not result in clinical symptoms and may be picked up only on screening studies of stool. This type of bleeding is not stressed in this chapter, and discussion is limited to GI bleeding that produces clinical signs and symptoms that bring patients to medical attention.

Acute upper and lower GI bleeding are common, with upper GI bleeding resulting in approximately 300,000 hospital admissions every year and lower GI bleeding accounting for 0.5% of all short-term hospital admissions. Acute GI bleeding may be seen in all age groups; however, the prevalence of different sources of bleeding varies greatly. In general, advanced age, with an associated increase in

Table 30-1. Associated Mortality from Upper GI Bleeding Related to Medical Comorbidity

CONDITION	MORTALITY (%)
Renal disease	29
Acute renal failure	64
Liver disease	25
Jaundice	42
Pulmonary disease	23
Respiratory failure	57
Cardiac disease	12.5
Congestive heart failure	28

comorbid illnesses, adversely impacts on the survival of patients with GI bleeding (Table 30-1). Despite recent advances in the diagnosis and management of acute GI hemorrhage, the mortality for all patients with acute GI bleeding has remained between 8% and 10% over many years. About 75% of all GI bleeding, regardless of its location and etiology, eventually stops. The rebleeding rate varies, depending on the bleeding lesion. Of the 25% of patients with continued bleeding and those who rebleed, more than 30% require surgical management, and around 30% die from bleeding or its complications. For these reasons, the goals of medical management of acute GI bleeding are:

1. Stabilize the patient with regard to hemodynamic parameters.
2. Determine the location of the bleeding.
3. Determine whether the patient is continuing to bleed.
4. Attempt to stop active bleeding.
5. Apply strategies to prevent rebleeding.

This simplified management plan has evolved into a technically demanding subspecialty that involves a multidisciplinary team, including an intensivist, a gastroenterologist, surgeons, and interventional radiologists. This chapter reviews the diagnostic and therapeutic workup of patients who present with acute GI hemorrhage, with an emphasis on the pathophysiology involved in their presentation.

CASE STUDY: *CONTINUED*

The patient's medical history was only significant for alcohol abuse, with no previous history of GI bleeding. Nine years earlier, during an evaluation for chronic epigastric pain, the patient had an upper GI series that demonstrated a 1.5-cm ulcer in the posterior portion of the bulb of the duodenum. This was treated with a histamine- (H_2-) receptor antagonist for a period of 2 months, and no further workup or therapy was given. The patient was not drinking at the time of diagnosis of his ulcer and was not taking any aspirin or NSAIDs. Currently, other than ibuprofen, the patient was taking no medications and had no known drug allergies. His family history was negative for liver disease, IBD, GI malignancy, neoplasms, or bleeding disorders. The patient was married and had two children who were alive and well. He worked as a bartender and had a 60-pack year-long smoking history. During binges, he drank up to 1 quart of hard liquor and a six-pack of beer a day for periods up to 1–2 weeks. He had been through alcohol counseling and detoxification on three separate occasions. Review of systems was negative for nausea and vomiting, preceding melena, weight loss, fevers, chills, or jaundice.

On physical examination in the emergency room, he was diaphoretic, his pulse was 120/min with a systolic blood pressure of 90 mm Hg after receiving 4 L of crystalloid. On sitting upright, his blood pressure fell to 70 mm Hg, and his systolic pulse rose to 140/min. His skin demonstrated normal turgor with pallor. He had no gynecomastia, no spider angiomata, no palmar erythema, and no Dupuytren's contractures. In addition, there were no cutaneous vascular lesions noted. Mucous membranes were dry with no oropharyngeal lesions. Ocular examination was normal. His neck was supple without peripheral adenopathy; his lungs were clear; and his cardiac examination revealed a rapid regular rate with a 1/6 systolic murmur heard at the apex. His abdomen was soft and flat. There were hyperactive bowel sounds and tenderness in the midepigastrium without evidence of peritonitis. There was no arterial bruit or venous hum. His liver was slightly enlarged and was felt three fingerbreadths beneath the right costal margin and had a smooth texture. There was dullness to percussion in Traube's space, and his spleen tip could be felt on inspiration and deep palpation of the left upper quadrant. His peripheral pulses were intact, and his neurologic examination was nonfocal. Rectal examination demonstrated dark, clotted blood in the vault. Blood work returned with notable values of a hemoglobin of 4 with a hematocrit of 14%; WBC count and differential were normal; and serum electrolytes were normal. BUN was 40 with a creatinine of 1.1. Serum amylase was elevated at 290 IU/L. Liver enzymes were abnormal with a serum AST of 103 IU/L and a serum ALT of 62 IU/L. Alkaline phosphatase was 143 IU/L, and bilirubin was 1.9 mg/dl with a conjugated fraction of 1.4 mg/dl. Prothrombin time was normal with an INR of 1.1; albumin was 3.8 g/dl. The platelet count was low at 100,000. Lavage through a nasogastric (NG) tube returned clear gastric contents with a small amount of undigested food. The tube was then removed. The patient was admitted to medical ICU with a presumptive diagnosis of lower GI bleeding.

Initial Assessment of Acute Upper GI Bleeding

The most important step in the initial management of patients with acute GI hemorrhage involves performing a rapid assessment of the degree of volume loss and initiating fluid resuscitation (Table 30-2). Thus the initial directed physical examination should assess for hemodynamic instability. Vital signs should be taken both in the supine and prone positions to assess for orthostatic changes. The initial assessment of the patient described in the clinical case demonstrated tachycardia and hypotension in the supine position; thus, this patient was in shock with circulatory collapse. This occurs when individuals have lost about 50% of their circulating blood volume. If normal vital signs are established in a supine position, vital signs should be taken in an upright position. An increase in heart rate greater than 15 beats/min or a fall in systolic blood pressure greater than 15 mm Hg defines orthostasis and can be seen in patients who have lost up to 25% of their circulating blood volume. Additional physical findings that suggest impending circulatory collapse include poor skin turgor and cold, clammy skin, which results from peripheral vasoconstriction, a reflex compensation for decreasing central filling pressures. Aggressive fluid resuscitation and transfusion of blood products is key to the survival of patients with acute GI bleeding and circulatory collapse.

Two large-bore, short intravenous catheters placed in the antecubital veins of the arm provide a rapid and convenient method for fluid resuscitation. Intravenous crystalloid solutions of normal saline or lactated Ringer's solution should be administered at a rapid rate. During the initial intravenous line placement, a sample of blood should be drawn to type and cross-match the patient for transfusion with

Table 30-2. Initial Assessment Parameters of GI Bleeding

HISTORICAL INFORMATION

Hematemesis
Hematochezia
Passage of maroon or melenic stools
Prior history of GI bleeding
History of liver disease and portal hypertension
History of bleeding disorders
History of medication use (NSAIDs, particularly aspirin or warfarin)
History of recent procedures or surgery (e.g., postpolypectomy bleeding)
History of chronic renal disease (platelet dysfunction)

KEY PHYSICAL EXAMINATION FINDINGS

Tachycardia, hypotension, and shock
Orthostatic changes
Cold, clammy skin

Characteristics of blood in stool found on rectal examination
Stigmata of chronic liver disease
Mucocutaneous telangiectasis
Abdominal tenderness and bowel sounds

KEY LABORATORY EVALUATION

BUN:creatinine ratio
Complete blood count
Coagulation profile
Typing and cross-matching of blood

KEY DIAGNOSTIC STUDIES

Nasogastric tube lavage
Endoscopy
Angiography
Nuclear scintigraphy

RBCs and to obtain any laboratory values that are deemed important, including a hematocrit, which can be determined within minutes in the emergency department. It should be stated at this point, however, that all laboratory data play a secondary role in the initial management of GI bleeding. The hematocrit measures the percentage of RBCs to plasma and is a poor marker for volume status in severe, life-threatening bleeding. Whole blood loss results in an equal loss of plasma and RBCs, and patients with massive, rapid exsanguination can die with a normal hematocrit. Over time, as extracellular fluid is recruited into the intravascular space, RBCs become selectively diluted, and subsequently the hematocrit falls. This compensation, however, may take hours. Other blood work that may be useful includes platelet count, prothrombin time (PT), BUN, and creatinine. Once a patient has been stabilized hemodynamically, a directed history can be taken and physical examination performed to determine the source of the GI bleeding and direct further workup.

Locating the Source of Bleeding

Hematemesis is defined as vomiting blood. The blood may be bright red, or it may appear similar to coffee grounds, a term that describes the appearance of blood that has been denatured by gastric acid. Obviously, hematemesis is a powerful historic feature that strongly supports upper GI bleeding. However, some patients may bleed from their upper GI tract (esophagus, stomach, or duodenum) and may not present with hematemesis. For this reason, placement of a NG tube with sampling of the gastric contents represents a rapid and highly effective mechanism for determining the location of bleeding. This is best performed in a cooperative patient in the upright position once fluid resuscitation has been initiated. The NG tube is lubricated and passed slowly and gently through the nose, and the patient is asked to swallow this tube along with sips of water. By injecting a small volume of air while auscultating over the gastric contour, one can hear a rush of air to ensure that the tube has been placed in the GI tract. Following this, a 60-ml syringe is used to aspirate gastric contents. If gross blood is seen, the tube can be left in place and lavage initiated to facilitate visualization of the gastric mucosa during subsequent endoscopy and determine the volume and extent of hemorrhage. If no gastric contents are returned, small amounts of water may be instilled and gastric suction repeated.

In an unstable or uncooperative patient or one whose mental status is such that he or she may not be able to protect the airway, elective intubation should be considered. This is particularly important in patients with massive hematemesis who are at risk for aspirating blood. If the NG aspirate is clear or demonstrates obvious gastric contents (undigested food), one cannot entirely exclude an upper GI source. Patients with duodenal bleeding may demonstrate pyloric scarring or spasm, which prevents the reflux of duodenal contents into the stomach. Up to 16% of patients with upper GI bleeding will have a clear NG lavage.

The presence of bile in the NG lavage suggests communication between duodenal contents and gastric contents and greatly increases the diagnostic accuracy of the NG lavage. This point is well illustrated in the clinical case.

Another key historical feature in the workup of patients with GI hemorrhage involves the quantity and characteristics of the stool, which are strongly dependent on the site and extent of GI bleeding and the bowel transit time. *Melena* describes the black, tarry, loose, malodorous stool that is formed from the bacterial degradation of hemoglobin in patients who have blood in the GI tract. Its presence suggests bleeding from the upper GI tract or small bowel; however, it is also seen in patients with right colonic bleeding and slow bowel transit. Conversely, massive bleeding from an upper GI source that traverses rapidly through the bowel can present as a bright-red rectal bleeding (hematochezia), as demonstrated in the clinical case. "Currant jelly" stool or maroon stool may accompany a small bowel or right colonic bleed. Red blood marbled into normal formed brown stool suggests a bleed in the left colon. Bright-red blood that coats the outside of a normal brown stool, drips freely into the toilet, or is seen on the toilet paper suggests an anorectal source. Obviously, a digital examination to sample the stool in the rectal vault and to palpate for gross abnormalities, including impaction and rectal masses, is a crucial part of the initial assessment of patients with acute GI bleeding.

Initial blood work may also help localize bleeding. Blood represents a large protein load in the GI tract, and patients with bleeding from the upper GI tract manifest an elevated BUN:creatinine ratio. A ratio greater than 25 is highly suggestive of upper GI bleeding and may be used as an independent indication for evaluating the upper GI tract, regardless of the characteristics of the stool on presentation or the findings of the NG aspirate. The patient in the clinical case had a BUN:creatinine ratio of 40.

The initial history and physical examination are performed once fluid resuscitation has been initiated and should focus on key issues that help determine the diagnostic workup over the next several hours. With respect to the history, certainly the physician should determine the onset of the bleeding, whether there were any previous episodes of bleeding, and whether there is associated abdominal pain. Upper quadrant pain in association with bleeding can be seen with ulcer disease, gastritis, and ischemic bowel. Lower quadrant pain and bleeding may be associated with IBD, colonic ischemia, or infectious diarrhea. Rectal pain may be associated with anal fissures or thrombosed hemorrhoids. The patient's age is important in determining the cause and location of the bleeding. Disease entities that cause bleeding are greatly influenced by the age of the patient, with ischemia, angiodysplasia, and neoplasia much more prevalent in the elderly. Medical history is clearly important. Patients with liver disease are at risk of portal hypertensive bleeding. Patients with preexisting IBD may bleed from this condition. Patients with peptic ulcer disease (PUD) may have recurrences.

Patients with collagen vascular or other rheumatologic disease may have associated vasculitis that predisposes to GI bleeding.

Patients should be thoroughly questioned regarding their medication intake. Ingestion of aspirin and other NSAIDs puts the patient at risk for GI bleeding. The presence of anticoagulants should also be investigated. Finally, family history of a bleeding diathesis should be elicited. With respect to the patient's habits, a smoking history is important because it is associated with PUD as well as the development of GI malignant neoplasms. Alcohol intake may be associated with liver disease, Mallory-Weiss tears, and chronic pancreatitis, all of which may contribute to the cause of bleeding. The patient in the clinical case had a history of PUD, NSAID use, alcohol abuse, and pancreatitis, all of which may directly or indirectly induce GI bleeding.

The focused physical examination should look first for stigmata of volume loss and hydration status. The turgor of the skin and moisture of the mucous membranes may help determine whether a patient is volume depleted. Vital signs should be measured and blood pressure checked when the patient is both lying down and standing. Examination of the skin should look for cutaneous lesions associated with GI hemorrhage, such as hereditary telangiectasia. Cutaneous stigmata of chronic liver disease, including palmar erythema, spider angiomata, gynecomastia, testicular atrophy, Dupuytren's contractures, caput medusae, splenomegaly, and jaundice, are key features. The cutaneous lesions associated with IBD, including erythema nodosum and pyoderma gangrenosum, should be investigated. Examination of the abdomen focuses on the presence or absence of bowel sounds, evidence of peritonitis, or evidence of splenomegaly, hepatomegaly, arterial bruits, or venous hums. The presence of abdominal scars from previous surgery should be noted. Finally, digital rectal examination determines whether there is melena in the rectal vault, bright-red blood, maroon stool, fecal impaction, rectal mass, hemorrhoids, or fissures. This directed history and physical examination can be accomplished in a matter of minutes.

Notes

Aspirin and other NSAIDs are commonly used over-the-counter medications that can cause GI ulceration and bleeding.

CASE STUDY: CONTINUED

The patient was typed and cross-matched and received 6 units of blood; his hematocrit rose to 30% following transfusion. His hemodynamic status improved, and he became normotensive with no orthostatic changes. A CT scan of the abdomen demonstrated evidence of pancreatitis with pancreatic edema and peripancreatic fat stranding. There was no evidence of pancreatic necrosis. The spleen was enlarged, and there was evidence of splenic vein thrombosis. Perisplenic and perigastric varices were seen. The liver appeared enlarged and hypodense, which is consistent with fatty infiltration. There were no mass lesions noted and no intraperitoneal or retroperitoneal air. The stomach was distended, and there was a large air-contrast fluid level.

Gastroenterology consultation was obtained. An urgent upper endoscopy demonstrated a normal esophagus with no evidence for varices or ulcerations. The gastroesophageal junction was normal with no evidence for a Mallory-Weiss tear. The stomach was entered, dilated, and filled with residual radiologic contrast and fluid, which was then aspirated. A detailed examination of the gastric mucosa demonstrated small varices in the fundus with no stigmata of recent or impending hemorrhage. There was no evidence of portal hypertensive gastropathy. The antrum was normal with no vascular ectasia. The pylorus appeared scarred and narrowed. It was traversed with difficulty, and a 2-cm ulcer crater with a visible vessel was found in the posterior duodenum. No active bleeding was seen. After 8 ml 1:10,000 epinephrine were injected in a circumferential fashion around the ulcer base, cautery was applied, using a bipolar probe set at 15 watts, for a total of 60 seconds in six 10-second applications. Antral biopsy specimens were taken for a CLO test, which turned positive immediately, indicating the presence of *Helicobacter pylori*.

Secondary Diagnostic Evaluations

At this point in the patient's presentation, it is crucial to determine whether the bleeding is occurring in the upper or lower GI tract. If the patient gives a history of melena, the NG lavage shows blood or coffee grounds material, the digital rectal examination exhibits melena, or the BUN:creatinine ratio is greater than or equal to 25, the possibility of upper GI bleeding should be strongly considered and an urgent endoscopy performed.

The particular roles of endoscopy for diagnosis and therapy are addressed in the sections that follow on specific causes of bleeding. In general, endoscopy has evolved into a powerful diagnostic and therapeutic tool, which has recently been demonstrated to change the patient outcomes in upper GI hemorrhage, decreasing the need for surgery, the number of blood transfusions, and the length of stay in the hospital and improving overall survival. An upper endoscopic examination can result in (1) a lesion found and treated successfully, (2) a lesion found that cannot be treated endoscopically, (3) no lesion found but evidence of blood in the upper GI tract, or (4) no lesion found and no stigmata of recent or impending bleeding. Each of these circumstances may prompt further investigations, and early consultation with surgeons and interventional radiologists is crucial to the optimal management of patients with both upper and lower GI bleeding.

In the absence of criteria for upper endoscopy, diagnostic modalities to evaluate the lower GI tract are slightly more problematic. Fecal matter throughout the colon must be evacuated to evaluate the colon thoroughly for potential sources of bleeding via an endoscopic route. If a patient is having bright-red rectal bleeding, anoscopy or flexible sigmoidoscopy can be performed quickly in the emergency room to rule out a rectal or perirectal source. If the patient is hemodynamically stable, the physician may leave a NG tube in place and prepare the patient with a cleansing solution to allow visualization of the colon 4–6 hours later. A polyethylene glycol solution is typically used at a rate of 1 L every 30 minutes. A prokinetic agent (such as metoclopramide) can be administered intravenously to facilitate bowel transit and increase the rapidity of the cleansing. Once stool and clotted blood have been expelled from the colon with the use of purging agents, a colonoscopy can be safely and effectively performed at the patient's bedside.

If the patient is hemodynamically unstable, an angiography may be performed to help localize the site of bleeding. In this procedure, the mesenteric arterial tree is approached from a femoral artery puncture, and selective catheterization of branches of the superior mesenteric and inferior mesenteric arteries can be performed to look for extravasation of contrast in the bowel lumen. Treatment of bleeding colonic lesions with transcatheter embolization or administration of vasoconstricting agents (such as vasopressin) can provide temporary or definitive management of lower GI bleeding. Less commonly, these approaches can be used to treat upper GI bleeding, accessing the celiac artery and its branches. If patients are hemodynamically stable and no lesions are found at colonoscopy but bleeding is continuous or intermittent, a nuclear-tagged RBC study can be performed. In these studies, the patient's RBCs are labeled with a radioactive agent and then reintroduced into the bloodstream. Extravasation of the radiographic material into the bowel lumen can be monitored with a scintigraphic camera. These studies require bleeding at a rate of 0.1 ml/min and thus are fairly sensitive. However, they suffer from poor localization, and many have questioned their clinical utility in an acute setting.

There is no role for barium radiography in the acute management of upper or lower GI bleeding. The barium coats the colonic mucosa and most frequently does not reveal mucosal lesions that are associated with bleeding. Furthermore, there is no therapeutic potential, and the presence of the radiopaque barium may even obscure the lesion and prevent the endoscopist from treating it or the interventional radiologist from pursuing angiography.

Early surgical consultation is important; however, it must be emphasized that mortality from operative interventions for GI bleeding is profoundly increased in those patients in whom an exact and accurate localization of the bleeding has not taken place preoperatively. Thus, every effort should be made to localize bleeding before sending patients for surgical management. PUD that has not responded to endoscopic therapy or has perforated must be managed surgically. Portal hypertensive bleeding may require shunt surgery, although transjugular intrahepatic portal systemic shunt (TIPSS) has greatly diminished the incidence of emergency shunt surgery. Colonic surgery for bleeding diverticula and neoplastic lesions of the large and small bowel may be required.

Table 30-3. Major Causes of GI Bleeding

UPPER GASTROINTESTINAL BLEEDING	LOWER GASTROINTESTINAL BLEEDING
Peptic ulcer disease	Angiodysplasia
Portal hypertension (varices and portal hypertensive gastropathy)	Diverticular bleeding
Esophagitis and gastritis	Hemorrhoids
Mallory-Weiss tears	Neoplasms and polyps
Mucosal damage related to nonsteroidal anti-inflammatory drugs	Acute occlusive and nonocclusive intestinal ischemia
Angiodysplasia	Inflammatory bowel disease
Watermelon stomach	Meckel's diverticulum
Aortoenteric fistulas	Infectious disease
Dieulafoy's malformation	Solitary rectal ulcer
Acute occlusive and nonocclusive intestinal ischemia	
Neoplasms	

Specific Causes of Upper GI Bleeding

Individual lesions that cause GI bleeding are discussed in detail next (Table 30-3).

PUD

Ulcers are one of the most common causes of upper GI bleeding. Typical peptic ulcers may be found in the lower esophagus, the stomach, and, most often, in the duodenum. Ulcer formation occurs when there is an imbalance in the homeostatic factors responsible for injury to the GI mucosa and the natural host defenses of the mucosa. Hydrochloric acid (HCl), produced by the parietal cells in the stomach, was the earliest factor recognized as capable of damaging the lining of the upper GI tract and leading to ulcer formation. However, the quantity of acid that is normally produced by individuals is insufficient to produce ulceration in the absence of factors that impair the natural mucosal defense mechanisms. Hypersecretors of acid, such as patients with gastrin-producing tumors (Zollinger-Ellison syndrome), develop multiple ulcers. A variety of physical stresses can both increase acid production and inhibit natural mucosal defenses and thus increase the incidence of ulcers (Table 30-4).

Table 30-4. Causes of Stress Ulcers

HIGH RISK	MEDIUM RISK	LOW RISK
Major burns	Major cardiothoracic surgery	Long-term mechanical ventilation
Major trauma	Sepsis	Acute renal failure
Severe head injuries	Acute mechanical ventilation	Hepatic failure

H. pylori has been strongly associated with the formation of duodenal ulcers. About 95% of patients with a duodenal ulcer and 75% of patients with gastric ulcers have *H. pylori* infection. Medical therapy for PUD (see Chapter 11), including H_2-receptor antagonists and proton pump inhibitors together with antibiotics to eradicate *H. pylori*, facilitates the healing of ulcers but should not be considered as therapy for acute bleeding in patients with PUD. Ulcer recurrence can be reduced by medical therapy once the acute bleeding has resolved and the ulcer is healed. Antibiotic therapy directed at *H. pylori* also greatly diminishes the risk of ulcer recurrence and the long-term risks of rebleeding from PUD. The patient in the case study had a previous duodenal ulcer and *H. pylori* infection. Thus, antibiotic therapy was crucial in his subsequent management. Finally, the ingestion of aspirin and other NSAIDs, many of which are purchased over the counter and taken for common aches and pains, are a common cause of both direct mucosal injury and impaired mucosal defenses.

A number of factors impact on the survival and outcome of patients with peptic ulcer bleeding, including the patient's age, the presence of comorbid illness (see Table 30-1), the location and size of the ulcer, the number of transfusions required, and the presence or absence of high-risk stigmata in the ulcer. Active bleeding coming from an ulcer base with a visible vessel when seen during endoscopy represents the highest-risk stigmata. Although bleeding may stop spontaneously, rebleeding should be expected in about 80% of cases, and the presence of active bleeding warrants endoscopic intervention. This intervention may include the injection of vasoconstrictive substances, such as epinephrine; the injection of sclerosing agents, including absolute alcohol; or the application of thermal energy using a bipolar probe or heater probe. Placement of vascular clips over bleeding vessels at endoscopy is also being studied.

The bleeding source of ulcers usually occurs when the acute inflammatory process invades small arterioles that run in the submucosa, resulting in active bleeding. If the body's hemostatic mechanisms control and arrest this acute episode of bleeding, a "visible vessel" may be seen protruding from the ulcer base on subsequent endoscopy. This visible vessel actually represents an adherent thrombus lying over the vessel and, if encountered during endoscopy, also represents a high-risk lesion; about 50% of patients rebleed unless active intervention is taken. Again, injection therapy or thermal therapy applied to visible vessels reduces the incidence of rebleeding. It is not uncommon to find a large clot overlying an ulcer base. If no active bleeding is seen coming from underneath, it is unclear whether active intervention should be undertaken to remove the clot and treat any underlying stigmata in the ulcer base. A flat, pigmented spot on an ulcer base represents further evidence of healing in a patient who has had an upper GI hemorrhage from PUD. The incidence of rebleeding from this lesion is lower than 10%; thus, endoscopic intervention is not justified. Finally, the risk of rebleeding from an ulcer with a clean,

H. pylori is a bacterium that infects the upper GI tract and is associated with gastric and duodenal ulcers.

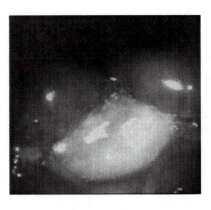

Fig. 30-1. A Large Gastric Ulcer with a Clean Base

flat, white base is less than 5%, and endoscopic intervention and perhaps further hospitalization are not required when such a lesion is encountered at endoscopy (Figure 30-1).

Ulcers caused by NSAIDs may be seen anywhere in the GI tract, including the small intestine and colon; however, they are most commonly found in the stomach. The endoscopic stigmata associated with peptic ulcers can be seen with NSAID ulcers, and the indications for treatment are the same. Avoidance of NSAIDs, if possible, along with acid reduction therapy is the mainstay of medical management. Ulcers that defy endoscopic management or that rebleed after endoscopic management should be considered high risk and may be indications for subsequent therapy with angiography or surgery.

Because of the risk of potential malignancy, all patients with gastric ulcers at the time of endoscopy should have a follow-up endoscopy in 8 weeks after treatment to document healing of the ulcer.

PORTAL HYPERTENSIVE BLEEDING

The pressure in any closed system is directly proportional to the resistance and flow in that system. Portal hypertensive GI bleeding results when portal blood trying to return to the right heart is interrupted. As portal pressure rises, the elevated portal pressure opens collateral pathways to return to the right heart. These collateral pathways lie in proximity to the GI mucosa; as these collateral vessels dilate with increasing pressure, the wall tension increases, and these vessels may rupture and bleed massively. The most common cause of portal hypertension is cirrhosis of the liver. In the process of cirrhosis, the normal vascular spaces within the liver that provide low resistance to portal blood flow are altered as a result of changes in their endothelial lining and fibrosis of the hepatic parenchyma. These physiologic alterations increase resistance to flow and circulating volume. In addition, hemodynamic alterations in cirrhosis increase the splanchnic blood flow. Collateral vessels then develop, resulting in the formation of esophageal varices and gastric varices (Figure 30-2). Noncirrhotic portal hypertension can be seen in patients with schistosomiasis, Budd-Chiari syndrome, and

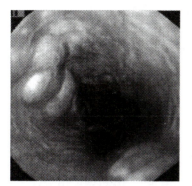

Fig. 30-2. Esophageal Varix with Active Bleeding

portal or splenic vein thrombosis resulting from mechanical obstruction of portal venous flow without underlying liver disease.

Splenic vein thrombosis, as seen in the case study, is most often caused by extension of direct inflammation in patients with acute or chronic pancreatitis or pancreatic malignancy. It may also be seen in patients with a hypercoagulable state. In this condition, blood is directly shunted through the short gastric venous system to produce gastric varices in the absence of esophageal varices. The finding at endoscopy of isolated gastric varices in a patient with upper GI bleeding indicates splenic vein thrombosis, particularly in the absence of underlying liver disease. Splenectomy is the treatment of choice in these patients when surgery is an option. In some patients with portal hypertension, blood may be rerouted through the hemorrhoidal vein system, and rectal varices may present with massive hematochezia. Finally, intra-abdominal varices may present as GI bleeding, particularly at sites of previous bowel anastomosis.

Portal hypertensive bleeding, most notably from esophageal varices, is usually massive and catastrophic. Such bleeding accounts for one-third of all deaths in cirrhotics, and the mortality rate for first variceal hemorrhages is around 20% in patients with preserved hepatic synthetic function and 60% for patients in liver failure. Therapy for bleeding esophageal and gastric varices is directed at eradicating the varices and lowering the portal pressure. Hemodynamic studies have demonstrated that variceal bleeding does not occur until the hepatic venous portal pressure gradient exceeds 12 mm Hg. Pharmacologic agents used to lower portal pressure include somatostatin and vasopressin, the latter used with nitroglycerin to avoid systemic side effects and augment its effects on portal pressure. Both agents decrease splanchnic blood flow and lower portal pressure. Therapeutic maneuvers to lower portal pressure include emergency shunt surgery (creation of a portosystemic conduit) or TIPSS placed by angiography.

Endoscopic treatment of variceal bleeding includes injection sclerotherapy and now more often band ligation. During injection sclerotherapy, sclerosing agents are injected into and around varices to cause vascular thrombosis and scarring in the adjacent tissue. This

therapy has been shown to be highly effective but is associated with local and systemic complications in nearly one-third of patients. Band ligation is a technique in which rubber bands are placed around the bleeding varices, which are sucked into a channel at the tip of the endoscope. These bands cause immediate thrombosis of the varices and then fall off over a period of 3–7 days. This technique has proven to be as effective as sclerotherapy, resulting in good control of acute bleeding in up to 90% of patients with many fewer complications compared with sclerotherapy. Once bleeding has been controlled, patients return for endoscopy at defined intervals and have any remaining varices electively eradicated by one of the above-mentioned techniques.

In addition, pharmacologic therapy with oral beta-blockers and nitrates may prevent rebleeding in patients who have presented with acute variceal bleeding and also may prevent the first episode of bleeding in patients with large esophageal varices. Shunt surgery may be considered for patients with recurrent bleeding and preserved liver function, whereas liver transplantation is reserved for patients with recurrent bleeding and poor liver function. For patients with active variceal bleeding failing endoscopic therapy, placement of a Sengstaken-Blakemore tube may be performed pending definitive treatment with TIPSS or surgery. The principle of pressure or tamponade to stop bleeding is the basis for this treatment modality; however, it is associated with a high complication rate.

MALLORY-WEISS TEAR

A Mallory-Weiss tear is a linear disruption in the gastric mucosa located high in the stomach on the gastric side of the gastroesophageal junction. The mechanism of injury is thought to be traumatic, that is, from retching-induced prolapse of the gastric mucosa into the esophagus. However, a history of antecedent retching is elicited only in 50% of patients with Mallory-Weiss tears. These lesions are more frequently seen in patients who abuse alcohol. They may be visualized at endoscopy, typically with the scope turned in a retroflexed position. Although they may bleed profusely, their natural history is fairly benign. Endoscopic therapy with injection or thermal agents may be applied, and angiography and surgery are rarely needed.

VASCULAR LESIONS OF THE UPPER GI TRACT

A variety of vascular lesions may be seen in the upper GI tract and are associated with acute upper GI bleeding. Most often, these are angiodysplasias in elderly individuals and may be found in the stomach or duodenum at endoscopy. They are best treated by thermal ablation. Gastric antral vascular ectasia is an interesting vascular lesion that is found most commonly in patients with collagen vascular diseases or chronic liver diseases. The ectatic vascular lesions take on a linear appearance, longitudinally directed from the pylorus and involving the distal stomach. These red strips look like the stripes on a watermelon, and thus this lesion has been called watermelon stomach

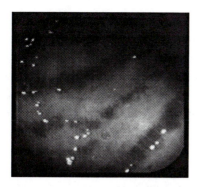

Fig. 30-3. Watermelon Stomach in a 50-Year-Old Woman with Scleroderma

(Figure 30-3). These lesions may be treated successfully with endoscopic thermal ablation using contact probes or lasers. Surgical antrectomy may be required in difficult cases.

True arteriovenous malformations, or hemangiomas, are rare lesions responsible for upper GI bleeding and may also be treated endoscopically. Dieulafoy's malformation is a relatively uncommon cause of massive upper GI arterial bleeding. The source of bleeding is a normal arteriole that, relative to its size, is running too close to the GI mucosa. The mechanism responsible for the mucosal damage that leads to rupture of these "caliber-persistent arteries," with subsequent massive bleeding, is unclear, but the lesions may be more commonly seen with a history of alcohol intake or NSAID consumption. The hallmark of Dieulafoy's lesions is rapid, abrupt bleeding that stops spontaneously. Bleeding can be massive, and patients frequently present in shock. Most often, on endoscopic evaluation, no mucosal abnormalities are noted. If endoscopy is performed during active bleeding and blood in the stomach can be evacuated to facilitate complete visualization, active arterial bleeding is usually seen spurting from a mound of normal mucosa. Occasionally, a mound of mucosa with an adherent clot or a small crater (so-called volcano sign) may be encountered. If one is lucky enough to see one of these lesions, they are amenable to endoscopic treatment. It is difficult to visualize these lesions angiographically unless they are actively bleeding. Once again, angiographic therapy can be undertaken if the lesions are recognized. Wedge resections of the stomach and, in extreme cases, total gastrectomies have been performed. Furthermore, Dieulafoy's lesions, although most often seen in the proximal stomach, have been reported almost anywhere in the GI tract and may be responsible for both upper and lower GI bleeding.

Specific Causes of Lower GI Bleeding

DIVERTICULOSIS

Diverticula are herniations of the colonic mucosa through defects in the muscularis layer resulting in the formation of pseudodiverticula. This condition is very common and is found in 50% of individuals over the

Endoscopy can accurately diagnose and treat most upper GI bleeding lesions and many lower GI bleeding lesions. Endoscopic management has improved patient outcomes for bleeding from peptic ulcers and for variceal bleeding.

age of 60 on a Western diet but is rare in countries with high-fiber diets (e.g., Africa). For this reason, despite the fact that only 5% of patients with diverticular disease bleed significantly, diverticulosis represents one of the most common causes of lower GI bleeding in the United States. Although diverticula are most common in the left colon, bleeding is seen most often from diverticula in the right colon. Bleeding occurs as a diverticulum expands and involves the lining of small arterioles running adjacent to it. Thus, bleeding is usually arterial and brisk. Most of these episodes stop spontaneously, but recurrent bleeding may occur.

The diagnosis of diverticular bleeding is usually inferred when the evaluation of a patient with acute lower GI bleeding fails to confirm another source of bleeding. On occasion, bleeding directly from a diverticulum is seen at the time of colonoscopy. Recent studies indicate that bleeding can be treated endoscopically with injection or thermal methods as described for peptic ulcer bleeding. A bleeding site may be seen during angiography, and it is inferred that the source is diverticular on the basis of the caliber of the artery and the absence of subsequent lesions discovered during colonoscopy. These lesions can be treated angiographically with transcatheter embolization or transcatheter administration of vasoconstricting substances. Recurrent diverticular bleeding is an indication for surgical resection of the involved colon. Once again, accurate localization of the bleeding site is critical to optimize the outcome of surgery. Diverticulosis may be seen in the small intestine with subsequent bleeding. This is quite rare, but when seen, it is most common in the jejunum. Like colonic bleeding, this bleeding is painless, but it is more difficult to diagnosis than colonic diverticular bleeding because of the inaccessibility of most of the small bowel to endoscopic approaches.

ANGIODYSPLASIA

Angiodysplasias are vascular lesions of the colon represent a common source of significant lower GI bleeding, accounting for 6% of all cases. These lesions may be found in up to 6% of the population and are most frequently diagnosed at colonoscopy, where they appear as spiderlike vascular prominences, occasionally with a visualized feeding arteriole or draining vein. When these lesions are large enough, they can be visualized with angiography. Light thermal ablation at colonoscopy represents the most effective treatment. Active bleeding during angiography can be controlled with embolization. These lesions may also be seen in the upper GI tract and small intestine and can be treated with thermal ablation. Medical management of these lesions with oral estrogen preparations with or without progesterone is not effective. Most commonly these lesions present as painless chronic blood loss, but occasionally they bleed significantly.

HEMORRHOIDS

Hemorrhoids occur in more than 50% of individuals in the United States, and bleeding internal hemorrhoids represents the most common cause of all lower GI bleeding in adults. Hemorrhoids present with scant hematochezia, but occasionally they bleed massively. A number of theories have been proposed as to the pathogenesis of hemorrhoids, but none has been validated. Recurrent hemorrhoidal bleeding can be treated conservatively with topical anti-inflammatory agents and increased fiber in the diet. Rubber-band ligation can be performed on internal hemorrhoids, as can injection sclerotherapy, cryosurgery, electrocoagulation, laser ablation, and photocoagulation. Finally, excisional surgery may be required.

IBD

Both ulcerative colitis and Crohn's disease commonly cause mucosal injury that results in GI blood loss; however, the requirement for transfusion and the presentation as hemodynamically significant GI bleeding are relatively uncommon, occurring in about 5% of cases. Bleeding usually subsides with the rapid institution of aggressive medical therapy; however, profuse bleeding has been considered an indication for surgery.

Less common causes of inflammatory or immune GI bleeding include vasculitis, diversion colitis, infectious diarrhea, and graft-versus-host disease. These entities are reviewed separately and are beyond the scope of this chapter.

MECHANICAL INJURY

Lower GI bleeding may occur following endoscopic manipulation, including biopsies and removal of polyps. Most of these lesions can be treated during endoscopy, if they are immediately recognized following the procedure or during follow-up endoscopy if bleeding has been delayed.

The solitary rectal ulcer syndrome is a benign, chronic ulcerative disease involving the internal lateral wall of the rectum. There is a close association with mechanical trauma from rectal prolapse. These lesions present with painful bowel movements (dyschezia) and associated rectal bleeding. They may be diagnosed at endoscopy and may be treated with topical agents, including anti-inflammatory medications delivered via enema, or operative resection for refractory cases.

NSAID intake may also be associated with lower GI bleeding, most commonly in the small intestine but occasionally in the colon.

VASCULAR INSULTS

Arterioenteric fistulas are an uncommon cause of massive GI bleeding. These most often occur in the duodenum following aortic graft surgery but may be seen more distally in the GI tract. They may cause catastrophic, fatal bleeding and can be treated with emergent surgical repair if recognized early by endoscopy, CT scan, or angiography.

Mesenteric ischemia may present with GI bleeding. These patients usually have pain out of proportion to physical findings. Small bowel ischemia is often fatal and can present with GI bleeding described as currant jelly stool. If an elderly patient with vascular disease presents with abdominal pain out of proportion to the physical findings associated with lower GI bleeding, urgent surgical evaluation should be considered with or without preceding angiography.

Colonic ischemia may also present with lower GI bleeding. These patients are not as systemically ill as patients with small bowel ischemia, and most resolve spontaneously, with less than 50% requiring surgical management.

NEOPLASMS

Malignant neoplasms of the GI tract, either primary or metastatic, can present with significant GI bleeding. At colonoscopy, colonic tumors can be visualized. Tumor bleeding is best controlled by surgical excision of the involved bowel. Metastatic tumors with a high proclivity for GI tract metastasis and hemorrhage include melanoma and renal cell cancers, although a variety of primary malignant neoplasms can also present in this manner (Figure 30-4). Endoscopic treatment of these lesions is usually ineffective, and surgical extraction or angiographic embolization are the best treatments.

LESS COMMON LESIONS

As in upper GI bleeding, Dieulafoy's malformation, true arteriovenous malformations, and portal hypertensive bleeding may be encountered in the colon and small bowel. Their diagnosis may be more difficult because of the time required for colonic cleansing, and endoscopic treatment is less commonly reported. Finally, Meckel's diverticulum is the most common congenital abnormality of the GI tract, with an incidence that ranges up to 4%. Fifty percent of these diverticula contain heterotopic tissue, the most common being gastric mucosa, which is found in over 60% of cases. This gastric mucosa is active and can produce acid, with resulting ulceration and bleeding in the adjacent mucosa. Bleeding is the most common presentation of a Meckel's diverticulum in children and is seen most frequently in the first 2 years of life. The diagnosis is based on a high index of clinical

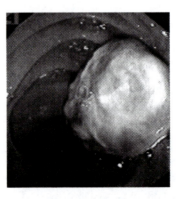

Fig. 30-4. Renal Cell Cancer Metastasized to the Small Bowel, Presenting with Massive GI Bleeding

suspicion and is confirmed at angiography or suggested by using a technetium pertechnetate scan, which demonstrates heterotopic gastric mucosa in the right lower quadrant. Surgical resection represents definitive therapy.

Summary

GI bleeding is a common medical condition that requires a multidisciplinary team approach (Figure 30-5). Initial management involves assessment and correction of acute volume depletion. Next, localization of the bleeding is critical. Endoscopy has evolved into a powerful tool, not only in diagnosing upper and lower GI bleeding lesions but also in applying therapy. Endoscopic treatment of peptic ulcer bleeding and esophageal variceal bleeding has improved patient outcome. Angiographic techniques offer a complementary approach to endoscopic evaluation, and early input from surgeons is critical to determine the need for and timing of operative interventions.

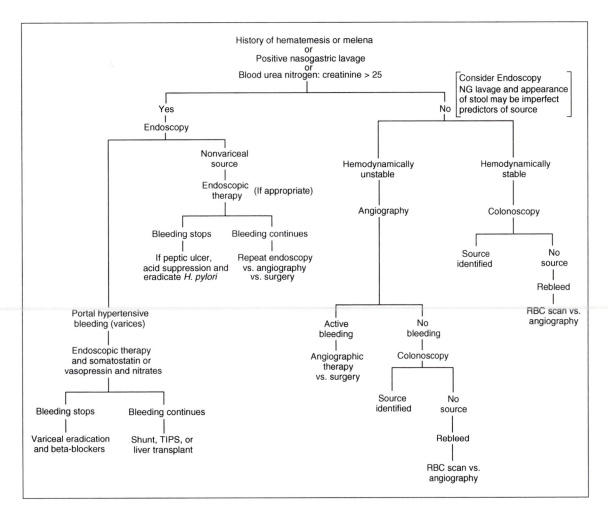

Fig. 30-5. Algorithm for Management of Gastrointestinal Bleeding

RBC = red blood cell; TIPS = transjugular intrahepatic portal systemic shunts.

*R*EVIEW *Q*UESTIONS

Directions: For each of the following questions, choose the one best answer.

1 Which of the following statements regarding colonic diverticulosis is *true?*

A It involves true diverticula containing all layers of the colonic wall.
B Diverticula are more often found in the right colon.
C Diverticular bleeding is more often seen in the right colon.
D It is rare in the United States.

2 GI bleeding is best managed by a(n)

A gastroenterologist.
B surgeon.
C interventional radiologist.
D multidisciplinary team.

3 Which of the following statements regarding GI bleeding is *true?*

A The hematocrit is always abnormal early in the course of an acute GI bleed.
B A clear aspirate from a NG tube ensures that the patient is not having an upper GI bleed.
C *H. pylori* is an infectious agent that is associated with peptic ulcers.
D Portal pressure rises in patients with cirrhosis may lead to variceal bleeding and is due to increased vascular resistance and decreased circulating plasma volume.

4 Which of the following statements concerning bleeding from esophageal varices is *true*?

   A Bleeding is often minimal and does not necessarily require blood transfusions.
   B Variceal bleeding is not affected by the hepatic venous pressure gradient.
   C Treatment may include sclerotherapy, banding, transjugular intrahepatic portal systemic shunts, or surgery.
   D The mortality rate of a first variceal bleed is 20% in patients with liver failure.

References

Beejay U: Acute gastrointestinal bleeding in the intensive care unit. The gastroenterologist's perspective. *Gastroenterol Clin North Am* 9(2): 309–336, 2000.

Besson I, Ingrand P, Person B, et al: Sclerotherapy with or without octreotide for acute variceal bleeding. *N Engl J Med* 333:555–560, 1995.

Cappell MS: Management of gastrointestinal bleeding induced by gastrointestinal endoscopy. *Gastroenterol Clin North Am* 29(1):125–167, vi–vii, 2000.

Comar KM: Portal hypertensive bleeding. *Gastroenterol Clin North Am* 32(4):1079–1105, 2003.

Huang CS: Nonvariceal upper gastrointestinal bleeding. *Gastroenterol Clin North Am* 32(4):1053–1078, 2003.

Jensen DM, Machicado GA: Colonoscopy for diagnosis and treatment of severe lower gastrointestinal bleeding. Routine outcomes and cost analysis. *Gastrointest Endosc Clin N Am* 7:477–498, 1997.

Jensen DM, Machicado GA, Jutabha R, et al: Urgent colonoscopy for the diagnosis and treatment of severe diverticular hemorrhage. *N Engl J Med* 342:78–82, 2000.

Laine L: Non-steroidal anti-inflammatory drug gastropathy. *Gastrointest Endosc Clin N Am* 6:489–504, 1996.

Laine L, Cook D: Endoscopic ligation compared with sclerotherapy for treatment of esophageal variceal bleeding. A meta-analysis. *Ann Intern Med* 123:280–287, 1995.

Laine L, Peterson ML: Bleeding peptic ulcer. *N Engl J Med* 331:717–727, 1994.

Luketic VA: Esophageal varices. I. Clinical presentation, medical therapy, and endoscopic therapy. *Gastroenterol Clin North Am* 9(2):337–385, 2000.

Luketic VA: Esophageal varices. II. TIPS (transjugular intrahepatic portosystemic shunt) and surgical therapy. *Gastroenterol Clin North Am* 29(2):387–421, vi, 2000.

Miller LS, Barbarevech C, Friedman CS: Less frequent causes of lower gastrointestinal bleeding. *Gastroenterol Clin North Am* 23:20–52, 1994.

Reinus JF, Brandt LJ: Vascular ectasias and diverticulosis. *Gastroenterol Clin North Am* 23:1–20, 1994.

Savides TJ: Therapeutic endoscopy for nonvariceal gastrointestinal bleeding. *Gastroenterol Clin North Am* 29(2):465–487, vii, 2000.

Walsh JH, Peterson WL: The treatment of *Helicobacter pylori* infection in the management of peptic ulcer disease. *N Engl J Med* 333:984–991, 1995.

Answers and Explanations

Chapter 1

1. **The answer is C.** Hepatocellular carcinoma is the leading cause of cancer death worldwide and is related to the endemic occurrence of hepatitis. Colon cancer is the second leading cause of cancer mortality in the United States.

2. **The answer is D.** Nearly one-third (33%) of all cancers in the United States originate in the GI tract. Colon cancer is the second leading cause of cancer death in this country.

3. **The answer is A.** The fundus and body serve a reservoir function and regulate the speed of emptying of liquids. The mixing and grinding food and regulation of the speed of emptying solids are functions of the antrum. The pylorus separates the stomach from the small intestine and prevents postprandial duodenogastric reflux.

4. **The answer is C.** The villi are located in the small intestine. The main functions of the small intestine are absorption and secretion. The functional unit of the small intestine is the villus. In the human species, the cells lining the villi are renewed every 5–6 days. In celiac disease, the villi are flattened, resulting in decreased absorption capacity and subsequent diarrhea.

5. **The answer is B.** Proximal small bowel disorders such as celiac disease may affect absorption of vitamins, iron, and magnesium, whereas disorders of the terminal ileum, such as Crohn's disease, may result in vitamin B_{12} deficiency.

6. **The answer is C.** The enteric nervous system is an intrinsic, semiautonomous network of nerves that mediates specific events controlled by reflex responses. The enteric nervous system is an impressively large system and contains many more neurons than the spinal cord. Its cell bodies can reflexively control complex functions in the absence of input from the autonomic or voluntary nervous system. The myenteric plexus and Meissner's plexus contain the cell bodies of the enteric nervous system. The most abundant class of transmitters in the enteric nervous system and neuroendocrine cells are regulatory peptides. Each peptide may have a multitude of effects, depending on the site tested. Regulatory peptides may be released as neurotransmitters, paracrine transmitters, or hormones.

Chapter 2

1. **The answer is A.** The initial inflammatory reaction that develops in a patient who has appendicitis is often difficult to localize and presents one of the greatest challenges general surgeons and gastroenterologists see in clinical practice. As the appendix becomes distended, afferent nerves in the mesentery become activated, and the patient becomes more clearly aware that the pain is localized to the right lower quadrant. This enhanced recognition of location occurs through somatic neural pathways traveling through the spinothalamic tract. Autocrine control mechanisms are those mechanisms that feed back to the same cell that released a transmitter. A classic example of this is the release of somatostatin by mucosal endocrine cells and its feedback to

itself to further reduce secretion of somatostatin. Another example of paracrine-type secretion is the increased secretory response in the mucosal injury that is mediated by the release of cytokines and transmitters from mucosal immune cells that have been activated by mucosal injury. An example of this is the increased secretion of hydrochloric acid by parietal cells that are stimulated through the release of histamine by mucosal mast cells. Local injury can also result in distention of the lumen, which will result in proximal contraction and distal relaxation to induce a peristaltic sequence. These sequences are reflexively controlled by the release of neurotransmitters in the enteric nervous system. In contrast to these three types of local control mechanisms, classic hormonal release by cells in the digestive tract is effective in controlling events that require the participation of several organs over long distances. A typical example of this is the response of the gallbladder, pancreas, and stomach to a meal containing fat induced by the release of CCK. The small intestine, sphincter of Oddi, and pylorus are all influenced by CCK.

2. **The answer is C.** CGRP as well as substance P are important neurotransmitters in the afferent neurons that innervate the GI tract and carry nociception to the CNS via the dorsal root ganglia. The vagal motor complex is involved with relaxation of the upper and lower esophageal sphincters but not with sphincters below the esophagus. Relaxation of the sphincter of Oddi is mediated by the hormonal release of CCK and by reflex-mediated release of NO by intrinsic neurons. Rectal distention can lead to a conscious sensation of distention through the pelvic nerve and the spinal cord and result in local neural reflex to cause relaxation of the anal sphincters through the myenteric plexus. The superior mesenteric ganglion plays little role in this response. As with the internal anal sphincter, the final mediators of lower esophageal sphincter relaxation are intrinsic neurons in the myenteric plexus that release NO. Although nerves in the submucosal plexus may exert influences on motor control by way of afferent pathways, they do not directly affect circular or longitudinal muscle function.

3. **The answer is B.** NO-containing neurons originating in the myenteric plexus are the key neurons to control relaxation of enteric sphincters and muscles. However, these nerves are not known to mediate sensory information. Eighty percent of all vagal nerves are afferent nerves passing to the CNS through the nodose ganglion. CGRP and substance P are important transmitters mediating sensory information through spinal afferent pathways that pass through the dorsal root ganglion to the spinal cord lamellae. These pathways include the spinothalamic tract, which also carries information from mesenteric neurons that surround GI organs (not the femoral nerve).

4. **The answer is C.** Enteroglucagon is an important trophic hormone in the small intestine. Disorders of malabsorption and those associated with the resection of the small intestine result in an increased release of enteroglucagon from mucosal endocrine cells in the ileum. Gastrin is another very important trophic hormone. Motilin, secretin, and somatostatin have not been shown to be trophic hormones.

5. **The answer is A.** One of the best described physiologic roles of somatostatin is to inhibit further release of gastrin in the presence of adequate acid in the stomach. In general, somatostatin serves as an inhibitory transmitter throughout the digestive tract. It has been shown to inhibit the secretion of materials from the stomach and small and large intestines, to inhibit hormone release, and when released as a neurotransmitter from nerves in the myenteric plexus, to relax GI muscles. Amylase secretion is stimulated by the release of CCK from endocrine cells in the duodenal mucosa. Cycles of motor activity during fasting that are seen in the small intestine and stomach are initiated by the hormone motilin, which is released from duodenal enteroendocrine cells. The inhibition of upper digestive motility and secretion by the presence of excess nutrients in the ileum is known as the ileal brake. A key transmitter in this response is PYY.

6. **The answer is A.** The inhibition of further gastrin release is mediated by somatostatin released from paracrine cells in the gastric mucosa. NO is the key transmitter involved in the relaxation of circular muscles distal to distention as part of the peristaltic reflex and relaxation of the anal sphincter to permit defecation. NO is not involved in contraction or the pelvic floor reflex.

7. **The answer is A.** Regulatory peptides do not have branching side chains. They are categorized into families by their amino acid homology, not by function. Posttranslational processing greatly influences the potency of neuropeptides by changing the length of the peptide chain or adding sulfated bonds that alter their three-dimensional structure. Regulatory peptides have a great diversity in the number of amino acids in the chain length.

8. **The answer is D.** Under most circumstances, the effects of VIP are similar to those of NO. The effect of VIP and NO on the sphincter of Oddi is to cause relaxation that permits the bile in the gallbladder to be released into the duodenum. The inhibition of pancreatic secretion and intestinal motility in response to excess food in the ileum is known as the ileal brake and is mediated by PYY not NPY. Under the usual fight-or-flight reflex, sympathetic transmitters cause inhibition of GI motility; this does not occur during digestion. Somatostatin is a most important inhibitory mediator of gastrin release, and the key role for NO is to cause relaxation of the lower esophageal sphincter.

Chapter 3

1. **The answer is C.** The earliest effects are on the enterocytes of the small intestinal mucosa, the cells primarily responsible for absorption. Both transporters and glycocalyx enzymes are affected. Other deficiencies may occur later in the disease, when mucosal destruction would also eliminate enteroendocrine cells, not cause enzymatic defects. This later decline in the number of enteroendocrine cells results in decreased pancreatic secretions, although the pancreatic ducts remain normal. Diarrhea is common but is due to impaired mucosal absorption of water more than muscle contractions. The bacterial population of the colon may be slightly decreased as a result of diarrhea but is not an early defect.

2. **The answer is B.** Vitamin B_{12} is absorbed through the cooperation of the stomach and the distal ileum. Parietal cells of the gastric glands secrete intrinsic factor, which binds and protects vitamin B_{12} from digestion. Significant damage to the gasteric mucosa from atrophy or ulceration can decrease the production of intrinsic factor. Herniation of the cardiac stomach through the diaphram would not result in a significant loss of intrinsic factor. The vitamin B_{12}–intrinsic factor complex then binds to specific receptors in the mucosa of the distal ileum, where it is taken up by endocytosis and released at the base of the epithelial cells into the circulation. Surgical removal of even the final 15 cm of the ileum severely impairs the ability to reabsorb vitamin B_{12}. Bacterial infections can physically block access of vitamin B_{12}–intrinsic factor complex to its receptor.

3. **The answer is D.** The H^+-K^+-ATPase pump is stored within cytoplasmic vesicles until neural or hormonal stimulation occurs, at which time the transporter is inserted into the canalicular apical surface. K^+ only shuttles in and out of the apical end of the parietal cell and is not trasported at the base of the cell. H^+ and Cl^- are pumped out of the apical end of the cell by two separate mechanisms; there is not a joint H^+-Cl^--ATPase. Blood pH tends to be buffered by the release of bicarbonate ions out of the base of the parietal cell; there should not be a leakage of H^+ into the bloodstream. Carbonic anhydrase in the parietal cell catalyzes the conversion of carbon dioxide and water to HCO_3^- and H^+, not the opposite.

4. **The answer is A.** Brunner's glands secrete alkaline mucus to neutralize the acidic chyme. They are abundant in the submucosa of the duodenum. Whereas Paneth cells and goblet cells would be present in the duodenum, Paneth cells are also found in other segments of the small intestine, and goblet cells are found throughout the small and large intestines; therefore, these two cell types would not serve as diagnostic features for the duodenum. Peyer's patches characterize the ileum; surface mucous cells characterize the stomach.

Chapter 4

1. **The answer is C.** Striated muscles are found in the lower digestive tract in the external anal sphincter. Striated muscles are also found in the UES and in the proximal one-third of the esophagus. There are no striated muscles, however, in the LES. Striated muscles, like smooth muscles, depend on calcium to induce

a contraction. Although smooth muscles are generally considered involuntary muscles, some smooth muscle functions can be influenced voluntarily. These include contractions of the smooth muscle regions of the esophagus, induced by swallowing, emptying the stomach of air through belching, and voluntary initiation or inhibition of bowel movement.

2. **The answer is C.** Slow waves occur more frequently than contractions because not every slow wave is associated with activation leading to a contraction. Only during phase III of the IMMC is every slow wave likely to be associated with a contraction. At other times contractions are considerably less frequent than slow waves. Slow waves are not generated by cells in the submucosal plexus. The submucosal plexus contains intrinsic neurons. The frequency of slow waves remains constant throughout the day under normal circumstances and certainly is not altered by the presence or absence of contractions. Finally, it is important to remember that slow waves are first seen in the digestive tract in the midcorpus of the stomach. There are no slow waves recorded under usual circumstances in the esophagus or fundus.

3. **The answer is C.** During stimulation of the sympathetic nervous system, such as occurs in a fight-or-flight situation, the digestive system is shut down. Under ideal circumstances the sphincters then would close and reduce the flow between luminal organs. Adrenergic stimulation of the sphincters through norepinephrine therefore induces sphincteric contraction.

   Only the UES and external anal sphincter contain striated muscles. All other GI sphincters are smooth muscles. Anatomically, sphincters represent a thickening of the circular (not longitudinal) muscle. In some muscles, such as the pyloric sphincter, this is readily apparent; in others, such as the LES, this can only be detected with a dissecting microscopic and quantitative assessment. One of the important functions of sphincters is to retard the flow of air and fluids in a retrograde direction. Not all sphincters prevent this completely. Specifically, the retrograde flow of luminal contents from the duodenum into the stomach is only partially reduced by the pyloric sphincter. Likewise, the LES is commonly associated with reflux of materials from the stomach into the esophagus, including both air (belch) and gastric acid (reflux or heartburn). The distinction between normal and abnormal reflux across the LES then requires quantitative assessment or the presence of complications of acid reflux.

4. **The answer is B.** Phase III of the IMMC is important in the emptying of solid material from the stomach and upper digestive tract to the colon and in reducing the overall bacterial count in the small intestine. An absence of phase III of the IMMC has been associated with small intestine bacterial overgrowth. The initiation of phase III is through the release of motilin by mucosal endocrine cells in the duodenum. This initiates the activity front in the stomach and duodenum. Progression through the jejunum and ileum, however, is dependent on opioid neurotransmitters. Phase I is a resting phase during which there is little movement of material out of the digestive tract, particularly the stomach. Phase II is a mixing phase, which is indistinguishable from a fed pattern. Certainly, it would be uncommon to record a high frequency of retrograde contractions under either circumstance. The IMMC terminates in the distal ileum or the ileocecal sphincter. The IMMC, however, does not progress into the colon.

Chapter 5

1. **The answer is C.** Although histamine increases intracellular cAMP, gastrin and ACh cause an increase in parietal cell intracellular Ca^{2+} concentration. The effect of both intracellular Ca^{2+} and cAMP increase is to stimulate activity of H^+-K^+-ATPase, which results in increased H^+ output from the cell. A Cl^- channel is not the key regulatory site for HCl formation. Somatostatin works to inhibit acid secretion. Although parietal cells secrete high concentrations of H^+, they are protected from this acid bath by a layer of mucus in which HCO_3^- is present. As a consequence of this mucous layer, the pH at the level of the cell is nearly neutral.

2. **The answer is E.** In both pancreatic and bile ducts, through increases in cAMP, secretin activates both Cl^-–HCO_3^- exchangers and Cl^- channels to increase the output of alkaline fluid. HCO_3^- channels per se

have not been identified in pancreatic or biliary duct epithelial cells, though HCO_3^- is permeable to anion (Cl^-) channels.

3. **The answer is B.** Cotransporters and exchangers do not require energy and are involved in facilitated diffusion. Pumps require energy, usually ATP, to move ions up their electrochemical gradient. Ion channels are often phosphorylated to become open, but once opened, ions passively move down their electrochemical gradients.

4. **The answer is A.** As the flow of saliva is increased, so is the concentration of Na^+, Cl^-, and HCO_3^-; K^+ concentration is decreased.

5. **The answer is E.** The protein product of the CFTR gene is a cAMP-dependent Cl^- channel expressed in a variety of epithelial cells. Ion movement through this channel modulates the concentration of salt in the sweat of patients with cystic fibrosis, but the channel itself is not secreted. In addition to being present in pancreatic duct, airway, and intestinal cells, CFTR is also found in the liver uniquely expressed in bile duct cells. CFTR is not a digestive enzyme, but by secreting alkaline fluid provides a hospitable environment for digestive enzymes to be effective.

6. **The answer is A.** Decreased NO release activates mast cells, which release various compounds, among them PAF. PAF, in turn, stimulates filtration secretion to increase fluid into the lumen of the intestine through intercellular pathways not directly involving ion channels. However, ion channels can be activated to increase secretion via effects on prostaglandins and neurotransmitters. This, too, is in response to decreased (not increased) NO release. Mucosal mast cells also require activation to promote increased intestinal secretion.

7. **The answer is D.** 5'-AMP is released by various leukocytes; among them, eosinophils are an important source. Following the conversion of 5'-AMP to adenosine, adenosine binds to adenosine receptors to increase intracellular cAMP concentrations to activate cAMP-dependent Cl^- secretion. The conversion to adenosine takes place extracellularly, and the effect on intracellular concentrations of cAMP is in response to the binding of adenosine to its receptor. C is incorrect because the ecto-5'-nucleotidase does not produce extracellular cAMP but adenosine.

Chapter 6

1. **The answer is E.** This patient has no evidence of problems with digestion or absorption, which excludes choices A, B, and C. Colon cancer is also possible but unlikely, given the degree of weight loss with a normal CT scan (which should identify spread to the lymph nodes or liver), absence of anemia, and a normal stool guaiac test. Her stable weight for the past 2 months also argues against cancer, although this should remain a concern. This patient was suffering from postmenopausal depression, with loss of appetite and a dry mouth from her antidepressants, making it difficult to swallow. After hormonal replacement and a change in antidepressents, her appetite and energy returned, and she regained her lost weight.

2. **The answer is E.** The main goal in treating viral diarrhea is to replace fluids and electrolytes. Distilled water fails to replace the electrolytes lost. The sodium chloride solutions are too high in sodium and would fail to be absorbed, further dehydrating the patient. The honey water, like distilled water, lacks electrolytes. Excellent over-the-counter rehydration solutions that contain optimal carbohydrate-to-sodium concentrations are now available. These solutions are effective in preventing dehydration even in prolonged bouts of viral diarrhea.

3. **The answer is B.** Fatty acid and fat-soluble vitamin absorption occurs in the upper small intestine. Lipase is not absorbed. Bile acids are absorbed in the distal ileum. Usually, over 100 cm of the terminal ileum must be lost before bile salts are no longer absorbed. If less than 100 cm of the terminal ileum are resected, some of the bile may pass into the colon and cause diarrhea.

4. **The answer is A.** Colipase is synthesized in the pancreas as procolipase in a 1:1 ratio with pancreatic lipase. Colipase is activated in the small intestine by trypsin. Colipase enhances the activity of lipase, which is secreted in the active form, but it is not an absolute requirement. Other lipases are unaffected by colipase.

5. **The answer is D.** If you missed this question, you should reread the entire chapter.

Chapter 7

1. **The answer is B.** Bile salts are absorbed mainly in the distal ileum. Surgical removal or disease activity of the distal ileum can result in bile salt malabsorption. Bile salts increase active colonic anion secretion, thereby causing a secretory diarrhea with a stool osmolar gap of less than 50 mOsm/L. Choice A is incorrect because a secretory diarrhea results in an osmotic gap of less than 50 mOsm/L. Choices C and D are incorrect because bile acids induce a net secretion of fluid in the colon, resulting in a decrease in the osmotic load. Osmotic diarrhea results from the presence of nonabsorbable solutes in the intestinal lumen, which increase the intralumenal osmotic load, thereby increasing the stool osmolar gap.

2. **The answer is C.** Intestinal epithelial cells demonstrate functional polarity with active transport at one cell surface and passive at the other. The end result is a net transcellular transport of a given solute. Intestinal epithelial cells are joined together by tight junctions, when in part regulate the passage of solute across the epithelium. The movement of ions across the apical membrane of the epithelial cell requires the presence of specialized channels, pumps, or carriers, and the unique transport properties of a particular intestinal segment are determined by the specitic transport proteins within the epithelial cell membrane and the characteristics of the adjoining tight junctions.

3. **The answer is B.** Large quantities of urinary Cl^- enter the colon and are absorbed in part by enhanced apical absorption through the Cl^-–HCO_3^- exchanger. This promotes excess HCO_3^- and K^+ secretion. A high serum level of Cl^- (hyperchloremia) and low serum K^+ (hypokalemia) result. The net excretion of the base HCO_3^- leads to a net metabolic acidosis. Excess NaCl absorption would not lead to the observed metabolic derangement, and excess urinary HCO_3^- is not typical.

4. **The answer is D.** Patients with long-standing diabetes can develop autonomic neuropathy with loss of sympathetic absorptive stimulation. Clonidine, an α_2-agonist, can alleviate the diarrhea through sympathetic stimulation. Somatostatin inhibits the activity of several secretagogues, including VIP and serotonin, and is useful in treating patients with VIPoma and the carcinoid syndrome but not patients with the diarrhea associated with diabetes. Magnesium sulfate is a nonabsorbable solute that would worsen the diarrhea. Corticosteroids lead to an increase in Na^+ absorption and would not be used to treat the underlying disorder in diabetic diarrhea.

5. **The answer is C.** VIP, prostaglandins, and the enterotoxin of *V. cholerae* are all intestinal secretagogues. However, somatostatin stimulates net intestinal absorption by inhibiting the effects of multiple intestinal secretagogues, including VIP and serotonin.

6. **The answer is D.** In addition to the anti-inflammatory effects, stimulation of Na^+ absorption throughout the intestinal tract probably contributes to the antidiarrheal effects of glucocorticoids seen in inflammatory bowel disease. Rehydration with NaCl would correct the underlying dehydration resulting from the diarrhea but would not lessen the diarrhea itself. Glucocorticoids do not inhibit HCO_3^- secretion, and the activity of the amiloride-sensitive Na^+ channels in the distal colon is stimulated by mineralocorticoids.

Chapter 8

1. **The answer is B.** Blood flows into the liver via both the hepatic artery and portal veins. On reaching the hepatic sinusoids, blood is filtered of its cellular elements and the protein-rich plasma enters the spaces of Disse.

2. **The answer is D.** Although proper drug detoxification requires an intact cell with its full complement of organelles, the smooth endoplasmic reticulum is primarily responsible for drug metabolism. The nucleus helps regulate cellular activity. The Golgi apparatus is involved in lipid metabolism. Mitochondria perform oxidative phosphorylation.

3. **The answer is A.** The liver begins embryologically as a solid mass of hepatocytes but during fetal and early infancy is remodeled into sinusoids one or two cells thick. Under conditions of active regeneration following

certain forms of liver injury, the cell plates may increase to as many as five or six cells thick. This would, however, only occur during the active phase of liver regeneration. Hepatocytes arranged in plates that are as thick as five or six cells should be carefully evaluated for neoplastic change based on loss of normal or physiologic growth control.

4. **The answer is C.** The liver is unique among the body's organs by virtue of its dual blood supply: (1) a high-pressure, highly oxygenated hepatic artery component and (2) a low-pressure, relatively deoxygenated portal vein component. Therefore choices A, B, and D are incorrect.

5. **The answer is D.** The liver is an organ of conditional renewal capable of dramatic regeneration following tissue injuries. Although all cellular constituents of the liver are capable of regeneration to varying degrees, the intrinsic architecture must be preserved to enable cellular regeneration to recover the normal status of the organ. The refined Rappaport model recognizes three zones of liver parenchyma. The liver has a dual blood supply, via the hepatic artery and portal vein. In cirrhosis, there is scarring and fibrosis, and the normal histology is not maintained.

6. **The answer is D.** As in the clinical case, hepatocytes situated around the central veins are the most vulnerable to the effects of hypoxia. The vulnerability is related to the position furthest from the portal tract and therefore supplied by blood relatively desaturated in oxygen.

7. **The answer is C.** Bile is a complex fluid highly saturated in cholesterol, phospholipid, and bile salts. Precipitation of gallstones is most likely to occur in the gallbladder, where all these constituents become very concentrated. The blood supply is via the cystic artery. In the gallbladder, isotonic absorption of sodium bicarbonate and chloride concentrates the bile. Other functions include release of bile in response to cholecystokinin, moderation of pressure in the hepatobiliary system, bile acidification, and absorption of some organic components of bile.

8. **The answer is C.** Blood enters the linear parenchyma via the portal tracts, resulting in a periportal zone of hepatocytes richly supplied by oxygen and a pericentral zone of oxygen-poor liver cells. Good correlation between histology and physiology follows the concept of liver acinus that is centered on the portal tract. The common bile duct is formed when the right and left hepatic ducts are formed. This structure is extrahepatic. The ampulla of Vater protrudes into the duodenum as the papilla. The ligamentum teres connects the liver to the anterior body wall.

Chapter 9

1. **The answer is C.** Although HMG CoA reductase is the rate-limiting enzyme in the synthesis of cholesterol, 7α-hydroxylase is the enzyme that determines how much cholesterol is converted to bile acids. The other two enzymes are part of carbohydrate metabolism.

2. **The answer is A.** Bilirubin is a bright red-brown substance that contributes color to bile. Taurocholic acid, glucuronidated steroid hormones, and mixed inorganic ions are present in bile but contribute no color.

3. **The answer is B.** As in the patient in the case study, even moderate obesity can cause steatosis. Neither progesterone nor vitamin A therapy has been shown to correlate with the development of fatty liver; however, estrogen administration does. Heavy alcohol use can also cause steatosis. However, steatosis is usually reversible if the causes are withdrawn.

4. **The answer is B.** CCK and an increase in the ionic content of bile encourage contractility, and the sphincter of Oddi relaxes to permit delivery of bile to the duodenum.

5. **The answer is C.** About 20% of the gallbladder contents are delivered during the interdigestive period, and this is coordinated with the MMC. This partial removal of bile is thought to help inhibit gallstone formation by mixing the contents of the gallbladder regularly. The sphincter of Oddi permits this delivery by partial relaxation. Cholestasis does not affect the delivery during the interdigestive period, nor does the distention of the gallbladder.

6. **The answer is B.** Neither fluid nor trypsin in the duodenum has any effect on the delivery of bile, but the presence of dietary lipids in the duodenum will stimulate bile delivery. Answer A is incorrect because the gallbladder contracts and the sphincter of Oddi relaxes.

7. **The answer is C.** Cholestyramine binds tightly the bile salts, preventing their ileal uptake by the entero-hepatic circulation and permitting them to be excreted in the feces. The strategy of this therapy is that the liver is then forced to convert more cholesterol to bile salts to replace that lost from the body. Although some bile pigments (answer B) could be bound to the agent, this would not affect the cholesterol level because cholesterol is not a precursor of bile pigments. This agent may affect motility slightly by providing bulk, but this would not be a factor in reducing cholesterol.

Chapter 10

1. **The answer is C.** Progesterone is a hormone that relaxes smooth muscle cells. The LES is a sphincter that is composed of smooth muscle cells. Therefore, progesterone produces LES relaxation. There are two types of postganglionic neurons that affect the LES. One of these is acetylcholine (ACh), and its function is to stimulate or contract smooth muscle cells such as the LES. Thus, ACh increases LES pressure. The other postganglionic neuron releases noncholinergic nonadrenergic inhibitory neurotransmitters, which cause smooth muscle relaxation. VIP and NO are two of these neurotransmitters.

2. **The answer is A.** All of the mechanisms listed contribute to or exacerbate GER. An incompetent LES is associated with spontaneous reflux; this, however, is seen in only a small number of patients with GER and is usually only noted in patients with severe esophagitis. Likewise, poor peristalsis is most often seen in patients with severe esophagitis. An amplitude of only 30 mm Hg is required for the peristaltic wave to prevent retrograde movement. Gravity also functions to prevent reflux in patients with weak peristalsis. Although delayed gastric emptying can contribute to reflux, it is rarely the primary underlying mechanism responsible for the reflux episode. Intragastric pressures can increase as a result of reduced gastric emptying. This will increase the pressure gradient across the LES, which will allow movement of the gastric contents across the sphincter into the esophagus. This mechanism is more important after a very large meal and in certain disease states, such as diabetes and scleroderma. In most individuals, the gastric cavity can accommodate a considerable increase in volume without a rise in intragastric pressure. Thus transient LES relaxations have been found to be the most important cause of GERD in healthy individuals and in those with esophagitis.

3. **The answer is B.** Endoscopy is the best test for detecting mucosal disease, including esophagitis and Barrett's esophagus. Only 60% of patients with clinically significant GER have evidence of mucosal disease, thereby limiting endoscopy's sensitivity in the detection of GER. Esophageal manometry evaluates the motility of the esophagus, including LES pressures and esophageal peristalsis. However, many patients with GER have normal LES pressure and esophageal peristalsis. Barium esophagography provides a visual image of the esophagus and is best used in the detection of structural lesions. During the fluoroscopic part of the examination, an episode of reflux may be detected. Individuals with reflux do not reflux continuously throughout the day, and this test only evaluates a specific point in time. It is highly likely that a patient will not experience a reflux episode during the specific testing period. However, 24-hour pH monitoring measures the pH in the esophagus around the clock for one day. This length of time should include most of the patient's usual daily activities. Furthermore, this test allows an association to be made between the symptoms reported by the patient at a specific point in time with the pH at that same point in time. Therefore, it is the best test for diagnosing the presence or absence of GER.

4. **Answer is C.** The LES is not hypotensive; it may be hypertensive but this is not required for diagnosis. Achalasia is most commonly seen in those 20–60 years of age; it is uncommon in children. On manometry on typically sees aperistalsis and incomplete relaxation of the LES. The esophagus may be dilated when viewed on barium studies.

5. **Answer is D.** The atypical manifestations of reflux include: hoarseness, globus hystericus, chronic throat clearing, cough, and asthma.

Chapter 11

1. **The answer is D.** The only mechanism listed in the question that stimulates acid secretion in the prandial phase of gastric acid secretion is the thought, sight, smell, and taste of food.
2. **The answer is C.** Many mucosal aggressive factors have been discussed in the literature, including pepsin, bile, alcohol, tobacco, caffeine, NSAIDs, and *H. pylori*. However, it has become clear that the most important aggressive factor at this time is *H. pylori*. This is the most common infection of humans in the world today and has been clearly shown to play an important role in the pathogenesis of ulcers.
3. **The answer is C.** Although all of the agents listed in the question have been used in the treatment of PUD, they have different mechanisms of action, costs, and dosing schedules. The drugs that have the greatest power to neutralize acid are PPIs. Although PPIs are important in treating PUD, cost and other factors must be taken into account, so that these are not necessarily the first-line therapy for all patients with PUD.
4. **The answer is C.** Although truncal vagotomy may be quite helpful, there are many complications that can occur from this surgery. Pancreatic basal enzyme secretion can actually decrease; there is a loss of the gastrocholecystic reflex; and postvagotomy diarrhea can occur. Somatostatin-producing tumors do not occur postvagotomy.
5. **The answer is C.** One or more ulcers involving the stomach and duodenum in the absence of a gastric or small intestine malignancy is the most appropriate definition of PUD when used in clinical medicine. Ulcers often involve more than just the mucosa and submucosa. PUD is considered a benign process so that if gastric cancer is present, it is not PUD. Stress plays no role in the production or definition of PUD.

Chapter 12

1. **The answer is E.** Antitreponemal antibody and ACE are tests for syphilis and sarcoidosis, respectively. Ferritin may be low secondary to iron deficiency but is not diagnostic. Antireticulin antibody alone is not very sensitive; however, if antigliadin antibody and antiendomysial antibody were also performed and are positive, the sensitivity approaches 95%. HLA typing, although difficult to obtain, can be very helpful. More than 95% of celiac disease patients have HLA-DQ2 molecule.
2. **The answer is C.** The patient has a fairly classic history for Whipple's disease. Although rare, occulomasticatory myorhythmia is diagnostic for Whipple's disease, as are the PAS-positive macrophages with rod-shaped inclusion bodies. The biopsy results in A are what one would expect to see in celiac disease. The presence of a thickened basement membrane in B is seen in tropical sprue. Eosinophilic infiltrate in D is seen in eosinophilic gastroenteritis.
3. **The answer is D.** This patient, with her history of travel to India, megaloblastic anemia, and diarrhea, most likely has tropical sprue. Although choice A may be helpful because lactase deficiency is often present, it does not treat the enteric colonization that is thought to be a factor in the development of tropical sprue. Choice B would be therapy for celiac disease and choice C for Whipple's disease.
4. **The answer is B.** Crohn's disease is associated with an increased risk of adenocarcinoma of the small intestine, particularly the ileum. Celiac disease is a risk factor for both T cell lymphoma and adenocarcinoma, although the tumors in celiac disease usually occur in the jejunum rather than in the ileum. Whipple's disease, small intestine bacterial overgrowth, and necrotizing enterocolitis do not have a strong association with malignancy.
5. **The answer is E.** Carcinoid disease most often involves the ileum. The classic syndrome of flushing, diarrhea, and abdominal pain appears when there is metastatic disease. The stellate pattern for the involved arteries is most commonly seen in carcinoid syndrome. Choices A through D do not present with this classic triad of symptoms. Arteriogram for adenocarcinoma often shows a hypovascular mass with encasement of tumor vessel. Non-Hodgkin's lymphoma and leiomyosarcoma are not reported to have a classic arteriogram picture. Ischemia will cause narrowing or constriction of a vessel.

6. **The answer is B.** This patient presented with a classic history for intestinal ischemia. Only an arteriogram is considered the gold standard for making this diagnosis, which must be made as quickly as possible to save as much bowel as possible. Although the other tests may be helpful in contributing to the diagnosis, they are not considered conclusive. An abdominal x-ray might show thumbprinting, an indication of bowel wall edema. Edema may also be seen on an abdominal CT scan. An elevated amylase, an electrolyte profile consistent with metabolic acidosis, and a CBC demonstrating leukocytosis are suggestive but not diagnostic for ischemia. An abdominal sonogram with Doppler may give an indication of venous and arterial flow, but an arteriogram is more sensitive and therefore the diagnostic test of choice.

7. **The answer is C.** The patient presents in young adulthood with obstipation and urologic symptoms. In addition, her biopsy is classic for a primary visceral myopathy, particularly when considered with her urinary symptoms. Finally, her manometry is consistent with a myopathy. Late scleroderma and dermatomyositis would have the same manometry results but a different clinical picture. Familial visceral neuropathy would have a biopsy that showed a degeneration or decreased numbers of nerve fibers. Small bowel manometry would show incoordination or disorganization in motor activity. Diabetes mellitus is a neuropathic disorder and would cause a similar manometric response.

Chapter 13

1. **The answer is C.** Pain of chronic pancreatitis is often difficult to control. In patients with small-duct disease, pancreatic enzyme supplements often ameliorate abdominal pain. Pain improvement is due to enhanced feedback inhibition of pancreatic enzyme secretion by minimizing release of CCK and other pancreatic secretagogues and therefore putting the pancreas to rest. Further therapeutic interventions (choices A, B, and D) are attempted if patients fail more conservative treatment.

2. **The answer is A.** The most common cause of chronic pancreatitis in children in the United States is cystic fibrosis. The sweat chloride test would be the appropriate next step for diagnosing cystic fibrosis. More invasive procedures should be performed only if less invasive testing is not diagnostic.

3. **The answer is B.** Obstruction of CBD may be caused by pancreatic pseudocyst, acute inflammation, or retroperitoneal fibrosis. CBD obstruction develops in 5%–10% of patients, who then present with jaundice, right upper quadrant pain, or cholangitis. Ascending cholangitis is treated with antibiotics and relief of obstruction. ERCP allows for diagnostic and therapeutic intervention by assessing the etiology of obstruction as well as potential for therapeutic intervention to relieve obstruction. An admission to the ICU would be appropriate after relief of the obstruction. An uncomplicated ulcer would not present with fever and obstructive liver function tests. Pancreatic carcinoma is in the differential for etiology of obstructive cholangitis, but it is less likely than pseudocyst.

4. **The answer is B.** Appropriate treatment and evaluation of mild gallstone pancreatitis involves supportive measures, resting the pancreas, and assessing for the presence of cholelithiasis, choledocholithiasis, or dilated CBD, which may be due to an obstructing stone impacted at the ampulla. Emergent ERCP for stone extraction is indicated in severe gallstone pancreatitis. ICU monitoring is not indicated for acute mild pancreatitis. The presentation is atypical for pseudocyst.

5. **The answer is A.** The serum amylase level in hyperlipidemia-induced pancreatitis may be normal because the elevated triglycerides may interfere with its measurement. A clue to the diagnosis is that serum may appear turbid as a result of high concentration of triglycerides. Diluting the serum decreases interference of triglycerides with amylase measurement. Management of hyperlipidemic pancreatitis involves lowering triglyceride level and supportive measures. Emergent ERCP is not indicated in acute pancreatitis secondary to hypertriglyceridemia. Repeating undiluted amylase will be false negative again. Endoscopy will not help with the diagnosis of acute pancreatitis.

6. **The answer is A.** Cholangitis is a possible complication of acute pancreatitis. Cholangitis can occur with bacterial infection of an obstructed bile duct. In acute pancreatitis, bile duct obstruction may be due to gallstone,

pseudocyst, or inflammation in the head of the pancreas. Emergent ERCP to relieve obstruction (via stone extraction or stent placement) is indicated in patients with cholangitis. Initiation of antibiotics is important, but common bile duct obstruction must be relieved to treat the infection and ascending cholangitis. Clinical presentation and laboratory findings are most consistent with ascending cholangitis rather than infected pancreatic necrosis.

7. **The answer is B.** Drug-induced pancreatitis is a diagnosis of exclusion. Other possible causes of pancreatitis need to be considered and appropriately evaluated. Treatment involves stopping the culprit medication and supportive measures. ERCP will not assist in diagnosis or management of uncomplicated drug-induced pancreatitis. Amylase isoenzymes are not indicated in drug-induced pancreatitis.

8. **The answer is B.** Recognition of other medical problems that may have similar presentation to pancreatitis is important. Free air on abdominal x-ray is diagnostic for perforated bowel and is managed with surgical intervention and antibiotics. All of the other choices would be inappropriate in the management of this patient that needs acute surgical intervention. Although diverticulitis may result in perforation, this patient is more likely suffering from perforated ulcer. ERCP is not the treatment for perforated viscus.

Chapter 14

1. **The answer is B.** Fecal incontinence may be associated with a history of trauma to the anorectal area, including surgical trauma and obstetric trauma. Certain neurologic disorders, such as multiple sclerosis, may be associated with fecal incontinence. Back injuries affecting the sacral spine may result in a neurologic etiology of fecal incontinence. Patients with diabetes may have incontinence associated with sphincter abnormalities as well as sensory deficits. The other diseases listed are not associated with incontinence; in fact, hypothyroidism often results in constipation.

2. **The answer is C.** A scintigraphic examination, that is, a nuclear medicine scan called a gastric emptying test, would be the most appropriate test in the clinical situation described. A barium swallow evaluates only the esophagus. Upper GI endoscopy may show retained food in the stomach but does not document gastric emptying delay physiologically.

3. **The answer is C.** Abdominal pain associated with a change in stool frequency is part of the Rome II criteria, listed in Table 14-2.

4. **The answer is E.** Functional disorders lack biochemical and histologic markers, and consequently they are often difficult to diagnose and treat. Organic disease, on the other hand, may be a structural or physical abnormality that may be identified by a study, such as endoscopy or a radiologic test. Both organic disorders and functional disorders are very real. Functional disorders do not represent psychosomatic problems; however, there may be psychologic factors involved in the way patients deal with the disorder. This can also be true for organic diseases.

5. **The answer is D.** Ileal propulsive waves are more common in patients with IBS as compared to normal controls. There is a lower rectosigmoid distention threshold for pain, the MMC periodicity is shorter, and the rectal compliance to balloon distention is lower in IBS patients.

6. **The answer is D.** CIP may be associated with anti-PCNA in scleroderma. Many CIP patients are subject to surgery without cause because CIP is difficult to differentiate clinically from mechanical obstruction. The etiology of CIP is not known.

Chapter 15

1. **The answer is D.** M cells are specialized epithelial cells overlying the Peyer's patches. They sample intraluminal antigens and then transport these antigens to the Peyer's patches, where they are presented to cells with MHC class II antigens, which then present the antigens to lymphocytes. M cells themselves do not possess class II antigens and therefore cannot function as antigen-presenting cells.

2. **The answer is A.** Intraepithelial lymphocytes are mostly T lymphocytes, which bear CD8 receptors. They function mainly as cytotoxic-suppressor cells, and their numbers greatly increase during disease states, such as celiac disease or graft-versus-host disease. These cells are regionally specific and are thought to play a role in controlling mucosal abnormalities.

3. **The answer is A.** Secretory IgA is initially present in a monomeric form. It is then bound to the J chain and transported across the epithelial cell, where it is bound to secretory component, endocytosed, and then excreted into the lumen. The SC is only partially cleaved and acts to prevent degradation of secretory IgA. Secretory IgA does not activate complement. Its main function is to prevent adherence of bacteria to epithelial cells and decrease colonization.

4. **The answer is B.** Mast cells and nerves in the gut are often closely positioned. Release of neuropeptides such as VIP, substance P, and somatostatin can activate mast cell degranulation with the release of histamine.

5. **The answer is D.** The mucosal barrier is made up of both immunologic and nonimmunologic components. Nonimmunologic components include bile, mucus, gastric acid, gut flora, peristalsis, and tight junctions of the epithelial cells. Macrophages are a nonspecific immunologic component of the mucosal barrier and act by phagocytosis of foreign antigens. Secretory IgA is a specific mucosal antibody that is secreted by the mucosal surface, and IL-1 is a cytokine that activates various parts of the immune system.

6. **The answer is B.** Skin testing is a simple and sensitive method for the detection of specific mast cell–bound IgE antibodies in a patient suspected of a mild food allergy where anaphylaxis is not expected. A positive skin test can then be confirmed with an oral food challenge in such patients. In patients with a suspected anaphylactic reaction, RAST or ELISA testing can be done using the patient's serum. Cytotoxicity food allergy testing is of no proven benefit in the evaluation of food allergy.

Chapter 16

1. **The answer is D.** The correct answer indicates that you are considering toxic megacolon in the diagnosis. The patient should be given no medications prior to diagnosis. Opiate antidiarrheals may in fact accelerate the course of toxic megacolon. As always, as the very first step, it is important to assess the patient's hemodynamic status and implement any necessary resuscitative measures, such as fluid repletion.

2. **The answer is B.** Primary sclerosing cholangitis is characterized by fibrosing inflammation and may lead to bile duct obliteration, biliary cirrhosis, and hepatic failure. Primary biliary cirrhosis is not an extraintestinal manifestation. There are four types of arthritis associated with IBD: peripheral arthritis, spondylitis, sacroiliitis, and hypertrophic osteoarthropathy. Erythema nodosum and pyoderma gangrensoum are the two main skin lesions associated with IBD.

3.–7. **The answers are: 3-B, 4-B, 5-D, 6-B, 7-A.** Crohn's disease is a transmural disease with involvement of all of the layers of the GI tract wall. In contrast, UC is a mucosal disease. The *only* time that UC is transmural is in the setting of toxic megacolon when the inflammation progresses to involve deeper layers. This is a severe manifestation of the disease. Even in moderate UC, disease remains a mucosal process.

Because of the transmural nature of Crohn's disease, fistulas or abnormal connections may form between loops of bowel or between the small or large intestine and other organs (such as vagina or bladder) or skin.

Surgery is not the initial treatment of choice for either disease. Medical management should be considered first. Indications for surgery include perforation, complicated bleeding, complete obstruction, advanced toxic megacolon, cancer, or failure to respond to medical therapy.

The presence of granulomas is pathognomonic for Crohn's disease. These granulomas are rarely seen, however, and their absence do not preclude the diagnosis of Crohn's.

Chapter 17

1. **The answer is A.** *H. pylori* infection is associated with 80% of gastric ulcers and 95% of duodenal ulcers in the absence of NSAIDs. A positive result on serologic testing indicates only that the patient has been

exposed to the organism in the past, not the presence of ulcers. Residence in developing countries is a risk factor for ulcers, and treatment will reduce the recurrence.

2. **The answer is D.** The treatment of choice is metronidazole. The best means by which to diagnose *Giardia* is to detect *Giardia* antigen in the stool. It is unclear how *Giardia* causes diarrhea. It is likely multifactorial. *Giardia* is not an invasive organism.

3. **The answer is A.** CMV esophagitis is extremely uncommon except in patients who are immunosuppressed. *Cryptosporidium* and *E. coli* 0157:H7 outbreaks have been reported in Wisconsin and Washington, respectively. Schistosomiasis is among the most common infectious diseases in the world.

4. **The answer is B.** Antibiotics are the most common risk factors for *C. difficile* colitis infection.

5. **The answer is C.** Antibiotic therapy for *E. coli* has not been proven to reduce the severity of disease and the likelihood of developing hemolytic uremic syndrome. Fluoroquinolones are the treatment of choice for shigellosis. Metronidazole is the treatment of choice for giardiasis. Metronidazole and vancomycin are effective against *C. difficile*.

Chapter 18

1. **The answer is D.** HAV transmission is greatest when it is shed in the feces. This occurs most notably during the 3–4-week incubation period, before symptoms appear and before medical attention is sought. Once individuals seek medical attention and are symptomatic, they are usually no longer infective.

2. **The answer is A.** Most cases of HAV go unnoticed; it is generally indolent and confers lifelong immunity. Worldwide, HAV is generally a childhood illness and is almost universal in developing areas. Although icteric forms of HAV do occur, it does not commonly present this way. HAV is transmitted by the fecal–oral route but not by sexual contact. It resolves within weeks to months of illness.

3. **The answer is B.** HBV has the greatest morbidity and mortality, with a lifetime risk of HCC in infected Asians approaching 50%. Of those people living in Sub-Saharan Africa and the Far East, 5%–20% are HBsAg-positive. It is thought that this is a result of the high prevalence of maternal–fetal transmission. HAV, HDV, and HCV have a much lower worldwide morbidity and mortality.

4. **The answer is C.** HBsAg denotes active infection. This occurs during the 4–6-week incubation period, followed by a rise in anti-HBc. When the HBsAg level falls, anti-HBs then rise. The period between active infection and antibody formation is called the window period, during which only anti-HBc can be measured. HBcAg is not a clinically useful marker because it does not circulate freely in the blood. IgG anti-HBc generally denotes past infection.

5. **The answer is B.** HDV is a defective virus and is highly infectious. It depends on HBsAg to replicate in humans. It can only occur in patients infected with HBV as either a coinfection or a later superinfection in an already infected patient. Only HDV requires the helper function of HBV.

6. **The answer is A.** Unlike HBV, HCV does not incorporate into the host's genome. HCV replication has been documented in the liver but has not been confirmed in extrahepatic sites. Antibodies are made against the virus, but they do not appear to play a role in viral clearance. The high rate of mutation of the virus is felt to be the key factor leading to persistence of HCV infection.

7. **The answer is D.** HGV is considered an "innocent bystander," and treatment with IFN is currently not the standard of cure. Although treatment with IFN only cures HCV in up to 20% of patients, attempts to eradicate the virus is reasonable in those most likely to respond (noncirrhotic, compliant patients).

8. **The answer is C.** HEV is generally a self-limited illness, often occurring as outbreaks in endemic areas. For unknown reasons, pregnant women who contract HEV are at risk for fulminant hepatitis and death. Although maternal–fetal transmission of HBV is very high, especially in developing areas, it is not commonly associated with fulminant hepatitis. HGV has not been shown to be of particular concern in pregnant women infected with the virus.

Chapter 19

1. **The answer is D.** This patient has hemochromatosis. The disease is likely due to inappropriately high intestinal absorption of iron. Untreated, this disease may progress to irreversible liver disease. Phlebotomy should be initiated to prevent the development of end-stage complications. Other family members should be studied.

2. **The answer is D.** This patient has Wilson's disease. The disorder is autosomal recessive. The genetic defect is on the long arm of chromosome 13. The primary defect in Wilson's disease is not related to ceruloplasmin. Ceruloplasmin levels are usually low to absent. Lowering copper stores does improve clinical symptoms in most patients.

3. **The answer is C.** Hemochromatosis, Wilson's disease, and α_1-antitrypsin deficiency are inherited in an autosomal recessive pattern. To have the disease, the offspring would have to inherit the affected gene from each parent. If each parent is *Bb*, then the chance of inheriting the disease as *bb* is 25%.

4. **The answer is C.** Approximately one-tenth of ingested iron is absorbed from the GI tract. Iron is absorbed in the proximal small bowel. It is transported from the site of absorption bound to transferrin, which can carry only two atoms of iron per molecule. In the liver, it is taken up by ferritin, which is capable of holding thousands of atoms per molecule.

5. **The answer is B.** Copper is absorbed in the proximal small bowel. In contrast to iron absorption, as much as 60% (25%–60%) of ingested copper is absorbed. Very little copper circulates in the free state. In fetal life almost all of the body's copper is in the liver, whereas the adult liver contains only 8% of the total stores.

6. **The answer is A.** There is no specific therapy for liver disease in α_1-antitrypsin deficiency. The α_1-antitrypsin gene is located on chromosome 14. (The genetic defect for Wilson's disease is on chromosome 13.) The Pi type correlates poorly with the severity of liver disease. Liver transplant is curative, because α_1-antitrypsin is primarily synthesized in the liver.

Chapter 20

1. **The answer is B.** This is a classic presentation of PBC. The liver function tests are purely cholestatic and would not be consistent with an active HBV infection. Ceruloplasmin, which would be unusual given the patient's age and the predominanace of cholestasis, is useful in ruling out Wilson's disease. An ERCP would be useful to rule out any obstructive biliary lesions; however, given the inherent risk of this procedure, it should only be performed when the diagnosis is still unclear following further workup. A CT scan of the abdomen would be reasonable if further workup did not reveal the answer.

2. **The answer is E.** Fat-soluble malabsorption can occur in PBC, resulting in vitamin A deficiency, which can cause night blindness. Vitamin E deficiency also can occur, but this usually causes a neurologic abnormality, affecting the posterior columns, which manifests as ataxia and loss of proprioception. A slit lamp examination would not be helpful. Although copper accumulation can occur in the eyes of patients with chronic cholestatic diseases, such as PBC, this usually does not affect the vision. A Schirmer test is used to test for dry eyes, which although common in PBC, would not affect night vision.

3. **The answer is E.** This patient has symptoms and signs that are consistent with hepatitis, in particular AIH. A laparoscopic cholecystectomy should not be performed without evidence of gallstone disease. The pattern of injury on the liver function suggests that this is hepatocellular injury, so an ERCP is not the first diagnostic test of choice. An AMA is more useful in diagnosing PBC, which usually presents with a liver injury pattern that is more cholestatic in nature. Although eating disorders are common in this age group, elevated liver injury tests suggest other etiologies of the patient's symptoms.

4. **The answer is C.** The subsequent workup with liver biopsy, viral hepatitis serologies, ceruloplasmin, and ANAs is appropriate for the workup of apparent chronic hepatitis.

5. **The answer is A.** This is a patient with a history of ulcerative colitis who appears to have a clinical picture consistent with bacterial cholangitis, a complication of primary sclerosing cholangitis. To address this possibility, blood culture and liver function tests would be useful. A slit lamp examination to look for Kayser-Fleischer rings can be used to aid in the diagnosis of Wilson's disease, but in patients with chronic cholestatic diseases such as PSC, copper accumulation can occur in the absence of Wilson's disease.

Chapter 21

1. **The answer is C.** Sodium retention resulting from the increased activity of the renin-angiotensin system leads to water retention and contributes to the formation of ascites. Reversal of this mechanism by using an aldosterone antagonist is a useful first-line approach to treating ascites. Loop diuretics are usually added when aldosterone antagonists are ineffective but may be started concurrently. Thiazide diuretics and carbonic anhydrase inhibitors are not very effective in patients with significant ascites and are associated with many electrolyte abnormalities that may complicate the management of the patient's disease.

2. **The answer is B.** β-Adrenergic blockers are effective in treating the hyperdynamic state associated with portal hypertension and have been shown to decrease the complication rate from variceal bleeding. β-Adrenergic blockers are titrated, using the blood pressure and heart rate to obtain maximal clinical benefit. β-Adrenergic blockers typically cause constriction in vasculature innervated by β_2 receptors. β-Adrenergic blockers do not affect the afferent arterioles in the renal vasculature. Contractile myofibroblasts are sensitive to vasodilators, not β-blockers.

3. **The answer is C.** This patient's agitation is a manifestation of her hepatic encephalopathy. In the acute setting, osmotic cathartic agents like lactulose are effective in reducing the circulating ammonia content. Protein restriction has a role in the prevention of hepatic encephalopathy but is not effective in the acute setting. Diuresis does not reduce the ammonia content and is not effective. Sedative drugs like benzodiazepines should not be used in the management of encephalopathy, because they may exacerbate symptoms by binding to the benzodiazepine receptor in the brain, which has been shown to play a role in the pathogenesis of hepatic encephalopathy.

4. **The answer is C.** Ballooning of the hepatocytes is a dynamic lesion associated with alcoholic liver disease, which contributes to increased sinusoidal pressures and leads to portal hypertension. Abstinence can reverse the ballooning changes and decrease portal pressure. Collagen deposition in the spaces of Disse is a fixed lesion and will not regress with abstinence. Portal flow is not a significant factor in alcoholic liver disease. Portal vein thrombosis is associated with cirrhosis but typically does not regress spontaneously.

5. **The answer is B.** The most appropriate next step is to determine the precipitating factors that may have contributed to the patient's new onset of hepatic encephalopathy, including infections such as SBP, GI bleeding, drug ingestion, and hypokalemia. Although the patient may need more aggressive diuretic therapy after infection has been ruled out, the acute treatment of hepatic encephalopathy does not include aggressive diuretic use, which may occasionally worsen hepatic encephalopathy. Ultrasound of the abdomen may be useful at a later time to evaluate the cause of worsening ascites after infection has been excluded, but it is not useful for the initial evaluation of hepatic encephalopathy. Lumbar puncture and EEG may be useful for the evaluation of confusion to exclude meningitis and seizure disorders, but it is not useful in the initial evaluation of hepatic encephalopathy.

Chapter 22

1. **The answer is C.** Drugs and bacterial infections cause intrahepatic cholestasis, as does Byler's disease. Gallstones in the common duct cause physical blockage of the duct, rather than within the liver cells, as do the others listed.

2. **The answer is B.** UDPGT conjugates bilirubin by adding one or, more commonly, two residues of glucuronic acid. This renders the bilirubin soluble. The other enzymes are present in the canalicular membrane but are not involved in the mechanism of the disease.

3. **The answer is C.** Given the age of the patient, it is likely that he is taking some medication that interferes with conjugation of bilirubin. His total and direct bilirubin should be measured and liver function tests performed. His alcohol consumption history should be taken. A liver biopsy should not be done at this point, because other tests should provide important information. Stones may be retained and can still form, even in the absence of a gallbladder, often as a result of changes in bile composition, infection, or scarring from surgery. Such stones may be in smaller ducts, so the negative finding on the common bile duct does not mean that stones are an impossibility. However, the most likely cause in this patient is drug-induced cholestasis.

Chapter 23

1. **The answer is A.** The standard treatment of acute cellular rejection is intravenous administration of large doses of corticosteroids, such as methylprednisolone. If the rejection episode does not respond to corticosteroids, OKT3 is often used. Some investigators have reported the use of tacrolimus as rescue therapy in patients on cyclosporine-based immunosuppression.

2. **The answer is D.** Foam cell arteriopathy is the histologic hallmark of chronic rejection. However, it is seen in only a minority of patients. Portal and periportal hepatitis and venular endotheliitis are commonly seen in acute cellular rejection. Small bile-duct loss is also a characteristic feature of chronic rejection; however, it should be demonstrated in at least 50% of the portal areas, and at least 20 portal areas should be available for examination.

3. **The answer is B.** Massive hepatocyte necrosis typically occurs in hyperacute rejection. Acute cellular rejection characteristically shows the triad of nonsuppurative cholangitis, endotheliitis, and portal and periportal hepatitis. Arteritis may also be seen, but endothelial foam cells are not present. Lobular infiltration with polymorphs is not a typical feature of acute rejection.

4. **The answer is C.** T cells expressing CD8 markers recognize the alloantigens and initiate the immune response. CD4-positive cells are also involved in graft recognition; however, they interact with self–class II MHC. B cells are not directly involved in the recognition of alloantigens, and natural killer cell activity is not MHC-restricted.

5. **The answer is A.** Both cyclosporine and tacrolimus act predominantly by blocking the transcription of the IL-2 gene. The inhibition of IL-2 expression suppresses the inflammatory response. Cyclosporine combines with the intracellular protein cyclophillin, which blocks IL-2 expression; this does not cause lysis of T cells. It does not directly affect B cell proliferation or T cell purine synthesis.

Chapter 24

1. **The answer is A.** Fatty liver is very common in alcoholics and may even be induced by short-term heavy use of alcohol. Diabetes may occur in some alcoholics who have extensive pancreatic damage but is not as common as fatty liver. Absorption of water-soluble vitamins is decreased. Elevations of serum transaminases are not usually remarkably high unless viral hepatitis is also present.

2. **The answer is D.** The ADH enzyme removes H from CH_3CH_2OH, converting it to acetaldehyde and transferring the H to NAD^+ to generate NADH. Zinc is an integral part of the structure of the enzyme. Both of these nutrients are often deficient in alcoholics. The other cofactors are not involved in this enzymatic reaction.

3. **The answer is C.** Although fatty liver appears to be the first stage of liver damage during chronic alcohol consumption, it does not necessarily lead to cirrhosis or alcoholic hepatitis, particularly when good nutrition is present. Females who are alcoholics are at a significantly higher risk than males for developing cirrhosis.

4. **The answer is A.** Because the liver's secretion of protein in general and clotting factors in particular is reduced in alcoholics, the ability of the blood to clot is reduced, and an increased prothrombin time occurs. Esophageal varices often form as consequence of portal hypertension secondary to liver damage. Thyroid storm is not caused by alcohol abuse, although the function of the thyroid can be disrupted. Although dietary deficiencies occur, they are not usually life-threatening.

5. **The answer is A.** Pancreatitis is very common in alcoholics. B is incorrect because loss of peripheral fat and muscle is common. Although increased gastric acid secretion and delayed gastric emptying are common in alcoholics, there is no evidence that there is an increased risk for oral and esophageal cancer in alcoholics, especially in those who smoke. D is not correct because alcoholics are often deficient in clotting factors.

6. **The answer is C.** Peroxidation of membrane lipids occurs due to free radicals generated during alcohol metabolism. These membrane changes are not due to vitamin deficiencies. Mitochondria are larger than normal in the livers of alcoholics, thought to be in response to reduced ATP levels, and the smooth endoplasmic reticulum is significantly increased, because secretion from the liver cell is impaired and proteins appear to be retained in that subcellular fraction.

Chapter 25

1. **The answer is D.** A comprehensive history should be obtained and physical examination performed. All of the other choices have a role in the evaluation of abdominal pain, but they are secondary to a good history and physical examination. Although the initial symptoms may be classic for one diagnosis, there are many causes for them. Pain is often a symptom, not a disease entity in its own right. For example, if further questioning revealed a strong family history of myocardial infarction for men in their early 40s, the clinical workup would have different priorities from those for another patient with similar presenting symptoms.

2. **The answer is A.** Visceral pain tends to be poorly localized and vague in quality and is mediated at the spinal cord level. It is often associated with a local reflex arc, and both intensity and quality of the stimulus can have a varying effect on the severity of resultant pain. Somatic pain on the other hand is well localized, sharp, and definite. It is mediated at higher (cortical) levels, and pain is usually well correlated with the intensity of the stimulus. Pain sensation is transmitted via the celiac plexus as part of the reflex arc. The limbic system may have a role in interpretation of pain sensation as related to time of day and circadian cycle. However, it has not been demonstrated as having a direct role in pain states.

3. **The answer is C.** The concept of secondary gain is one in which a particular state (i.e., chronic pain) or behavior pattern is prolonged because it has brought with it other benefits that may not be continued if the initial condition is resolved. Examples include increased attention, compensation or disability benefits, access to a health care support system, and access to potentially habit-forming or addictive medications. Not all secondary gain behavior is antisocial or undesirable, but its role in chronic pain states cannot be ignored.

4. **The answer is D.** Surgical and anesthetic plexus therapy, as well as narcotic analgesics, are accepted therapeutic modes in appropriate patients suffering from chronic abdominal pain. Alternative modes may be employed either as an adjuvant to block therapy or alone as circumstances (i.e., general patient condition and wishes) permit. Some patients either do not want or cannot receive invasive intervention. Antidepressants have been proven to enhance the quality of life or, in combination with invasive block, increase the perceived effectiveness of the procedure. They do enhance appetite and can help break the cycle of despondency often noted with chronic pain states. There is little recognized role for antipsychotics outside of their approved usage for mental illness in chronic pain patients. Muscle relaxants and biofeedback have been shown to be more effective in relieving pain arising from musculoskeletel sources then that from visceral organs.

5. **The answer is B.** Maximum local anesthetic doses are usually calculated in mg/kg of body weight. Gender is often factored in as it relates to body weight. However, markedly obese or cachectic patients may have local anesthetic dosage adjusted slightly with regard to their ideal body weight and overall physical condition. Class of drug (amide or ester) is significant with regard to metabolic and elimination pathways but in itself does not affect clinical effectiveness. It, as well as pH and pKa can be important determinants in how rapidly a local anesthetic diffuses toward the intended site of action across tissue planes. Local anesthetics

work by blocking the transmission of an action potential along a nerve axon. This occurs in all nerve tissue, whether it is located in the central nervous system, peripheral nervous system, cardiac conduction system, or intestinal neural plexus. Side effects of local anesthetics are extensions of their clinical functions. For example, unintended cardiac conduction blockade from local anesthetics is considered a side effect, whereas control of arrhythmia by the same mechanism is a therapeutic goal.

Chapter 26

1. **The answer is D.** The total blood volume in the patient described in the case study is increased, and the total plasma volume is increased. Hepatic blood flow is unchanged, and the total renal blood flow is increased. The ratio of hepatic blood flow to cardiac output is decreased because of the increase in cardiac output.

2. **The answer is C.** Increased blood pressure, peripheral edema, and proteinuria are not common occurrences in every pregnancy. This is not a cholestatic problem. These findings are consistent with preeclampsia by definition: hypertension, edema, and proteinuria. Essential hypertension would not present this way, especially in a patient who has a recent history of normal blood pressure.

3. **The answer is C.** This patient has developed the HELLP syndrome. There is evidence of hemolysis on the smear, and the low haptoglobin is consistent with hemolysis. The clinical presentation of intrahepatic cholestasis also usually occurs in the third trimester. Symptoms include pruritus, dark urine, light stools, and jaundice. In acute fatty liver of pregnancy, symptoms include anorexia, nausea, vomiting, malaise, epigastric pain, headache, and progressive jaundice. In severe cases oliguria, GI bleeding, somnolence, or coma ensue. Viral hepatitis usually presents with malaise, fatigue, jaundice, and fever.

4. **The answer is C.** The bile acid pool size is increased. There is decreased enterohepatic circulation and increased percentage of cholic acid. The stasis of bile does promote the formation of gallstones.

5. **The answer is C.** The most common cause of acute diarrhea in the pregnant patient is an infectious pathogen. Ulcerative colitis and Crohn's disease may initially present during pregnancy but are not the most common causes of diarrhea. Cholecystitis would normally present with right upper quadrant pain, not acute diarrhea, as the main manifestation even in the nonpregnant patient.

6. **The answer is A.** Viral hepatitis is the most common cause of jaundice in the pregnant patient. Acute cholecystitis may not even present with jaundice. Patients with autoimmune liver disease may become pregnant, but they are not often jaundiced. In fact, patients with decompensated liver disease rarely are able to conceive. For this reason as well, alcoholic liver disease is not the most common cause of jaundice in pregnancy.

7. **The answer is C.** Progesterone is a mediator of lower esophageal sphincter relaxation. Gastric acidity is a major factor in determining the severity of aspiration pneumonitis in patients who require anesthesia during delivery and are at high risk for aspiration. Prevention should therefore include increasing the gastric pH. Nonsystemic therapy with antacids appears to be both safe and effective in pregnancy. Antacids, may, however interfere with iron absorption. The safety of H_2 blockers in pregnancy has not been studied in a prospective manner, but clinical experience suggests that pregnant women and their infants are not at increased risk for problems. However, the most conservative approach is usually initiated, and initial treatment should consist of lifestyle modification with antireflux precautions, avoiding those foods that tend to decrease lower esophageal sphincter pressure (e.g., chocolate, peppermint) and that may irritate the esophageal mucosa, eating smaller meals, and not eating before lying down. Head-of-bed elevation should be recommended.

8. **The answer is A.** Bulking agents, such as fiber, may be recommended and are safe during pregnancy. Lubricants such as mineral oil should be avoided for routine use because decreased absorption of fat-soluble vitamins may result. Castor oil should be avoided in pregnancy because it may initiate uterine contractions. Cascara sagrada has been reported to result in loose stools in the newborn.

Chapter 27

1. **The answer is B.** The *p53* gene inactivation is felt to be a late event in the pathogenesis of CRC. A is incorrect because although *ras* mutations are believed to be early events, allelic deletion of the *APC* gene may precede it. C is incorrect because the *APC* gene is involved in both FAP and sporadic colorectal carcinoma. D is incorrect because the *DCC* gene is a tumor suppressor gene.

2. **The answer is B.** One of the characteristics of the transformed cell is to participate in autocrine growth regulation, which may permit the cell to grow in the absence of extrinsic growth factors. Transformed cells are anchorage independent and have a lack of density-dependent contact inhibition; therefore, they pile up on each other in multiple layers and have the property of tumorigenicity but not mutagenicity.

3. **The answer is C.** Clonal expansion occurs when a cell develops a series of mutations that confers a growth advantage to that cell, subsequently leading to malignancy. The concept of multistep tumor formation suggests that tumors develop as a result of multiple genetic alterations, making choice A false. Knudson's hypothesis states that loss of *both* alleles of a tumor suppressor gene is required to develop malignancy. It is the activation of oncogenes and the inactivation of tumor suppressor genes that leads to malignancy.

4. **The answer is C.** The rate of a cell's proliferation is determined by intrinsic and extrinsic regulation. The cell cycle does not determine the differentiation of the cell. The G0 phase may be the longest phase in cells that have a long resting phase. The cell is only briefly tetraploid just prior to cell division; most of the time, the cell is diploid.

5. **The answer is D.** This is the classic presentation for HNPCC, where affected patients have a strong family history of colon cancer presenting at an early age with a predisposition for the right colon. There is also an association with cancers of the endometrium, stomach, and urinary tract in these families. FAP is associated with thousands of polyps, with all affected patients developing colon cancer unless prior colectomy is performed. Li-Fraumeni syndrome is a condition with an inherited germline mutation of the *p53* gene. An inherited K-*ras* mutation syndrome has not been described. Also, K-*ras* is an oncogene and not likely to be associated with a family cancer syndrome.

6. **The answer is C.** When dysplasia is found, patients with Barrett's esophagus should undergo close surveillance; monitoring at 2-year intervals is inadequate. An esophagectomy for low-grade dysplasia, however, would not be warranted because an understanding of the natural history of low-grade dysplasia is unclear. The patient must be informed that he has a permalignant condition and will require close observation.

Chapter 28

1. **The answer is D.** Omeprazole is a potent inhibitor of acid secretion because it inhibits the final step of acid production in the parietal cell by irreversibly binding to the proton pump, the H^+-K^+-ATPase enzyme. This makes all prior events in the parietal cell "null and void." Omeprazole has no effect on the receptors for ACh, histamine, or gastrin, and it does not stimulate somatostatin production by the parietal cell.

2. **The answer is B.** All patients with a documented history of ulcer disease should be checked for infection with *H. pylori* and treated if positive because eradication decreases the risk of recurrent ulcer disease. Although maintenance therapy with H_2-receptor antagonists is also effective for decreasing the recurrence of PUD, it is no longer cost-effective to do so. Therefore, there is no role for famotidine, cimetidine, or omeprazole in this patient if he is infected with *H. pylori*.

3. **The answer is B.** Both domperidone and metoclopramide inhibit gastric dopamine receptors, thereby inhibiting gastric relaxation. Metoclopramide also inhibits dopamine receptors in the CTZ, thereby acting as an antiemetic. Cisapride facilitates ACh release in the myenteric plexus, thereby causing contraction of gastric and duodenal muscle. In this manner, it accelerates gastric emptying in patients with gastroparesis. Erythromycin stimulates motilin receptors.

4. **The answer is A.** Sorbitol acts physiologically by reaching the colon unchanged, where it is metabolized by colonic bacteria to short-chain fatty acids that increase stool osmolarity, thereby drawing fluid into the lumen and increasing stool volume. It does not cause any damage to the colon and is not associated with habituation. The most common adverse effect of sorbitol is bloating, as a result of the production of gas by the colonic bacteria. Bisacodyl, castor oil, and phenolphthalein are all stimulant laxatives that can cause damage to the myenteric plexus and metabolic abnormalities resulting from their effects on electrolyte secretion. Mineral oil is a lubricant laxative that is also associated with risks, including malabsorption of fat-soluble vitamins, aspiration pneumonia, and pruritus ani from fecal leakage.

5. **The answer is E.** Motion sickness is a cause of nausea and vomiting involving primarily the vestibular apparatus. The predominant vestibular pathways involve cholinergic and histaminergic input to the vomiting center. Transdermal scopolamine and meclizine would be the best options to inhibit vestibular input selectively. Unlike meclizine, which is an antihistamine with drowsiness as an adverse effect, transdermal scopolamine, an anticholinergic, has the advantage of not causing sedation, which is important for the safety of the taxi driver and his passengers, let alone other drivers or pedestrians! Metoclopramide has multiple adverse CNS effects, which can present a problem to a driver, and prochlorperazine, a phenothiazine, has broad effects on the CTZ and vomiting center that are probably not necessary in a patient with motion sickness.

Chapter 29

1. **The answer is B.** A stressed patient requires approximately 30 kcal/kg/d to maintain lean body mass. For a 60-kg woman, this is 1800 kcal/d.

2. **The answer is D.** The indications for parenteral nutrition can be generally summarized into three categories: malabsorption, such as in Crohn's disease or celiac disease; conditions producing small bowel obstruction; and enterocutaneous fistulas with an output of more than 500 ml/day. Patients have the right to refuse necessary medical treatment after being informed of the risk of refusing the treatment; however, no family should ever be told that parenteral nutrition is an acceptable substitute for enteral nutrition when the family simply does not wish insertion of a feeding tube.

3. **The answer is A.** Elemental diets are fiber-free diets that consist of simple sugars, fats, amino acids, and sometimes di- or tripeptides. Because of the free amino acids they contain, they are normally unpalatable and are best suited for administration via a feeding tube. They are used in cases where the patient has a limited surface area available for nutrient absorption, such as in short bowel syndrome.

4. **The answer is C.** Kwashiorkor is defined as protein malnutrition in the face of adequate nonprotein caloric intake. It is not usually seen in patients who are able to tolerate and can afford a typical Western diet. Hospitalized patients are normally supplied with a diet that provides adequate protein intake. Colonic obstruction normally produces marasmus (protein-calorie malnutrition) by rendering the patient incapable of maintaining any enteral intake.

5. **The answer is B.** Gluconeogenesis requires the provision of three-carbon molecules for the synthesis of glucose. In humans, fatty acids can be broken down only into two-carbon fragments and therefore cannot be used for gluconeogenesis. Soluble fibers are not normally absorbed by the intestine and therefore do not provide substrate for gluconeogenesis. Trace elements, such as chromium, are necessary for the proper uptake of glucose by cells but do not provide materials for gluconeogenesis. In the face of glucose deficiency, the body breaks down visceral and somatic protein stores to provide the three-carbon substrates needed.

6. **The answer is A.** An enteral diet is indicated in any patient in which adequate functioning small bowel is present to absorb the necessary nutrients. Enteritis, bowel obstruction, and malabsorption all impair the ability of the bowel to absorb nutrients and may make nutrition by the enteral route impractical or impossible.

Chapter 30

1. **The answer is C.** Diverticula contain only the mucosal layer protruding through the muscularis and thus are pseudodiverticulum. These lesions are more common in the left colon but are more likely to bleed from the right colon. Diverticulosis is very common in the United States and may relate to the Western diet, which is low in fiber.

2. **The answer is D.** GI bleeding is best managed by a multidisciplinary team consisting of an intensivist, a gastroenterologist, a surgeon, and an interventional radiologist.

3. **The answer is C.** The hematocrit represents the percentage of RBCs in the serum and only falls once redistribution of fluid occurs into the space. Up to 16% of patients with duodenal bleeding will have negative NG aspirates, presumably due to pylorospasm and no retrograde flow of blood into the stomach. Over 90% of duodenal ulcers are associated with *H. pylori* infections. Eradication of *H. pylori* hastens ulcer healing and decreases recurrence. Pressure is proportional to resistance × flow. In cirrhosis, vascular resistance is increased at the level of the hepatic microcirculation. In addition, flow is increased due to an increased circulating volume.

4. **The answer is C.** Treatment may include all of the modalities mentioned in option C and may also include pharmacologic agents to decrease portal pressure. Bleeding from varices is usually massive. Hemodynamic studies have demonstrated that variceal bleeding does not occur until the hepatic venous pressure gradient exceeds 12 mm Hg. The mortality rate for first variceal bleeding is about 20% in patients with preserved liver function but 60% for those with liver failure.

Appendix

Normal Lab Values*

CHEMISTRIES

Sodium	135–145 mEq/L
Potassium	3.5–5.1 mEq/L
Chloride	98–106 mEq/L
Bicarbonate	22–29 mEq/L
BUN	7–18 mg/dL
Creatinine	0.6–1.2 mg/dL
Glucose	70–115 mg/dL
Calcium	8.4–10.2 mg/dL
Phosphate	2.7–4.5 mg/dL
Magnesium	1.3–2.1 mg/dL
Anion gap	7–16 mEq/L
Osmolality	275–295 mOsm/kg
Protein	6.0–8.0 mg/dL
Albumin	3.5–5.5 g/dL
Total bilirubin	0.2–1.0 mg/dL
Dir. bilirubin	0.0–0.2 mg/dL
Lipase	10–140 U/dL
Amylase	25–125 U/dL
SGOT/AST	7–40 U/L
SGPT/ALT	7–40 U/L
GGT	9–50 U/L
AlkPhos	38–126 U/L
Uric Acid	2.0–6.9 mg/dL
LDH	120–240 U/L
Free T_4	0.71–1.85 ng/dL
TSH	0.32–5.00 μIU/mL

HEMATOLOGY

WBC	$4.5–11.0 \times 10^3/\mu$L
RBC	$3.8–5.7 \times 10^6/\mu$L
Hemoglobin	13.5–17.0 g/dL
Hematocrit	39–50%
MCV	80–96 fL
MCH	27–33 pg/cell
MCHC	32–36% hgb/cell
Platelets	$150–400 \times 10^3/\mu$L
RDW	11.0–16.0%
Segs (Neuts)	35–73%
Lymphocytes	15–52%
Monocytes	4–13%
Eosinophils	1–3%
Basophils	0–1%

URINALYSIS

Color	<yellow>
Turbidity	<clear>
Specific Gravity	1.003–1.035
pH	4.5–8.0
Ketones	<negative>
Protein	<negative>
Blood	<negative>
Glucose	<negative>
Nitrite	<negative>
Leukocyte Esterase	<negative>
Osmolality	50–1400 mOsm/kg
Sodium	40–220 mEq/day
Potassium	25–125 mEq/day

COAGULATION

PT	12.3–14.2 sec
PTT	25–34 sec
Bleeding Time	2–7 min
Thrombin Time	6.3–11.1 sec
Fibrinogen	200–400 mg/dL
INR (International Normalized Ratio)	1.0

* There may be specific number variations from one laboratory to another.

Index

Azotemia, 258t, 482
Azotorrhea, 267

B cells. *See* Lymphocytes, B
B vitamins. *See specific B vitamins*
Bacteremia, 408
Bacterial overgrowth, 232–233, 233t, 319
Bacterial toxins. *See* Toxins
BALT (bronchial patches), 294f
BAO (basal acid output), 208
Barbiturates, 444
Barium studies, 181, 243, 315–317, 330
  contraindicated for GI bleeding, 557
Baroreceptors, 125
Barrett's esophagus, 178t, 181, 195,
    502–503
Basal acid output (BAO), 208
Basal electric rhythm, 68
Basophils, 87
Bell's palsy, 178t
Belsey Mark IV procedure, 185, 197
Benadryl, 531, 531t
Bentiromide test, 269, 269t
Benzamides, 530
Benzodiazepines, 409t, 410, 445t, 530f
  antagonists, 410
Bernstein test, 196
Beta-blockers, 562
Bethanechol, 531t
Bicarbonate (HCO$_3^-$)
  chloride-bicarbonate (Cl$^-$-HCO$_3^-$)
      exchanger, 83, 84, 85f, 119,
      121, 121f
  and H$^+$ secretion in stomach, 82, 211
  in saliva, 80, 81f, 95
  secretion by intestine, 86, 127
  secretion by pancreas, 30, 84
  in stomach, 49, 49f, 81, 83, 518
  transport, 120–121, 121f
Bile, 5, 39–40, 70, 100, 134, 136
  composition of, 158–159, 159t
  concentration of, 161
  flow, 419
  functions of, 159–160
  gallbladder bile, 159, 162
  in GI disorders, 192, 209
  hepatic bile, 159, 162
  in lipid digestion, 107–108, 108f
  pigments, 159
  reflux, 419
  storage of, 100, 161
  synthesis/secretion of, 158, 417–419
Bile acids, 100, 101, 108, 158, 159t,
    417–419
  bile acid-dependent/independent flow,
      158, 418
  binding by antacids, 518
  binding resin, 393
  decreased by alcohol use, 448, 448t
  deficiency, 543
  enterohepatic circulation and, 160
  itching. *See* Pruritis
  synthesis of, 156, 156f, 157f, 164t
Bile ducts, 6, 46f, 80, 139
  canals of Hering, 139, 142, 146

carcinoma of, 321
common (CBD), 160, 162
  obstruction of, 270
ductopenia, 393
embryology of, 38t, 39
innervation of, 160
obliteration/loss of, 321, 430t, 433
obstruction of, 258, 272
secretion, 84–85, 85f, 134
  aquaporin channel, 85f
  inhibition of, 85
stones in, 419t
Bile salts, 83, 86, 98t, 100, 102, 107
  deficiency of, 319
  as intestinal secretagogue, 123t, 128
  malabsorption, 116t
  micelles, 107, 108f, 109, 161
Biliary atresia, 421t
Biliary cirrhosis. *See* Cirrhosis,
    primary biliary
Biliary glycoproteins, 158
Biliary stenting, 389f
Biliary tract, 160–161
  motility, regulation of, 161–163
Biliary tree, 146–147, 158
  bacterial infection of, 164, 164t
Bilirubin, 6, 16, 152, 158, 159, 159t. *See
    also* Jaundice
  detoxification of, 418
  elevation in hepatitis E, 364
  elevation in PSC, 394
  encephalopathy, 421
  and gallstones, 163–164, 164t
  hyperbilirubinemia, 418, 419t, 420–423,
      421t, 423
  metabolism, 415–418, 420–423, 421t
Bilirubin uridine diphosphate-
    glucuronosyltransferase
    (UDPGT), 158, 163, 418,
    420–421, 421t
Billroth I and II surgeries, 213f, 233t
Bisacodyl, 526t, 528
Bismuth, colloidal, 216
Bismuth subsalicylate, 479
Bleeding, gastrointestinal, 319, 409t, 448,
    448t, 548–568
  algorithm for management of, 567f
  lower GI, 549
    causes of, 558t, 563–567
    rebleeding, 550, 559–560, 562
    treatments for, 557, 561–567
  upper GI, 549–563
    causes of, 558–563, 558t
    initial assessment of, 552–553, 552t
    locating the source of, 553–555
    secondary diagnostic evaluations,
      556–557
  variceal, 405–406
Blood
  coagulation proteins, 155t
  hematopoiesis, 39, 136
Blood urea nitrogen. *See* BUN
Bombesin, 162, 204, 207–208
Bone marrow transplantations (BMT), 328
Borborygmi, 106f

Botulinum toxin (botox), 185–186
Bowel, small. *See* Intestine, small
Bradycardia, 512
Bradykinin, 300
Brain, 449t
Brain-gut axis, 17, 33
Branched-chain amino acids, 447, 541
Bromosulfophthalein, 417
Bronchiectasis, 320t, 322
Bronchitis, 320t, 322
Brunner's gland, 55, 55f, 235t
Budd-Chiari syndrome, 483, 560
Budesonide, 323
Bulimia, 528
Bulk agents, 526, 526t
BUN (blood urea nitrogen), 225t
  BUN:creatinine ratio, 554, 556
Bupivacaine, 463t, 466
Burn patients, 211
Burr cells, 482–483
Butyrophenones, 530, 531, 531t
Byler's disease, 419t, 422

C-cells, 26
C-fibers, 19
Cadherins, 493, 499
Caffeine, in peptic ulcer disease, 209
Cajal, interstitial cells of, 69–70
Calcineurin inhibitors, 434, 435
Calciosomes, 67
Calcitonin, 26, 123t
Calcitonin gene-related peptide (CGRP),
    18, 26
  in gastric reflexes, 19
Calcium (Ca^{2+}), 29, 451t, 509, 510f
  absorption in small intestine, 101, 102
  antacids as source of, 216
  Ca^{2+}-calmodulin complex, 29, 67,
      86, 126f
  channels, 66–67, 243
  hypercalcemia, 252t, 258t, 266
  hypocalcemia, 258t
  intracellular signaling mechanisms, 80,
      82f, 123t
  intracellular storage of, 67
  in muscle contraction, 66, 66f
  and resting membrane potential, 29, 66
Calcium carbonate, 215–216, 519
Calcium oxalate, 16
  stones, 321
Calculi, 320t
Calmodulin, Ca^{2+}-calmodulin complex, 29
Calories, nutritional requirements for, 540
CAMP. *See* Cyclic adenosine
    monophosphate
Campylobacter, 128, 329t, 342
Canals of Hering, 139, 142, 146
Cancer, 488–504
  adenocarcinoma, 181, 502–503
  adenoma-carcinoma sequence,
      497–498, 498f
  adenomatous polyps, 494, 498f
  aneuploidy, 502–503
  Barrett's esophagus, 178t, 181, 195,
      502–503

Cancer (*Continued*)
  and bleeding, 557, 558t, 566, 566f
  carcinogens, 489, 499f
  carcinoids, 236–237, 236t, 515–516
  cell characteristics, 493
  cell growth regulation, 491–492, 491t
  cell replication cycle, 490–491, 490f
  chromosomal alterations in, 489,
    502–503
  colorectal. *See* Colorectal cancer
  endocrine tumors, 122
  gastrinoma, 116t
  and gene expression, 492–493, 492f
  genetic predisposition for, 489–490, 496
  hepatocellular carcinoma, 2, 360,
    427, 428
  neuroendocrine tumors, 31, 32
  oncogenesis, 493–495, 503
    clonal expansion, 494
    multistep tumor formation, 494, 495
  and radiation injury, 80–81
  of small intestine, 234–240, 235t, 236,
    236f, 236t
    adenocarcinomas, 234–236, 236t
    carcinoids, 236–237, 236t
    leiomyomatous tumors, 234–240, 236t
    lymphomas, 235t, 236t, 237–239, 238t
  tumor suppressor genes, 494, 496–497,
    496f, 499, 499f, 503
  VIPoma, 116t, 122, 127, 129
Candida, 198, 329–330, 329t
Cannabinoids, 530f, 532
Caput medusae, 405, 555
Carbohydrates
  digestion/absorption, 95, 101, 103–105,
    104f, 451t
  metabolism, hepatic, 152–153, 153f, 154f
  nutritional requirements for, 542
Carbon dioxide (CO_2), 49, 49f
Carbon tetrachloride, 442
Carbonic acid, 49, 49f
Carcinoids, 236–237, 236t, 515–516. *See
  also* Cancer
Carcinoma. *See* Cancer
Cardiac region of stomach, 4, 47–48
Caries, dental, 81, 95, 96
Carnitine deficiency, 482
Carotene, 229
Carotid baroreceptors, 125
Carriers, of electrolytes, 79, 117
Casanthranol, 526t
Cascara, 526t
  sagada, 478
Castor oil, 478, 526t, 528
Cataracts, 320, 320t, 434t
Catecholamines, 127
Catapres, 284t
CBD. *See* Common bile duct
CCK. *See* Cholecystokinin
CCK-gastrin family of regulatory peptides,
  26t, 30–31
CD antigens, 291–292, 296, 297, 429
CECT (contrast-enhanced computer
  tomography) scans, in assessment

of pancreatitis, 253, 255, 257,
  258f, 259t, 260f
Cecum, 5, 57, 57f
  embryology of, 38t
Celiac disease, 7, 98t, 102, 110, 221–228,
  244t, 245
  and cancers, 226–227, 235, 236t
  clinical presentation, 225–226
  complications of, 226–227
  diagnosis of, 224–225, 306
  and inflammation, chronic, 299
  and nutrient absorption, 537
Celiac ganglion, 18, 141, 160, 529f
Celiac plexus, 46, 160, 204, 460
  block, 463t, 464–469
    in pancreatitis, 272
    permanent, 466–469
    temporary, 466
    under CT guidance, 466f, 467f, 468f
Cell adhesion, 493, 499
Cell-cell communications, 13–23
  across gap junctions, 70
  autocrine, 13, 14f, 32
  brain-gut axis, 17–19, 33
  endocrine, 13–14, 14f, 15, 16, 23–25, 32,
    123t, 205, 205f
  in gastric acid secretion, 509, 510f
  neurocrine, 13, 14, 14f, 23, 32, 123t,
    205, 205f
  paracrine, 13, 14f, 23, 25, 32, 87–88,
    123t, 205, 205f
Cell cycle, 490–491, 490f
Cell death, 145
Cell growth, 17, 491–492, 493
Cell proliferation, 493
Cellular rejection, 430–432, 430t, 431f
Cellulose, 103, 104f
Central nervous system (CNS), 7–8, 13
  brain-gut axis, 17–22, 33
  effects of alcohol on, 449t
Cephalic phase of digestion, 82
Cephalosporin, 346
Cerebral palsy, 421
Ceruloplasmin, 155t, 375, 375f,
  376–377, 376t
CFTR. *See* Cystic fibrosis transmembrane
  conductance regulator
CGMP. *See* Cyclic guanosine
  monophosphate
CGRP. *See* Calcitonin gene-related peptide
Chagas' disease, 182, 186–187, 244t, 245
Channels. *See* Ion channels
Charcot-Leyden crystals, 232
Chemoreceptor trigger zone (CTZ), 521,
  529–532, 529f
Chenodeoxycholic acid, 128, 158
Chewing, 96, 447
CHF. *See* Congestive heart failure
Chief cells, 49–50, 81, 83, 212
  secretion of pepsinogen, 96, 203, 509
Chloramphenicol, 346
Chloride (Cl^-)
  channels, 67, 79, 84, 85f, 119
    antagonists, 67
    and diarrhea, 87, 88

GABA binding and, 411f
  and intestinal secretion, 86
  and H^+ secretion in stomach, 82
  and pancreatic secretion, 84
  and resting membrane potential, 29
  in saliva, 80, 81f
  secretion of, 119, 120f
  sodium-potassium-chloride (Na^+-K^+-Cl^-)
    cotransporter, 80, 81f
  in stomach lumen, 48, 49, 49f
  transport, 119, 120, 265
Chloride-ATPase pumps, 48
Chloride-bicarbonate (Cl^--HCO_3^-)
    exchanger, 83, 84, 85f, 119,
    121, 121f
Chlorpromazine, 418t, 419t, 445t, 531t
Chlorthalidone, 252t
Choking, 447
Cholangiocarcinoma, 321, 389t, 395
Cholangiopancreatography (ERCP)
  in cholestasis, 420
  in pancreatitis, 252t, 257, 268, 271–272
  in primary sclerosing cholangitis,
    394–395, 395f, 396
Cholangitis
  and hepatic allograft rejection, 430t, 431
  infectious, 395
  primary sclerosing (PSC), 385, 389t,
    394–396, 395f
    associated diseases/disorders
      hyperbilirubinemia, 421t, 423
      inflammatory bowel disease, 318,
        320t, 321, 394
      maldigestion/malabsorption,
        98t, 226
      ulcerative colitis, 389t, 394
    autoantibodies in, 386t, 388
    and cholestasis, 419t
    clinical features of, 389t
    diagnosis of, 389t, 394–395, 395f, 396
    and HLA genotypes, 386
    treatment of, 389t, 395–396
Cholecystectomy, 5, 163, 484
Cholecystokinin (CCK), 18, 23, 24t, 25,
  84, 99
  actions of, 22t, 50t, 158, 160, 161, 162
  family of regulatory peptides, 26t, 30–31
  and gallbladder contractions, 418
  posttranslational processing of, 27
  release, control of, 97
  secretion by enteric endocrine cells, 24, 25
  stimulation of acid production, 205, 207
  stimulation test, 269, 269t
  and swallowing/achalasia, 184
Choledochal cyst, 421t
Choledocholithiasis, 419t
Cholelithiasis, 321
Cholera, 86–87, 128, 129, 336
Cholescintigraphy, 162
Cholestasis, 391–392, 416, 542
  cellular alterations in, 418–419, 418t
  extrahepatic/intrahepatic, 419–420
    causes of, 419t
    treatment of, 420
  familial forms of, 422

and hepatic allograft rejection, 430t, 432f
  in pregnancy, 422, 481
Cholesterol, 107, 108f, 163, 164t, 484
  as component of bile, 158, 159t
  elimination by liver, 152
  hypercholesterolemia, 380, 394
  metabolism of, 156–157, 156f, 157f
  stones, 163, 164t, 484
Cholesterolesterase, 107f, 108
Cholestyramine, 5, 164t, 221
  resin, 283
  resin therapy, 422
Cholic acid, 158, 448
Chromium, 539t
Chronic intestinal pseudo-obstruction (CIP), 285–286
Chylomicrons, 108, 108f
Chyme, 51, 55, 97, 101
Chymotrypsin, 267
Chymotrypsinogens A and B, 99
Cigarette smoking. See Tobacco
Cimetidine, 12, 83, 97, 214, 509–513
  adverse effects of, 511–512
  and alcohol use, 444, 445t, 448
  chemical structure of, 511f
  in pregnancy, 476
CIP. See Chronic intestinal pseudo-obstruction
Circular muscle, of GI tract, 43, 45
Cirrhosis, 2, 3t, 320t, 321, 560, 561
  ascites in, 406
  cryptogenic, 321
  and hepatitis B, 360
  of liver, 140, 145, 148, 372, 373, 396
    and alcohol, 444–445, 446, 447
    hemodynamic changes in, 407
    liver transplant for, 427
  primary biliary (PBC), 98t, 164t, 385, 389t, 391–394
    associated diseases, 393
      cholestasis, 419t
        hyperbilirubinemia, 421t, 423
        inflammatory bowel disease, 321
    autoantibodies in, 386–388, 386t
    clinical features of, 389t, 391–392
    complications of, 393–394
    diagnosis of, 389t, 391–393
    and HLA genotypes, 386
    treatment of, 389t
Cisapride, 521t, 522f, 524, 531t
Clarithromycin, 524
Cloaca, embryology of, 41
Clonidine, 123, 127f, 244t, 284, 284t
Clonorchis, 163
Clostridium
  botulinum, 185–186
  difficile, 220, 329t, 345
  perfringens, 242
Clotting factors, 448t
CMV. See Cytomegalovirus
CNS. See Central nervous system
CoA. See Acetyl coenzyme A
Cobalamin. See Vitamin B$_{12}$
Cocaine, 241

Codeine, 127, 127f, 445t
  in pain relief from neoplasia, 463t, 465
Coelom, 135
Coenzyme A. See Acetyl coenzyme A
Colchicine, 127f, 221, 447
Colipase, 107–108
Colitis
  Crohn's, 319, 322
  diversion, 565
  γ-enterocolitis, 229, 242
  infectious, 315, 339–347, 340f, 341f
  ischemic, 315
  necrotizing enterocolitis (NEC), 242
  pain of, 459
  pancolitis, 318–319
  proctocolitis, 324
  radiation, 315
  ulcerative (UC), 124, 128, 299, 313–314, 565
    association with primary sclerosing cholangitis, 389t
    complications of, 319, 394
    crypt abscesses in, 314, 314f
    diagnosis of, 315–317, 315f, 316f
    endoscopic photograph of, 315f
    in pregnancy, 479–480, 479t
    pseudopolyps in, 316–317
    treatment of, 322–325, 323t
    versus Crohn's disease and IBD, 310–325, 313f, 313t
Collagen vascular disorders, 231, 241, 244t, 554, 562
Collagenous sprue, 226
Collagens, 141
Colloidal bismuth, 216
Colon, 4f, 5. See also Colitis
  ascending, 4f, 5, 38t, 57, 57f
  colectomy, 324, 394, 498
  descending, 4f, 5, 38t, 57f, 58
  embryology of, 38t, 40–41
  fluid absorption, 114–115, 115f
  hepatic flexure, 57f
  histology of, 31, 58–59, 59f
  ischemia of, 566
  melanosis coli, 528
  obstruction of, 258
  sigmoid, 4f, 5, 38t, 57f
  slow wave frequency, 68t
  strictures of, 258
  tonic contractions of, 70
  toxic megacolon, 317–318, 318f, 319, 348
  transverse, 4f, 5, 38t, 57, 57f
Colonoscopy, 557, 564, 567t
  contraindicated for toxic megacolon, 318
Colorectal cancer (CRC), 489–490, 497–502
  hereditary nonpolyposis colorectal cancer (HNPCC), 500–501
  mismatch repair (MMR) genes, 500–502
  tumorigenesis model, 494, 498–500, 499f
Coma, 482
Common bile duct (CBD), 160, 162
  obstruction of, 270
Compazine, 531, 531t

Complement fixation, 293
Compliance, 403
Conditioned responses, 8
Confusion, mental, 214
Congestive heart failure (CHF), 241
Conjunctivitis, 343
Connective tissue diseases, 189–190
Constipation, 3t, 464–465, 477–478, 532
Constrictor muscles, 172
Contraceptives. See Oral contraceptives
Contractions, gastrointestinal, 64–74. See also Motility
  electrical properties of smooth muscles, 68–70, 68t, 69f
  excitation-contraction coupling, 65, 66, 66f
  interdigestive migrating motor complex (IMMC), 73–74
  intermittent transient relaxations (TLESRs), 71
  mechanisms of, 65–68
  multiorgan patterns of, 73–74
  muscle types involved in, 65–66
  patterns of, 68, 70–74
  peristalsis, 72–73
  phasic, 67, 70, 71, 72–73
  regulation of, 68–70
  retrograde, 72, 74
  segmentary, 72
  slow waves, 68–69, 68t, 69f
  tonic, 67, 70–72
  in vomiting, 64, 74–75
Contrast-enhanced computer tomography scans. See CECT scans
Copper, 148
  deficiency, 539t
  metabolism, 374–378, 375t, 376t
  overload, primary. See Wilson's disease
  overload, secondary, 374–375
  toxicity, 377
Corneal ulcerations, 320, 320t
Coronary ligament, of liver, 136f
Corticosteroids, 322–323, 323t. See also specific corticosteroids
  in alcoholic hepatitis, 447
  in immunosuppression, 430t, 434, 434t, 436
Cotransporters of electrolytes, 79, 80, 81f, 86, 120
COX-2 inhibitors, 210, 518
Cranial nerves
  in swallowing, 171
  in vomiting, 529f
CRC. See Colorectal cancer
CREST syndrome, 189–190
Cricopharyngeal achalasia, 71t
Cricopharyngeus muscle, 172
Crigler-Najjar syndromes, 421–422, 421t
Crohn's disease, 7, 98t, 102, 124, 128, 233t, 235
  clinical features of, 312–313, 313f
  complications of, 319
  diagnosis of, 315–317, 315f, 316f
  fistulas in, 315, 319, 324
  and gallstones, 164

Dysphagia, 96, 177–192, 447. *See also* Swallowing
  acid suppression treatment, 517
  classification of, 177–178, 178t
  diagnosis of, 189–192, 198
  esophageal, 180
  etiologies of, 181–182
  fiber optic endoscopic examination of swallowing safety (FEESS), 191
  transfer, 177–178
Dyspnea, 231
Dystonia, 531

Ecchymosis, 225
ECG. *See* Electrocardiogram
ECL cells. *See* Enterochromaffin-like (ECL) cells
Eclampsia, 481–482
Eczema, 303
EGF. *See* Epidermal growth factor
Eicosanoids, 124
Elastase, 267
Elderly patients, 214
  and pain, 462
Electrocardiogram (ECG), 68
Electrogastrogram, 69
Electrolyte management, 113–129
  electrolyte balance, 5, 86
  movement, 79
  secretion, 77–89
  transport, 114–118, 129
    active/passive transport, 114, 116
    regulation of, 121–129, 122f, 123t
    specific ion, 118–121, 118f, 120f, 121f
Elemental diets, 543
Emboli, 241, 320t, 322
Embryology, of GI tract, 37–41, 38f, 38t. *See also specific organs*
Emetic center, 529, 529f. *See also* Vomiting
Emollient laxatives, 526t, 527–528
Emotion, 8
Encephalopathy
  hepatic, 408–411, 409t, 447, 449t
  Wernicke's, 449t
Endocarditis, 229, 231
Endocrine cells, 13, 14f, 16
Endocrine hormone pathway. *See* Cell-cell communications, endocrine
Endocrine pancreas, 5
Endocrine system
  and chronic alcohol ingestion, 449t
  of GI tract, 23–25
  neuroendocrine tumors, 31
Endocrine tumors, 122
Endoscopic retrograde cholangiopancreatography (ERCP). *See* Cholangiopancreatography (ERCP)
Endoscopic ultrasound (EUS), 268
Endoscopy
  in celiac disease diagnosis, 224
  in IBD, 312, 313t, 315t
  in treatment of GI bleeding, 556, 559–563, 567t

Endothelial cells, 87, 139–140, 402, 402f
  spaces of Disse, 139, 141–142, 406
Endotheliitis, 430t, 431, 431f
Endotoxins. *See* Toxins
Enflurane, 445t
Enkephalins, 26t, 127, 204
ENS. *See* Enteric nervous system
Entamoeba histolytica, 329t, 347–348, 479
Enteral nutrition, 543–544, 544t
Enteric nervous system (ENS), 7, 8, 14
  anatomy of, 19–20, 122
  electrophysiologic characteristics of, 20–21
  enteric hormones, 8
  intrinsic control of the GI system, 19–22, 33, 123–124
  neurotransmitters in, 8, 21–22, 33
Enteritis, 537, 544t
  gastroenteritis, eosinophilic, 78, 88–89, 98t, 102, 232
  regional. *See* Crohn's disease
Enterobacter cloacae, 228
Enterochromaffin-like (ECL) cells, 23, 32, 129, 509, 510f
  in carcinoid tumors, 515–516
Enteroclysis, 315–316
Enterocolitis, 229, 242
Enterocytes, 52f, 53, 58, 108f
  activated, 87, 87f
Enterocytozoon bieneusi, 338
Enteroendocrine cells, 14, 31, 50, 50t
Enteroglucagons, 17, 22t, 24t, 26, 30
  glycentin, 26t, 30
  oxyntomodulin, 26, 26t, 30
  and reflex slowing of motility, 31
  secretin-VIP family, 26t, 30
  secretion by enteric endocrine cells, 24
  stimulation of HCl production, 205
Enterohepatic circulation, 157, 160
Enterokinase, 99, 101
Enteromegaly, 186
Enterotoxigenic diarrhea, 87, 115, 128
Enterotoxins, 54, 115, 128
Enterovirus, 354
Enzymes. *See also specific enzymes*
  pancreatic exocrine function, 5
  secretion by duodenum, 5
Eosinophilic gastroenteritis, 78, 88–89, 98t, 102, 232
Eosinophils, 87, 88, 290
Epidermal growth factor (EGF), 145, 169, 491, 495, 518
Epiglottis, 74
Epinephrine, 127, 542
  in enteric nervous system, 21
Episcleritis, 320, 320t
Epistaxis, 225
Epstein-Barr virus, 252t
Erb's palsy, 479
ERCP. *See* Cholangiopancreatography
Ergotamines, 241–242
Erosions, of GI lining, 208
Erythema, 300
  nodosum, 320t, 555
  palmar, 444t

Erythematosus, 244t
Erythromycin, 32, 521t, 524, 525, 531t
Escherichia coli, 86–87, 123t, 128, 329t, 344
  0157:H7, 344
  in tropical sprue, 228
Esomeprazole, 214, 513–514, 514f, 517t
Esophageal body, 168–169, 169f
Esophagitis, 83, 178t, 194–195, 196, 198
  bleeding from, 558t
  Candida, 329–330, 329t
  CMV, 329t, 330–331
  HSV, 329t, 331–332, 331f
  reflux, 299
  ulcerative, treatment of, 512–513, 516, 517t
Esophagography, 190–191
Esophagus, 3, 43–44. *See also* Esophagitis; Gastroesophageal reflux disease; Swallowing
  adenocarcinoma of, 195
  alcohol effects on, 447, 448t
  anatomy of, 43–44
  Barrett's, 178t, 181, 195, 502–503
  carcinoma of, 181, 489
  corkscrew/rosary bead, 188t
  diffuse esophageal spasm (DES), 187–188, 188t
  dysphagia of, 180–186, 183f, 184f
  embryology of, 38t, 39
  esophagectomy, 187
  histology of, 44–45, 44f
  infections of, 328–332, 331f
  innervation of, 8, 18
  lower sphincter (LES) of. *See* Sphincter, lower esophageal
  manometry of, 174–176, 175f, 176f, 182, 187–188, 188t, 191–192, 197t
  motility disorders, 188–189, 188t
  neurotransmitters in, 21
  non-GERD-related esophageal mucosal disease, 197–198
  peristalsis of, 65, 67, 173, 174–176, 176f, 193t, 194
  sigmoid, 184f
  spasm of, 67, 178t, 187–188, 188t
  stricture of, 447
  in swallowing, 168–178, 180–186, 183f, 184f
  upper sphincter (UES) of. *See* Sphincter, upper esophageal
  varices of, 447, 448t, 560, 561f
Estradiol-binding globulin, 155t
Estrogens
  and arterial occlusion, 240–241
  and cholestasis, 418t
  and gallstone formation, 163, 164t
ET-OH. *See* Alcohol, ethyl
Ethanol. *See* Alcohol, ethyl
EUS. *See* Endoscopic ultrasound
Exchange carriers, 79
Exons, 492, 492f
Extracellular matrix, 141, 492–493

Spleen, 7, 401f, 420
  embryology of, 40
  hyposplenism, 226
  splenectomy, 561
  splenomegaly, 555
Splenic flexure, 57f
Splenic vein thrombosis, 561
Spondylitis, 320, 320t
Sprue
  celiac. *See* Celiac disease
  collagenous, 226
  nontropical. *See* Celiac disease
  tropical, 98t, 102, 227–229
Src genes, 495
Starch, 103
Steatorrhea, 100, 102, 221, 229, 230, 448
  idiopathic. *See* Celiac disease
  in pancreatitis, 267, 272
Steatosis, 157, 164, 446. *See also* Fatty liver
  and inflammatory bowel disease, 321
Stellate cells, 140, 372, 402f
Stem cells, in gastric glands, 52
Stenosis, 263
Stents, 396
  biliary, 458
Steroid hormones, 127f, 156. *See also*
    Corticosteroids; Estrogens
  and cholestasis, 419t
  therapy for autoimmune liver diseases,
    389t, 395–396
Sterols, 156f
Stimulant laxatives, 526t, 528
Stomach, 4, 4f, 35–51, 203f. *See also*
    Gastritis; Peptic ulcer disease
  acid secreting (parietal) cells, 17, 203,
    204–206, 205f, 206f
  alcohol effects on, 448, 448t
  anatomy of, 45–46, 46f, 203, 203f
  antrum of, 4, 30, 46, 46f, 96–97,
    203–204, 203f, 206f
  body of, 46, 46f, 48, 96, 203f
  cancer of, 489
  cardiac region of, 4, 47–48
  curvatures of, 39, 46f
  digestion in, 81–83, 94f, 96–98,
    203–204, 203f
  distal, 97–98
  embryology of, 38t, 39
  fundus of, 4, 46, 46f, 48, 96, 203, 203f
  gastrectomy, 21, 97, 518
  gastric glands, 48–51
  gastric pits, 47, 81, 83, 203
  gastroenterostomy, 212
  histology of, 46–51, 47f
  infections of, 332–333
  innervation of, 8, 18, 204
  maximal acid output (MAO) of, 212
  mucosa of, 46–51, 47f
  pH maintenance in, 81, 83
  proximal, 96–97
  pylorus of, 4, 31, 46, 46f, 51, 96
    digestive functions, 97, 203–204, 203f
    pyloric glands, 203–204
    pyloroplasty, 212
  ulcers, treatment of, 514, 517, 517t

Stool osmolality, 116
Strangulation, in small bowel ischemia, 240
Streptomyces tsukubaensis, 435
Streptozocin, 237
Stress, 8
Stretta system, 197
Strictures
  of esophagus, 447
  of intestine, 258, 316, 319, 324–325
  strictureplasty, 324–325
Strongyloides, 221, 232
Submucosa, 42–43, 42f
  of anus, 60, 61f
  of esophagus, 45
  of intestine, 52f, 59f, 295f
Submucosal gland, 42f
Submucosal plexus (Meissner's plexus), 8,
    14f, 19, 42f, 204
  and fluid/electrolyte transport, 123
Substance P (SP), 18, 25, 123t, 204
  and activated mast cells, 297
  and GI contractions, 73
  neuromedin family, 26t
Sucralfate, 216, 519
Sucrase, 101
Sucrose, 103
Sugars, 103
Sulfasalazine, 323–324, 323t, 479
Sulfonamides, 253t
Sulfur (S), and copper metabolism, 377
Superior mesenteric vein, 401, 401f
Superoxides, 124
Surcralfate, 476
Swallowing, 45, 167–198. *See also*
    Gastroesophageal reflux disease
  anatomy of swallowing mechanism,
    168–173, 169f
  control of, 7, 170–171, 170t
  dysphagia, 96, 177–192, 447
  esophageal body, 168–169, 169f
  esophageal manometry, 174–176, 175f,
    176f, 191–192
  neural innervation, 170–171, 172
  odynophagia (painful swallowing),
    194, 198
  physiology of, 173–174
  process of, 171–173
  sphincters involved in, 168–176,
    175f, 176f
Sympathectomy, 463t, 467, 469
Sympathetic nervous system, 14, 18,
    122–123
Symporters (cotransporters), 79
Synovitis, 320
Syphilis, 334
Systemic lupus erythematosus, 244t,
    245, 387

T cells. *See* Lymphocytes, T
Tachycardia, 216, 253, 443, 524, 532, 552t
Tachykinins. *See* Substance P
Tachyphylaxis, 464
Tacrolimus, 430t, 434, 434t, 435–436
Taeniae coli, 57, 57f, 59f
Tagamet. *See* Cimetidine

Tardive dyskinesia, 523, 531
Taste, 80, 81
TATA gene sequence, 492, 492f
TCA cycle, 153f, 154f, 156f
  effects of alcohol on, 444
Technetium pertechnetate, 567
Teeth, 95
  dental caries, 81, 95, 96
Tegaserod, 282–283
Telangiectasia, 190, 552t, 555
TENS. *See* Transcutaneous electrical
    stimulation
Teratogenic substances, 479
Testicular atrophy, 449t, 555
Testosterone, 449t
Testosterone-binding globulin, 155t
Tetracycline, 198, 215, 229, 346
Tetrahydrocannabinol, 530f, 532
Tetrodotoxin, 67
TGF-α, 145
TGF-β, 145
Theophylline, 512
Thiamine (vitamin B$_1$), 108–109, 109f
  deficiency, 449t, 450, 451t
Thiazide, 252t
Thoracic duct, 142
Thoracotomy, 185
Thorazine, 531t
Threonine phosphorylation, 491, 491t
Thrombocytopenia, 434t, 436, 483, 512
Thrombosis
  and allograft rejection, 430, 433
  in inflammatory bowel disease, 320t, 322
  mesenteric arterial, 241
  splenic vein, 561
  in treatment of variceal bleeding, 561–562
  vascular, 258t
  and vascular resistance, 404
Thrush. *See* Candida
Thymus, 300, 385
Thyroid, antithyroid drugs, 419t
Thyroid-binding globulin, 155t
Thyroid disease, association with primary
    biliary cirrhosis, 393
Tight junctions, 116–117
  and inflammation, 124
  in liver, 139
TIPS (transjugular intrahepatic
    portosystemic shunt), 406, 410,
    557, 561, 562
TLESRs. *See* Intermittent transient
    relaxations
TNF. *See* Tumor necrosis factor
Tobacco
  in peptic ulcer disease, 209
  and small bowel ischemia, 241
Tolbutamide, 444, 445t
Tolerance
  immune, 433–436
  oral, 300–301
Tolypocladium inflatum Gams, 435
Tongue, 38t
Tonic contractions, 67, 70–72
Tonsils, 38t
Torticollis, 523

Total parenteral nutrition (TPN), 256, 317, 419t, 420, 423, 543, 545. *See also* Nutrition
Toxic megacolon, 317–318, 318f, 319, 348
Toxins
    bacterial endotoxins, 86, 87, 123t, 128, 242
    botulinum toxin (botox), 185–186
    Clostridium perfringens, 242
    enterotoxins, 54, 115, 128
    Escherichia coli, 86–87, 123t
    excretion of, 100
    Vibrio cholerae, 86–87, 115, 116t, 123t, 128
    Yersinia, 123t
TPN. *See* Nutrition, total parenteral
Trace element deficiencies, 538, 539t
Transaminases, 390, 532
Transamination reactions, 153, 154f
Transcortin, 155t
Transcription, gene, 492
    regulatory proteins, 495
Transcutaneous electrical stimulation (TENS), 469
Transderm Scop (scopolamine), 531t
Transfer dysphagia, 177–178
Transferrin, 155t, 371, 372t, 539t
Transformed cells. *See* Cancer, cell characteristics
Transforming growth factor (TGF)-α, 491, 495
Transglutaminase antibody, 110, 225
Transit rates, 6, 64, 72
Transmitters. *See* Neurotransmitters
Transplants
    bone marrow (BMT), 328
    graft-versus-host disease (GVHD), 299
    liver. *See* Liver, orthotopic transplantation of
Transport of water/electrolytes
    active transport, 114, 117
    overview, 114–118, 129
    passive transport, 114, 117
    regulation of, 121–129, 122f
    specific ion transport, 118–121, 118f, 120f
Transporters, 82, 85f, 104, 118–121, 120f
Traube's space, 551
Trehalase, 101
Trehalose, 103
Treitz, ligament of, 256, 544, 549
Tremor, 434t, 435, 436
Treponema pallidum, 329t, 334
Tricarboxylic acid cycle. *See* TCA cycle
Tricyclics, 445t
Trigeminal nerve, 171, 172
Triglycerides
    digestion of, 107–108, 108f, 159–160
    hydrolysis of, 107f
    metabolism of, 156–157, 156f
Trimethoprim-sulfamethoxazole, 231, 339, 343, 346
Tropheryma whippelii, 229–230
Tropical sprue, 98t, 102, 227–229
Trypanosoma cruzi, 186–187

Trypanosomiasis, 186
Trypsin, 53, 99, 265, 267, 267t, 269, 269t. *See also* α₁-antitrypsin
Trypsinogens I–III, 99
Tubuloalveolar glands, 55
Tubulovesicular system, 48
Tumor necrosis factor (TNF), 297, 434t
    antibody to, 323t, 324
Tumor suppressor genes, 494, 496–497, 496f, 499, 499f, 503
Tumorigenicity, 493. *See also* Cancer
Turner's sign, 253
Tyrosine phosphorylation, 491, 491t

UC. *See* Colitis, ulcerative
UDPGT (uridine diphosphate-glucuronosyltransferase), 158, 418, 420–421
    deficiency, 421t
UES. *See* Sphincter, upper esophageal
Ulcerative colitis (UC). *See* Colitis, ulcerative
Ulcers, 83, 208–209, 226. *See also* *Helicobacter pylori*; Peptic ulcer disease
    acid suppression, in treatment of, 514, 517, 517t, 519
    bleeding of, 448, 448t, 554
    Cushing's ulcer, 209
    duodenal, 514, 517, 517t, 519
    gastric, 71t, 81–82, 83
    of mouth, 434t, 436
    solitary rectal, 558t, 565
    stress, causes of, 558t
Umbilical blood flow, 135
Urea cycle, 153–154, 154f, 444, 444t
Urecholine, 531t
Uremia, 529
Urethra, embryology of, 38t
Uridine diphosphate-glucuronosyltransferase. *See* UDPGT
Urinary bladder, embryology of, 38t
Urinary retention, 465
Ursodeoxycholic acid, 393, 396, 446
    as treatment for pruritis, 417
Urticaria, 303
Uveitis, 320, 320t

Vagotomy, 163, 212–214, 213f, 525
Vagus nerve, 8, 18, 33, 43–44, 46
    in embryological stages, 39
    innervation of gallbladder/biliary ducts, 160
    innervation of stomach, 96, 204, 205f
        stimulation of acid secretion, 82, 82f, 207
        stimulation of mucus secretion, 83
    innervation of swallowing, 171
Valproic acid, 253t
Valves of Kerkring. *See* Plicae circulares
Vancomycin, 345
Variceal bleeding, 405–406
Vascular adressins, 297
Vasculitis, 226, 320t, 565

Vasoactive intestinal polypeptide (VIP), 22t, 25, 26, 30, 84, 123t, 128
    and activated mast cells, 297
    concentration needed for activity, 122
    functions of, 50t, 73, 162, 171, 204
    inhibition of, 127
    nitric oxide (NO), interactions with, 72, 73
    as secretagogue, 125f
    secretin-VIP family, 26t, 30
    VIPoma, 116t, 122, 127, 129
Vasoconstriction, 241–242, 557
Vasodilation, 407
Vasopressin, 242, 557
Vectoral flow, 79
Verapamil, 127f
Vestibular system, 529–530, 529f, 530f
Vibrio cholerae, 86–87, 115, 116t, 128, 329t, 336
Villi of small intestine, 52, 52f, 53, 55, 56f
    absorption by, 5, 101, 115
    atrophy of, 110, 224, 303, 304f, 448, 448t
    contractions of, 16
    microvilli, 52f, 53, 86, 101, 115
    transport properties of, 116–117
VIP. *See* Vasoactive intestinal polypeptide
VIPoma, 116t, 122, 127, 129
Viruses, 349–350. *See also* Hepatitis, viral
    adenovirus, 222, 329t, 335
    cytomegalovirus (CMV), 198, 252t, 329t, 330–331, 349
    DNA, 489
    herpes simplex (HSV), 198, 329t, 331–332, 331f, 484
    and infections of GI tract, 329t, 330–332
    RNA, 489
    rotavirus, 329t, 335
Visceral afferent neurons, 18–19
Vitamin A, 108–109, 109f, 229
    deficiency of, 393, 450, 451t
Vitamin B₁ (thiamine), 108–109, 109f
    deficiency of, 449t, 450, 451t
Vitamin B₂ (riboflavin), 451t
Vitamin B₆ (pyridoxine), 451t
Vitamin B₁₂, 45
    absorption of, 83, 96, 101, 109, 229, 319
    deficiency of, 7, 83, 102, 229, 319
    and intrinsic factor, 45, 48, 56, 83
    supplements, postgastrectomy, 97
Vitamin C, 109, 451t
Vitamin D, 102, 109, 228, 229, 451t
    malabsorption of, 393
Vitamin E, 102, 109, 446
    deficiency of, 393
Vitamin K, 16, 109, 228
    deficiency of, 393, 451t
Vitamins, 108–109. *See also specific vitamins*
    absorption of, 5, 7, 101, 543
    and malabsorption disorders, 225, 228–229
    deficiencies of, 101, 228, 538, 539t
    fat-soluble, 101, 107, 108–109, 109f
        deficiencies of, 393
    metabolism of, 160

CPSIA information can be obtained at www.ICGtesting.com
Printed in the USA
242168LV00001B/4/A

9 781593 771812